ALLE ZEIT WACH
SJ
1842

Neurology

Proceedings of the XIIIth World Congress of Neurology Hamburg, September 1–6, 1985

Edited by

K. Poeck H.-J. Freund H. Gänshirt

With 113 Figures and 86 Tables

Springer-Verlag
Berlin Heidelberg New York Tokyo

Editors

Prof. Dr. KLAUS POECK
Abteilung Neurologie, R.W.T.H.
Pauwelsstraße, 5100 Aachen, FRG

Prof. Dr. HANS-JOACHIM FREUND
Neurologische Universitätsklinik
Moorenstraße 5, 4000 Düsseldorf, FRG

Prof. Dr. HEINZ GÄNSHIRT
Neurologische Universitätsklinik
Voßstraße 2, 6900 Heidelberg, FRG

ISBN-13:978-3-642-70009-5 e-ISBN-13:978-3-642-70007-1
DOI: 10.1007/978-3-642-70007-1

Library of Congress Cataloging in Publication Data. World Congress of Neurology (13th : 1985 : Hamburg, Germany). Neurology : Proceedings of the XIIIth World Congress of Neurology, Hamburg, September 1–6, 1985.
Includes bibliographies and index. 1. Neurology–Congresses. I. Poeck, Klaus. II. Freund, H.-J. III. Gänshirt, H. (Heinz), 1919– . IV. Title. [DNLM: 1. Neurology–congresses. W3 WO538X 13th 1985n / WL 100 W926 1985n] RC327.W625 1986 616.8 86-6753
ISBN-13:978-3-642-70009-5 (U.S.)

2125/3130-543210

World Federation of Neurology

President:	R. L. Masland, USA
First Vice-President:	Sir John Walton, United Kingdom
Vice-Presidents:	E. Csanda, Hungary
	S. Katsuki, Japan
	C. Loeb, Italy
	M. Mustafa, Egypt
	A. Spina-Franca, Brazil
Secretary Treasurer General:	J. F. Toole, USA
Joint Secretary Treasurer General:	P. Juul-Jensen, Denmark

XIIIth World Congress of Neurology

Honorary Presidents:	H. J. Bauer, Federal Republic of Germany
	L. van Bogaert, Belgium
	M. Critchley, United Kingdom
	P. van Gehuchten, Belgium
	W. A. den Hartog Jager, The Netherlands
	R. Jung, Federal Republic of Germany
	S. Katsuki, Japan
	S. Refsum, Norway
	A. Subirana, Spain
	K.-J. Zülch, Federal Republic of Germany
President:	K. Poeck, Aachen
Vice-President:	H. Gänshirt, Heidelberg
Secretary General:	H.-G. Mertens, Würzburg
Secretary:	G. Brune, Münster
Treasurer:	K. Schimrigk, Homburg/Saar
Chairman of Program Committee:	H. J. Freund, Düsseldorf
Assistant Secretary:	W. Hacke, Aachen
Assistant Treasurer:	H. Zeumer, Aachen
Members:	R. Ch. Behrend, Hamburg
	P. A. Fischer, Frankfurt
	W. D. Heiß, Köln
	H.-Ch. Hopf, Mainz
	D. Janz, Berlin
	D. Seitz, Hamburg
	M. Wolter, Berlin

German Neurological Society

President:	K. Poeck, Aachen
Vice-President:	P. A. Fischer, Frankfurt
Secretary:	W. Firnhaber, Darmstadt
Treasurer:	E. Volles, Seesen

Contents

3 Neuroepidemiology and Clinical Trials

Neuroepidemiology

Clinical Trials

4 Neuroimaging

List of Contributors

You will find the addresses at the beginning of the respective contribution

On the Dynamics Between Growth and Decline in the Aging of Intelligence and Memory

P. B. BALTES and R. KLIEGL [1]

The view of aging and old age predominantly held in Western societies is one of general decline in capacity and efficiency. Older persons are judged to be less efficient, less adaptive, and less intelligent than younger adults. In addition to scientific evidence such as that collected in opinion surveys (e.g., [22]), the view of aging as decline is also evident in cultural products of art [28], as well as in everyday communications in the mass media. The image of old age as a period of decline seems deeply embedded in the social fabric of society.

Counterexamples to this view of aging as decline are considered exceptions to the rule. Individuals undoubtedly exist who perform extraordinary mental and physical feats in old age. Aside from well-known artists such as Pablo Casals, or the pianists Vladimir Horowitz and Arthur Rubinstein, consider the 75-year-old who has run the 42-km marathon in about 3 h 15 min, a time not easily reached by most young adults. Exceptions from aging as universal and inevitable decline, although they do not alter our general view, are important to note because they serve to challenge the boundaries of the "normal" and suggest the value of re-examining the limits of reality. Indeed, the search for the limits and plasticity of aging is the essence of our own research approach. In the area of intelligence, for instance, we are interested in understanding the conditions and range of reserve capacity or plasticity that older individuals hold in intelligence and cognitive functioning.

The view of aging as decline, or decline view, also characterized the beginning of psychological research on aging. During the last decade or so, however, the situation has changed. One much-debated question in the psychology of aging has become whether psychological aging is indeed solely a phenomenon of gradual, cumulative, and inevitable decline. Here, this debate will be illustrated in one research area – the study of intelligence and memory.

What is the scientific evidence on the aging of intelligence and memory? Recent decades have witnessed a number of new findings that challenge the stereotype of general and universal decline [5, 7, 9, 29, 31, 47]. Four lines of research are particularly relevant:

[1] Max Planck Institute for Human Development and Education, Lentzeallee 94, 1000 Berlin 33, Federal Republic of Germany.

Neurology
Ed. by K. Poeck, H. J. Freund, and H. Gänshirt

1. On the nature of aging of each of the several abilities that constitute the provinces of intelligence
2. On interindividual variability and cultural change in intellectual aging
3. On the plasticity (reserve capacity) of intellectual functioning in old age
4. On maximum limits of intellectual functioning

Together, these lines of research have opened a new window on the aging of intelligence and related cognitive functions.

Different Intellectual Abilities Age Differently

Most research on intelligence in adulthood and old age has employed standardized psychometric tests of intelligence. Such intelligence tests are based on a multiability structural conception of intelligence. Intelligence is not seen as a single ability; rather, it is conceived of as a system of multiple abilities. To view intelligence as a system of clusters of mental abilities permits the possibility that different abilities can age differently, in the same manner as different organs of the human body show different rates of aging [14, 20, 43].

In fact, the possibility that distinct intellectual abilities age differently is part of a major psychometric theory of intelligence developed by Cattell and Horn [12, 26, 27]. The central feature of the Cattell-Horn theory of intelligence relevant to considerations of aging is the distinction between two large clusters of intellectual abilities, fluid intelligence and crystallized intelligence. Fluid intelligence deals with the "content-free" basic processes of information processing and reasoning; another shorthand description of it would be that it represents the basic architecture or the basic "mechanics" of intellectual functioning. In order to minimize the role played by cultural content, fluid intelligence is assessed by efficiency of problem-solving with material that is novel or overlearned. Crystallized intelligence, on the other hand, refers to a cluster of subabilities that deal with content- and knowledge-based elaboration of reasoning. Crystallized intelligence, or the "pragmatics" of intelligence, is typically measured by tasks involving language, interpersonal communication, social intelligence, and cultural knowledge. Professional expertise and wisdom are exemplars of crystallized intelligence [16, 17].

What about the life-span developmental fate of fluid and crystallized intelligence, the mechanics and the pragmatics of intelligence? The theory postulates that fluid and crystallized intelligence show rather different trajectories of aging (Fig. 1). The initial course up to early adulthood is identical: both ability clusters show an upward trend. Beginning in middle adulthood, their aging differs markedly. Fluid intelligence is expected to exhibit a fairly early and regular aging loss. Crystallized intelligence, by contrast, is expected to continue growth during adulthood and show stability into old age.

It is now argued that age functions can best be identified when tested at "limits" of performance or reserve capacity: performing tasks under conditions of stress, of a high degree difficulty, or demanding extensive practice (expertise) (Fig. 2). In psychology, testing-the-limits – similar but not identical to stress testing in medicine – may become the chosen method of identifying aging changes both in the basic sci-

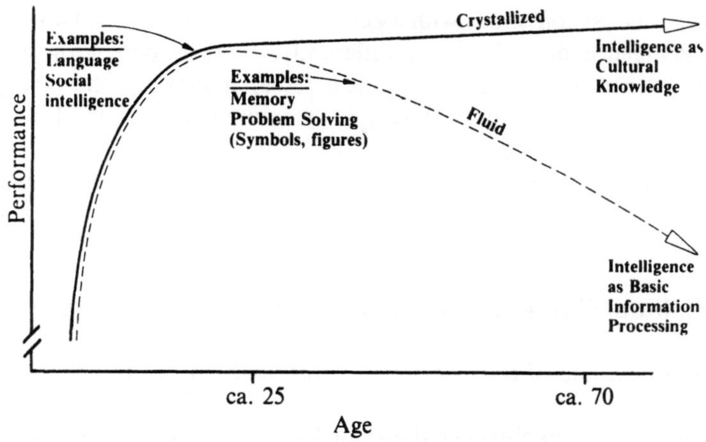

Fig. 1. Postulated developmental trajectories of fluid and crystallized intelligence. (After [12, 26])

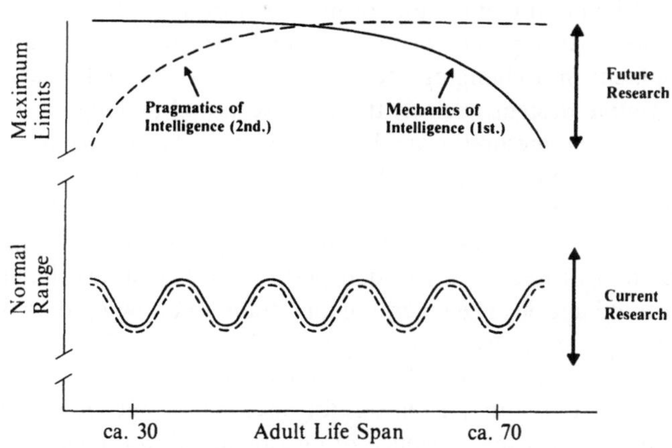

Fig. 2. Testing-the-limits and the aging of the mechanics vs. the pragmatics of intelligence. Age changes affect functioning within the normal range less than at the limits. (After [7])

ence laboratory and in clinical practice [2, 7, 29, 46]. This topic is discussed in more detail later in this paper.

Why should fluid and crystallized intelligence differ so dramatically in their life-span developmental course? According to the theory, fluid intelligence reflects primarily the biological integrity of neurophysiological functioning and brain status. Because these foundations of fluid intelligence are susceptible to biological aging and neurological trauma over the course of life, fluid intelligence is predicted to decline with age, beginning in early adulthood. Crystallized intelligence, by contrast, is largely the manifestation of accumulated experience and cultural learning. As experience and learning continue throughout the life span, crystallized intelligence is expected to show an increase into late adulthood.

The Cattell-Horn theory, then, with its differing courses of aging for fluid and crystallized intelligence, is one of the first examples of the idea that intellectual aging is not synonymous with a general loss of functioning. Different ability clusters of intelligence do indeed age differently; there is both growth and decline during adulthood and old age. Empirical research supports the theory [27, 36]. Whereas most individuals show losses in measurements of fluid intelligence beginning around age 30–40, many individuals equally maintain their level of functioning in crystallized-type measurements, such as on a test of language knowledge, up to age 70.

Cultural Change and Interindividual Variability in Aging

The next line of research involves the study of cultural change and interindividual variability. This research has produced two other findings which demonstrate that the aging of intelligence does not follow a fixed course of continual and universal decline. The findings are a substantial degree of variation in the aging of intelligence (a) between persons and (b) between generations or birth cohorts.

The finding of cultural or historical variation in intelligence was possible because of the development of new research designs better suited to capture age development in a changing society. Whereas traditional research used simple age-comparative designs such as the cross-sectional or longitudinal method, since the late 1960s new methods have been developed that incorporate historical variations into these designs [4, 32, 39]. In part, this development of more complex aging designs occurred because simple cross-sectional and longitudinal studies did not produce the same outcomes. For decades, cross-sectional results had confirmed the expected pattern of loss of intellectual performance with age, beginning in early adulthood around age 30. The emerging longitudinal follow-up data did not show the same decline pattern: instead, in longitudinal studies, individuals up to age 60 or so exhibited little change in intellectual functioning.

One of the major reasons for discrepancy between cross-sectional and longitudinal studies is the existence of historical, cultural change. For these reasons the desired methodology is one in which age and generational or so-called birth cohort membership can be varied simultaneously. This is achieved by the application of so-called sequential strategies which consist of successions of cross-sectional and/or longitudinal studies as shown in Fig. 3.

Using such sequential strategies, Schaie and his colleagues began in 1956 what is now perhaps the classic study on adult and old-age development of intelligence; a study that has revolutionized our conceptions of the aging of intelligence. The study began with 500 subjects and has been continuously expanded at 7-year intervals, involving, as of 1984, a 28-year follow-up of more than 2000 subjects measured repeatedly on a large battery of intelligence tests [40, 41]. Control groups measured at longer intervals are also included (Fig. 4).

Two findings of Schaie's research program are highlighted here: the results on (a) interindividual variability and (b) historical change.

Interindividual Variability. A first major finding in Schaie's research is that of sizeable variability in the overall course of intellectual aging between individuals. Consider, for example, the onset of aging loss as illustrated in Fig. 5. Depending upon

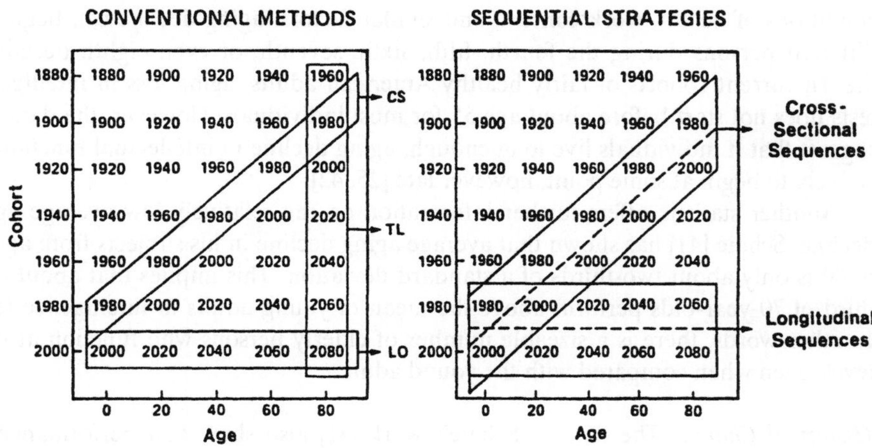

Fig. 3. Cohort-sequential strategies. (After [4, 39])

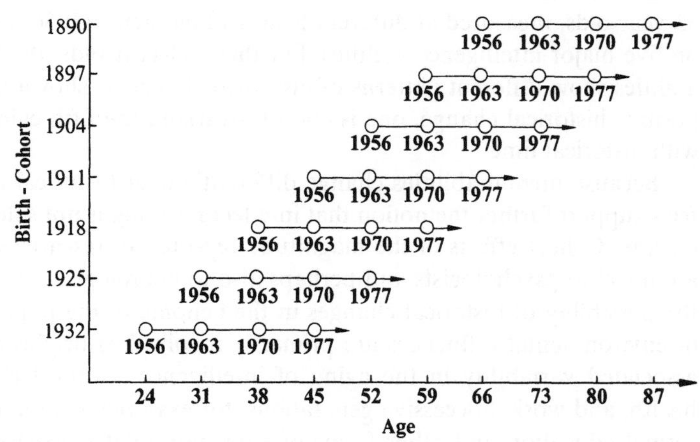

Fig. 4. Sequential strategy of Schaie's study of adult and old-age intelligence [41]

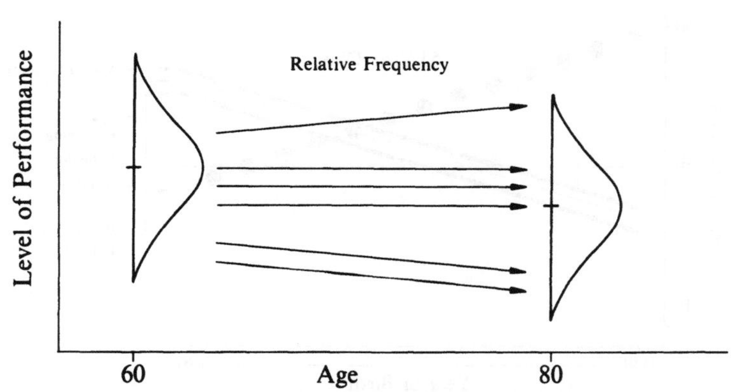

Fig. 5. Substantial individual differences in the course of intellectual aging from age 60 to 80. (After [5])

conditions of health, work context, and similar factors, aging decline can begin for different persons during the fourth, fifth, sixth, seventh, or even eighth decade of life. In current cohorts of fairly healthy American adults, aging loss in intelligence tests does not start before about age 55 for most individuals. However, the data still suggest that if individuals live long enough, aging decline in intellectual functioning is likely to begin at some point, however late [25, 42].

Another statistic offers further information on the relatively low average aging decline. Schaie [41] has shown that average aging decline in his subjects from age 60 to 80 is only about two-thirds of a standard deviation. This implies that about one-third of 70-year-olds perform above the mean of young adults in intelligence tests. In other words, there is a sizeable number of elderly persons who function at high levels even when compared with the yound adult.

Historical Change. The data of Schaie's work [41] also show that performance on intelligence tests does not only change with age, but also with history. Cohort or historical differences between age levels can be as large as longitudinal aging changes within the same cohort. Consider, for example, the findings for one age group, say 53-year-olds, measured at different historical moments (1956, 1963, 1970, 1977, etc.) on five major intelligence abilities. For these 53-year-olds, the five different mental abilities show different patterns of historical change as shown in Fig. 6. Three show positive historical change, one is cohort-invariant, the fifth evinces negative change with historical time.

Because mental abilities change differently over historical time, such cohort effects support further the notion that intellectual aging is not solely a phenomenon of decline. Cohort effects of the magnitude reported in research on adult intelligence are novel to psychologists and perhaps also to neurologists. In our view, aside from the possibility of historical changes in the genome of the population, three clusters of environmental influences are primarily involved as origins of cohort effects and associated variability in the aging of intelligence: cultural changes in education, health, and work. Successive generations, for example, exhibit on the average more formal education and other forms of education-related experiences, such as those

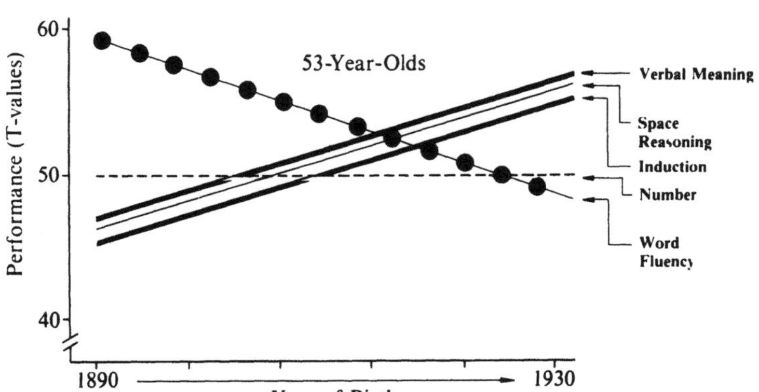

Fig. 6. Historical change: simplified trends representing the average performance of 53-year-olds from different birth cohorts, as estimated by Schaie [41], based on time-lag comparisons

associated with the introduction of television. Many other facets of everyday life show sociocultural change that may be related to level and rate of intellectual functioning. At present, however, it is not yet possible to specify which of the factors are responsible for the cohort changes observed in intellectual aging.

Cognitive Intervention Research on Plasticity in Old Age

The results presented thus far describe what, in one Western cultural context and at a few historical moments, the aging of psychometrically measured intelligence looks like. The central finding is great variability and openness in level and course, between abilities as well as between individuals and historical cohorts. The aging of intelligence is not a rigidly fixed phenomenon that can be captured by simple age designs. No single cohort-specific or ability-specific study tells the final story on the aging of intelligence [4, 35, 38, 39].

Does variability between individuals have a counterpart in plasticity within one individual? The inquiry into variability of intellectual performance within the same person, i.e., plasticity or reserve capacity, has been the direction of our own recent research [10, 29]. We ask whether the variability in level of intellectual performance obtained in descriptive cohort and age comparisons can be simulated as plasticity in single individuals.

Psychological Evidence

One of our central resulting research questions is the following: Is it possible to elevate the level of intellectual performance of elderly individuals by an amount comparable to the one reported either as aging loss or as the difference between same-age persons from different cohorts? To resolve this issue we provide older individuals with added learning experience and practice in intellectual functioning.

Training of Intelligence Test Performance. Meanwhile, some ten cognitive training studies with a total of about 1000 older persons have been completed in our laboratories, in the United States at the Pennsylvania State University (with Sherry L. Willis) and at the Max Planck Institute for Human Development and Education in Berlin (with Freya Dittmann-Kohli). Each of the studies extended over a period of about 1 year [8, 10, 47]. Study participants are between 60 and 80 years of age and above average in health and education. We estimate that our participants, both country and city dwellers, represent perhaps 50%–75% of the 60- to 80-year-olds living in rural Pennsylvania and in Berlin.

In most studies, the training program consists of five to ten training sessions distributed over 1–2 months. Cognitive training focuses on that cluster of intelligence that according to theory and data is sensitive to aging loss, i.e., fluid intelligence. During training, reasoning problems similar to those contained in tests of fluid intelligence are explained, solutions are practiced, and corrective feedback is given.

The results of these various practice and learning studies are highly consistent. As is illustrated in Fig. 7 taken from Baltes et al. [8], older individuals benefit markedly from exposure to cognitive activity. In tests similar to the training focus, per-

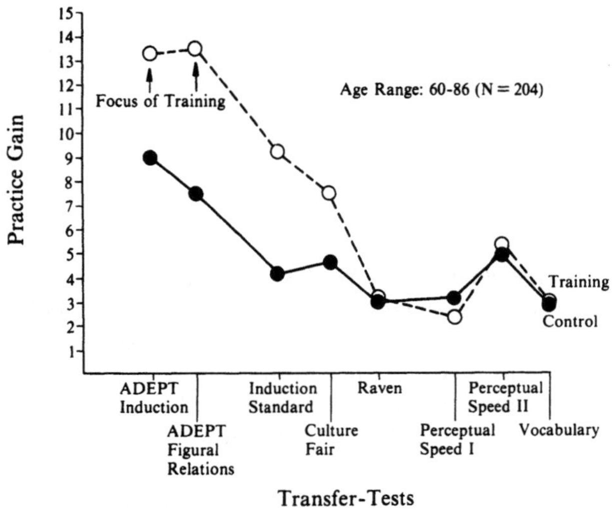

Fig. 7. Results from a cognitive training study conducted in Berlin [8]. The content focus of training was the two major subabilities (figural relations, induction) that constitute fluid intelligence. Training effects were measured by a battery of intelligence tests which differed increasingly (*l* to *r*) from focus of training in the requisite factual and procedural cognitive skills

formance gain is about one standard deviation: an amount rather similar to the aging loss reported in descriptive longitudinal research on this age range [41]. In addition, the training gain is maintained at all occasions studied following the practice sessions, i.e., up to 6 months following the intervention. The evidence for transfer from the abilities trained to other clusters of intelligence, however, is moderate. As might be expected, transfer to training is restricted of tests of intelligence tapping the same ability as that trained.

More refined analyses of test performances also show that trained older adults not only increase their average level of test performance, but are also more accurate (i.e., show fewer errors) and are able to solve more difficult problems than before the training program. Another important finding is that the large majority of participants in our research seem to profit from practice and training. Participants are classified into subgroups by, e.g., subjective health status, age, level of education, initial level of test performance or IQ, but these subgroups do not differ substantially in amount of training gain.

Training of Memory. During the last year we have extended our research on intellectual plasticity and reserve capacity to the area of memory [30]. Our training focus is on memory tasks (such as the well-known digit span) that require subjects to repeat strings of digits or words. Without training, typical subjects are able to repeat four to eight digits or a similar number of words in the correct order (3-1-5-0-8, etc., house-car-family-telephone, etc.).

Using theories of cognitive psychology and memory [13, 18], we have developed training modules that permit subjects to achieve record-like performances. These training programs extend over 30–50 individual sessions. Thus far, we have worked with 15 healthy elderly people in the age range 67–78. In terms of IQ, these subjects are above average. However, they were not selected because they are particularly gifted in memory functioning. In the course of the training programs we engineer an expert memory system that involves the acquisition and combination of three components: working memory, a declarative knowledge system about digits, and a mnemonic strategy (Method of Loci) of encoding and retrieving [30].

As with our research on training psychometric intelligence, in this research on reserve capacity of memory our elderly subjects also prove capable of demonstrating remarkable gains in performance. After 30 sessions of memory training, all elderly subjects can repeat – under self-paced conditions of about 20-s presentation intervals between words – at least 30 words in the correct order after one presentation of the list of words (Fig. 8). As to digit strings, all elderly persons studied so far are able to repeat – again under self-paced presentation rates of about 20-s intervals – strings of digits as long as 40 after they have been presented only once. Our best elderly person can repeat a string of 120 digits with a presentation rate of 8-s;

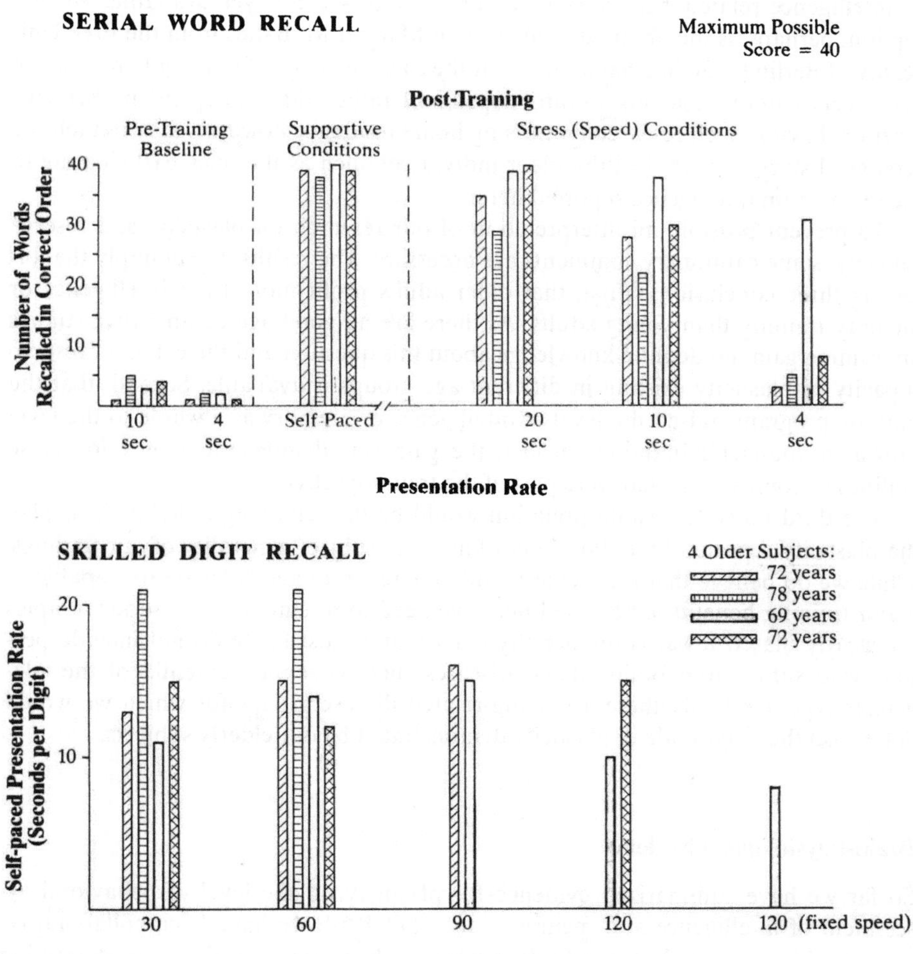

Fig. 8. Research on reserve capacity: performance of four elderly subjects in word span and digit span. (From [45])

on the surface, at least, an amazing performance for a 70-year-old. Note that presenting a string of 120 digits at an 8-s presentation rate takes 16 min.

These memory task performances by elderly people are of such magnitude that they can be classified as approaching the performances of expert mnemonists [18]. Thus the findings suggest that, as in the area of psychometric intelligence, many elderly people have a reserve capacity of memory functioning extending far beyond our everyday and scientific conceptions of what the aging of memory is like.

One missing piece of the puzzle is whether the everyday world of many older persons is indeed one that generates intellectual atrophy, due to lack of experiences and demands conducive to high intellectual performance. Based on casual observation and sociological analyses of role changes following retirement, this seems a reasonable assumption. A major tenet of the sociology of old age is that aging brings with it a loss of social role and involvement, but careful, direct observations of intelligence-related behaviors of older persons are not yet available. An exception, perhaps, is the observational work of Margret M. Baltes from the Free University of Berlin [1, 3]. She has shown that the social ecology of nursing homes is one that steers elderly residents toward dependent rather than independent, self-sufficient behavior. Such research on nursing home residents, however, may not tell the ecological story of fairly healthy older individuals such as the ones participating in the research on intelligence reported here.

To prevent possible misinterpretation of our research on plasticity and reserve capacity, some cautionary comments are necessary. The results do *not* imply the following three conclusions. First, that older adults profit more from intelligence or memory training than young adults. As there are no good age-comparative studies on training gain, no definite knowledge about this question and the extent of reserve capacity or plasticity existing in different age groups is available. Second, that the training programs raised the level of intelligence or memory as a whole to the level shown in younger adulthood. In fact, the gain was demonstrated only for those abilities or components that were part of the training activity.

The third possible misinterpretation would be that all aging individuals display the plasticity reported here. We do not know the subject generality of our findings. While we do believe that most elderly individuals up to age 80 or so are capable of major training benefits as reported here, we need to re-emphasize that our samples are clearly biased towards the healthy elderly and most likely do not include persons who suffer from brain-related diseases such as senile dementia of the Alzheimer type. Certainly there are aging-related disease groups for which we would not expect the magnitude of plasticity demonstrated by our elderly subjects.

Brain-Physiological Evidence

So far we have summarized evidence for plasticity on the level of behavioral assessment of intelligence and memory. Since fall 1984, we have been collaborating with the Max Planck Institute for Neurological Research at Cologne in examining whether the psychological plasticity of intellectual functioning observed in many elderly people has a correlate or counterpart in physiological brain functioning [24]. This collaboration involves the use of positron emission tomography (PET). PET scanning of radiolabelled fluorodeoxyglucose permits the in vivo assessment of cerebral glucose utilization in the brain. It also provides an imaging technique to display the regional distribution of glucose metabolism in various parts of the brain [23, 37].

To date we have studied 20 elderly subjects (ages 68–80): ten participated in 30 sessions of memory training as described above and ten formed a control group. PET scan measures were taken twice, before and after training, approximately 3 months apart. Departing from the usual PET scan procedure, in which scans are performed while subjects are in various resting states, our subjects worked silently on a long memory task for the 40-min measurement period. This strategy allows great control over what subjects do during PET scan.

Three of our research questions are: (a) Does an intensive 30-session memory training produce changes in the metabolic rate of glucose in the brain? (b) If an effect of memory training on brain glucose metabolism is obtained, is it evident only if subjects engage in the specific memory activities trained or is it evident also when other memory activities are performed? (c) If an effect is obtained, is it general to the whole brain or region-specific?

The evidence collected thus far is encouraging. Memory-trained subjects evince a higher level of glucose consumption, about 10% higher than control subjects, in one specific area of the brain (lentiform nucleus: globus pallidus and putamen). Thus the preliminary answer seems to be that continued memory practice can indeed result in a higher level of brain energy metabolism in the elderly – at least in situations when memory functions are called upon. We are currently examining more systematically whether, in addition to the effect in the area of the lentiform nucleus, there are other regional effects in the sense of a continuum of transfer.

We need to be careful not to overestimate and overgeneralize the significance of the findings reported. However, our findings on metabolic brain plasticity fit into another line of research reported over the last few years by others. Evidence is building up that development and growth of the normally aging brain extends into old age [19, 33]. Once, many thought that the brain was fixed in structure and connectivity by the time of early adulthood. Diamond and her colleagues [15] at Berkeley, however, have shown that there seems to be new dendritic growth in the cortex of elderly rats if stimulated through environmental enrichment. Research by Lynch [34], in a similar vein, suggests that growth and deterioration of brain structures exist conjointly throughout the life course. However, according to Lynch the overall proportions of growth and deterioration of brain structures, as measured for instance in dendritic growth following injury, changes across the life span. In old age, growth continues but is reduced in relative magnitude.

Our assumption from a distance is that clinical neurologists may have been more aware of the possibility of further growth in brain structure in old age than psychologists, biochemists or physiologists. What else could lie behind the kind of recovery and compensatory responses often found in elderly patients after sudden brain damage? However, clearer and more direct laboratory demonstration of such growth processes in old age may represent a new level of insight and knowledge about the matter.

In any case, having the special opportunity of speaking as psychologists to a world congress of neurology, we would like to highlight the value and possible excitement of interdisciplinary work. We consider this joint program between two Max

Planck Institutes a rare opportunity. It was possible rapidly to interconnect two recent developments that hold much promise in two otherwise fairly separate disciplinary areas, the bioneurological and the behavioral sciences. Specifically, we were able to combine PET scan methodology, on the one hand, with cognitive-science type psychology on the other.

Age Differences and Testing-the-Limits

Let us return to the psychology of the aging of intelligence and comment further on another research strategy called testing-the-limits. Increasingly, psychologists join in the argument that more sensitive measures of development and aging are available if one tests people at limits of performance [2, 7, 21, 29, 46].

As to aging, for instance, the one definitional criterion scientists agree upon is that aging brings with it increased vulnerability and reduction in system adaptivity [14, 43]. These can both be most easily estimated at limits of performance. Moreover, it is expected that differences between comparison groups, such as age groups, are magnified at the limits.

In our own research on the aging of intelligence and memory, we use testing-the-limits primarily for three purposes. First, it permits study of the extent of reserve capacity or plasticity. Second, it allows at the same time for identification of constraints on plasticity including constraints on intellectual advances in old age. Third, it permits the systematic study of compensatory processes if limits are reached [7, 29, 30].

Consider the two-ability theory of intelligence mentioned earlier. If one takes wisdom as an exemplar of the crystallized "pragmatics" of intelligence [44] and memory for digits as a typical task of the fluid "mechanics" of intelligence, age differences in tasks for these two are expected to be fairly small at baseline, i.e., there is much overlap in the age distributions within the normal or nontrained range of performance. As one moves subjects toward maximum limits or peaks of performance, as can be accomplished through the application of training procedures, the expectation is that the overlap in the age distributions can be reduced. The idealized expectation is that in the end, nonoverlapping age distributions would result, in the present example with opposite directionality for wisdom vs memory for digits (Fig. 9).

For the case of memory for words and digits (a fluid intelligence task), we have conducted such testing-the-limits work on age differences. The outcome, as shown in Fig. 10, is supportive of our expectation. At baseline, subjects of different ages and ability levels differ very little from each other. At limits or peaks of performance, however, arrived at by training subjects and then increasing level of difficulty (speeding up presentation rate), subject differences – including age differences – are magnified. At limits of performance we expect also to be in a better position to study the problem that intrigues us most: the dynamics of growth and decline. How do subjects behave when and if they reach a threshold of performance? In this context, the first author and his colleagues have identified a process called "selective optimization with compensation" as an adaptive strategy prototypical of successful aging [5, 6, 7, 17].

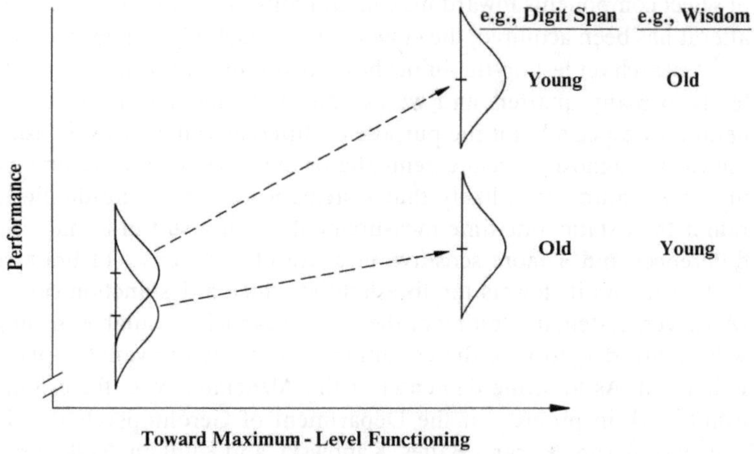

Fig. 9. Unravelling overlap in age-performance distribution by means of testing-the-limits: wisdom vs. digit span

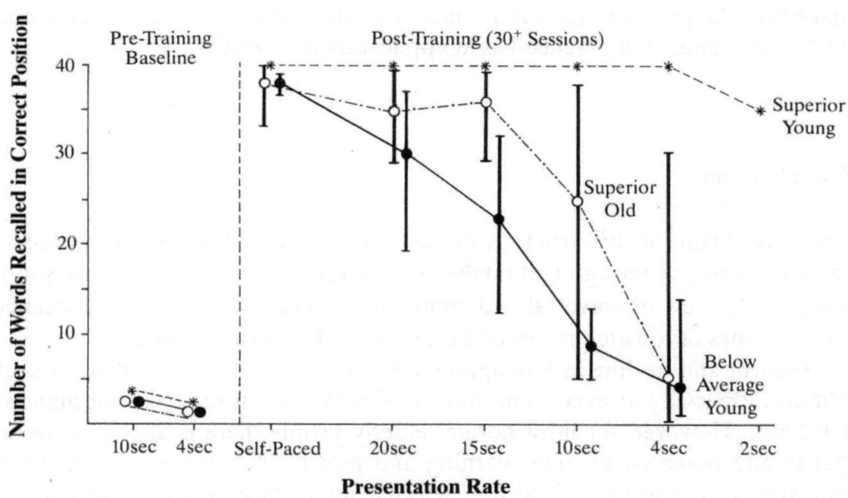

Fig. 10. Age differences are magnified at limits: sample case of skilled memory for words, for three groups. (From [30])

There is much similarity, of course, between our approach of testing-the-limits and methods of stress and adaptivity testing in biology and medicine [2, 14, 20]. However, it seems on the surface that there are also differences in emphasis. Testing-the-limits as we use it is not restricted to one-time static assessments or small variations in treatment. Rather, based on a theoretical analysis of the mechanisms at hand (e.g., memory), we engineer extensive intervention programs, identify progress in select components toward maximum limits of performance, and also test whether, after it has been acquired, the system deconstructs if components are removed [29].

Research on testing-the-limits has broad ramifications. Its possible usefulness extends to many quarters and we assume that similar assessment strategies exist in neurology especially for the purpose of differential diagnosis; consider, for instance, the early diagnosis of senile dementia or the assessment of reserve potential following brain injury. It is likely that systematic use of testing-the-limits procedures – rather than static, one-time measurement – will result in a magnification of group differences and a more sensitive measure of early onset of brain-related diseases. Testing-the-limits lowers the threshold at which a dysfunction can be identified [2]. Moreover, systematic testing of the reserve capacity available to subjects or patients will permit diagnosis of the conditions and range of available plasticity to a given individual. As to senile dementia of the Alzheimer type, for example, there is relevant work in progress at the Department of Gerontopsychiatry at the Free University of Berlin. Margret Baltes, Kanowski, and Kühl and colleagues are examining whether testing-the-limits approaches result in early and more effective diagnosis of Alzheimer-type diseases.

In the long run, the development of such testing-the-limits procedures will be most powerful if theoreticians and practitioners cooperate closely. In psychology, in any case, this is one of the examples where advances in theory and practice seem to make such cooperation imperative: theory-guided analysis of the model of behavior on the one hand, with practice-based application on the other.

Conclusions

The core theme of this article is the search for the real limits, as opposed to the imagined ones, of the aging of intelligence and memory. Contrary to the simple and widely-held view of universal and cumulative decline, the evidence associated with the four lines of research reviewed turned out to be more complex.

Growth and decline in intelligence exist conjointly. Certainly there is decline in old age, especially at maximum limits of functioning in the basic mechanics of intelligence. However, for most normal elderly people there is also great reserve capacity and potential for new learning and growth in those aspects of intellectual functioning that are practiced and selected for further development and specialization. If provided with cognitive enrichment and practice, most elderly people up to age 75 or so are capable of remarkable gains and peaks of intellectual performance, including in those areas of functioning, such as memory, where the typical expectation is one of early and regular decline. Not unlike the Roman god Janus, with his two faces looking in opposite directions and thus at different aspects of life, intellectual aging represents a dynamic between growth and decline. As we move toward old age, this dynamic between growth and decline is likely to increase and become the central drama of life.

This new window on the aging of intelligence was opened by the invention of a new set of methodologies. We have singled out two. First, the advent of cohort-sequential strategies which expanded simple cross-sectional and longitudinal methods to include variation of historical time or cohort. Second, the systematic use of theory-guided intervention and testing-the-limits procedures.

Testing-the limits in particular makes the dynamic between growth and decline most conspicuous. It has not only generated new evidence on remarkable reserve capacity or plasticity of the elderly, but in its search for peaks or maximum limits on performance it has also emphasized the other side of the coin, i.e., the boundary conditions of plasticity. At limits, both positive and negative aspects of aging may be enlarged or accentuated. Moreover, it is in limits of performance that we may have a new research tool available for early diagnosis of aging-related pathologies as well as for the study of compensatory processes following loss of functioning.

It is in the nature of the present evidence that psychological aging is conditioned by the biocultural context in which aging takes place and by what individuals do as they age. It is important, therefore, to bear in mind that the forms of intellectual aging reported here support the conclusion that what we happen to observe in our descriptive research on the natural history of the aging of intelligence is but a sample of what is possible in principle (see also [11]). Existing limits in a given society or in given science are not absolute or necessary ones. In this sense, the search for the range and limits of intellectual plasticity has not only suggested new approaches in the scientific study of psychological aging. It has also opened up new social vistas on what the aging of intelligence could be like if conditions were different.

Summary

In this paper, four lines of research on the aging of intelligence and memory are reviewed: research on (a) differential aging of subabilities, (b) intersubject variability and historical change, (c) plasticity and reserve capacity, and (d) limits of functioning. The nature of intellectual aging is not a simple movement toward loss of functioning. Rather, growth and decline interact in complex ways. Aging loss is most likely to occur at maximum limits of the basic mechanical operations of intelligence. Growth can exist in those aspects (the "pragmatics" of intelligence) in which individuals practice and engage in further evolution of knowledge systems. Testing-the-limits is presented as a methodological strategy by which mechanisms of positive and negative changes of cognitive aging can be identified. Suggestions are also offered for the use of testing-the-limits procedures in biomedical work such as research on senile dementia of the Alzheimer type.

References

1. Baltes MM (1982) Environmental factors in dependency among nursing home residents: a social ecological analysis. In: Wills TA (ed) Basic processes in helping relationships. Academic, New York, pp 405–425
2. Baltes MM, Kindermann T (1985) Die Bedeutung der Plastizität für die klinische Beurteilung des Leistungsverhaltens im Alter. In: Bente D, Coper H, Kanowski S (eds) Methoden zur Objektivierung pharmakotherapeutischer Wirkung. Springer, Berlin Heidelberg New York Tokyo, pp 171–184 (Hirnorganische Psychosyndrome im Alter, vol 2)

3. Baltes MM, Reisenzein R (1986) The social world in long-term care institutions: psychological control toward dependency? In: Baltes MM, Baltes PB (eds) The psychology of control and aging. Erlbaum, Hillsdale, pp 315–343
4. Baltes PB (1968) Longitudinal and cross-sectional sequences in the study of age and generation effects. Hum Devel 11:145–171
5. Baltes PB (1984) Intelligenz im Alter. Spektrum der Wissenschaft 5:46–60
6. Baltes PB, Baltes MM (1980) Plasticity and variability in psychological aging: methodological and theoretical issues. In: Gurski G (ed) Determining the effects of aging on the central nervous system. Schering, Berlin, pp 41–66
7. Baltes PB, Dittmann-Kohli F, Dixon RA (1984) New perspectives on the development of intelligence in adulthood: toward a dual-process conception and a model of selective optimization with compensation. In: Baltes PB, Brim OG Jr (eds) Life-span development and behavior, vol 6. Academic, New York, pp 33–76
8. Baltes PB, Dittmann-Kohli F, Kliegl R (in press) Reserve capacity of the elderly in aging-sensitive tests of fluid intelligence: replication and extension. Psychology and Aging
9. Baltes PB, Schaie KW (1976) On the plasticity of intelligence in adulthood and old age: where Horn and Donaldson fail. Am Psychol 31:720–725
10. Baltes PB, Willis SL (1982) Plasticity and enhancement of intellectual functioning in old age: Penn State's adult development and enrichment project (ADEPT). In: Craik F, Trehub SE (eds) Aging and cognitive processes. Plenum, New York, pp 353–389
11. Brandtstädter J (1984) Personal and social control over development: some implications of an action perspective in life-span developmental psychology. In: Baltes PB, Brim OG Jr (eds) Life-span development and behavior, vol 6. Academic, New York, pp 1–32
12. Cattell RB (1971) Abilities: their structure, growth, and action. Houghton Mifflin, Boston
13. Chase WG, Ericsson KA (1982) Skill and working memory. In: Bower GH (ed) The psychology of learning and motivation, vol 16. Academic, New York
14. Coper H, Jänicke B, Schulze G (1985) Biopsychological research on adaptivity across the life-span of animals. In: Baltes PB, Featherman DL, Lerner RM (eds) Life-span development and behavior, vol 7. Erlbaum, Hillsdale, pp 207–232
15. Connor JR Jr, Diamond MC, Johnson RE (1980) Aging and environmental influences on two types of dendritic spines in the rat occipital cortex. Environmental Neurology 70:371–379
16. Dittmann-Kohli F, Baltes PB (1986) Toward a neofunctionalist conception of adult intellectual development: wisdom as a prototypical case of intellectual growth. In: Alexander C, Langer E (eds) Beyond formal operations: alternative endpoints to human development. Oxford University Press, New York (in press)
17. Dixon RA, Baltes PB (1986) Toward life-span research on the functions and pragmatics of intelligence. In: Sternberg RJ, Wagner RK (eds) Practical intelligence: origins of competence in the everyday world. Cambridge University Press, New York (in press)
18. Ericsson KA (1985) Memory skill. Can J Psychol 39:188–231
19. Finch CA (1985) Modulation of aging processes in the brain. In: Bergener M, Ermini M, Stähelin HB (eds) Thresholds in aging. Academic, London, pp 175–188
20. Fries JF, Crapo LM (1980) Vitality and aging. Freeman, San Francisco
21. Guthke J (1982) The learning test concept – an alternative to the traditional static intelligence test. German Journal of Psychology 6:306–324
22. Harris DB (1975) The myth and reality of aging in America. National Council on Aging, Washington
23. Heiss D, Phelps ME (eds) (1983) Positron emission photography of the brain. Springer, Berlin Heidelberg New York Tokyo
24. Heiss WD, Pawlik G, Wienhard K, Beil C, Kliegl R, Smith J, Heckhausen J, Baltes PB (1986) PET demonstrates effect of memory training on cerebral energy metabolism. Max Planck Institute for Neurological Research, Cologne/Max Planck Institute for Human Development and Education, Berlin
25. Hertzog C, Schaie KW (1985) Stability and change in adult intelligence: I. Analysis of longitudinal covariance structures (unpublished manuscript, Pennsylvania State University)

26. Horn JL (1978) Human ability systems. In: Baltes PB (ed) Life-span development and behavior, vol 1. Academic, New York, pp 211–256
27. Horn JL (1982) The aging of human abilities. In: Wolman BB (ed) Handbook of developmental psychology. Prentice-Hall, Englewood Cliffs, pp 847–870
28. Joerissen P, Will C (1983) Die Lebenstreppe: Bilder der menschlichen Lebensalter (Catalog of an art exhibit). Rheinland-Verlag, Cologne
29. Kliegl R, Baltes PB (1986) Theory-guided analysis of mechanisms of development and aging through testing-the-limits and research on expertise. In: Schooler C, Schaie KW (eds) Cognitive functioning and social structures over the life course. Ablex, Norwood (in press)
30. Kliegl R, Smith J, Baltes PB (in press) Testing-the-limits, expertise, and memory in adulthood and old age. In: Klix F, Hagendorf H (eds) Proceedings of symposium in memoriam Hermann Ebbinghaus. North-Holland, Amsterdam
31. Labouvie-Vief G (1985) Intelligence and cognition. In: Birren JE, Schaie KW (eds) Handbook of the psychology of aging, 2nd edn. Van Nostrand Reinhold, New York
32. Labouvie EW, Nesselroade JR (1985) Age, period, and cohort analysis and the study of individual development and social change. In: Nesselroade JR, von Eye A (eds) Developmental and social change: explanatory analysis. Academic, New York, pp 189–212
33. Lerner RM (1984) On the nature of human plasticity. Cambridge University Press, New York
34. Lynch GS (1983) Aging and brain plasticity. Invited address (Div 20), 91st annual convention of the American Psychological Association, Anaheim, California, Aug 1983
35. Nesselroade JR, von Eye A (eds) (1985) Developmental and social change: explanatory analysis. Academic, New York
36. Nesselroade JR, Schaie KW, Baltes PB (1972) Ontogenetic vs. generational components of structural and quantitative change in adult cognitive behavior. J Gerontol 27:222–228
37. Phelps ME, Mazziota JC (1985) Positron emission tomography: human brain function and biochemistry. Science 228:799–809
38. Riley MW (1973) Aging and cohort succession: interpretation and misinterpretations. Public Opinion Quarterly 37:35–49
39. Schaie KW (1965) A general model for the study of developmental problems. Psychol Bull 64:92–107
40. Schaie KW (1979) The primary mental abilities in adulthood: an exploration in the development of psychometric intelligence. In: Baltes PB, Brim OG Jr (eds) Life-span development and behavior, vol 3. Academic, New York, pp 67–115
41. Schaie KW (ed) (1983) Longitudinal studies of adult psychological development. Guilford, New York
42. Schaie KW, Hertzog C (1983) Fourteen-year cohort-sequential analysis of adult intellectual development. Dev Psychol 19:531–543
43. Shock NW (1977) System integration. In: Finch CE, Hayflick L (eds) Handbook of the biology of aging. Van Nostrand Reinhold, New York
44. Smith J, Dixon RA, Baltes PB (1986) Expertise in life planning: a new approach to investigating aspects of wisdom. In: Commons M, Sinnott JD, Richards FA, Armon C (eds) Beyond formal operations II: adult cognitive development. Praeger, New York (in press)
45. Smith J, Kliegl R, Kramer D, Baltes PB (1986) Skilled memory: a method for studying reserve capacity (to be published)
46. Wiedl KK (1984) Lerntests: nur Forschungsmittel und Forschungsgegenstand? Zeitschrift für Entwicklungspsychologie und Pädagogische Psychologie 16:245–281
47. Willis SL (1985) Towards an educational psychology of the adult learner. In: Birren JE, Schaie KW (eds) Handbook of the psychology of aging. Van Nostrand Reinhold, New York

1 The Dementias

Clinical Aspects of the Dementias

Historical Overview of the Dementias

S. HOYER [1]

Among other characteristic symptoms, forgetfulness is prominent in dementia. It may be speculated that Adam and Eve's forgetting of God's admonition not to eat from the tree of knowledge is the first documentation of mild presenile dementia (*Genesis* iii) as is nicely demonstrated in the painting by Lucas Cranach *Das Paradies* (Paradise). However, the use of the term "dementia" to describe impairment of the previously intact intelligence first became common in the middle of the last century. It was Esquirol [3] who provided a definition of "démence senile". Intelligence, on the other hand, had been defined as the totality of physical substrate and processes of thought and its use in the practical and theoretical tasks of life [13].

Historically, infirmity was attributed to the aging process in general as was pointed out as early as 2600 B.C. by Ptahhotep who had been the vizier of King Isesi in the 5th dynasty of the Old Egyptian Kingdom: "... the heart, void, recalls not the past..." [8]. This and other notions of those times and the following centuries, indicate that the heart and not the brain was considered as the organ of the mind.

The identification of the brain as the organ of thinking and feeling was ingeniously performed by Hippocrates (ca. 460–370 B.C.) although the original idea that the brain might be the organ of the mind obviously derived from Alkmaeon who lived about 100 years before Hippocrates.

However, it was Hippocrates who formulated very clearly in Caput VII of his *De Morbo Sacro* that the brain is the organ of the mind and emotions:

"Unde cerebrum, tum functiones sanas... Ac nosse homines convenit, no aliunde nobis voluptates, lactitias, risus, et jocos, quam hinc contingere, itemque dolores, molestias, tristitias, et ejulatus. Hacque, parte praecipue sapimus et intelligimus, et videmus, et audimus, et turpia, et honesta cognoscimus, malaque et bona; itemque, quae jucunda sunt, et injucunda, partim quidem consuetudine discernimus, partim vero utilitate percipimus. Hac etiam parte voluptates et molestias temporibus dignoscimus, neque eadem nobis platent. Eademque ipsa parte et insanimus et deliramus, terroresque et metus; partim quidem noctu, partim etiam interdiu nos circumstant, insomniaque et errores intempestivi, et curae non convenientes, indeque rerum praesentium ignoratio, desuetudo, et imperitia nobis proveniunt. Atque hacc omnia ex cerebro nobis contingunt, cum minime sanum..." In English translation:

[1] Department of Pathochemistry and General Neurochemistry, University of Heidelberg, 6900 Heidelberg, Federal Republic of Germany.

Neurology
Ed. by K. Poeck, H. J. Freund, and H. Gänshirt

One should know that the brain is not only the source of pleasure, joy, laughter and jest, but also of pain, sorrow, grief and tears. Particularly through it, we think and grasp, see and hear, and discriminate turpitude from honesty, the bad from the good. And also, we distinguish customarily pleasant and unpleasant events. We learn to distinguish in particular between pleasure and grief even if this is unpleasant. In the same way, we become insane and delirious, feel terror and fear by night or by day. From this derives sleeplessness and untimely errors, inconvenient anxiety, ignorance of present events and illiteracy. All this comes from the brain if it is not healthy.

And Hippocrates continued:

"Intelligentiae autem cerebrum internuntius est" – It is the brain which is the mediator of intelligence and "Quidam autem, nos corde sapere, dicunt, quodque ipsum tristitiam et curam sentit. Verum non ita se res habet..." – It is also said that we are wise by means of our heart which also feels despondency and anxiety. However, this is not true.

Thus, Hippocrates may be regarded as the founder of the neurosciences.

In contrast to Hippocrates, Aristotle (384–322 B.C.), who was a disciple of Plato, believed that the heart was the location of intelligence and mind. His school was an influential one so that the ideas of Aristotle and Hippocrates existed side by side over several centuries.

The great Greco-Roman physician Galen (ca. 129–200 A.D.) continued the thinking of Hippocrates on mind, intelligence and brain and added the relation between emotion and somatic symptoms. It was Galen who transmitted the most comprehensive and significant medical knowledge from the Greek to the Roman culture. Here it was widely distributed until the end of the Roman Empire. The idea that mind is located in the brain was then lost and the mind was transferred from the brain to the heart for more than 1500 years.

Profound reverence for the erudition of the Greek and Roman medical schools induced the Arabs to translate the manuscripts of Hippocrates and Galen, and to enrich them with their own experience. In this respect, Avicenna (980–1037 A.D.) is especially noteworthy. It was thanks to Arab medicine that the knowledge of Hippocrates and Galen was not lost, but, when retranslated into Latin, formed the basis of scientific medicine in Renaissance Europe. However, progress in medicine developed in an ambivalent way. Insanity and amentia were not regarded as diseases or even disabilities of the brain. People suffering from such symptoms were considered to be possessed by the devil or other demons. Clearly, such ideas would not have been taken seriously as descriptions of diseases of organs other than the brain.

Although the scientific level of medical knowledge of mental function and dysfunction was underdeveloped at that time, there was nevertheless popular awareness of aging in general and insanity in particular. The old desire of humanity not to suffer from infirmity, but to maintain eternal youth found its expression in Lucas Cranach's painting *Der Jungbrunnen* (The Fountain of Youth). Insanity in its most grotesque form was figuratively represented by Hieronymus Bosch's "Narrenschiff" (The Ship of Fools).

The neglect of the brain in medical science is also apparent in the simplicity of the graphic representation of the brain ventricles drawn by Leonardo da Vinci in contrast to his very thorough and exact drawings of muscles, vessels, bones, etc.

The ignorance of normal and abnormal brain function and thus of brain diseases, and the general abhorrence of mental disability, accounted for the fact that people suffering from those diseases, irrespective of their cause, were placed in lunatic asylums, often in chains and in company with criminals, as shown in paintings by Francisco Goya and William Hogarth. It was thus a great step forward when in 1784 the first special house for mentally diseased people was established in the context of a general hospital. This was the *Narrenturm* in Vienna, popularly termed *Kaiser Josephs Gugelhupf.*

In the first edition of the *General Psychopathology,* Karl Jaspers [5] pointed out that the history of psychiatry may be divided into

1. The history of the care of the insane and the establishment of mental homes
2. The history of leading authorities in this field
3. The history of scientific psychiatry

These points may also hold true for the history of the dementias.

After the pioneering work of Philippe Pinel who, in September 1793, freed the mentally disabled of the Bicêtre in Paris by the removal of their chains, five outstanding neuropsychiatrists formulated the basis of the modern view of dementia:

Jean Etienne Dominique Esquirol (1772–1840)
Wilhelm Griesinger (1817–1868)
Theodor Meynert (1833–1892)
Emil Kraepelin (1856–1926)
Alois Alzheimer (1864–1915)

As was mentioned earlier, Esquirol was the first to define senile dementia. His main work, however, was to draft the major legislation on nursing and accommodation with dignity of mentally diseased people in 1838.

When Griesinger became the head of the Charité hospital in Berlin in 1865, he started to increase the significance of scientific medicine in general and of psychiatry in particular which had just begun to emancipate itself from philosophy. He defined psychiatric diseases as disorders of the brain, and insanity as a symptom. Griesinger was the first to recognize the fundamental difference between diffuse and focal processes of organic brain diseases. Based on anatomical findings, he repeatedly mentioned that the most important and most constant variation in mentally diseased people could be found in cortical disorders.

Beside Griesinger, Meynert can be regarded as the founder of scientifically orientated psychiatry. He was most concerned to free scientific psychiatry from speculation and pure empiricism. Like Griesinger, he was convinced that neuropsychiatric disorders are caused by the diseased brain. He suggested that functional disturbances, e.g. brain blood flow variations in and between grey and white matter, may play a major role in the genesis of brain disorders [9]. Griesinger and Meynert thus renewed the ideas of Hippocrates and extended them to cover diseased states of the brain.

Based on this neuroanatomical and neurofunctional dynamic concept of brain diseases, Kraepelin began his fundamental work on the classification of psychiatric illnesses, a classification which was accepted worldwide as a foundation of biologically orientated scientific psychiatry. In a systematic approach, he distinguished between insanity due to arteriosclerosis on the one hand and presenile and senile insanity on the other. This view has not lost its topicality even today. Although

Perusini reported in 1910 [10] that for clinical and histological reasons the presenile type of dementia is more severe than the senile type, the distinction between presenile and senile types of dementia as used by Kraepelin was based on other than purely medical and scientific grounds. In the 1880s, laws on health insurance and old age pensions became effective in Germany, and it was decided that the latter should begin at the age of 65 years – the starting point of the senium.

In 1902, Kraepelin asked Alois Alzheimer to join him in Heidelberg. At that time, Alzheimer had worked in the Community Hospital for the Insane and Epileptics (*Städtische Heilanstalt für Irre und Epileptiker*) in Frankfurt/Main for 14 years. Here he met Franz Nissl who markedly influenced Alzheimer's neuropathological work. In 1903, Alzheimer moved from Heidelberg to Munich where he stayed until 1912. This was his most scientifically fruitful period. In 1912, he was asked to accept the chair of nervous diseases at the University of Breslau. However, in 1912, Alzheimer contracted a sepsis from which he never recovered. He died of insufficiencies of the heart and kidney in 1915.

At the 37th Meeting of Southwest German Neuropsychiatrists, held in Tübingen from the 3rd to the 4th of November 1906, Alzheimer reported *Über eine eigenartige Erkrankung der Hirnrinde.* He was the second speaker in the afternoon session, and its protocol notes that there was no discussion after his presentation. Alzheimer described the morphological changes of a 51-year-old female patient who had been admitted to the hospital in Frankfurt/Main where he had worked formerly. The patient suffered from severe memory disturbances, disorientation and focal symptoms such as aphasia. The patient died 4½ years after admission, and her brain was sent to Alzheimer for neuropathology. He found arteriosclerosis of the large brain vessels, an uniform brain atrophy without any macroscopic foci, and, using Bielschowsky's silver staining technique, remarkable changes of the neurofibrils which had replaced the neurons. He assumed a chemical change of the fibrils which survived the death of the neuron, and he concluded a peculiar brain disease from the neuropathological changes. This first description of a disorder which would later bear his name was then published in 1907 [1].

In 1911, Alzheimer [2] reported on a 56-year-old man who had been admitted into the Munich Psychiatric Clinic. The patient suffered from severe memory disturbances, disorientation, and inability to take care of himself. With steady progression of the disease, the patient had died in 1910. The neuropathological examination did not show any arteriosclerosis of the brain vessels, but regression disturbances. The frontal, parietal and temporal gyri of both hemispheres were found to be markedly atrophic and the sulci were widened. No softening of the cortex or white matter could be observed. Microscopically, numerous plaques were present frontally, but in an enormous amount parietally and temporally, mostly in the second and third cortical layers. Alzheimer emphasized that he was unable to find a single cell which showed the degeneration of fibrils he had described before. And he also stressed that senile dementia and arteriosclerosis of the brain are different brain diseases, as manifested by the presence of the senile plaques first described by Redlich [12] and later by Fischer [4] and Perusini [10] among others.

Alzheimer's excellent clinical and morphological work, his clear description of similarities and differences in neuropathology correlated with clinical symptomatology was the basis for classifying organic brain disorders such as presbyophrenia or Korsakoff's syndrome, Pick's disease and Alzheimer's disease itself. It was Kraepelin who first used this term, on page 627 of the 8th edition of his *Psychiatrie* in 1910 [7]. Kraepelin continued to use this classification in the later editions of his book so that it became known and accepted worldwide.

The merit of Alzheimer and his contemporaries cannot be overestimated. Their ideas on Alzheimer's disease are still valid and have been confirmed by many findings from modern research in morphobiology, metabolism and other important fields. Nevertheless, great uncertainties remain regarding the aetiology, pathobiochemistry and successful treatment; the number of people suffering from this disease is high and may increase in the future. Therefore, the words of Robert Koch [6] who established the aetiology of tuberculosis may be modified to apply to Alzheimer's disease. If the number of people who suffer from a disease is the measure of the significance of that disease, then Alzheimer's disease surpasses all the other organic brain diseases. Common medical care has thus reason enough to address its attention to such a terrible disease.

References

1. Alzheimer A (1907) Über eine eigenartige Erkrankung der Hirnrinde. Allg Z Psychiatr 64:146–148
2. Alzheimer A (1911) Über eigenartige Krankheitsfälle des späten Alters. Z Gesamte Neurol Psychiatr 4:356–385
3. Esquirol JED (1838) Des maladies mentales considérées sous les rapports médical, hygiénique et médico-légal. Ballière, Paris
4. Fischer O (1907) Miliare Nekrosen mit drusigen Wucherungen der Neurofibrillen. Eine regelmäßige Veränderung der Hirnrinde bei seniler Demenz. Monatsschr Psychiatr Neurol 22:361–372
5. Jaspers K (1913) Allgemeine Psychopathologie. 1st edn. Springer, Berlin Heidelberg New York, p 326 (9th edn. 1973)
6. Koch R (1882) Die Ätiologie der Tuberkulose. Vortrag Physiolog Ges Berlin 24. 3. 1882. In: Sudhoff K (ed) Klassiker der Medizin. Barth, Leipzig, pp 10–38
7. Kraepelin E (1910) Psychiatrie. Ein Lehrbuch für Studierende und Ärzte, 8th edn vol II, Part I. Barth, Leipzig, pp 593–632
8. Lichtheim M (1973) The old and middle Kingdoms. In: Ancient Egypt Lit 1. University of California Press, Berkley, p 63
9. Meynert T (1884) Psychiatrie. Braunmüller, Wien
10. Perusini G (1910) Über klinisch und histologisch eigenartige psychische Erkrankungen des höheren Lebensalters. Nissl-Alzheimer's Arbeiten 3:297–358
11. Pierer JF (1806) Hippocratis opera, vol II, Sectio V, De Morbo Sacro Liber. Caput VII. Literarisches Comtoir, Altenburg, pp 475–492
12. Redlich E (1898) Über miliare Sklerose der Hirnrinde bei seniler Atrophie. Jahrb Psychiatr Neurol 17:208–216
13. Schneider K (1958) Klinische Psychopathologie, 5th edn. Thieme, Stuttgart, p 63

The Descriptive Epidemiology of the Dementias

D. W. K. Kay[1]

Introduction

As has long been known, dementia is an important cause of admission of elderly patients to psychiatric hospitals. In addition, many demented persons are to be found in nonpsychiatric facilities such as geriatric hospitals, nursing homes and communal homes of various kinds. But are these merely the tip of an iceberg? Only community surveys in which each person has an equal chance of being identified can provide unbiased information about the incidence and prevalence of dementia in a population and the characteristics of those affected. In this paper I shall try to describe what epidemiological surveys have revealed.

The Prevalence of Moderate/Severe Dementia

During the past 25 years there have been over 20 studies [1] reporting prevalence rates of dementia among persons aged 60 or 65 years and over in the community at large. Usually, rates are given for different degrees of severity, such as "mild, moderate and severe", "mild and severe", or even "mild to moderate, and severe". Such categories are not found in the official classifications, are seldom rigorously defined by authors, and add to the difficulties of comparing results.

Moderate and severe dementia corresponds more or less to dementia as seen in clinical cases. The criteria proposed by Roth [2], or the definitions given in the *International Classification of Diseases* or in the 3rd edition of the *Diagnostic and Statistical Manual of the American Psychiatric Association,* are usually adopted. In a few studies standardised interviews have been used [3, 4]. A computerised diagnostic system "Agecat" has been developed [5] to complement the Geriatric Mental State used in the US-UK Diagnostic Project [3].

For such cases the reported rates range from under 1% to about 7%. However, the majority lie between 3% and 5% (Table 1, first column). The right-hand column shows the overall rates, when mild dementia (second column) was included. These are generally over 11%, but some are as low as 4%–5%. Mild dementia is discussed later, and the following paragraphs refer to moderate/severe dementia.

---

[1] Prudhoe Hospital, Prudhoe, Northumberland, NE42 5NT, Great Britain.

Neurology
Ed. by K. Poeck, H. J. Freund, and H. Gänshirt

Table 1. Number of studies reporting prevalence rates of dementia within the stated range

Rate (%)	Moderate/severe	Mild	All degrees
< 2	3	2	0
2– 3	4	1	0
3– 4	6	0	0
4– 5	4	1	3
5– 6	2	2	0
6– 7	3	0	0
7– 9	1	1	1
10–14	0	4	4
≧15	0	1	4
Total	23	12	12

Do Regional Differences Exist?

Do these wide variations in reported rates of dementia reflect real differences between studies and regions? The fact is, the surveys differ in many ways and very few can be strictly compared with each other.

The different aims of the investigators determine the size and choice of the target or "at risk" population, the age group to be studied and whether or not institutions are included in the survey. There are, for example, surveys of complete, delimited populations, as in Lundby, Sweden [6] and Samsö, Denmark [7], probability samples as in New Haven [8] and Newcastle [9], age-stratified samples as in Hobart [4] and Glasgow [10], and two early studies of isolated general practices. The New Haven study of the elderly is part of a large-scale epidemiological survey concerned with psychiatric morbidity throughout the age range, while those in Glasgow, Hobart, Japan [1], Mannheim [12], Newcastle and Moscow [see 12], and the US-UK Cross-National Geriatric Study [3], were concerned only with the elderly. The surveys in Stockholm [13] and in Turku, Finland [14], focused exclusively on dementia.

The "target population", which provides the denominator for the calculation of rates, may be based on census returns for a large, defined population (perhaps 100000 people), or on the other hand it may consist of just a few hundred persons chosen from electoral rolls or general practitioners' lists, or identified from house visits. The resulting morbidity rates may refer to point or period prevalence.

The effect of individual factors is not always apparent. However, population rates derived from hospitalisation data [13] or based on cases ascertained by the community survey method [14] tend to be low, i.e. <1% to about 2%. In this method, information is first obtained from various sources, and only those persons who are reported to be affected are personally examined.

In contrast, in the interview method the aim is to individually locate and personally interview every person in the target population. Using this method, four or five times as many moderately or severely demented persons are found to be living in private households as in institutions [12]. This method is, however, limited to fairly small samples, and a combination of both methods gives the best estimate of the

Table 2. Age-specific prevalence rates for moderate/severe dementia

Place		Age range (years)				
		65–69	65–74	70–79	75+	80+
		Rate (%)				
Newcastle	[9]	2.3		3.9		22.0
Glasgow	[10]		1.6		7.2	
Japan	[11]	1.9		6.5		16.2
Lundby[a]	[6]	0.9+		5.1		21.8
Samsö[a,b]	[7]	0		1.9		13.2
Hobart	[4]			2.5		7.8

[a] Includes institutions; + 60–69
[b] Community survey method

number of demented persons in a population, and their distribution between private houses and institutions.

Choice of Diagnostic Criteria. The choice of stringent diagnostic criteria appears to account for some of the lower rates reported. These rates are informative, in that they suggest that at least 2% of the age group 70–79 and 5% of the over-80s, are unable to provide even for their basic personal needs, owing to dementia [15].

With few exceptions [3], regional comparisons of the prevalence of dementia using identical methods of sampling and diagnosis lie in the future. However, the marked regional variation in the rate of certification of dementia as a cause of death in the United Kingdom [16] provides prima facie evidence for the existence of an environmental agent. The uneven clustering of unrelated cases observed in the Edinburgh survey of presenile dementia [17] also supports this possibility. The remarkable geographical concentration of cases with the Guam parkinsonism dementia complex is of course well documented. However, apart from familial occurrence in some pedigrees, and the susceptibility to the disease of persons with Down's syndrome, risk factors for Alzheimer-type dementia have not yet been established.

Age Specific Prevalence Rates. One thing at least is clear: the prevalence of dementia increases with age (Table 2). Under the age of 60, the prevalence is about 0.1% [14]; in the age group 60–69, under 2%; in those aged 70–79, 2%–6%; and at ages over 80, the rate is usually 15%–20% [4, 6, 7, 9–12]. The prevalence increases markedly after the age of 80. The higher figures in each age group were obtained with the interview method.

The Incidence of Dementia

Now prevalence is a function of both incidence and duration. It follows that the age-specific increase in the prevalence of dementia could be due to an accumulation of survivors rather than to increasing incidence of new cases [18]. Studies of incidence are therefore of great interest, but are difficult to carry out, since the same population must be assessed in the same way on two (or more) separate occasions. So far, few such studies have been reported [15, 19].

Age-Specific Incidence. The best-known study was begun in 1946 in Lundby, Sweden, by Essen-Möller [6]. A delimited population of 2500 persons of all ages, was reexamined twice, after 10 and again after 15 years, by Hagnell and colleagues [19]. New cases of dementia were identified both from personal interviews and from other sources of information, employing clinical criteria.

In Lundby [19], the annual incidence increased throughout the senium. It was about 0.4% between the age of 60 and 69, and increased to about 5% after the age of 80. The increase occurred in both sexes. This high rate of incidence is being reproduced in the Baltimore Longitudinal Study [20].

Cumulative Incidence of Dementia. Hagnell [19] also calculated the cumulative probability of becoming demented at various ages, assuming survival. This was about 3% by the age of 70, 15% by 80, and 40% by the age of 90. After 90, there were too few survivors for probability calculations to be made, but new cases continued to appear. In the Baltimore study the cumulative incidence for senile dementia alone is 29% by age 85 [20]. These rates are higher than previously reported [13] and need to be confirmed. They are, for instance, of the same order as the rates reported in first-degree relatives of unselected Alzheimer patients.

Changes of Incidence Over Time. Hagnell reported that the incidence of dementia had decreased from the first to the second period. A falling incidence of strokes has been reported elsewhere, but in Lundby both vascular and senile dementia were reduced [19]. The causes are conjectural.

Clinicopathological Diagnosis

Clinical Findings. In the Turku population, senile and presenile dementia of Alzheimer type accounted for over half the cases and vascular dementia for 36%. Parkinson's disease, trauma and alcohol-related diseases in that order were the commonest other causes, which together comprised only 12% of the total [14]. These cases were thoroughly investigated, but in community studies as a rule the accepted criteria for senile dementia (insidious onset, progression and exclusion of other causes by appropriate investigations) are difficult to satisfy and differential diagnosis is unreliable. Bearing this in mind, senile dementia of Alzheimer type has formed 26%–80% of the total in studies in Europe and the United States, while in Japan relatively more vascular and other non-Alzheimer dementias are reported [11]. This merits further study. In Lundby, the incidence rates for senile and vascular dementia were similar [19].

Autopsy Findings. Unfortunately, pathological diagnosis is hardly ever available in survey research. However, in a series of routine autopsies carried out at the University Medical Center, Michigan, Alzheimer-type changes were found to increase continuously after 71 years of age [21]. In 13% of persons over 65, and in 54% of persons over 85, these changes were sufficiently severe to qualify the case pathologically as Alzheimer's disease.

In an autopsy series of demented, elderly patients reported from Newcastle, all of whom died in institutions, Alzheimer-type changes alone were found in 64%, a mixed picture in 12%, multiple infarcts alone in 11%, and 3% were due to other causes. In 10% the brain was normal. The autopsy findings so far available support clinical opinion that Alzheimer-type dementia is the predominant dementia of old age.

Mild Dementia and the Use of Rating Scales

Autopsy series on so-called mild dementia have not been reported. Mild dementia is an ill-defined condition, and its connotations are still unclear. The reported prevalence rates vary from 4% to an exceptionally high rate of 50% in one study [11]. The next highest rate is 15% [7]. The percentage of cases with mild dementia varies from less than 40% to 80% of all cases of dementia.

Follow up studies in Denmark [23] and the United Kingdom [24] suggest, however, that mild dementia is heterogeneous. Only a minority of cases appear to be early cases of progressive dementia. The remainder are associated with a variety of mental and physical disorders. Moreover, the boundary between what is normal and what is pathological is particularly unclear at advanced ages, where normative data are scanty. More detailed descriptions and agreed definitions of mild dementia are highly desirable.

Seeing that in the general population dementia does not present as an all-or-none entity, some investigators have adopted a dimensional approach using rating scales, instead of or in addition to clinical diagnosis. Scales which have been used in this way include the Rational Scale of Dementia [3, 4] and the Mental Status Questionnaire [25], both used in the US-UK Cross-National Project, the Short Portable Mental Status Questionnaire in North Carolina [26], the Mini-Mental State Exami-

Table 3. Age-specific rates of dementia in the community, using rating scales

Reference	Place	Scale	Age (years)	*n*	Rate (%)
Weissman et al. [8]	New Haven	MMSE	65–74	1016	1.1
			75–84	770	4.3
			85+	202	16.8
Gurland et al. [3]	New York	RSD	70–79	218	5.0
			80+	83	15.7
Kay et al. [4]	Hobart	RSD	70–79	158	4.4
			80+	116	12.1
Clarke et al. [27]	Leicester	CAS	75+	1073	1.6

MMSE, Mini-Mental State Examination; RSD, Rational Scale of Dementia; CAS, Cognitive Assessment Scale nation in New Haven [8] and Hobart [4], and the Cognitive Assessment Scale in Leicester, England [27]. The score distributions obtained are skewed, but unimodal, and show no obvious discontinuities separating normal from abnormal. When cut-off points are applied, age-specific rates are obtained which, with one exception [27], are similar to those reported using diagnostic categories (Table 3).

These scales need to be modified for use in the community to increase their sensitivity. Some of them test only a limited area of cognition. The cut-off points may need to be adjusted for subjects' educational level [25, 26]. In short, as Cooper and Bickel point out in their review of population screening for dementia [28], the use of rating scales in the community is still in the experimental stage.

Do Sex Differences Exist?

Women form the majority of demented persons over the age of 80, and in institutions [14], but this is due at least in part to demographic and social factors. However, in New Haven, among persons aged over 80 living at home, rates of dementia were higher in women than in men [8]. Since a rating scale was used in this study, this difference could be put down to educational disadvantage among the women. Another explanation may be that women survive for a longer period in a dependent state than men [see 8], which would tend to increase the prevalence of aged women with dementia. As regards incidence, in Lundby no sex difference was observed either for senile or vascular dementia [19].

Dementia and Dependency

The epidemiology of dementia should encompass its social consequences. Studies of elderly persons at home [10] and in institutions (Kay and Holding, unpublished work), in which dementia and dependency on others in everyday tasks were separately assessed, showed that about 75% of persons who were unable to care for their basic personal needs were severely demented, while 70% of the severely demented were profoundly dependent. Dementia as a symptom of stroke or Parkinsonism greatly increased dependency; and in the presence of dementia common conditions such as arthritis, cataract or obesity became unmanageable.

Demographic Gerontology

How will demographic and social trends affect the elderly in the future? The fact that dementia is a disease of old age makes the age structure of future populations a critical factor. Projections are notoriously uncertain, but everyone who will be aged 65 or over in the year 2050 has already been born. Hence (if mortality remains constant) the numbers of the old and very old who will be alive in the next half century can be predicted with some confidence. For example, by the year 2020, the number of persons in the world aged 65 years or over will be more than doubled, and the number over 80 almost trebled. In Europe, the over-65s will increase by 50%, while the over-80s will increase by nearly 100% [29]. These projections make it realistic to speak of a "coming epidemic of dementia".

However, the relative numbers of the young, middle-aged and elderly will depend on the birth rate. Whatever the birth rate, the labour force will remain fairly constant in size. But the percentage of young will determine what resources remain over for the care of the old.

The outlook for men and women is not the same. About 35% of women in developed countries are now living to be 85 years old, compared with about half that percentage of men. The male : female ratio after the age of 60 will continue to decrease. The proportion of elderly widows living alone will continue to increase.

Conclusions

In conclusion, there are sound reasons for thinking (a) that over the next 50 years, the age group in which dementia is most prevalent will increase disproportionately; (b) that dementia is a major cause of dependency in the aged; (c) that women will be specially at risk, both for dementia and for institutional care. Finally (d), even small differences in the rates imply large differences in the total number of persons who are affected in a population. Therefore, methods of identifying and rating dementia in the community need to be improved so that its incidence and prevalence can be more precisely determined, regional differences properly evaluated and its social consequences adequately assessed.

References

1. Henderson AS, Kay DWK (1984) The epidemiology of mental disorders in the aged. In: Kay DWK, Burrows G (eds) Handbook of studies on psychiatry and old age. Elsevier, North Holland, pp 53–88
2. Roth M (1964) The natural history of mental disorders in old age. J Ment Sci 101:281–301
3. Gurland B, Copeland J, Kuriansky J, Kelleher M, Sharpe L, Dean LL (1983) The mind and mood of aging. Croom Helm, London
4. Kay DWK, Henderson AS, Scott J, Wilson J, Rickwood D, Grayson DA (1985) Dementia and depression among the elderly living in the Hobart community: the effect of the diagnostic criteria on the prevalence rates. Psychol Med 15:771–788
5. Copeland JRM, Dewey ME, Griffiths-Jones HM (1986) A computerised psychiatric diagnostic system and case nomenclature for elderly subjects: GMS and AGECAT. Psychol Med 16:89–99
6. Essen-Möller E, Larsson H, Uddenberg CE, White G (1956) Individual traits and morbidity in a Swedish rural population. Acta Psychiatr Scand [Suppl] 100:1–160
7. Nielsen J (1962) Geronto-psychiatric period-prevalence investigation in a geographically delimited population. Acta Psychiatr Scand 38:307–330
8. Weissman MM, Myers JK, Tischler GL, Holzer CE, Leaf PJ, Orvaschel, Brody JA (1985) Psychiatric disorders (DSM-III) and cognitive impairment in the elderly in a U.S. urban community. Arch Gen Psychiatry 41:959–967
9. Kay DWK, Bergmann K, Forster EM, McKechnie AA, Roth M (1970) Mental illness and hospital usage in the elderly: a random sample followed up. Compr Psychiatry 11:26–35
10. Broe GA, Akhtar AJ, Andrews GR, Caird FI, Gilmore AJJ, McLennan WJ (1976) Neurological disorders in the elderly at home. J Neurol Neurosurg Psychiatry 39:362–366
11. Kaneko Z (1975) Care in Japan. In: Howells JG (ed) Modern perspectives in the psychiatry of old age. Bruner/Mazel, New York, pp 519–530

12. Cooper B, Sosna U (1983) Psychische Erkrankung in der Altersbevölkerung. Eine epidemiologische Feldstudie in Mannheim. Nervenarzt 54:239–249
13. Larsson T, Sjögren T, Jacobson G (1953) Senile dementia. Acta Psychiatr Scand [Suppl 167] 39:136
14. Mölsä PK, Marttila RJ, Rinne UK (1982) Epidemiology of dementia in a Finnish population. Acta Neurol Scand 65:541–552
15. Åkesson H (1969) A population study of senile and arteriosclerotic psychoses. Hum Hered 19:546–566
16. Gardner MJ, Winter PD, Barker DLJP (1984) Atlas of mortality from selected diseases in England and Wales 1968–1978. Wiley, Chichester
17. Whalley LJ, Holloway S (1985) Non-random geographical distribution of Alzheimer's presenile dementia in Edinburgh, 1953–76. Lancet March 9:578
18. Mortimer JA, Schuman LM, French LR (1981) The epidemiology of dementing illness. In: Mortimer JA, Schuman LM (eds) The epidemiology of dementia. Oxford University Press, New York, pp 132–154
19. Hagnell O, Lanke J, Rorsman B, Öhman R, Öjesjö L (1983) Current trends in the incidence of senile and multi-infarct dementia. A prospective study of a total population followed over 25 years; the Lundby study. Arch Psychiatr Nervenkr 233:423–438
20. Sluss TK, Gruenberg EM, Kramer M (1981) The use of longitudinal studies in the investigation of risk factors for Senile Dementia – Alzheimer type. In: Mortimer JA, Schuman LM (eds) The epidemiology of dementia. Oxford University Press, New York, pp 132–154
21. Miller F de W, Hicks SP, D'Amato CJ, Landis JR (1984) A descriptive study of neuritic plaques and neurofibrillary tangles in an autopsy population. Am J Epidemiol 120:331–341
22. Blessed G (1984) Clinical features and neuropathological correlations of Alzheimer type disease. In: Kay DWK, Burrows GD (eds) Handbook of studies on psychiatry and old age. Elsevier, North Holland, pp 133–143
23. Nielsen J, Homma A, Björn-Henriksen T (1977) Follow-up 15 years after a geronto-psychiatric prevalence study. Conditions concerning death, causes of death and life expectancy in relation to psychiatric diagnosis. J Gerontol 32:554–561
24. Bergmann K, Kay DWK, Foster E, McKechnie AA, Roth M (1971) A follow up study of randomly selected community residents to assess the effects of chronic brain syndrome and cerebrovascular disease. In: Psychiatry, part 2. Excerpta Medica International Congress Series no 274. Excerpta Medica, Amsterdam, pp 856–865
25. Gurland BJ (1981) The borderlands of dementia: the influence of sociocultural characteristics on rates of dementia in the senium. In: Miller NE, Cohen GD (eds) Clinical aspects of Alzheimer's disease and senile dementia. Raven, New York, pp 61–80
26. Pfeiffer E (1975) A short portable mental status questionnaire for the assessment of organic brain deficit in elderly patients. J Am Geriatr Soc 23:433–440
27. Clarke M, Clarke S, Odell A, Jagger C (1984) The elderly at home: health and social status. Health Trends 16:3–7
28. Cooper B, Bickel H (1984) Population screening and the early detection of dementing disorders in old age. Psychol Med 14:81–95
29. World Health Organization (1982) World Health Stat Q 35:3–4

Clinical Presentation of the Dementias

G. BLESSED[1]

Dementia can arise at any age. Rare before middle life, when its onset constitutes a personal tragedy for the sufferer and his/her immediate family, it is most commonly found among the very old, where the syndrome and its consequent deficits must be differentiated from those, often similar in form, produced by the ageing process.

Dementia often develops insidiously and its precise onset may be difficult to determine unless circumstances bring an old person with incipient dementia under scrutiny. Thus an admission to hospital for an intercurrent illness, a family holiday in unfamiliar surroundings or the death of a spouse may be events which bring dementia to light. Sometimes these events have called for psychological adjustments to a rapidly changing situation, and it can be argued that the deteriorating brain's reduced reserve of cognitive skill is overwhelmed by this need for rapid adaptation. But it is equally possible that such events simply bring old people, who otherwise lead fairly undemanding lives, under scrutiny which reveals their deficits. Often such events are described as having *caused* the dementia: "She started to fail after her husband died suddenly." While the possible causative nature of such major life events should not be denied, and justifies further research, it is clearly tempting to exaggerate their importance; for they offer plausible explanations for an otherwise bewildering human condition. The same considerations apply to abruptness of onset. This has been shown to be more commonly associated with dementias of vascular aetiology than those based upon diffuse neuronal disorders. Thus Hachinski [1] allocates 'abrupt onset' a weighted score of 2 for vascular aetiology, and in the recently published NINCDS[2]: ADRDA criteria for the recognition of Alzheimer's disease [2], sudden apoplectic onset makes the diagnosis of 'probable' Alzheimer dementia 'unlikely' or at best 'uncertain'. However, slowly evolving disorders can be *noticed* abruptly by patients and their relatives alike, and if a subject suffering from early Alzheimer's disease collapses, or faints, or suffers a transient ischaemic attack and subsequent scrutiny reveals the hitherto unsuspected dementia, it is tempting to assume a vascular aetiology because of the combination of acute onset plus the presumed 'vascular' nature of the associated episode.

[1] Brighton Clinic, Newcastle General Hospital, Westgate Road, Newcastle-upon-Tyne, NE4 6BE, Great Britain.

[2] National Institute of Neurological and Communicable Disorders and Stroke: Alzheimer's Disease and Related Disorders Association.

Neurology
Ed. by K. Poeck, H. J. Freund, and H. Gänshirt

Clinical Symptoms of Dementia

These are set out in certain definitions of dementia. Ignoring those which are insufficiently detailed to form an adequate basis for clinical diagnosis, I will concentrate upon two, those of Roth and Myers [4]:

1. A memory disturbance taking the form of defective registration of new impressions.
2. An impairment of intellect resulting in defective grasp, reasoning and learning ability. Disorientation for time and place is a characteristic outcome of severe impairment of memory and intellect.
3. A coarsening of personality. There is deterioration of social conduct and personal appearance. The emotions become labile, often blunted, and their range narrows.

And of the Royal College of Physicians of London (1981) "Dementia is the global impairment of higher cortical function including memory, the capacity to solve the problems of day to day living, the performance of learned perceptuo-motor skills, the correct use of social skills and control of emotional reactions, in the absence of gross clouding of consciousness. The condition is often irreversible and progressive." These definitions identify certain key clinical features of dementia and I would like to concentrate on five of these.

1. Reduced ability to register and recall new material
2. Impairment of grasp, reasoning and learning, including the incapacity to solve the problems of day-to-day living
3. Disorientation (for time, place and persons)
4. A coarsening and blunting of the personality
5. A deterioration in the performance of learned perceptuo-motor skills, of social conduct, personal appearance and self-care skills.

These features can be explored by measurement: by testing of individual patients, by rating scales completed by observers of the patients' usual behaviour, or by a combination of both methods. In the following demonstrations, deficits have been measured in 128 elderly people who attended a psycho-geriatric assessment centre and were followed up to autopsy. Of this group, 66 members proved to have Alzheimer's disease of the brain at autopsy, and 62 to have normally aged brains (using criteria established by Tomlinson et al. [11]).

Registration and Recall of New Material

The ability to register a name and address and recall it five minutes later was tested (modified Roth-Hopkins test [6]). The results are shown in Fig. 1.

There are important differences between the two groups. Even limited memory skill is rare in subjects with Alzheimer's disease. However, total failure on this test is also shown by nearly half the subjects with 'normal' brains. Reducing the 'normal' cases to clinical diagnostic categories it can be seen (Table 1) that those who do badly are predominantly cases of acute confusion or clinical cases of dementia unassociated with major disease of the brain.

However, impairments of memory are relatively common in both elderly depressives and cases of late paraphrenia, with 20% of such cases failing to score at all on this test.

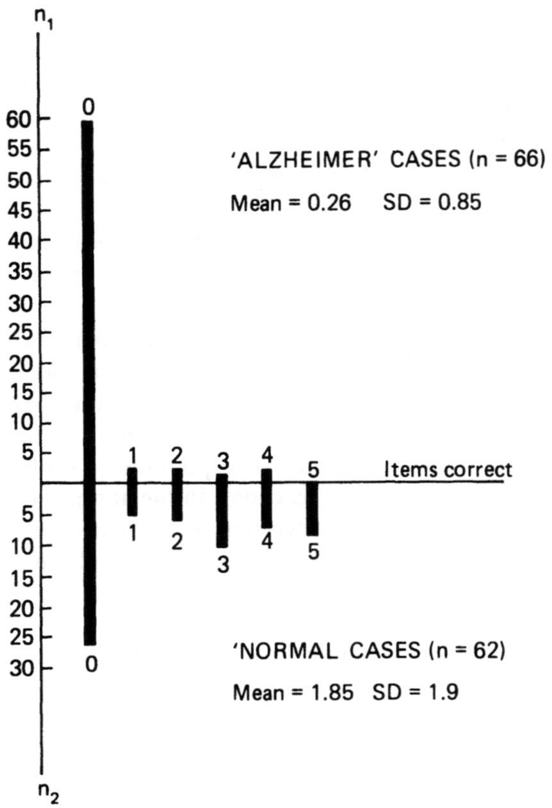

Fig. 1. Name and address recall at 5 minutes

Table 1. Name and address recall at 5 minutes; 62 patients with pathologically 'normal' brains

Diagnosis	*n*	Mean score	Std. Dev.
Acute confusion	19	0.95	1.43
Dementia	8	0.88	1.64
Depression [a]	24	3.04	1.78
Schizophrenia [b]	6	1.8	2.14
Mixed cases (OBS/FBS)	3	0.33	0.58
Others	2	–	–

[a] 4 cases failed to score
[b] 2 cases failed to score

Impaired Cognitive Functioning

Observers completed a scale rating cognitive items according to 'dementia score' [6].

In this case the differences are more striking and the overlap between scores allocated to the Alzheimer patients and controls is much smaller; moderate impairment or greater (score 4 or 4+) was found in only 19.3% of the cases with normal brains compared with 94% of the Alzheimer cases. None of the depressed patients were judged to be moderately impaired.

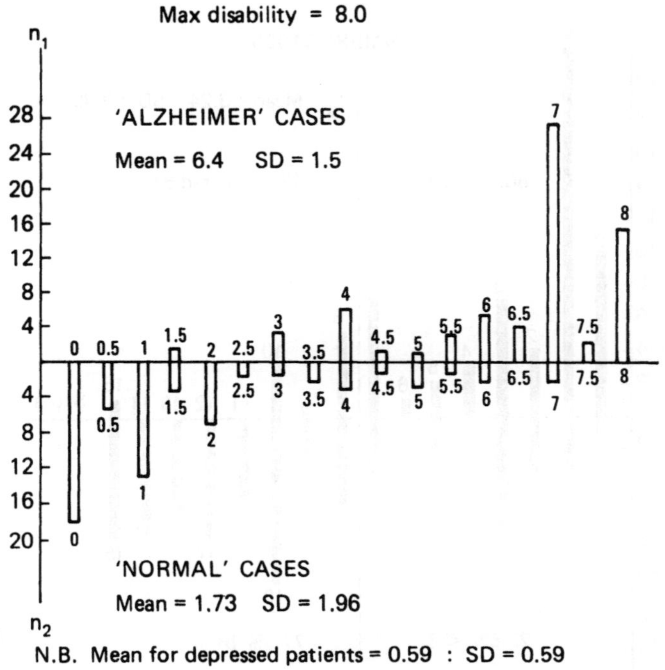

Fig. 2. Cognitive decrease reported by relatives

Orientation

The first 15 items of a modified Roth-Hopkins test were applied [6].

Again, mean scores differed considerably, with a cut-off score based upon 50% impairment successfully separating the two groups in over 75% of cases. Nevertheless, one pathologically proven case of Alzheimer's disease obtained a full score on this test (Fig. 3)!

Personality Deterioration

Observers completed a scale rating personality items by 'dementia score'.

In the results, although a significant difference in mean levels of personality decline exists, differences between Alzheimer and normal cases are smaller than for any of the measures previously considered. The reason for this may be twofold. First, personality change in old people, produced by Alzheimer's disease, may be attributed by relatives to the effects of ageing; secondly, some personality change is frequently wrought by psychiatric disorders other than dementia – notably depression and schizophrenia. Consequently, the development of perceptible personality deterioration may be a less reliable marker for Alzheimer's disease in old people than disorientation or perceived cognitive decline (Fig. 4).

Perceptuo-Motor Skills and Habits

Patients were rated on feeding, dressing and continence items according to 'dementia score'.

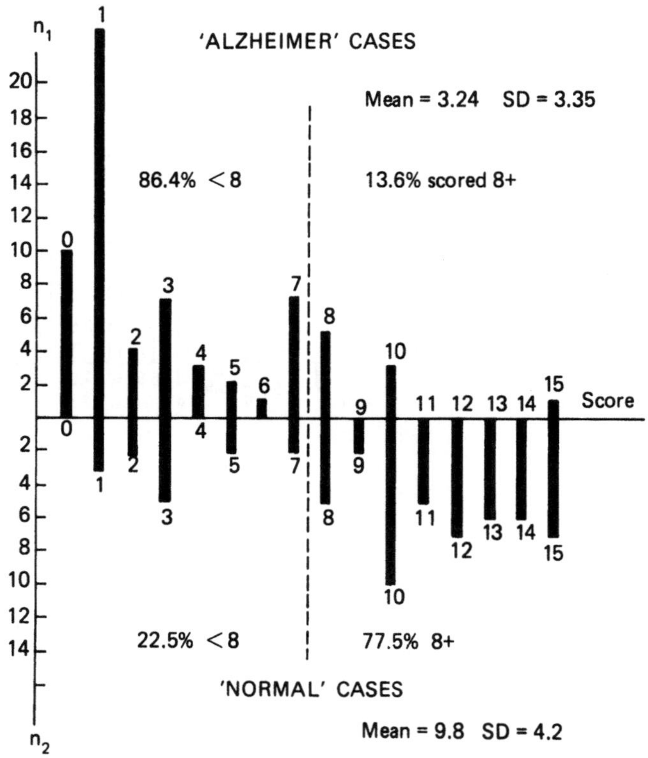

Fig. 3. Orientation

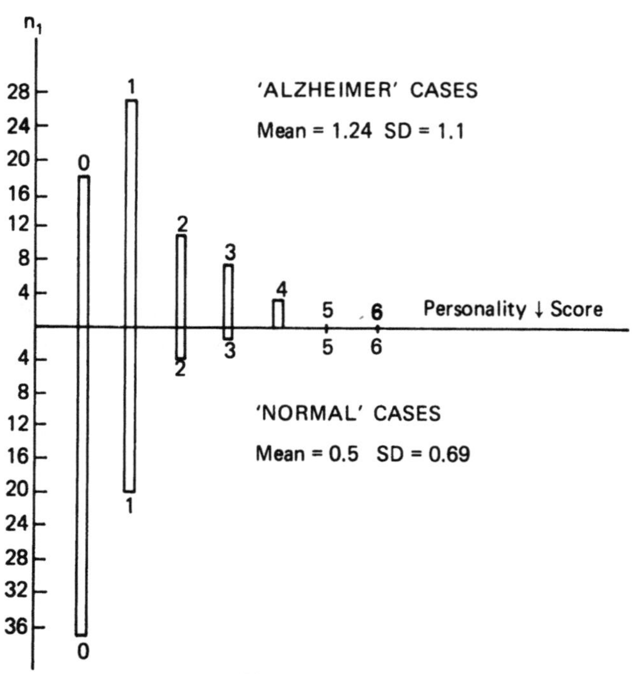

Fig. 4. Personality deterioration

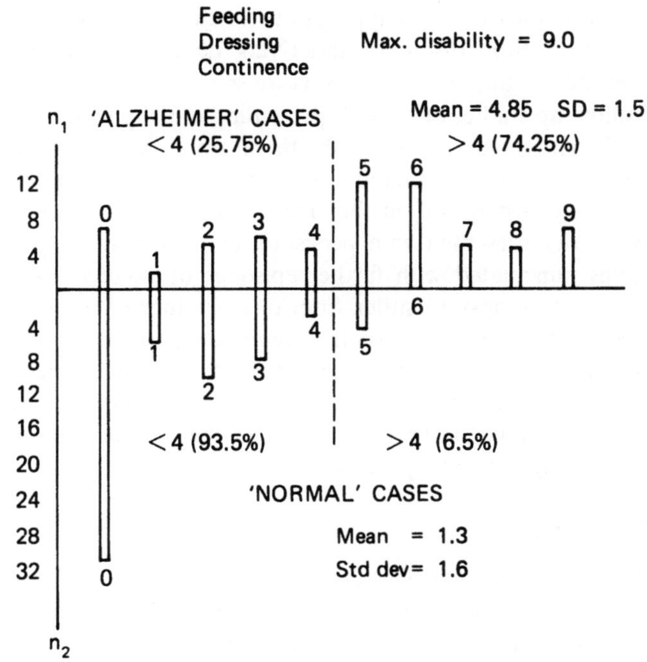

Fig. 5. Decline in habits reported by relatives

The separation achieved by this test is comparable to that found in the orientation and cognitive decline measures. However, clinically less severe cases of Alzheimer's disease may retain good habitual functions. Conversely, serious deterioration of habits can sometimes be found in cases with functional psychiatric disorders in old age – this is particularly true of depressive illness.

Summary of Clinical Symptoms

Although the five features examined are all described as 'typical' for dementia, the results reported suggest that, using pathologically proven Alzheimer's disease as the paradigm of dementia, some are more typical than others. Memory impairments and personality change emerge as those which show the greatest overlap with other psychiatric disorders encountered in the senium, while loss of skills and habits, disorientation and cognitive decline emerge as the more reliable markers, at least for dementia of Alzheimer type.

Exclusion Criteria: Their Use in Diagnosis

Clouding of Consciousness

There seems to be universal agreement that a diagnosis of dementia should never be made in the clouded patient. In the author's view such a statement is perfectly valid for pure research but inappropriate for clinical practice, for there is nothing inherent in the cerebral disorders underlying dementia which protects the patients from episodes of impairment of consciousness. Indeed, the reverse is likely to be true. Follow-up studies of patients presenting initially with acute confusional states [7] reveal that whereas at 6 months there are striking differences in prognosis between cases of senile dementia and acute confusion, at 2 years the differences are less apparent. Furthermore, in the small number of cases presenting as acute confusion who later presented with persisting or progressive cognitive decline (albeit sometimes punctuated with further episodes of clouded consciousness), all have been found at autopsy to suffer from one or other of the two common varieties of dementia [5]. Thus it appears that demented patients can and do become clouded and may present to clinics with acute confusional states which remit, leaving a residue of dementia. Only longitudinal observations of such cases over weeks or months, with retesting of cognitive function after the clouding has subsided, will reveal the underlying dementia process.

Depression

This is another important exclusion criterion. Again, it must be applied intelligently, for stroke and multiple infarction dementia are known to be associated with clinical depression and early cases of Alzheimer type dementia may also suffer a period of depression which may be of a severity to demand psychiatric treatment. Nevertheless, depression is the commonest 'forger' of the clinical picture of dementia, as Post [8], Marsden and Harrison [9] and Ron et al. [10] have shown. It follows that when dementia and depression co-exist in a patient, the diagnosis of dementia must always remain in doubt while the depression remains, and there is need for even more careful clinical evaluation of such cases. Ron et al. have also shown that EEG findings, studies of the structural integrity of the brain using air or computed tomography scan screening and psychological testing of such cases can clarify the diagnosis.

Two other strategies may be helpful. The first is again serial observation with retesting after the depression has cleared with treatment. The second depends upon an evaluation of the severity of the two components in a 'mixed' case. Severe depression with mild dementia is likely to be primarily an affective disorder, while severe dementia with mild or fluctuating depression, dementia.

Physical Disease

Roth [3] urged caution in making a diagnosis of senile psychosis in an old person suffering from physical ill health, and the NINCDS: ARDRA criteria suggest "absence of specific disorders that in and of themselves could account for the progressive deficits in memory and cognition". While cardiac dementia, dialysis dementia and the dementias of B_{12} deficiency, hypothyroidism and other medical disorders are well documented, it is impracticable to exclude all cases who present with dementia in whom physical disease can be detected on careful screening. Indeed, the majority of demented elderly subjects will have at least one physical disease in addition to their dementia, and unless these are recognised causes of dementia, they should not be used as a means of excluding the diagnosis. The author's unpublished observations reveal that the main significance of physical disease is for the longevity of the demented patient, with the healthiest specimens surviving longest. Of great importance in contemporary practice is the possibility that the patient might be taking drugs prescribed in some cases for long inactive medical conditions, which may be inducing cognitive decline without detectable clouding of consciousness. All patients presenting with dementia need a careful review of their current medication with withdrawal of any treatments not justified by their present medical health status, followed by a period of cognitive rehabilitation and retesting before a firm diagnosis is made.

Inconsistent Features of Dementia

I wish to focus on just three of those less constant features, aphasia, apraxia and agnosia. These 'parietal lobe' deficits can occur concurrently, and except in cases of vascular dementia it is uncommon to find one of them present in isolation, though the others may be detectable only on careful testing of neocortical skills. Speech/language disturbance, acalculia, constructional apraxias and dysgraphic handicaps slowly evolving in a demented patient free from the stigmata of multiple stroke disease are diagnostic of Alzheimer's disease in over 90% of cases [5].

Summary

The clinical features of dementia may not be confined to patients with progressive cerebral disease. They can be found to some extent in normal aged people, and particularly in those with other psychiatric disorders such as acute confusion, depression and schizophrenia. In discriminating between dementia and other psychiatric disorders, some clinical features are more reliable than others, but none is totally reliable.

Exclusion criteria may be of value in refining diagnostic accuracy of dementia for research purposes, but they should be applied carefully and sparingly if the numbers of patients admitted to a cohort for study is to be kept acceptably high, and if the cohort so defined is to have relevance for clinical practice. In the author's view, where exclusion seems necessary because of the concurrence of dementia with acute confusion, depression or serious physical disease, longitudinal observation with appropriate treatment will often clarify the true diagnosis.

Of the less typical features of dementia, the neocortical deficits – aphasia, apraxia, agnosia – appear to be the most reliable markers for the presence of Alzheimer's disease, but they are frequently absent in very aged demented subjects who nevertheless prove to have Alzheimer's disease at post-mortem.

References

1. Hachinski VC et al. (1975) Cerebral blood flow in dementia. Arch Neurol 32:632–637
2. McKhann G et al. (1984) Clinical diagnosis of Alzheimer's disease: report of the NINCDS:ADRDA work group under the auspices of the Department of Health and Human Services Task Force on Alzheimer's disease. Neurology 34:939–944

3. Roth M (1955) The natural history of mental disorders arising in the senium. J Ment Sci 101:281–301
4. Roth M, Myers DH (1969) The diagnosis of dementia. Br J Hosp Med March 1969:705–717
5. Blessed G (1980) Clinical aspects of the senile dementias. In: Roberts PJ (ed) Biochemistry of Dementia. John Wiley, Chichester pp 1–14
6. Blessed G, Tomlinson BE, Roth M (1968) The association between quantitative measures of dementia and of senile change in the cerebral grey matter of elderly subjects. Br J Psychiatry 114:797–811
7. Blessed G, Wilson ID (1982) The contemporary natural history of mental disorder in old age. Br J Psychiatry 141:59–67
8. Post F (1975) Dementia, depression and pseudodementia. In: Benson DF, Blumer D (eds) Psychiatric aspects of neurologic disease. Grune and Stratton, New York, p 99–120
9. Marsden CD, Harrison MJG (1972) Outcome of investigation of patients with presenile dementia. Br Med J 2:249–252
10. Ron MA, Toone BK, Garralda ME, Lishman WA (1979) Diagnostic accuracy in presenile dementia. Br J Psychiatry 134:161–168
11. Tomlinson BE, Blessed G, Roth M (1970) Observations on the Brains of Demented Old People. J Neurol Sci. 11:205–242

The Evolution of the Diagnosis of Dementia: Past, Present, and Future

R. KATZMAN[1] and C. KAWAS[2]

It is perhaps surprising to note the improvement in differential diagnosis of dementing illnesses that has occurred in the past several years. Less than a decade ago a number of retrospective studies had reported a 30%–50% error rate in diagnosis of dementia [4, 17], whereas in the past 2 years the error rate has been reduced to 15%–20% [20]. A significant achievement; but an important gap yet to be closed.

The apparent delay in the development of an adequate differential diagnosis had its roots, perhaps, in the fact that this topic has not always been the favorite enterprise of neurologists. In the 1885 edition of Gowers' *Diseases of the Nervous System* (a text 1356 pages long), only 16 lines are spent on "senile dementia" and only one page on general paresis. Of course, many of the degenerative diseases of the brain had not yet been discovered. But lack of interest persisted. In the 1951 edition of Walshe's text (*Diseases of the Nervous System*), there is still no description of the differential diagnosis of dementia, no description of Alzheimer's disease, no description of dementia as associated with subacute combined degeneration, and only three pages on general paresis. Merritt's and Brain's texts began a more systematic coverage of these diseases. It is only in the past decade that this topic has become fully accepted and adequately described in the majority of neurological texts. One can only speculate on the cause of this lack of interest. Had dementia simply been abandoned to psychiatrists (most of whom – with notable exceptions – were themselves not interested), was dementia simply considered to be part of normal aging, or had the localizationist interests of neurologists become so great that generalized affections of the brain had to be ignored?

Our current understanding of the clinical entity, dementia, can be traced back to the pioneering work of Roth in recognizing that mental illness in the elderly was due to multiple and separable disorders, one of which was dementia, and that differentiating such disorders was critical toward understanding prognosis. Alzheimer's disease accounts for 50%–55% of the cases of dementia; vascular disease for another 20%–25%. However, the clinician must also consider over 60 additional disorders which may cause dementia [5, 9–11]. The latest addition to this list has been AIDS;

[1] Department of Neurosciences, UCSD, La Jolla, CA 92093, USA.
[2] Baltimore Aging Study, Frances Scott Key Hospital, Baltimore, MD, USA.

Neurology
Ed. by K. Poeck, H. J. Freund, and H. Gänshirt

the HTLV III virus has been identified in brains of patients who manifest dementia and pyramidal tract signs [7, 19].

There is now a generally accepted formal definition of dementia contained in the 1980 edition of the *Diagnostic and Statistical Manual of the American Psychiatric Association* (DSM III) [1]. The definitions in DSM III of dementia, depression, and amnestic syndrome have played a role in improving diagnostic accuracy. Dementia, as defined in DSM III, requires the presence of both intellectual decline and impaired functioning; a critical aspect of the definition is that memory plus other areas of cognition must be altered; and the patient must be alert, without a fluctuating level of awareness.

Particular emphasis has been paid by a number of authors to "pseudodementia," that is, depression presenting as memory and related problems [3, 24]; in fact, in several of the retrospective series, this has been the major source of diagnostic error [4, 17]. It is our experience that using DSM III diagnoses for dementias and depression and recognizing that older individuals with unipolar or bipolar depressions may have secondary memory deficits (dementia in depression) permits the interested clinician to separate these syndromes with accuracy.

Diagnostic Workup

A consensus has also developed in the United States as to the diagnostic procedures appropriate for the diagnosis of dementia. The presence of dementia is established by history and mental status examination; neuropsychologic evaluation may be needed. The differential diagnosis of the sixty or more disorders that may be presented as dementia requires the history, physical and neurologic examination, and the following special procedures: CT; EEG; X-ray of the chest; and electrocardiogram. A blood count, biochemical screen, serologic test for syphilis, thyroid function tests, and vitamin B_{12} level are obtained where possible. With the availability of automated tests, these procedures have often been carried out before the dementia patient is referred to a neurologist. The yield today from the blood tests is small, perhaps providing a diagnosis in 1%–2% of the cases; but for that 1%–2%, these tests are very important since many of the conditions are treatable. Often a spinal tap and a neuropsychological evaluation is useful. Special procedures useful in evaluation of patients with suspected normal pressure hydrocephalus include monitoring of intracranial pressure, infusion tests, and isotope cisternography.

The Mental Status Test: Neuropsychological Evaluation

A development that occurred in parallel with the characterization of the dementia syndrome was the development of formal mental status tests. There is a direct line from Mayer-Gross' observations on the *Symptoms of organic brain disease* published in 1931 [13] and the 1937 Mayer-Gross and Guttman *Schema for the examination of organic cases* [14] to the three tests most widely used in current dementia research – the Folstein et al. mini mental status; the Blessed et al. orientation information concentration test; and the Mattis dementia rating scale [2, 12, 22]. All three of these tests are sensitive, reliable, and validated against external measures. The Folstein and Blessed scales are incorporated into the core battery of the federally funded Alzheimer Disease Research Centers in the United States.

Mayer-Gross's interest had been in identifying mental symptoms that differentiated generalized disease of the brain in contrast to focal disease, as well as the symptoms that differentiated organic from "functional" disorders. An interesting amalgam is now taking place. Neuropsychological tests that have developed in part in the tradition of behavioral neurology and in part in the tradition of psychologists interested in measuring mental functions have been added to the mental status tests as part of the core battery by the Alzheimer Centers in the United States. These neuropsychological tests are valuable in confirming the diagnosis of dementia, in following cognitive changes, and in differential diagnosis. They permit a more detailed account of loss of such specific functions as language, memory, and visuospatial skills. The test battery must be sufficiently broad in abilities and levels of skills tested to be usable with patients at different levels of dementia.

Neurologic Examination

Many neurodegenerative disorders may present as a dementia. The neurologic examination is crucial to the differential diagnosis of these conditions. In each of these disorders, except Alzheimer's or Pick's disease, prominent motor features will sooner or later establish the diagnosis. Since Pick's disease involves cortical degeneration in a specific pattern, the symptoms will be cognitive and include behavioral changes if frontal lobes are involved, and language if temporal lobes are the most afflicted. The diagnosis of Huntingtons' disease depends upon the presence of dysarthria and chorea as well as a dementia; moreover, a family history can usually be obtained in this dominant autosomal disorder. Parkinson's disease is readily identified by the tremor, posture, bradykinesia, and rigidity; progressive supranuclear palsy by the impairment of vertical eye movements and extrapyramidal features. Less frequently encountered disorders are the olivopontocerebellar and spinal cerebellar degenerations, adult form of metachromatic leukodystrophy, progressive myoclonus epilepsy, and Hallervorden-Spatz disease. Recently, we have seen several patients with amyotrophic lateral sclerosis who presented with dementia. Symptoms included marked personality changes due, perhaps, to frontal lobe involvement.

Computerized Tomography

The CT has been recognized from the time of its availability as the procedure of choice for the identification of mass lesions and adult hydrocephalus. It is important to note that pre-CT autopsy series such as that of Jellinger [8] indicate that 4%–5% of patients presenting with dementia have either brain tumors or subdurals, and 1%–2% have hydrocephalus.

Magnetic Resonance Imaging

The resolution of MRI scans carried out with a magnetic flux density greater than 1 T appears to be at least as good as that of fourth-generation CT scans. MRI has the added advantages of absence of artifact due to bone and better visualization of white matter changes. Visualization of anatomic landmarks is greatly enhanced, especially if scan time is increased. Hence, MRI may replace CT scan in the differential diagnosis of dementia if experience bears out its potentialities.

MRI and Vascular Dementia. MRI has a particular role to play in the diagnosis of vascular dementia since it is capable of identifying a high proportion of old infarct and lacunes. Tomlinson et al. [22] demonstrated that dementia occurs with multiple strokes when more than 50–100 g of cerebral hemisphere is destroyed. It should become possible to estimate the volume of tissue destroyed on MRI. If this turns out to be clinically feasible, then multi-infarct dementia will become an MRI diagnosis.

Binswanger's Disease. Rosen et al. [18] demonstrated that the CT picture of altered appearance of white matter was consistent with the pathologic demonstration of demyelination in hemispheral white matter in a patient with Binswanger's disease. This report has led to an increase in the number of patients diagnosed during life with this disorder. However, it is found that some elderly without the symptoms of Binswanger's disease show white matter attenuation; this has been termed the "leukoencephalopathy of normal aging." This phenomenon is accentuated on MRI. Adequate clinical pathologic studies have not been carried out. The need for correlation of clinical and anatomic features with the CT and MRI images, suggesting disease of white matter both in patients with symptoms and in normal elderly with abnormal white matter on scans, should be a high priority. A specific diagnosis based upon imaging may be possible; but if not, the nature of the white matter change in normal aging – a quite unexpected finding – needs to be defined.

Ischemic Score

While awating such studies, a most useful instrument is the Hachinski ischemic score. First devised upon the basis of clinical experience, later confirmed on the basis of a retrospective pathologic study. We currently have the opportunity of investigating the usefulness of the ischemic score in a prospective study of the development of dementia in 488 initially nondemented 80-year-olds. To date, 26 subjects have developed Alzheimer's disease, and 11 vascular dementia. Both the original Hachinski scoring system and the Rosen modification separated patients with Alzheimer's disease from those with vascular dementia, but many of the scores were borderline. However, these ischemic scores do not take into account CT data; in our series, 10 of the 11 subjects who developed vascular dementia had positive CT scans. Kawas has proposed a new scoring system which utilizes items from the original 13-item Hachinski system and, in addition, gives weight to the CT scan findings (Table 1). This scoring system proved to discriminate between the subjects in our study who developed Alzheimer's disease and those with vascular dementia.

Evoked Responses

Primary sensory systems remain intact in most dementing illnesses, with the obvious exceptions of subacute combined degeneration due to vitamin B_{12} deficiency and multiple sclerosis. Event-related potentials that are generated in association cortex

Table 1. Comparison of ischemic scores

	Hachinski	Rosen	Kawas[a]
Abrupt onset	2	2	2
Stepwise deterioration	1	1	1
Fluctuating course	2		
Nocturnal confusion	1		
Relative preservation of personality	1	1	
Depression	1		
Somatic complaints	1	1	
Emotional incontinence	1	1	
History of hypertension	1	1	
Associated arteriosclerosis	1		
History of stroke	2	2	2
Focal neurologic symptoms	2	2	2
Focal neurologic signs	1	1	2
CT (or MRI) evidence:			
Definite infarct			2
White matter change (Binswanger's)			1

[a] C. Kawas and R. Katzman (to be published)

might be expected to be a sensitive indicator of early dementia. The potential that has proven of most interest has been the P300, a positive potential with a latency of 300 ms in young adults, produced in response to infrequent or unexpected stimuli. There is no doubt that P300 is altered in Alzheimer patients as a group, compared with age-matched normal subjects. However, as with so many tests, it is not yet useful in individual cases, both because of normal variations and because of difficulty in obtaining these potentials in all subjects. Current investigations are directed toward identification of stimulus parameters that might improve the sensitivity and selectivity of this procedure.

Cerebral Blood Flow

CBF, determined by clearance of inhaled γ-emitting xenon, reflects the degree of dementia rather than the specific disease.

Alzheimer's Disease

Diagnostic Criteria and Peripheral Markers

A task force on Alzheimer's disease, established about 18 months ago by the U.S. Department of Health and Human Services, developed a new nomenclature with specific criteria for the diagnosis of Alzheimer's disease [15]. The term "definite Alzheimer's" is reserved for those instances in which there is histologic confirmation of the disorder. "Probable Alzheimer's" describes the patient whose clinical course and findings are characteristic: an insidious onset, continuous progression, and involvement of two or more areas of cognition in a patient who is otherwise healthy and alert, and in whom other disorders that might produce dementia have been ruled out. These criteria are similar to previously described research diagnostic criteria. The term "possible Alzheimer's" then covers the approximately 40% of Alzheimer patients who also have an atypical course – for example, patients who present with primary loss of one area of cognition.

Markers for Alzheimer's Disease

Perhaps the most important advance in the diagnosis of dementia would occur if a highly specific biochemical marker of this disease were found. Such a marker does not now exist. However, a variety of procedures other than cognitive measures will differentiate groups of Alzheimer patients from groups of normal subjects; e.g., atrophy on CT. Other inconsistent measures include P300 evoked response, degree of immunosuppression, CSF acetylcholinesterase, and choline uptake by red cells. Would a panel of such markers increase diagnostic accuracy? The authors doubt that it would, but this approach should be further explored.

Dementias of Unknown Cause

Our knowledge of dementing disorders is not complete. In several autopsy series, about 5% of the cases reported to have had dementia during life do not have evidence of pathologic changes at postmortem. The clinical course often resembles that of Alzheimer's disease. To what extent do these cases represent dementias of systemic or metabolic origin not properly worked up during life? To what extent do they represent neurodegenerative diseases whose anatomic or biochemical pathology has not yet been recognized?

Summary

Significant advances in the differential diagnosis of dementing illnesses have occurred in the last decade as clinical syndromes have been better defined, as the importance of clinical tools, including the mental status examination, has been appreciated, and as new technologies, especially the CT, have become available. A useful method of incorporating CT findings in the differential diagnosis of vascular dementia is described. Further advances are to be expected with the utilization of MRI. A major deficiency remaining is the lack of a specific peripheral marker of Alzheimer's disease.

References

1. American Psychiatric Association (1980) Diagnostic and statistical manual of mental disorders. American Psychiatric Association, Washington, D.C.
2. Folstein MF, Folstein SE, McHugh PR (1975) Mini-mental state: A practical method for grading the cognitive state of patients for the clinician. J Psychiatr Res 12: 189–198
3. Folstein MF, McHugh PR (1978) Dementia syndrome of depression. In: Katzman R, Terry RD, Bick KL (eds) Alzheimer's disease: senile dementia and related disorders. Raven, New York

4. Garcia CA, Reding MJ, Blass JP (1981) Overdiagnosis of dementia. J Am Geriatr Soc 29:407–410
5. Haase GR (1977) Diseases presenting as dementia. In: Wells CE (ed) Dementia, 2nd. ed. Davis, Philadelphia, pp 27–67
6. Hachinski V (1978) Cerebral blood flow differentiation of Alzheimer's disease from multi-infarct dementia. In: Katzman R, Terry RD, Bick KL (eds) Alzheimer's disease: Senile dementia and related disorders, vol. 7. Aging. Raven, New York, pp 97–104
7. Horoupian DS, Pick P, Spigland I, et al. (1984) Acquired immuno deficiency syndrome and multiple tract degeneration in a homosexual man. Ann Neurol 15:502–505
8. Jellinger J (1976) Neuropathological agents and dementia. Acta Neurol Belg 76:83–102
9. Katzman R (1984) Dementia. In: Appel SH, Wiley J (eds) Current neurology, vol 5. Wiley, New York, pp 91–116
10. Katzman R (1985) Clinical presentation of the course of Alzheimer's disease: the atypical patient. Interdisc Top Gerontol 20:12–18
11. Katzman R, Terry RD (eds) (1983) The neurology of aging. Davis, Philadelphia
12. Mattis S (1976) Mental status examination for organic mental syndrome in the elderly patient. In: Bellack R, Karasu B (eds) Geriatric psychiatry. Grune and Stratton, New York
13. Mayer-Gross W (1931) Some symptoms of organic brain disease. Arch Psychiatr Nervenkr 92:433–618
14. Mayer-Gross W, Guttmann E (1937) Schema for the examination of organic cases. J Ment Sci 83:440–448
15. McKhann G, Drachman D, Folstein M, Katzman R, Proce D, Stadlan EM (1984) Clinical diagnosis of Alzheimer's disease report of the NINCDS-ADRDA work group under the auspices of department of Health and Human Services Task Force on Alzheimer's disease. Neurology 34:939–944
16. NIA Task Force (1980) Senility reconsidered. Treatment possibilities for mental impairment in the elderly. Special communication. JAMA 244:259–263
17. Ron MA, Toone BK, Garralda ME, Lishman WA (1979) Diagnostic accuracy in presenile dementia. Br J Psychiatry 134:161–168
18. Rosen WG, Terry RD, Fuld PA, et al. (1980) Pathological verification of ischemic score in differentiation of dementias. Ann Neurol 7:486–488
19. Shaw GM, Harper ME, Hahn BH, et al. (1985) HTLV-III infection in brains of children and adults with AIDS encephalopathy. Science 227:177–182
20. Sulkava R, Haltia M, Paetau A, et al. (1983) Accuracy of clinical diagnosis in primary degenerative dementia: correlation with neuropathological findings. J Neurol Neurosurg Psychiatry 46:9–13
21. Terry RD, Katzman R (1983) Senile dementia of the Alzheimer type. Ann Neurol 14:497–506
22. Tomlinson BE, Blessed G, Roth M (1970) Observations on the brains of demented old people. J Neurol Sci 11:205–242
23. Wells CE (1977) Diagnostic evaluation and treatment in dementia. Wells CE (ed) Dementia, 2nd edn. Davis, Philadelphia, pp 247–273
24. Wells CE (1979) Pseudodementia. Am J Psychiatry 136:895–900

Brain Imaging in the Assessment of the Dementias

R. S. J. Frackowiak[1]

Introduction

To address the role of brain imaging in the diagnosis and management of the dementing illnesses demands, in 1985, a consideration of three major modalities: (a) X-ray computerised tomography (CT); (b) nuclear magnetic resonance imaging (MRI) and spectroscopy; and (c) emission computerised tomography with positron (PET) and single photon emitting isotopes (SPECT). This review will focus on questions of clinical importance and attempt to show how these imaging methods may contribute to providing answers to them.

Imaging

The field of brain imaging has developed rapidly since the first CT scans of the human brain were obtained in 1972–1973. CT has become a sophisticated, rapid, efficient, high-resolution method of surveying the structure of the brain based on the differential capacity of the constituent tissues to attenuate a beam of X-rays. The facility of use, ease of imaging interpretation, capacity to reconstruct images from a data set in different planes by software interpolation and above all sensitivity to treatable diseases of importance, have had direct clinical impact of major consequence. This is balanced only by the disadvantages of patient exposure to ionising radiation, low contrast between normal gray and white matter and the cost, which makes this a diagnostic tool available to only a small proportion of the world's population.

MRI is a relative newcomer to clinical imaging. This modality likewise allows analysis of cerebral structure in vivo and does so without the use of ionising radiation. The technique is highly sensitive to brain proton concentration, i.e. to fat and water content. Therefore, the gray/white contrast is greatly enhanced and bone adjacent to brain produces no artifacts on the images, an advantage of major importance in posterior fossa pathology and in assessing cortical atrophy. Disadvantages

[1] MRC Cyclotron Unit, Hammersmith Hospital, 150 Ducane Road, London W12 0HS, Great Britain.

Neurology
Ed. by K. Poeck, H. J. Freund, and H. Gänshirt

to date include cumbersome patient access to the imager, a long examination time, a much wider range of scanning parameters, the correct choice of which may be crucial to detecting or missing pathological change, and a disappointing lack of discrimination between various diseases of the brain, e.g. tumour from oedema from infarction. A number of these constraints may be resolved with technological development of instrument design and contrast enhancement with paramagnetic substances, as well as with increased experience of image production and interpretation.

PET has the capability of providing physiological, biochemical and pharmacological information *in vivo,* which at least in principle should complement structural information available from CT and MRI. This modality is also in a phase of rapid expansion. Tomographic scanners are presently being designed and built which have resolutions close to theoretical limits (2–3 mm), sensitivities which are orders of magnitude higher than first-generation clinical machines and temporal resolutions which permit very short time frame analyses of dynamic changes in tissue isotope tracer concentrations. It is instructive to remember that MRI functions on the basis of tissue proton concentration which is of the order 50 molar, whereas PET measures tissue tracer concentrations in the nanomolar or picomolar range. The variety of functions measurable with PET is also rapidly increasing. In addition to measurement of various aspects of cerebral energy metabolism, techniques are being reported which identify neurotransmitter pathways; e.g. dopaminergic [57, 73], opiate [33, 48], benzodiazepine [16], serotonergic [74]; measure basic physiological variables such as blood volume [163], haematocrit [55], pH [14, 65], blood-brain barrier permeability [56] and transport kinetics, amino acid metabolism [12] and the distribution of appropriately labelled pharmacological agents [48]. The further development of such techniques depends on appropriate advances in synthetic chemistry (though even now one-third of the pharmacopoeia is already amenable to labelling with positron emitters), and with respect to data interpretation, an improved appreciation of the metabolic fate of tracers and concomitant advances in kinetic modelling.

SPECT occupies a midground, without true quantitative potential, but perhaps able in the future to provide images of clinical importance if diagnostic, or unique patterns of appropriate tracer distributions can be recognised [36]. The principle advantages of this imaging modality are its comparatively lower cost and less demand for the multidisciplinary technical expertise required by the much larger scope offered by PET. The potential for nuclear magnetic spectroscopic analysis of the biochemistry of regions of brain in vivo in humans is largely speculative. Energy charge can be observed and pH measured with ^{32}P spectroscopy. Unfortunately the energy charge is the final common path of integrated cellular function which is maintained in most diseases until all the adaptive, interrelated biochemical pathways maintaining cellular energy balance have finally become exhausted and cell death is imminent. It is doubtful whether this variable alone will have any significant clinical impact in cerebral disease. However, proton as opposed to phosphorus spectroscopy may provide information on local concentrations of molecules which may function as transmitters or modulators. It is doubtful however, because of signal-to-noise considerations, whether the in vivo regional localisation or resolution will ever match the chemical resolving capacity of this technique.

Ageing and Atrophy

Can changes intrinsic to normal ageing be defined with these imaging modalities? The quantitation of cortical and cerebral atrophy has been a difficult task, and often the terms are used to convey a subjective interpretation of a CT image without objective measures and without reference to the range of "atrophic" change encountered in normal people of the appropriately matched age cohort. Post-mortem studies comparing brain volume with cranial capacity (which changes little with age) have shown a decline in normal subjects, with a loss of about 5% of brain volume into advanced old age [42]. This compares with a mean loss of 13.4% in patients with histologically proven Alzheimer's disease under 80 years of age. CT efforts at quantifying cerebral atrophy in vivo have centred on ventricular enlargement and widening of sulci and fissures [4, 47, 68]. Methods have been hampered by partial volume artifacts, but analyses of the reliability of linear, planimetric and more recently volumetric measurements have been published [34].

Cortical as opposed to generalised cerebral atrophy is more difficult to assess quantitatively because of the proximity of cortex to bone and the lack of good gray/white contrast. Methods such as measuring and summing the width of the four largest sulci have been proposed [49]. These have obvious shortcomings when CT scanning is used, but may be considerably easier and more accurately done on MRI scans. Other methods depend on computer analysis of the digital measures of density (CT numbers) which generate the CT image [45]. Cut-off points are defined in an attempt to distinguish between cerebral tissue, bone and CSF spaces. These techniques can give an approximation of volume if the physical size of image voxels is taken into account. There are also methods described which rely on the increase in surface area of the brain which will accompany the increased convolutions of the cortex consequent on atrophy, relating this to cranial capacity, again a measure that may be easier with MRI [71]. Such methods though sometimes computerised, automated and relatively easy to use, have gained little acceptance in clinical management. In terms of diagnostic sensitivity, patients with no cerebral atrophy and Alzheimer's disease as well as normal subjects with marked atrophy have been regularly reported, so that this does not constitute a diagnostic criterion of much importance. In this context, there is an interesting report which compared the CT scans of demented and nondemented patients which were apparently normal on visual inspection [61]. The analysis involved measuring the mean CT number in a large region of interest in white matter of the centrum semiovale. A significantly lower CT number was observed in the demented patients with no overlap between demented and nondemented groups. This work has been extended to include CSF volume as an additional discriminatory variable giving added diagnostic information [5]. No parallel MRI measurements, which might have greater sensitivity to white matter change have been reported. Of interest to research remains the observation by some workers of correlations between atrophy and neuropsychological tests of memory, orientation and other cognitive functions [24, 45, 47].

PET has concerned itself to date with defining the functional state of the normal ageing brain largely in terms of energy metabolism, though a recent report has suggested a decline in dopaminergic receptor numbers (imaged with methylspiperone ^{11}C) with age in normal males [74]. The picture as regards energy metabolism remains confused. There seems to be a mild but significant decline in cerebral blood flow (CBF) with age, but there is a wide variation within each age group and some overlap in the elderly between the brains of normal subjects and demented patients. Oxygen metabolism shows little or no decline from the third to the eighth decade [58, 62]. Glucose metabolism has been reported to show both no decline [23], and a significant decline [53] with normal ageing. The reasons for these discrepancies are not entirely clear, but may be methodological, or may relate to different criteria for the selection of normal subjects. A number of reports of local glucose metabolism measured in normal subjects suggest significant focal redistributions may occur, depending on the ambient degree and kind of sensory stimulation the subject is receiving when the physiological measurement is made [60]. Attempts at correlating neuropsychological test scores and glucose consumption rates have been reported, with no significant relationship noted [22].

The relative contributions of CT and PET information in normal ageing has been assessed. One report suggests structural atrophic changes without metabolic alterations and a lack of significant relationships between various structural and metabolic measures [20]. This observation is the converse of that found in patients with Alzheimer's disease [21]. These results are preliminary and require confirmation. The general conclusion at present is that the addition of physiological to structural data does not yet give information with sufficient sensitivity to be able to discriminate normal from pathological ageing in individual cases, though group discrimination is much more precise.

Dementia

The most important question is to ask whether there is a problem in the clinical diagnosis of the dementias and whether the expensive technology of imaging may reasonably be expected to improve the outcome in patients with this disease. It has been estimated that up to 40% of patients referred to a neurologist with a provisional diagnosis of Alzheimer's dementia may have some other primary disease [64], which may be structural and hence detectable with CT or MRI [59]. It is therefore valid to ask: (a) are the imaging modalities able to diagnose dementing illnesses? (b) can they discriminate between degenerative, vascular and other types of pathology? and (c) what is their role in evaluating disease mechanisms or monitoring management? The preceding section on atrophy and normal ageing indicates that a diagnostic approach centred on the image of structure as the only test is not tenable [17, 46]. It is clear that the major contribution of CT is in the exclusion of structural disease as a cause of dementia. This is occasionally the case with space-occupying lesions such as meningiomas, butterfly (transcallosal) gliomas, or other intrinsic tumours which because of their siting, growth characteristics, or the production of secondary hydrocephalus may produce a dementia-like syndrome.

Differential Diagnosis

The differentiation of vascular from degenerative dementias is of considerable importance in management. They are the two commonest causes of the dementia syndrome in clinical practice. The scope for preventing further cerebral damage by existing medical or surgical methods in vascular patients means that early diagnosis is of considerable practical importance to 15%–35% of those with dementia [70]. The differentiation can often be achieved clinically with considerable accuracy [40, 65]. CT and MRI are capable of showing structural change resulting from ischaemia, though CT can miss areas of partial cell loss due to diffuse ischaemic change. Potentially confusing in diagnosis is the finding of low attenuation by deep and periventricular white matter in apparently normal old people as well as in hypertensive patients suffering from progressive subcortical arteriosclerotic encephalopathy [39, 72]. MRI in 20 consecutive patients without evidence of structural disease on CT, over the age of 60, demonstrated change in deep white matter in one-third [9]. The incidence of hypertension, transient ischaemia, cardiac disease and emotional lability was high and all patients also showed evidence of lacunar infarction. The evidence is still sparse, but it seems that MRI is more sensitive to ischaemic change than CT, especially in white matter.

The detection of the syndrome of normal pressure hydrocephalus [1, 2] has become much less of an issue since the generally poor response to shunt therapy in the majority of cases has become evident [69]. Indeed, of those presenting with the classical syndrome, shunting, if helpful, usually improves gait with little effect on mental status. CT scanning criteria distinguishing hydrocephalus from cerebral atrophy have been proposed and include dilated temporal horns, an enlarged fourth ventricle and sulci of normal convexity [43, 44]. CSF metrizamide cisternography provides data on CSF pathways in a manner analogous to RISA cisternography, but gives no information on whether the hydrocephalus is compensated or progressive [41]. PET measurements of energy metabolism, recently reported, show no change in oxygen metabolism or blood flow in a well-defined population of patients before and after shunting [10]. Indeed, only in patients with acute obstructive hydrocephalus was any improvement in cerebral physiology noted.

The physiological changes detectable by PET consequent on Alzheimer's disease have been reported extensively [3, 25, 28, 30]. The decline of metabolic rates for oxygen and glucose is a universal finding. This is however a nonspecific measure of neuronal function. Any disease resulting in cell death will result in a decreased metabolic rate. The impairment of oxygen consumption in a group of demented patients with presumed Alzheimer's disease and multi-infarct dementia correlated with severity, but not type of dementia [28]. Focal patterns of impairment have been reported and appear to have some discriminant value [8, 28]. Patients with multi-infarct disease tend to show patchy defects of metabolism (and CBF), while early Alzheimer's disease is characterised by a focal emphasis in posterotemporal and parietal regions. More severe disease is accompanied by an additional impairment of frontal metabolism [28]. Similar observations have been made with respect to glucose metabolism [19, 30].

Observations with PET have extended to rarer forms of dementia. For example, in Huntington's disease caudate glucose metabolism is significantly depressed in early disease [54]. Observations in subjects at risk have differentiated two groups in those who show structural integrity of the caudate nuclei on CT. One is characterised by low and the other by normal metabolic activity [50]. The possibility of defining patients who will develop the Huntington syndrome is being pursued by follow-up studies. Patients with Huntington's disease are also being examined in relation to striatal dopamine storage capacity (with Dopa ^{18}F) and postsynaptic dopaminergic receptor populations (with methylspiperone ^{11}C) (Leenders et al., unpublished work). These ligands are therefore giving added information and specific composite patterns of diagnostic importance.

Patients with dementia and extrapyramidal features have also been investigated using PET techniques. Jakob-Creutzfeldt disease, which may present in this manner, shows no, or a few nonspecific changes on CT [35]. PET measurement of energy metabolism has been reported to show a pattern of dysfunction similar to that in Alzheimer's disease [32]. Parkinsonian patients with dementia show similar defects of energy metabolism [51], but also a marked defect in striatal dopamine storage and normal methylspiperone uptake (Leenders et al., in preparation). Patients with the clinically similar syndrome of dementia and progressive supranuclear palsy show a decline in striatal and frontal labelled bromospiperone binding [6], impaired dopamine storage (Leenders et al., in preparation) and a markedly and focally depressed frontal metabolism of glucose [18] and oxygen (Leenders et al., in preparation). CT can also be helpful in this latter condition, often showing midbrain atrophy and enlarged basal cisterns.

Differentiating dementia from the potentially treatable pseudodementia of psychiatric origin in the elderly is of major clinical importance. Structural information is of little help in differential diagnosis, though exclusion of structural disease and vascular changes may aid management. A report comparing whole brain glucose consumption in normal volunteers and those with various mood disorders showed no difference between patients with unipolar depression, and normal subjects [7]. However, patients with a bipolar illness in the depressed phase, or with psychomotor activity and a depressed mood had significantly lower rates. Though the numbers are small, there is an indication that information concerning this important differential diagnosis may be forthcoming from studies of energy metabolism [52].

Pathogenic Mechanisms

The contribution of PET to the management and understanding of the dementias has extended outside the confines of diagnostic information in the individual patient. The analysis of energy supply and demand relationships has demonstrated that both in degenerative and vascular dementia *chronic* ischaemic processes do not play a role in pathogenesis [28]. In a few cases of vascular dementia, associated with extensive extracranial vascular occlusion and stenoses, patients can be identified who are at greatly enhanced risk of acute ischaemic events. They show impairment and exhaustion of homeostatic reserve mechanisms which normally protect the brain from a failure of energy supply [27, 38]. These pathophysiological observations indicate the lack of rationale for the use of vasodilating agents in the treatment of demented patients [37], and indicate an albeit small subgroup which on physiological grounds, might benefit from prophylactic revascularisation surgery.

The objective assessment of treatment and monitoring of progression of disease, are amenable to study by PET, which seems more sensitive than measures of structural change in Alzheimer's disease [21]. Thus in 17 patients with Alzheimer's disease and 5 normal subjects, correlations between WAIS verbal and performance IQ scores and the cortical glucose metabolic rates in left parasylvian and right posterior parietal regions, respectively, have been described [15]. It has been suggested that a substantial decline in energy metabolism occurs in Alzheimer patients before cognitive decline becomes very evident. However, once symptomatic, small additional metabolic decrements are associated with marked deterioration in intellectual function [26]. This latter observation is open to some question as more linear correlations between energy metabolism and neuropsychological function have been demonstrated in Alzheimer's disease [28] and also the intellectual decline accompanying multiple sclerosis [11].

There are preliminary reports suggesting further directions in which functional PET imaging is developing which may be of diagnostic and possibly more fundamental importance in understanding dementia of the Alzheimer type. Central cholinergic mechanisms are being investigated with labelled choline [10], and analogues which select out specific aspects of choline and acetylcholine metabolism and kinetics (Eckernas et al., personal communication), this type of measurement if practicable, would be helpful in avoiding the necessity for biopsy in research protocols, allowing complete sampling of the brain and providing a means of serially measuring cholinergic function with treatment. Cerebral protein and amino acid metabolism have been investigated with methionine ^{11}C [13] and significant changes in posterior temporal, parietal and subsequently frontal metabolism in patients with dementia have been demonstrated.

Two preliminary reports comparing the relative merits in Alzheimer's disease of PET, MRI and CT have appeared recently. The results must be considered very preliminary. One report compares the three modalities in two patients [11]. The other more extensive series makes regional comparisons of CT and PET findings in 11 normal subjects and 9 patients with degenerative dementia [21]. Regional CT values did not discriminate between the two groups whilst PET with deoxyglucose ^{18}F showed a 21%–28% reduction in glucose utilisation in the patients with dementia compared with normal subjects, which correlated with cognitive decline.

Summary and Conclusions

We are able to diagnose dementia with considerable accuracy clinically in the majortity of cases [67]. The principal problem is detecting patients with pseudodementia, treatable structural disease and a significant vascular pathogenesis. From the preceding review it is clear that none of the imaging modalities can be said to constitute a single test for the positive diagnosis of Alzheimer's disease. The major role of CT and MRI is in excluding the treatable structural causes of dementia and detecting vascular change. However, the combination of Alzheimer and vascular changes – not infrequently seen pathologically [70] – remains difficult to distinguish. Functional measurement and imaging are beginning to demonstrate facets of neurochemistry of significance in differential diagnosis. Measurement of energy metabolism has elucidated some pathogenic mechanisms in multi-infarct disease and provides a tool of some considerable sensitivity for following cognitive dysfunction objectively. This will be of future importance in assessing treatment strategies effectively and economically in humans.

References

1. Adams RD, Fisher CM, Hakim S, Ojemann RG, Sweet WH (1965) Symptomatic occult hydrocephalus with normal cerebrospinal fluid pressure. N Engl J Med 273:117–126
2. Adapon BD, Braunstein P, Lin JP (1974) Radiologic investigations of normal pressure hydrocephalus. Radiol Clin 12:353
3. Alavi A, Ferris S, Wolf A, Reivich M, Farkas T, Dann R, Christman D, Fowler J (1980) Determination of cerebral metabolism in senile dementia using F-18-tomography. J Nucl Med 21:21
4. Albert M, Naeser MA, Levine HL, Garvey AJ (1984) Ventricular size in patients with presenile dementia of the Alzheimer type. Arch Neurol 41:1258–1263
5. Albert M, Naeser MA, Levine HL, Garvey AJ (1984) CT density numbers in patients with senile dementia of the Alzheimer type. Arch Neurol 41:1264–1269
6. Baron JC, Maziere B, Loch C, Sgouropoulos P, Bonnet AM, Agid Y (1985) Progressive supranuclear palsy; loss of striatal dopamine receptors demonstrated in vivo. Lancet 1:1163–1164
7. Baxter LR, Phelps ME, Mazziotta JC, Schwartz JM, Gerner RH, Selin CE, Sumida RM (1985) Cerebral metabolic rates for glucose in mood disorders: studies with positron emission tomography and fluorodeoxyglucose F18. Arch Gen Psychiatry 42:441–447
8. Benson DF, Kuhl DE, Hawkins RA, Phelp ME, Cummings JL, Tsai SY (1983) The fluorodeoxyglucose ^{18}F scan in Alzheimer's disease and multi-infarct dementia. Arch Neurol 40:711–714
9. Bradley WG, Waluch V, Brant-Zawadzki M, Yadley RA, Wycoff RR (1984) Patchy, periventricular white matter lesions in the elderly: a common observation during NMR imageing. Noninvasive Med Imageing 1:35–41
10. Brooks DJ, Beaney RP, Powell M, Leenders KL, Crockard HA, Thomas DGT, Marshall J, Jones T (1985) Studies on cerebral oxygen metabolism, blood flow and blood volume in patients with hydrocephalus before and after surgical decompression using positron emission tomography. Brain (in press)
11. Brooks DJ, Leenders KL, Head G, Marshall J, Legg NJ, Jones T (1984) Studies on regional cerebral oxygen utilisation and cognitive function in multiple sclerosis. J Neurol Neurosurg Psychiatr 47:1182–1191
12. Bustany P, Henry JF, DeRotrou J, Signoret P, Cabanis E, Zarifian E, Ziegler M, Derlon M, Crouzel C, Soussaline F, Comar D (1985) Correlations between clinical state and positron emission tomography measurement of local brain protein synthesis in Alzheimer's disease, Parkinson's disease, schizophrenia, gliomas. In: Greitz T, Ingvar DH, Widen L (eds) The metabolism of the human brain studied with positron emission tomography. Raven, New York, pp 241–249
13. Bustany P, Henry JF, Soussaline F, Comar D (1983) Brain protein synthesis in normal and demented patients – a study by positron emission tomography with C-L methionine. In: Magistretti PL (ed) Functional radionuclide imageing of the brain. Raven, New York, pp 319–326
14. Brooks DJ, Lammertsma AA, Beaney RP, Leenders KL, Buckingham PD, Marshall J, Jones T (1984) Measurement of regional cerebral pH in human subjects using continuous inhalation of $^{11}CO_2$ and positron emission tomography. J Cereb Blood Flow Metab 4:458–465
15. Chase TN, Fedio P, Foster NL, Brooks R, DiChiro G, Mansi L (1984) Wechsler adult intelligence scale performance: cortical localisation by fluorodeoxyglucose ^{18}F-positron emission tomography. Arch Neurol 41:1244–1247
16. Comar D, Maziere M, Gadot JM, Berger G, Soussaline F (1979) Visualisation of ^{11}C-flunitrazepam displacement in the brain of the live baboon. Nature 280:329–331
17. Damasio H, Eslinger P, Damasio AR, Rizzo M, Huang HK, Demeter S (1983) Quantitative computed tomographic analysis in the diagnosis of dementia. Arch Neurol 40:715–719
18. D'Antona R, Baron JC, Samson Y, Serdaru M, Viader F, Agid Y, Cambier J (1985) Subcortical dementia: frontal cortex hypometabolism detected by positron tomography in patients with progressive supranuclear palsy. Brain (in press)

19. De Leon MJ, Ferris SH, George AE, Christman DR, Fowler JS, Gentes C, Reisberg B, Gee B, Emmerich M, Yonekura Y, Brodie J, Kricheff II, Wolf AP (1983) Positron emission tomographic studies of aging and Alzheimer's disease. AJNR 4:568–571
20. De Leon M, George AE, Ferris SH, Christman DR, Fowler JS, Gentes CI, Brodie J, Reisberg B, Wolf AP (1984) Positron emission tomography and computed tomography assessments of the ageing human brain. J Comput Assist Tomogr 8:88–94
21. De Leon MJ, George AE, Ferris SH, Rosenbloom S, Christman DR, Gentes CI, Reisberg B, Kricheff II, Wolfe AP (1983) Regional correlation of PET and CT in senile dementia of the Alzheimer type. AJNR 4:553–556
22. Duara R, Grady C, Haxby J, Ingvar D, Sokoloff L, Margolin RA, Manning RG, Culter NR, Rapaport SI (1984) Human brain glucose utilisation and cognitive function in relation to age. Ann Neurol 16:702–713
23. Duara R, Margolin RA, Robertson-Tchabo EA, London ED, Schwartz M, Renfrew JW, Koziarz BJ, Sundaram M, Grady C, Moore AM, Ingvar DH, Sokoloff L, Weingartner H, Kessler RM, Manning RG, Channing MA, Cutler NR, Rapoport SI (1983) Resting cerebral glucose utilisation as measured with positron emission tomography in 21 healthy men between the ages of 21 and 83 years. Brain 106:761–775
24. Eslinger PJ, Damasio H, Graff-Radford N, Damasio AR (1984) Examining the relationship between computed tomography and neuropsychological measures in normal and demented elderly. J Neurol Neurosurg Psychiatry 47:1319–1325
25. Ferris SH, De Leon MJ, Wolf AP, Farkas T, Christman DR, Reisberg B, Fowler JS, MacGregor R, Goldman A, George AE, Rampal S (1981) Positron emission tomography in the study of ageing and senile dementia. Neurobiol Aging 1:127–131
26. Foster NL, Chase TN, Mansi L, Brooks R, Fedio P, Patronas NJ, DiChiro G (1985) Cortical abnormalities in Alzheimer's disease. Ann Neurol 16:649–654
27. Frackowiak RSJ (1985) Pathophysiology of human cerebral ischaemia studies with positron tomography and ^{15}oxygen. In: Sokoloff L (ed) Brain imaging and brain function. Raven, New York, pp 139–162
28. Frackowiak RSJ, Pozzilli C, Legg NJ, DuBoulay GH, Marshall J, Lenzi GL, Jones T (1981) Regional cerebral oxygen supply and utilisation in dementia: a clinical and physiological study with oxygen-15 and positron tomography. Brain 104:753–778
29. Friedland RP, Budinger TF, Brandt-Zawadzki M, Jagust WJ (1984) The diagnosis of Alzheimer-type dementia. A preliminary comparison of positron emission tomography and proton magnetic resonance. JAMA 252:2750–2752
30. Friedland RP, Budinger TF, Ganz E, Yano Y, Mathis CA, Koss B, Ober BA, Huesman RH, Derenzo SE (1983) Regional cerebral metabolic alterations in dementia of the Alzheimer type: positron emission tomography with (^{18}F) fluorodeoxyglucose. J Comput Assist Tomogr 7:590–598
31. Friedland RP, Mathis CA, Budinger TF, Moyer BR, Rosen M (1983) Labelled choline and phosphorylcholine: body distribution and brain autoradiography: concise communication. J Nucl Med 24:812–815
32. Friedland RP, Prusiner SB, Jagust WJ, Budinger TF, Davis RL (1984) Bitemporal hypometabolism in Creutzfeldt-Jacob disease measured by positron emission tomography with (^{18}F)-2-fluorodeoxyglucose. J Comput Assist Tomogr 8:978–981
33. Frost JJ, Wagner HN, Dannals RF, Ravert HT, Links JM, Wilson AA, Burns HD, Wong DF, McPherson RW, Rosenbaum AE, Kuhar MJ, Snyder SH (1985) Imaging opiate receptors in the human brain by positron tomography. J Comput Assist Tomogr 9:231–236
34. Gado M, Hughes CP, Danziger W, Chi D, Jost G, Berg L (1984) Volumetric measurements of the cerebrospinal fluid spaces in demented subjects and controls. Radiology 144:535–538
35. Galvez S, Cartier L (1984) Computed tomography findings in 15 cases of Creutzfeldt-Jacob disease with histological verification. J Neurol Neurosurg Psychiatry 47:1244–1246
36. Gemmell HG, Sharp PF, Evans NTS, Besson JAO, Lyall D, Smith FW (1984) Single photon emission tomography with ^{123}I-isopropylamphetamine in Alzheimer's disease and multi-infarct dementia. Lancet 2:1248
37. Gibbs J (1985) Cerebral blood flow and metabolism in dementia, with reference to the effects of pharmacological intervention. In: Trimble M (ed) New brain imageing techniques and psychopharmacology. Oxford University Press, Oxford (in press)

38. Gibbs JM, Wise RJS, Leenders KL, Jones T (1984) Evaluation of cerebral perfusion reserve in patients with carotid artery occlusion. Lancet 1:310–314
39. Goto K, Ishii N, Fukasawa H (1981) Diffuse white matter disease in the geriatric population. Radiology 141:687–695
40. Hachinski VC, Lassen NA, Marshall J (1974) Multi infarct dementia. A cause of mental deterioration in the elderly. Lancet 2:207–210
41. Hindmarsh T, Greitz T (1977) Hydrocephalus, atrophy and their differential diagnosis – CSF dynamics investigated by computer cisternography. In: Du Boulay GH, Moseley IF (eds) Computerised axial tomography in clinical practice. Springer, Berlin Heidelberg New York, pp 205–217
42. Hubbard BM, Anderson JM (1981) A quantitative study of cerebral atrophy in old age and senile dementia. J Neurol Sci 50:135–145
43. Huckman MS (1983) Normal pressure hydrocephalus: evaluation of diagnostic and prognostic tests. AJNR 2:385
44. Huckman MS, Fox J, Topel J (1975) The validity of criteria for the evaluation of cerebral atrophy by computed tomography. Radiology 116:85–92
45. Ito M, Hatazawa J, Yamaura H, Matsuzawa T (1981) Age related brain atrophy and mental deterioration – a study with computed tomography. Br J Radiol 54:384–390
46. Jacoby RJ, Levy R (1980) Computed tomography in the elderly: 2. senile dementia: diagnosis and functional impairment. Br J Psychiatr 136:256–269
47. Jacoby RJ, Levy R, Dawson JM (1980) Computed tomography in the elderly: 1. the normal population. Br J Psychiatry 136:249–255
48. Jones A, Pike V, Luthra S, Turton D, Brady F, Jones T, Turner P, Dickinson S, Herold S, Leenders K, Chamberlain D, Brooks D, Lammertsma A, Kensett M, Zanelli Y, Maziere B, Heather J, Frackowiak R, Rees L (1985) ^{11}C-diprenorphine and ^{11}C-meptazinol: new specific and non-specific probes for studying human opioid binding sites using positron tomography. J Cereb Blood Flow Metab 5 [Suppl] (in press)
49. Kohlmeyer K, Shamena AR (1981) The size of the lateral ventricles and cortical sulci in old age subjects with and without dementia. Neuroradiology 138:89–92
50. Kuhl DE, Markham CH, Metter EJ, Riege WH, Phelps ME, Mazziotta JC (1985) Local cerebral glucose utilisation in symptomatic and presymptomatic Huntington's disease. In: Sokoloff L (ed) Brain imaging and brain function. Raven, New York, pp 199–209
51. Kuhl DE, Metter EJ, Benson DF, Ashford JW, Riege WH, Fujikawa DG, Markham CH, Mazziotta JC, Maltese A, Dorsey DA (1985) Similarities of cerebral glucose metabolism in Alzheimer's and Parkinsonian dementia. J Cereb Blood Flow Metab 5 [Suppl] (in press)
52. Kuhl DE, Metter EJ, Riege WH (1985) Patterns of cerebral glucose utilisation in depression, multiple infarct dementia and Alzheimer's disease. In: Sokoloff L (ed) Brain imaging and brain function. Raven, New York, pp 211–225
53. Kuhl DE, Metter EJ, Riege WH, Phelps ME (1982) Effects of human ageing on patterns of local cerebral glucose utilisation determined by the (^{18}F) fluorodeoxyglucose method. J Cereb Blood Flow Metab 2:163–171
54. Kuhl DE, Phelps ME, Markham CH, Metter EJ, Riege WH, Winter J (1982) Cerebral metabolism and atrophy in Huntington's disease determined by ^{18}FDG and computed tomographic scan. Ann Neurol 12:425–434
55. Lammertsma AA, Brooks DJ, Beaney RP, Turton DR, Kensett MJ, Heather JD, Marshall J, Jones T (1984) In vivo measurement of regional cerebral haematocrit using positron emission tomography. J Cereb Blood Flow Metab 4:317–322
56. Lammertsma AA, Brooks DJ, Frackowiak RSJ, Heather JD, Jones T (1984) A method to quantitate the fractional extraction of rubidium-82 across the blood brain barrier using positron emission tomography. J Cereb Blood Flow Metab 4:523–534
57. Leenders KL, Herold S, Brooks DJ, Palmer AJ, Turton B, Firnau G, Garnett ES, Nahmias C, Veall N (1984) Presynaptic and postsynaptic dopaminergic system in human brain. Lancet 2:110–111
58. Lenzi GL, Gibbs JM, Frackowiak RSJ, Jones T (1983) Measurement of cerebral blood flow and oxygen metabolism by positron emission tomography and the ^{15}O steady-state technique: aspects of methodology, reproducibility and clinical application. In: Magistretti PL (ed) Functional radionuclide imaging of the brain. Raven, New York, pp 291–304

59. Marsden CD, Harrison MJG (1972) Outcome of investigation of patients with presenile dementia. Br Med J 2:249–252
60. Mazziotta JC, Phelps ME (1984) Human sensory stimulation and depriviation: positron emission tomographic results and strategies. Ann Neurol 15 [Suppl]: S50–S60
61. Naeser MA, Gebhardt C, Levine HL (1980) Decreased computerised tomography numbers in patients with presenile dementia: detection in patients with otherwise normal scans. Arch Neurol 37:401–409
62. Pantano P, Baron JC, Lebrun-Grandie P, Duquesnoy N, Bousser MG, Comar D (1984) Regional cerebral blood flow and oxygen consumption in human ageing. Stroke 15:635–641
63. Phelps ME, Huang SC, Hoffman EJ, Kuhl DE (1979) Tomographic measurement of cerebral blood volume with C-11 labelled carboxyhaemoglobin. J Nucl Med 20:328–334
64. Ron MA, Toone BK, Garralda ME, Lishman WA (1979) Diagnostic accuracy in presenile dementia. Br J Psychiatry 134:161–168
65. Rosen WG, Terry RD, Fuld PA, Katzman R, Peck A (1980) Pathological verification of ischaemia score in differentiation of dementias. Ann Neurol 7:486–488
66. Rottenberg DA, Ginos MZ, Kearfott KJ, Junck L, Dhawan V, Jarden JO (1985) In vivo measurement of brain tumour pH using [^{11}C]DMO and positron emission tomography. Ann Neurol 17:70–79
67. Smith JS, Kiloh LG (1981) The investigation of dementia: results in 200 consecutive admissions. Lancet 1:824–827
68. Schwartz M, Creasey H, Grady CL, Deleo JM, Frederickson HA, Cutler NR, Rapoport SI (1985) Computer tomographic analysis of brain morphometrics in 30 healthy men, aged 21 to 81 years. Ann Neurol 17:146–157
69. Symon L, Dorsch NWC (1975) Use of long term intracranial pressure measurement to assess hydrocephalic patients prior to shunt surgery. J Neurosurg 42:258–273
70. Tomlinson BE, Blessed G, Roth M (1970) Observations on the brains of demented old people. J Neurol Sci 11:205–242
71. Turkheimer E, Cullum CM, Hubler DW, Paver SW, Yeo RA, Bigler ED (1984) Quantifying cortical atrophy. J Neurol Neurosurg Psychiatry 47:1314–1318
72. Valentine AR, Moseley IF, Kendall BE (1980) White matter abnormality in cerebral atrophy: clinicoradiological correlations. J Neurol Neurosurg Psychiatry 43:139–142
73. Wagner HN, Burns DH, Dannals RF, Wong DF, Langstrom B, Duelfero T, Frost JJ, Ravert HT, Links JM, Rosenbloom SB, Lukas SE, Kramer AV, Kuhar MJ (1984) Imaging dopamine receptors in the brain by positron tomography. Science 22:1264–1266
74. Wong DF, Wagner HN, Dannals RF, Links JM, Frost JJ, Ravert HT, Wilson AA, Rosenbaum AE, Gjedde A, Douglass KH, Petronis JD, Folstein MF, Toung JKT, Burns HD, Kuhar MJ (1984) Effects of age on dopamine and serotonin receptors measured by positron tomography in the living human brain. Science 226:1393–1396

Neuropsychological Approach to Dementia

E. Capitani, S. Della Sala, and H. Spinnler [1]

Clinical neuropsychology (CN) is considered useful to the neurologist insofar as it can supply information on the plurisectorial cognitive incompetence which lends the mean characteristic to organic mental deterioration (OMD), i.e., dementia (D). The general aim of this paper is twofold: to discuss the diagnostic utility of studying OMD neuropsychologically, and to scrutinize which research goals may most appropriately be tackled using this approach.

Contributions of CN to Diagnosis

Since the early days of CN the neurologist has asked the neuropsychologist to confirm or deny the presence of OMD, diagnosed by the general practitioner with an error rate – depending on the stage of D – claimed to range from 10% to 50% (7). A formal answer should be given only by means of a collection of everyday behavioral variables (a standardized behavioral inquiry) and a psychometric (so-called cognitive) profile that supplies repeatable measures of the patient's residual cognitive resources. The test performances and inter-test discrepancies which may come to the fore are expected to help in solving several differential diagnostic questions, ranging from those of identifying *pseudodementia* in its broadest sense (psychiatric, i.e., purely depressive or psychotic; pharmacological, including alcohol; and extracerebral or metabolic) to those of *benign senile forgetfulness* (affecting more than half of the nondemented elderly) and of the neuropsychological sequelae of *focal brain lesions.* Yet, by far the most important and frequent problem specifically presented by the neurologist to the neuropsychologist is that of distinguishing between Alzheimer-type dementia (DAT) in its early stages and those modifications of information processing that can be enterely attributed to *normal aging* (possibly aggravated by poor education). Two traditional strategies can be applied: (a) carrying out at least one full retest after a 6-month interval and (b) comparing the patients scores with the test performance of the normal population on a warranted statistical basis. It is maintained [5] that in combination with a thorough neurological and CT examina-

[1] Neuropsychology Center and 1st Neurological Department of the University, S. Paolo Hospital, via di Rudini 8, 20142 Milan, Italy.

Neurology
Ed. by K. Poeck, H. J. Freund, and H. Gänshirt

tion, CN provides more precise information than the informal clinical approach. Actually, the error rate of "presumptive" (i.e., not histopathologically nor histochemically proven, but ascertained by means of a sufficiently long follow-up) diagnosis of DAT drops to under 10%. Thus the current tendency to overdiagnose DAT in the elderly [7] could possibly be avoided by CN's more cautious approach.

The identification of psychometric concordances and discrepancies within the cognitive profile of the patient at issue appears to be the most precise contribution which CN can make to neurological diagnosis (i.e., the identification of the dementing disease). It was thought that such information could *frame the principal nosographic entities* involving D (DAT, MID, NPH, etc.) *within a specific pattern of test results.* Particular reference is made to the diagnostic contrast between DAT and the growing group of subcortical D and pseudodementias. In this respect, however, CN is far from hitting the mark. The diagnostic contributions of clinical neurology and brain imaging (especially of CT) are in this case far greater, given the poor specificity presently achieved by the currently available test batteries, the still undefined conception of the variety of subcortical D [4], and the short-term variability of pseudodemential traits due to general metabolic disorders. Actually, the building up of test batteries suited to bring the cognitive features of subcortical D and pseudodementias to the fore and to provide reliable measures of the behavioral impairment also for severely demented patients is still under study. In our opinion, however, it is unlikely that future tests will achieve this goal. This pitfall reduces the effectiveness of CN in the neurological assessment of D. Even the nosographic diagnosis of DAT continues in fact to rest on the current exclusionary approach, being provided chiefly by clinical examination rather than by univocally defined CN variables.

CN, on the other hand, is presently able to contribute to the framing of test impairments due to D, possibly allowing identification of *specific neuropsychological patterns* within a given dementing disease. Restricting discussion to DAT patients, empirical evidence emerges for a relevant variability in the demential behavior, which mostly occurs during the early stages of the disease. Focusing the attention on DAT, the analysis of the taxonomy of its early features based purely on their neuropsychological characteristics, is reminiscent of over a century of work carried out by the students of aphasia. Yet the analogy with the classical (focal) aphasic syndromes should not be pushed too far. Given the merely temporary saving of certain parts of the cerebral hardware in some DAT patients, and the late global involvement in nearly all, one should abstain from proposing that neuropsychological onset syndromes (e.g., anomia) represent genuine variants of DAT. However, as for the subdivisions of aphasia due to a dominant hemisphere lesion, it is useful to study DAT patients analytically in order to pinpoint their pseudofocal features and to form relatively homogeneous experimental groups. It is our opinion that many of the inconclusive results obtained from some cognitive studies on DAT patients (particularly those at the beginning of the disease) could be traced back to the variability of the average sectorial scores due to the cognitive heterogeneity of D patients. This heterogeneity is particularly notable along the left/right (viz., verbal/spatial) hemispheric dimension [9]. Hence it is likely that the catch-all diagnosis of DAT also needs, at least for experimental purposes, a detailed neuropsychological onset specification.

As already pointed out, behavioral disorders in some DAT patients frequently take on *pseudofocal patterns*, which correlate fairly well with the topographical results of a lowered cortical metabolism [2]. The reference is to: (a) The relatively frequent *aphasic onset* [8], sometimes tallying with a congruent CT asymmetry pointing to a prevailing left perisylvian atrophy. This morphological and behavioral occurrence was noticed by Pick in 1892 and 1904 [12] in several cases of "senile dementia". Obviously, this should not imply the systematic substitution of the label "DAT" with "Pick's disease" in all neuropsychologically and CT asymmetric cases. (b) Those forms, also frequent, in which *global amnesia* consistently shows the traits of an almost pure syndrome over rather long periods (e.g., the first 2–3 years) and differentiation from limbic amnesia and from benign senile forgetfulness is difficult. (c) Those rather rare forms with prevailing *spatial disorders* simulating a right parietal syndrome [3] or with visuoagnosic traits. (d) The rare forms, sometimes called "prefrontal," which often display marked attentional and/or even preeminent psychiatric (apathetic or excited) features.

CN should also be in a position to provide information on the *evolution* of nosographic and neuropsychological forms of D by providing repeatable cognitive measures. Whereas it appears that demential features of those patients with an associated neurological characterizing trait (e.g., extrapyramidal signs) show a rather consistent trend to preservation through the progress of the disease [10], the prevailing neuropsychological pseudofocal features seem to fade over a period of 6–24 months. This emerges from our experience with 19 initial DAT patients (see below, "A Neuropsychological Study of 29 DAT Patients"). In connection with the longitudinal approach, it is worth emphasizing that longitudinal data produce a progressively hazier and even false pattern due to the selectivity of the dropouts: it is, in fact, the more severely deteriorated patients who become unsuitable for further testing.

Contribution of CN to Research

Research into psychological mechanisms suitable to explain the phenomenology of D in the most comprehensive and concise manner is still in its initial, and up to now inconclusive, stages. The results of the CN approach must in turn be correlated with the earliest hardware modifications; such information, however, is understandably very difficult to obtain in the early stages of D (with the notable exception of PET data). Some of the issues at stake are listed here on a very provisional basis only.

Is the Alzheimer structural deterioration of the brain liable to cause initial and more severe damage to a *specific facet of the psychological processing*, thus giving the opportunity to reconstruct the psychological deterioration starting from *a more or less basic defect?* It is often apparent that in the early stages patients use their cognitive instruments (i.e., grammar and syntax with access to lexicon impeded) appropriately, at least for some aspects, but nevertheless timing and control are already hampered. Henceforth the patients appear hesitant and overtly concerned, as if they were aware that their control functions no longer perform the role of optimizing the residual resources when they are compelled to face a new task. It is only in the later stages that instrumental abilities appear to deteriorate too. To our knowledge, however, this kind of cognitive progression is supported only by clinical impressions, not by formal experiments. Moreover, the occurrence of early pseudofocal features is at variance with the flow of progression described above. Generally speaking, one could take into consideration: (a) The impairment of those functions chiefly conceived as controlling the processing of information, i.e., attention, intelligence, and some aspects of memory. They could be linked to the "horizontal" connectivity of the cortex, with foci in the areas of supramodal convergence. Incidentally, the prefrontal, posterior-parietal, and perihippocampal areas are among those usually suffering the most severe degeneration in DAT. The role of the "central executive" in Baddeley and Hitch's model of "working memory" should be considered here, as it has seen to be particularly affected in DAT patients [1]. (b) Alternatively, the defect could be centered in more "instrumental" abilities linked to the "vertical" organization of the cortex, such as language, spatial cognition, perception, and other aspects of memory (see above discussion of the pseudofocal onset features). (c) Or, as would possibly seem more likely to a neurologist, both the aforementioned types of functions could be involved, but at different stages of D. By and large, this important issue remains unsettled.

Are there features which differentiate the psychological processes of a D patient from that of a normal elderly person, i.e., *is senile processing only quantitatively different from D processing?* When dealing with this recurrent query, it can be asked whether Gowers' "abiotrophic" hypothesis (selective aging of the brain) finds support in reliable cross-sectional researches carried out on elderly people, provided they are accurately selected for absence of any of the several cognitive risks outstandingly more frequent in the elderly than in young subjects. It is our feeling that the inconsistency met with in the cross-sectional answers to this basic issue stems from the interaction of a poorly predictable sample bias (viz., the higher prevalence of psychiatric and internal medical disorders among the elderly) and from the normal modifications of control functions of senile processing (e.g., reduced processing speed, lowered capacity to engage in more than one task contemporaneously, forgetfulness, and reduced ability to learn a new skill). Provided one is confident with a statistically warranted model linking a given test score to age, one can produce artificial scores belonging to healthy advanced ages and verify whether and when they differ significantly from those of much younger DAT patients (Capitani, Della Sala, and Spinnler, in preparation). Such an approach could fit the purpose to skip the burden and unwieldiness of long-lasting experiments in the longitudinal cohort approach. Our first, very provisional findings do not suggest a cognitive identity between, let's say, a 60-year-old Alzheimer's patient and a healthy, in other respects comparable 100-year-old.

It is clear that this list of questions could be lengthened. However, underlying all these queries is the lack of a *reference model* illuminating the psychological mechanism(s) which is capable of rendering understandable the ecological behavior, intertest variability, and rule of evolution of a D patient. What is meant here is a reference system proposing one or more basic psychological defects and interpreting the subsequent chain of defects leading to cognitive incompetence. The lack of a psychological model has fostered the predominantly piecemeal approach of CN studies and the persisting predominance of purely, often bewilderingly, descriptive surveys.

Use of Neuropsychological Tools

Diagnostic Procedure

The *diagnostic approach* to D should be carried out stepwise, i.e. using definite tools to exclude preestablished alternatives. Whichever disease is involved, observation of behavioral disorders in everyday life which cannot be completely traced back to already existing neurological or psychiatric disturbances, or to impaired arousal, should give rise to suspicion of OMD. The diagnostic steps include: (a) a standardized behavioral inquiry, including specific OMD-oriented everyday items (e.g., "demential episodes," "facade phenomena," disorientation) aimed at confirming OMD suspected from the general history: (b) a multifaceted test battery capable of measuring analytically the severity of OMD by the patient's residual psychological resources; and (c) a neurological component (clinical and instrumental) aiming at identifying the underlying brain disease (this also encompasses, by exclusion, the presumptive diagnosis of DAT).

The *diagnostic statement* should separately include: (a) the neuropsychological contribution, i.e., the statement as to whether the presence of OMD is certain, probable, or merely possible and whether it is mild, moderate, or severe (where the diagnosis is positive and the deterioration mild, efforts must be made to achieve a detailed cognitive profile); (b) the clinical-neurological contribution, i.e., the identification of the dementing disease; and (c) any information obtained from the brain of the dead patient on its structural modifications.

Test Battery

We deliberately avoid proposing a "new" series of tests assembled in yet another *neuropsychological battery*. Reference will be made only to those laboratory measures we consider unavoidable for CN assessment of OMD in its early stages, possibly also fitting legal requirements. Standardized tests should study: (a) memory, chiefly by means of an episodic test approach (according to the double dichotomy of verbal/nonverbal information and short-/long-term recall) – special issues are those of "working memory," serial position curve, memory for prose, autobiographical recall, and semantic and procedural memory; (b) control of information processing: attention, intelligence, and orientation; and (c) "instrumental" abilities: language, praxis, spatial cognition, and perception (at least in the visual domain). Many of the discriminative purposes of the detailed CN approach to D have not yet been submitted to strict verification in order to show its superiority to an informal, bedside diagnostic framing. Moreover, it is not unlikely that a survey of discriminant analyses may show that the power of distinguishing D patients from the normal elderly remains when only a handful of tests or even just composite scores are used. Apart from its strictly diagnostic use, such an approach (i.e., that of compact lists of heterogeneous items) would contribute only little to the understanding of D, depending on the unpredictable interaction between the neuropsychological features and the adopted test assembly. Since a detailed psychological model of the D process is lacking, it remains advisable to continue in an admittedly descriptive vein and to cast the psychometric net as wide as possible.

In connection with this issue, it must be said that although the administration of extensive and time-consuming tests meets prevailing research goals, the impact of CN on the assessment of a D patient appears to be limited to suggesting rational frames for diagnostic procedures and, to a much lesser extent, to providing self-sufficient diagnostic tools.

A Neuropsychological Study of 29 DAT Patients: Occurrence of "Selective" (Pseudofocal) Cognitive Impairments

This research gave rise to several *methodological problems,* most of which are common to the majority of cognitive studies of D and are therefore worth considering here in some detail.

Standardization of a Psychometric Tool

In order to obtain data capable of describing a D patient analytically, a certain amount of good luck in the choice of tests is necessary, as well as good judgement in achieving an accurate standardization of the tests by applying them previously to normal controls and by elaborating an adjustment procedure for the test scores, including at least age, education, and sex [6]. For a wide variety of tests we collected the performances of 321 healthy subjects through a joint project involving the M. Negri Institute, Milan, and 11 other Italian research institutes. The information obtained permitted adjustment of any new test score for the variables above through a linear covariance model. The adjusted score was then converted into a "0–4 equivalent score" according to the following procedure. Non-parametric one-tailed lower 5% tolerance limits (with 95% confidence) were the cut-off point between 0 and 1; subjects ranking above centile 50 scored 4. Points 1, 2 and 3 were intermediate between 0 and 4 on a quasi-interval scale. Of a sample of 321 normal subjects, 11% score 1 or less, 27% score 2 or less and 50% score 3 or less. This procedure allows to avoid the traditional single cutoffs, which are likely to lead to false-negative values (in highly educated young people) or to false-positive classifications (in poorly educated elderly people) [11].

Patients and Tests

Patients. Our continuous 2-year series of 124 D patients has been drawn from the outpatients attending the Neuropsychology Center of Milan University for suspected OMD. Criteria for the *presence of OMD* were strictly clinical and ecological, stemming from the answers obtained from a standardized behavioural inquiry which tackled such issues as everyday memory, language, perception, sleep, mood, and orientation. The at least 6-month worsening of suspected early demential traits such as "demential episodes" (topographic or physionomic impairments, dressing or ideational apraxia, confusional blackouts, and so on) were taken into account in diagnosis. Following these criteria, 31 (20%) of 155 patients sent for consultation were found not to be demented.

Diagnosis of DAT (irrespective of whether clinical onset was before or after 65 years) was presumptively made by exclusion of other dementing diseases, combining neurological, internal medical, psychiatric, neurosurgical, and CT findings. Invasive procedures were systematically avoided. Of the 124 D patients, 82 (66%) were labeled with a presumptive diagnosis of DAT.

DAT patients fitting the following *sociobiological constraints* were excluded from the survey, as their performance reliability was presumed to be aspecifically and unpredictably hampered by extra-D factors: (a) illiteracy; (b) institutionalization; (c) age over 70 years; and (d) suspicion of DAT not confidently confirmed after 6 months. Hence the number of suitable DAT patients dropped from 82 to 56. Moreover, in order to study patients who could be confidently considered capable of understanding all test instructions, behavioral constraints were chosen to select only *mildly or moderately deteriorated DAT/pts,* that is those with rather good orientation on formal inquiries, i.e., more than 75% in space, 70% on family members, 50% in time, and 50% on personal identity cues. Thus our DAT sample dropped further from 56 to 29 patients. This also shows how hard it is to extend the results drawn from a selected group of patients to the overall DAT population.

The DAT patients participating in the present study were aged 62.1 ± 5.2 years (range 51 to 70) and had 8.9 ± 5.5 years of education (range 3 to 17) and 2.0 ± 1.1 years of clinical illness (range 1 to 4); there were 16 women and 13 men.

Tests. The tests employed with the *aim of finding disproportionately (i.e., "selectively") deteriorated DAT patients* were grouped on prima facie and traditional grounds (chiefly left vs right hemisphere abilities and memory), into three four-test sets:
1. *Verbal tests* (L in Table 1): token test, semantically cued timed word production, timed free associations of words to a stimulus word, production of sentence starting from two nouns;
2. *Spatial-Perceptual tests* (S): constructional apraxia, meaningful rearrangement of fragments, Street's completion test, visual length discrimination on pairs of vertical segments;
3. *Memory tests* (M): forward serial verbal span for bisyllabic words, spatial (positional) span (Corsi's block-tapping device), Buschke-Fuld supraspan learning test (selective reminding procedure), spatial supraspan learning test (Corsi's device).

Analysis of Test Scores:

"Selective", "Less Selective", and "Homogeneous" Neuropsychological Deteriorations Within an Overall Deteriorated Cognitive Profile

Each original score was adjusted for age, education, and sex and then converted into a 0–4 score. By this procedure, performance discrepancies due to differences in test difficulty were ruled out. Functions like memory, language, and so on were considered impaired when among the scores of the corresponding four-test set there was at least one definite pathological score of 0 that was not counterbalanced by a score of 4 (above centile 50); scores of 1, 2, and 3 were intermediate on a quasi-interval score. A DAT patient was considered to be suffering selective deterioration when there was severe impairment in only one of the three four-test sets (L, S, M); less selective deterioration when there was impairment in two of the three sets; and homogeneous deterioration when impairment was found in all three of the sets.

Results and Conclusions

Table 1 presents the classification of the 29 DAT patients in the study group: (a) Fifteen (52%) had homogeneous deterioration (slight in four cases and severe in 11), thus following the traditional trend of global deterioration from the early stages of DAT. (b) Seven (24%) had a clearly outstanding cognitive impairment, in the verbal (n=3) and the memory (n=4) domain respectively (and none in the spatial-perceptual alone), and thus displayed a more selective cognitive deterioration. (c) The chief association of impairments always encompassed memory; six patients with language involvement and one with severe additional spatial-perceptual involvement. Length of illness, education, and sex do not play crucial roles in the cognitive grouping of these DAT patients. It is not altogether surprising that among the less selective cases there was no patient with severe impairment of both predominantly left (L) and predominantly right (S) hemisphere activities. Four of the nine patients with severe aphasic traits had unmistakable (CT-assessed) asymmetric perisylvian atrophy: neither this nor reverse morphological asymmetry was ever apparent in the other cognitive subgroups. If we look at the reverse information, namely what functions are less often severely involved, the classical pattern emerges, listing in first place spatial-perceptual performances (59% of patients), then language (31%), and last memory (24%).

These data come from a study which is still in progress and whose further aim is to ascertain whether or not evolution cancels out the cognitive selectivity of deterioration. Provisional data on 19 DAT patients with 6–24 months follow-up indicate that it does.

We believe that these findings argue strongly in favor of multifaceted assessment of the behavioral status of any DAT patient who is part of a research sample, as it is certain that cognitive impairment may appear strongly heterogeneous, particularly when a highly selected sample of patients in the first stages of D is under study. This may affect the statistical outcome of nearly all cognitive experiments on D patients.

Table 1. "Selective", "less selective", and "homogeneous" deterioration with respect to memory (M), language (L), and spatial-perceptual (S) functions in 29 DAT patients

Four-test set	No. of patients	Length of illness (years)
Selective deterioration: $n=7$ (24%)		
M	4	1.5 ± 0.6
L	3	2.0 ± 1.7
S	–	–
Less selective deterioration: $n=7$ (24%)		
M+S	1	4.0 ± 0.0
M+L	6	1.7 ± 0.8
L+S	–	–
Homogeneous deterioration: $n=15$ (52%)		
Severe	11	2.2 ± 1.0
Mild moderate	4	2.0 ± 1.4

References

1. Baddeley A, Della Sala S, Logie R, Spinnler H (1985) Working memory and dementia. Abstract, INS 8th European Conference, Copenhagen. J Clin Exp Neuropsychol 7: 139
2. Chase TN, Foster NL, Fedio P et al. (1984) Regional cortical dysfunction in Alzheimer's disease as determined by positron emission tomography. Ann Neurol 15 [Suppl]: 170–174
3. Crystal HA, Horoupian DS, Katzman R et al. (1982) Biopsy-proved Alzheimer disease presenting as a right parietal lobe syndrome. Ann Neurol 12: 186–188
4. Cummings JL, Benson DF (1984) Subcortical dementia. Review of an emerging concept. Arch Neurol 41: 874–879
5. Eisdorfer C, Cohen D (1980) Diagnostic criteria for primary neural degeneration of the Alzheimer's type. J Fam Pract 2: 553–557
6. Gade A, Mortensen EK (1985) The influence of age, education and intelligence on neuropsychological test performance. Pre-print, EBBS Workshop on Clinical Neuropsychology, Zürich
7. Garcia CA, Reding MJ, Blas JP (1981) Overdiagnosis of dementia. Ann Geriatr Soc 29: 407–410
8. Kirshner HS, Webb WG, Kelly MP, Wells CE (1984) Language disturbance. An initial symptom of cortical degenerations and dementia. Arch Neurol 41: 491–496
9. Koss E, Friedland RP, Ober BA, Jagust WJ (1984) Lateral asymmetry in cerebral metabolism: a prominent feature of Alzheimer-type dementia. Pre-print, INS 12th Annual Meeting, Houston
10. Mayeux R, Stern Y, Spanton S (1985) Heterogeneity in dementia of the Alzheimer type: evidence of subgroups. Neurology 35: 453–461
11. Parsons OA, Prigatano GP (1978) Methodological considerations in clinical neuropsychological research. J Consult Clin Psychol 46: 608–619
12. Pick A (1904) Zur Symptomatologie der linksseitigen Schläfenlappenatrophie. Monatsschr Psychiatr Neurol 16: 378–381

Clinical Management of the American Patient with Dementia

J. P. BLASS and B. A. LILLISTON[1]

Introduction

The major limitations on the clinical management of patients with dementias are biologic. Specifically, no way is now known to prevent, reverse, or even slow the neurobiologic ravages of Alzheimer's disease. Economic state, social structures, and values inevitably influence how societies choose to deal with the problems the dementing diseases create.

Biologic Aspects

The United States is a highly developed and relatively rich country with a strong tradition in science and technology. These characteristics are reflected in the usual United States approach to the biologic aspects of dementing illnesses.

Evaluation

In the United States, the conventional diagnostic evaluation of patients with dementing disorders is relatively thorough, even if the patients are very old [32]. Careful history, medical, neurologic and psychiatric examination, and neuropsychological testing are of course fundamental [17, 32]. Diagnostic laboratory studies typically include CT scan [15] or increasingly MRI scan, which may be particularly good at detecting strokes (in the t-2 weighted, spin echo mode). Positron emission (PET) and single-photon (SPECT) tomography remain research techniques [6]. Evaluation typically also includes EEG, EKG, chest film, complete blood count and urinalysis, vitamin B_{12} level, thyroid studies, and a screen such as the SMA-12 or SMA-25 [47]. Other studies are done when clinically indicated. Lumbar puncture tends to be reserved for specific indications [5]. In general, diagnostic brain biopsies are done in demented patients only for very special indications.

[1] Dementia Research Service, Burke Rehabilitation Center, Cornell University Medical College, White Plains, NY 14853, USA.

Neurology
Ed. by K. Poeck, H. J. Freund, and H. Gänshirt

Definitive diagnosis of dementing illnesses and specifically of "definite" Alzheimer's disease still requires neuropathologic confirmation [23, 32]. The diagnosis of progressive dementia can be made with more than 95% accuracy simply by waiting to be sure that it is present [34], but in most series the accuracy in predicting the autopsy findings is no better than 75%–85% [34]. The increasing evidence that Alzheimer's disease has a major genetic component [11] makes definitive diagnosis more important to the surviving descendents. The proportion of autopsies done in teaching hospitals in the United States is now low, typically less than 30%, and is much lower for people who die in nursing homes or at home. Nor are there enough neuropathologists to perform a complete neuropathologic examination on every demented individual who dies. Cheaper and more efficient diagnostic tests which correlate well with autopsy findings are badly needed.

A number of studies have reported incidences of 5%–15% of metabolic or other highly treatable conditions uncovered by such an evaluation [34]. Patients in whom an intercurrent illness precipitates reversible confusion often prove to have an underlying, but still progressive dementing illness [9, 29].

Psychiatric disease is more frequently underdiagnosed, particularly depression [28]. The reported incidence of depression in Americans over 65 varies from 4% to over 50%, depending on the diagnostic criteria and the populations studied [7, 28]. The misdiagnosis of depression as dementia (i.e., pseudodementia), appears relatively easy to avoid if robust simple tests of cognitive function are used, and patients are tested gently and without time constraints, in a language they understand [10]. The dexamethasone test adds little in elderly populations [26]. Depression is a frequent complication of stroke [18]. Speculations about the neurobiologic basis of this relationship include the possibility that vascular events in the middle cerebral artery distribution damage the outflow tracts of the serotonergic raphe nuclei and adrenergic locus ceruleus. A steady 15% of the patients referred to our subspecialty dementia service over the last 6 years proved to have depression rather than dementia at the time of their referral [34]. About half went on to develop frank dementia, most often vascular. There appears to be a distinct syndrome of a small stroke which leaves no significant sequelae evident on conventional neurologic examination, but does precipitate a depression, which of course does not protect against the occurrence of more strokes [35]. Over 20 years ago, Roth emphasized the coexistence of depression and dementia in older people and the gratifying results of treating the depressive component vigorously.

Why do such a "high-tech" evaluation of demented patients? The paucity of undetected or inadequately treated medical conditions, even in elderly demented patients, argues that conventional American "high-tech" medical care works well for those who have true access to it. High-technology medicine is widely admired and publicized in our consumer-oriented society. The families of the patients request and often demand a meticulous evaluation [20]. The feeling that everything reasonably possible has been done for a loved one can provide comfort, and the effort of going through such an evaluation can purge guilt. Physicians are trained to provide these services. Lawyers enforce a tort system that has severe sanctions for missing even untreatable illness and few rewards for keeping costs down. The evaluation described is not expensive compared with the high costs of hospitalization in the United States – perhaps 3–5 days' worth.

Treatment

The techniques used in the United States to help patients with dementing disorders are in general analogous to those for other incurable diseases. Treat intercurrent illness effectively, but gently. Provide symptomatic relief, using both pharmacologic and other medical tools as well as rehabilitation techniques. Provide counsel, do not abandon the patient and family, and be careful to do no harm. And, try to develop specific and effective therapies [8].

Activist American physicians tend to treat intercurrent illnesses which can make it harder to cope with the effects of brain disease. Treating bladder infections which can exacerbate incontinence or arrhythmias which can exacerbate confusion can help clinical adaptation without altering the neurobiology of the underlying dementing illnesses. Symptomatic relief most often involves both pharmacologic and "rehabilitative" techniques.

Controlled studies of psychopharmacologic agents in the dementias are few [22, 41]. They are also hard to interpret, because of the biologic variability in neurotransmitter and receptor loss, even in patients with the same diagnosis. The anticholinergic tricyclics can precipitate acute delirium in patients with relatively mild cholinergic defects (as in early Alzheimer's disease), and many clinicians now prefer to start with nontricyclic agents [24]. Monoamine oxidase B inhibitors have been reported to be successful in depressed older patients where treatment with other antidepressants has failed [25]. Electrocortical therapy has provided dramatic relief in patients refractory to medical therapy [1]. Doses of hypnotics needed to keep a demented patient asleep all night can cause "hangovers" [9]. A relatively small dose of an antihistaminic *when a patient awakens* often allows sleep through most of the rest of the night. Benzodiazapines and antipsychotics are widely used to limit anxiety, hallucinations, or delusions. Wandering can be a major problem which typically responds better to behavioral than to pharmacologic techniques.

An extensive literature on behavioral management of dementing illnesses includes such "how to" books as *The 36-Hour Day, Family Guide to Alzheimer Disease,* and *Living with the Patient with Intellectual Dysfunction.* The principle is to adapt the environment so that the patient can function satisfactorily in it. As these disorders progress, more profound alterations in the environment typically become necessary. The list of things that can be done would provide an anthropologist's source book on American society today.

Counseling and support for the whole family unit are recognized to be very important, i.e., "dementia is a family disease." Informal counseling is available through such support groups as the 102 local chapters of the Alzheimer Disease and Related Disorders Association [4]. Formal counseling can vary from periodic "venting" sessions with a sympathetic physician or other health care professional to formal psychotherapy and even pharmacologic support for anxiety or frank depression in the caretaker. Care of the caretaker is recognized to be an essential part of the outpatient management of the demented patient.

Research on new methods of treatment is vigorous [16, 21]. Particular emphasis has been placed on cholinesterase inhibitors and other cholinergic agents for Alzheimer's disease. While they appear to induce reproducible improvements in certain aspects of learning – particularly list learning – even in Alzheimer patients [14, 39], the clinical significance of these changes is more questionable [27, 43]. As the pendulum swings back from the emphasis on the cholinergic lesion in Alzheimer's disease to a view that several neurotransmitters are involved, emphasis is moving to an attempt to treat the fundamental cellular lesions. For instance, we and colleagues at Mount Sinai Hospital are involved in a trial of the calcium agonist 4-aminopyridine, based on experimental data implicating altered cellular calcium homeostasis in this disorder [19]. At least 25 double-blind, placebo-controlled studies indicate that ergot derivatives can lead to improvements of some test parameters in some demented patients, but the clinical significance of the changes is widely questioned [45]. Patients with multi-infarct dementia are routinely treated with antiplatelet agents, by analogy with treatment for stroke, but with little direct evidence that they alter the dismal prognosis of this malignant presentation of vascular disease [3].

The large number of victims of Alzheimer's disease and other dementias provide not only a population to be served, but also a market to be exploited. Standards of medical research in the United States are rigorous. Findings are not accepted unless replicated in tightly controlled, double-blind, placebo-controlled trials. The Food and Drug Administration has strict criteria before a compound can be investigated in humans, let alone marketed. On the other hand, in our market economy it is difficult to keep "harmless" nostrums from being peddled by people who are something between misguided and greedy. It is easier to regulate mainstream researchers than more marginal individuals.

Nonbiologic Aspects

Family and Personal Considerations

Families remain the major support of the sick elderly, even in the postindustrial United States [2, 36]. Families tend to be "nuclear," but the majority of older Americans live within half-an-hour's drive of at least one of their children [38]. Less than 20% of families said they could not care for their relative at home whatever financial support were available [40]. Both older parents and their children generally feel that the most desirable place for an older person to live is their own home and the least desirable an institution [36]. The 8% of the population over 65 who never married, or those with no surviving children, are far more likely to end up in nursing homes [38]. Indeed, whether or not a demented patient is institutionalized depends more on the coping skills of the family than on the "objective" condition of the patient [12, 46], the duration of illness [2], or the emotional quality of previous relationships [13].

Home Health Services

These vary significantly among communities, by necessity for such a large country and by design in a society committed to pluralism. Services in the home are available at several levels. In New York state, for example, *companions* typically have no specific medical – or other – training. They provide the supervision needed to keep the home environment safe and comfortable for individuals impaired in activities of daily living. *Homemakers* are licensed by the state to organize and manage household activities such as shopping and cleaning, but normally perform no health services. *Home health aides* are health care practitioners licensed by the State of New York after a training course. They assist with personal hygiene (including dental care), perform simple medical functions under the guidance of a nurse, and also do light housekeeping. Licensed practical nurses (LPNs) and registered nurses (RNs) are highly trained professionals who work in hospitals or nursing homes more often than in homes. Personnel are available from 4 to 24 hours a day, depending on needs and finances.

Respite programs in the United States are generally on one of two models. In one, health care professionals live in the home of the impaired person while the primary caretaker is gone for periods ranging from several days to a week. The other is a residential facility, where a demented person can reside for a short time. Respite programs are still too new and too few for formal studies to have been done.

Adult day care programs for the demented are growing rapidly and now number over 1000 [30, 33]. They generally include a family support group. Studies at the Burke Rehabilitation Center indicated that such a program aided the patients' and families' adaptation to the illness while (as expected) not altering the biologic course [33].

Institutionalization is in general a last resort for the elderly in the United States [36]. The reasons for admission are most often illness or other collapse of the major caretakers or overwhelming illness in the patient. Most patients are not abandoned when they enter institutions. In one survey, only 11% received no visitors, 76% received at least monthly, and 61% at least weekly visits [40].

Facilities are of several types. In New York state, *domiciliary* homes are basically boarding houses for those with relatively little disability. *Health-related facilities* (HRFs) have nursing supervision 8 hours a day and provide for medical and nursing services, as ordered by a physician. *Skilled nursing facilities* (SNFs) provide 24-hour nursing and medical care [44]. *Psychiatric hospitals,* including state facilities, can provide long-term care, but by regulation are only for patients whose major disabilities are judged to be psychiatric rather than cognitive.

Financial and Legal Aspects

The United States system of paying for medical care is a rapidly changing crazy-quilt of federal, state, local, individual, public, and private mechanisms, which has been reported to provide relatively comprehensive care with relatively little social class bias, at great expense [31]. Medical care for demented patients over 65 is easily reimbursed; custodial care is not (i.e., dementia has been "medicalized").

Medicare, Medicaid, and Private Insurance

Medicare and medicaid are mandated and largely funded by the federal government, but administered and partially funded by the states. The doctrine is that local control is more efficient in so large and heterogeneous a country. *Medicare,* the major program in the United States for funding acute and ambulatory care for the elderly and seriously disabled, specifically prohibits payment for most long-term or custodial care (Social Security Act, sec. 1862). *Medicaid* uses a means test set at poverty levels to determine eligibility (e.g., an income no more than $8000 a year and assets of $4200 for two in New York state). Medicaid does pay for the cost of home care and nursing homes if such services are sanctioned by a designated public health agency. Recipients specifically include elderly demented patients who have become impoverished by paying for the "custodial" services they needed to stay alive. In 1980, only 0.7% of nursing home and home health care expenditure was reimbursed by third party insurance carriers.

Financially as well as socially, families appear to be the major resource for patients with Alzheimer's disease and other dementias in the United States. The costs appear to be met largely by devoted spouses or children, who are willing to modify their own living arrangements and schedules to provide the space and care needed (i.e., the true economic costs are now hidden).

Legal Aspects

People with dementia characteristically lose the ability to care for their savings as well as themselves. In commercial as well as other areas, United States law includes both federal and state jurisdictions, the latter derived sometimes from Common and sometimes from Roman law, modified by legislation and precedent. The legal mechanisms to protect demented people are a burgeoning, lucrative legal subspeciality. King Lear would have been wise to transfer his wealth to Cordelia had he lived in the United States today, since the public purse (medicaid) pays for "custodial" care only for the impoverished.

Ethical Aspects

In the United States, a patient mentally competent to make an informed decision, and certified to be so by two licensed psychiatrists, has the right to accept or refuse even life-saving therapy [42]. For incompetent (e.g., demented) patients, the general rule is to respect what the *patient* would have wanted if mentally intact. Most patients have devoted families, and close consultations between them, physicians, and sometimes lawyers and hospital ethics committees seem to solve most problems satisfactorily and quietly [37]. The political debate to develop clearer guidelines continues.

Conclusion

The biology of Alzheimer's disease and other dementing diseases presents medical and social challenges to which societies necessarily respond in accord with their own characteristics. The systems for caring for patients with dementias, for funding their care, and for deciding how much care to give allow wide variations in the United States that may seem disorderly. They are in accord, however, with the United States emphasis on individual choice – on pluralism and autonomy rather than beneficence. A taste for technology and for research is often attributed to Americans. One can only hope that research will provide effective ways to treat or even prevent Alzheimer's disease and other dementias. Such technical means would revolutionize the care of these patients all over the world.

References

1. Alexopoulos GS, Shamoian CJ, Lucas J, Weiser N, Berger H (1984) Medical problems of geriatric psychiatric patients and younger controls during electroconvulsive therapy. J Am Geriatr Soc 32:651–654
2. Aronson M, Lipkowitz R (1981) Senile dementia, Alzheimer's type: the family and the health care delivery system. J Am Geriatr Soc 29:568–571
3. Barclay LL, Zemcov A, Blass JP, Sansone J (1985) Survival in Alzheimer's disease and vascular dementias. Neurology 35:834–842
4. Barnes R, Raskind M, Scott M, Murphy C (1981) Problems of families caring for Alzheimer patients: Use of a support group. J Am Geriatr Soc 29:80–85
5. Becker PM, Feussner JR, Mulrow CD, Williams BC, Vokaty KA (1985) The role of lumbar puncture in the evaluation of dementia. J Amer Geriatr Soc 33:392–396
6. Benson DF, Kuhl DE, Hawkins RA, Phelps ME, Cummings JL (1983) The fluorodeoxyglucose ^{18}F scan in Alzheimer's disease and multi-infarct dementia. Arch Neurol 40:711–714
7. Blazer D (1982) The epidemiology of depression. J Am Geriatr Soc 30:587–592
8. Blass JP (1981) Dementia. Med Clin North Am 66:1143–1160
9. Blass JP, Plum F (1983) Metabolic encephalopathies in older adults. In: Katzman R, Terry RD (eds) The neurology of aging. Davis, Philadelphia, pp 189–220
10. Breen AR, Larson EB, Reifler BV, Vitaliano PP, Lawrence GL (1984) Cognitive performance and functional competence in coexisting dementia and depression. J Am Geriatr Soc 32:132–137
11. Breitner JCS, Folstein MF (1984) Familial nature of Alzheimer's disease. N Engl J Med 311:192
12. Brody S, Poulshock W, Masciocchi C (1978) The family caring unit: a major consideration in the long-term support system. Gerontologist 18:556–561
13. Bromberg E (1983) Mother–daughter relationships in later life: the effect of quality of relationship upon mutual aid. J Gerontol Soc Work 6:75–92
14. Davis KL, Mohs RC, Tinklenberg JR (1979) Enhancement of memory by physostigmine. N Engl J Med 301:946
15. Drayer BP, Heyman A, Wilkinson W, Barrett L, Weinberg T (1985) Early onset Alzheimer's disease: an analysis of CT findings. Ann Neurol 17:407–410
16. Ferris SH, Reisberg B, Crook T, Friedman E, Schneck MK, Sherman KA, Corwin J, Gershon S, Bartus R (1982) Pharmacologic treatment of senile dementia. Ment Health Aging 19:475–481
17. Folstein MF, Folstein SE, McHugh PR (1975) A practical method for grading the cognitive state of patients for the clinician. J Psychiatr Res 12:189–198
18. Folstein MF, Maiberger R, McHugh PR (1977) Mood disorder as a specific complication of stroke. J Neurol Neurosurg Psychiatr 40:1018–1020
19. Gibson GE, Peterson C (1983) Amelioration of age-related deficits in acetylcholine release and behaviour with 4-aminopyridine. In: Algeri S, Gershon S, Grimm V, Tofano G (eds) Aging of the brain. Raven, New York, pp 337–348
20. Glosser G, Wexler D, Balmelli M (1985) Physicians' and families' perspectives on the medical management of dementia. J Am Geriatr Soc 33:383–391
21. Harbaugh RE, Roberts DW, Coombs DW, Saunders RL, Reeder TM (1984) Preliminary report: intracranial cholinergic drug infusion in patients with Alzheimer's disease. Neurosurgery 15:514–518
22. Helms P (1985) Efficacy of antipsychotics in the treatment of behavioral complications of dementia: a review of the literature. J Am Geriatr Soc 33:206–209
23. Heilig CW, Knopman DS, Mastri AR, Frey W (1985) Dementia without Alzheimer pathology. Neurology 35:762–765

24. Jarvik LE, Mintz J, Steuer J, Gerner R (1982) Treating geriatric depression: a 26-week interim analysis. J Am Geriatr Soc 30:713–717
25. Jenike MA (1985) Monoamine oxidase inhibitors as a treatment for depressed patients with primary degenerative dementia (Alzheimer's disease). Am J Psychiatry 142:763–764
26. Jenike MA, Albert MS (1984) The dexamethasone suppression test in patients with presenile and senile dementia of the Alzheimer type. J Am Geriatr Soc 32:441–444
27. Jotzkowitz S (1983) Lack of clinical efficacy of chronic oral physostigmine in Alzheimer's disease. Ann Neurol 14:690–691
28. Kramer M, German PS, Anthony JC, Von Korff M, Skinner EA (1985) Patterns of mental disorders among the elderly residents of eastern Baltimore. J Am Geriatr Soc 33:236–245
29. Larson EB, Reifler BV, Featherstone HJ (1984) Dementia in elderly outpatients: a prospective study. Ann Intern Med 100:417–423
30. Mace N (1984) Day care for demented clients. Hosp Community Psychiatry 35:979–994
31. Macrae N (1984) Health care international. Economist, April 28, pp 17–33
32. McKhann G, Drachman D, Folstein M, Katzman R, Price D, Stadlan EM (1984) Clinical diagnosis of Alzheimer's disease: Report of the NINCDS-ADRDA work group under the auspices of the Department of Health and Human Services task force on Alzheimer's disease. Neurology 34:939–944
33. Panella JJ, Lilliston BA, Brush D, McDowell FH (1984) Day care for dementia patients: an analysis of a four-year program. J Am Geriatr Soc 32:1–4
34. Reding MJ, Wigforss K, Brush D, Blass JP (1984) Follow-up of patients referred to a dementia service. J Am Geriatr Soc 32:265–268
35. Reding MJ, Haycox J, Blass JP (1985) Depression in patients referred to a dementia clinic: a three-year prospective study. Arch Neurol, in press
36. Shanas E (1979) Social myth as hypothesis: the case of the family relations of old people. Gerontologist 19:3–9
37. Stollerman GH (1984) Quality of life: treatment decisions and the third alternative. J Am Geriatr Soc 32:483–484
38. Streib G (1972) Older families and their troubles: familial and social responses. Fam Coordinator 1:5–19
39. Thal LJ, Fuld PA, Masur DM, Sharpless NS (1983) Oral physostigmine and lecithin improve memory in Alzheimer disease. Ann Neurol 13:491–496
40. Tobin S, Kulys A (1981) The family in institutionalization of the elderly. J Soc Issues 37:145–157
41. Thompson MG, Moran MG, Neis AS (1983) Psychotropic drug use in the elderly. N Engl J Med 309:134–137
42. Wanzer SH, Adelstein SJ, Cranford RE, Federman DD, Hook ED, Moertrel CG, Safar P, Stone A, Taussig HB, Eys JV (1984) The physicians responsibility toward the hopelessly ill. N Engl J Med 310:955–959
43. Wettstein A (1983) No effect from double-blind trial of physostigmine and lecithin in Alzheimer diseases. Ann Neurol 13:210–212
44. Wolff ML, Smolen S, Ferrara BS (1985) Treatment decisions in a skilled nursing facility. J Am Geriatr Soc 33:440–445
45. Yesavage JA, Tinklenberg JR, Hollister LE, Berger PA (1979) Vasodilators in senile dementia. Arch Gen Psychiatr 36:220–223
46. Zarit SH, Reever KE, Bach-Peterson J (1980) Relatives of the impaired elderly – correlates of feelings of burden. Gerontologist 20:649–655
47. Zemcov A, Barclay LL, Brush D, McDowell F (1984) Computerized data base for evaluation and follow-up of demented patients. J Am Geriatr Soc 32:801–842

Clinical Management in Europe of Patients with Dementia

C. G. GOTTFRIES [1]

Introduction

To make progress in the clinical care of dementia patients, a relevant subdividing of dementia disorders must be at hand. The subdividing now in use is based on findings partly from the beginning of this century. It can be assumed that this classification of dementias can be improved so as to offer a better base for the care of the patients and for treatment research. In this paper the present subdividing of dementias will be discussed. Aspects will also be given on treatment strategies based on structural and biochemical findings in brains from patients with dementias.

Structural Changes in the Brains from Patients with Dementias

Dementia research has been carried out along different lines. One line that has given fruitful results is postmortem investigations of the human brain. For some time neuropathologists have described the structural changes in brains from patients with dementias and our present subdividing is based on these findings.

The dementias are divided into two main groups, that is, patients with cerebrovascular disorders (CVD) and patients with primary degenerative disorders. In CVD with dementia it is assumed that the dementia is due to infarctions of the brain and therefore this dementia form is called multiinfarction dementia (MID) [13].

In the beginning of this century Alzheimer ([1], cited in [22]) described lesions, senile plaques, and fibrillary tangles, in the brain from patients with a presenile dementia and this disorder has now got his name, Alzheimer's disease (AD). The lesions he described can, however, be found also in other dementia disorders and in normal aging. Senile dementia (SD) is a dementia form which is assumed to be a primary degenerative disorder with onset at above the age of 65 years. As the Alzheimer lesions can be found also in senile dementia this dementia has been called

[1] Dept. of Psychiatry and Neurochemistry, St. Jörgens Hospital, S-422 03 Hisings Backa, Sweden.

Neurology
Ed. by K. Poeck, H. J. Freund, and H. Gänshirt

senile dementia of Alzheimer type (SDAT) and SDAT together with AD form the group Alzheimer dementias (AD/SDAT). In bringing these disorders together one assumes that the Alzheimer lesions delimit a homogeneous dementia group. This is, however, not yet proven and therefore from a scientific point of view it seems unwise to bring AD and SDAT into one group. Alzheimer lesions can also be found together with brain infarctions. This dementia group is called a "mixed group" and it is assumed that as well the Alzheimer lesions as the infarctions cause the dementia.

Investigation of structural changes in the brain has revealed white matter disturbances [3]. White matter changes in brains from patients with dementia disorders have been confirmed in investigations with nuclear magnetic resonance (NMR). The white matter changes are not found only in patients with AD and SDAT but also in patients with MID [16]. According to Brun [2], the changes are more pronounced in patients with a late onset of dementia and look like incomplete infarctions. This indicates that hypoxia may have etiological importance.

Biochemical Changes in the Brains from Patients with Dementias

Chia et al. [6] have reported evidence for myelin disorders in brains from patients with AD. Higher levels of malondialdehyde and conjugated dienes in white matter from diseased brains suggested that free-radical mediated lipid peroxidation might be the source of the increased myelin disorder.

In our own investigations of patients with AD, SDAT, and MID white matter changes have been studied [11, 12]. It is shown that in patients with AD/SDAT and MID there are reduced concentrations of myelin components. The levels seen in Fig. 1 are preliminary data from an ongoing investigation at our institute. As seen in

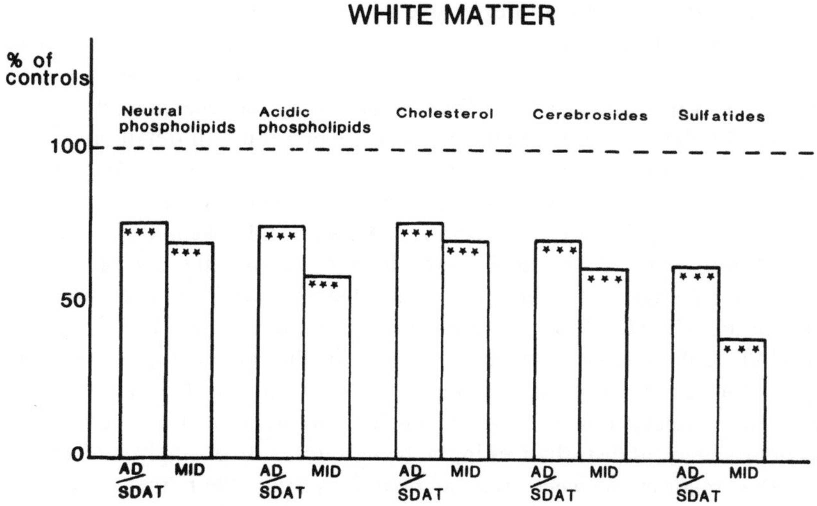

Fig. 1. White matter (centrum semiovale) changes expressed as percentage of controls ($n=21$), in a group of Alzheimer dementias ($n=22$) and a group of multiinfarction dementias (MID) ($n=9$). ***, $p<0.005$; group differences according to Student's t-test

the figure, neutral and acidic phospholipids, cholesterol, cerebrosides, and sulfatides are significantly reduced in AD/SDAT patients (n = 21) as well as in MID patients (*n* = 9) when compared with controls (*n* = 22). More detailed investigations must be performed in order to determine whether there are special patterns of myelin disturbances in the different dementia groups. The most severe decreases were, however, seen in the MID group.

The white matter changes may of course be the consequence of gray matter degeneration. However, it must also be assumed that the damage to the white matter has a more primary etiological importance for the dementia process eventually caused by disturbances in the blood circulation of the brain.

It is shown that patients with AD and SDAT have increased lactate concentrations in the cerebrospinal fluid (CSF) [9]. Also the lactate pyruvate ratio is increased which indicates that the demented patients may have suffered from hypoxia. Sourander et al. [21] have reported that patients with dementia have significantly increased sleep apnea attacks as compared with age-matched controls. In healthy elderly individuals, it is shown that there is a definite age effect with respect to apneas/hypoapneas during sleep. As well as number, duration of sleep apneas increase significantly in the seventies [20]. Could these sleep apneas be of importance for circulatory disturbances of the brain?

During the past two decades research concerning changes in the metabolism of neurotransmitters in brains from patients with dementia disorders has developed. It is obvious that in AD and SDAT there are several neurotransmitter systems in the brain that are disturbed (for review see [10]). In the UK and the USA the disturbed metabolism of acetylcholine (ACh) has been especially emphasized. It is obvious that the ACh system is severely disturbed and that these changes have behavioral consequences in the form of disturbed memory functions. There are, however, several reports indicating that also the monoaminergic neurotransmitters as well as some of the neuropeptides are deranged. From a clinical point of view it is also obvious that the severe and extensive clinical symptoms seen in the dementia disorders can not be explained only by a disturbance in one neurotransmitter system.

In our own investigation presented above, where myelin components were determined, also neurotransmitters, their metabolites, and enzyme activities were measured. The data are preliminary and will be presented in detail later. As is evident from Fig. 2, there are severe disturbances in the caudate nucleus in the two dementia groups: 5-hydroxytryptamine (5-HT), 5-hydroxyindolacetic acid (5-HIAA), dopamine (DA), homovanillic acid (HVA), and cholineacetyl transferase (CAT) are significantly reduced. In Fig. 3 the results from the investigation of the hippocampus are presented and again there are severe disturbances in both groups. Of interest is that in the AD/SDAT group there is highly significant and severely reduced activity of CAT in the caudate nucleus as well as in the hippocampus, while in the MID group the reduction of this enzyme is not significant in the hippocampus and only borders significance in the caudate nucleus. Apart from this difference, the pattern of neurochemical disturbances in the two groups is surprisingly similar.

The relation between the monoamines and their metabolites (HVA/DA, 5-HIAA/5-HT) may indicate that in the controls there is a reduced number of neurons as marked by low levels of DA and 5-HT, while the remaining neurons have an increased speed of turnover, as marked by nonreduced levels of metabolites

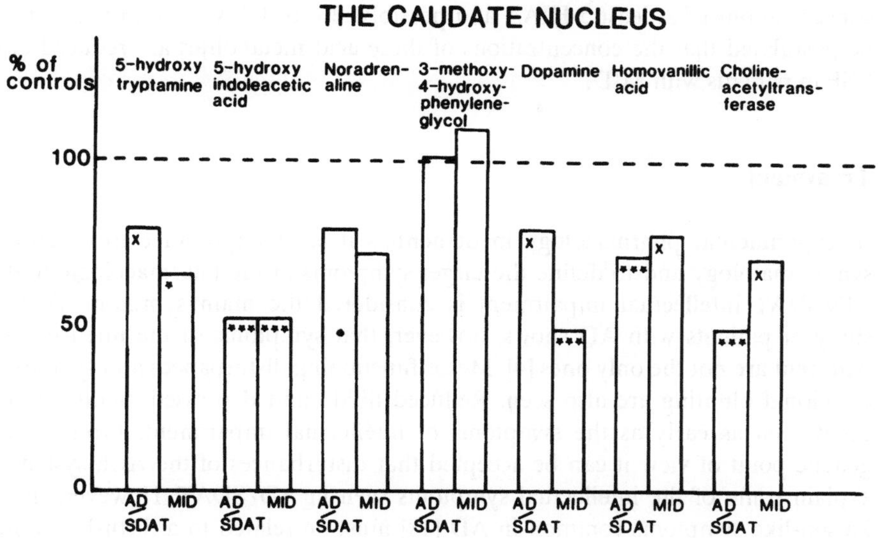

Fig. 2. Changes in the caudate nucleus expressed as percentage of controls ($n=21$), in a group of Alzheimer dementias ($n=22$) and a group of multiinfarction dementias (MID) ($n=9$). +, $p<0.10$; *, $p<0.05$; ***, $p<0.005$; group differences using Student's t-test

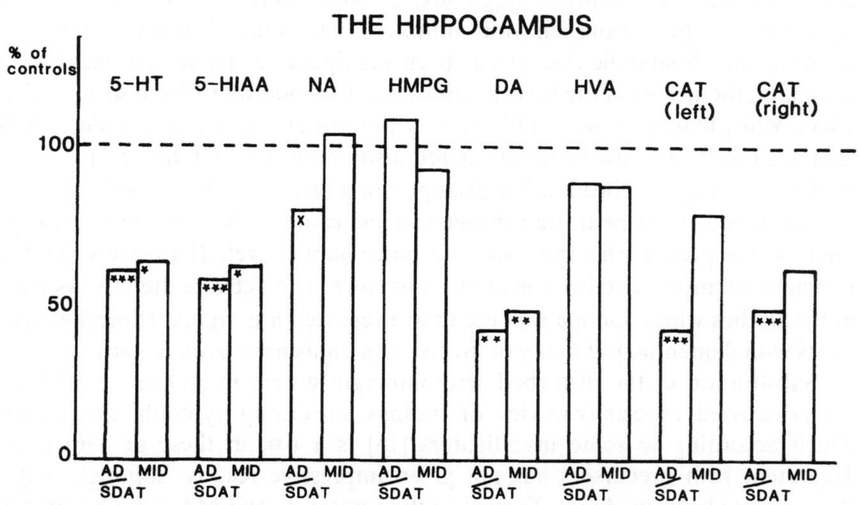

Fig. 3. Changes in the hippocampus expressed as percentage of controls ($n=21$), in a group of Alzheimer dementias ($n=22$) and a group of multiinfarction dementias (MID) ($n=9$). +, $p<0.10$; *, $p<0.05$; **, $p<0.01$; ***, $p<0.005$; group differences using Student's t-test

(HVA, 5-HIAA). In the Alzheimer brains also the metabolites were reduced, possibly indicating not only cell loss but also a neurochemical defect in the remaining neurons [5].

The study of acid metabolites in CSF is used in the diagnosis of dementia. Reduced levels of HVA and 5-HIAA are indicative of AD/SDAT (cf. [7]). In our present investigations, however, we can show that also patients with MID have reduced concentrations of at least 5-HIAA and possibly also of HVA in brain tissue. It must be postulated that the concentrations of these acid metabolites are reduced also in CSF in patients with MID.

Treatment

In experimental pharmacology in dementias it is of importance to describe the symptomatology and to define the target symptoms in the pharmacologic trials. In AD/SDAT intellectual impairment is considered the main symptom. A careful study of patients with AD shows, however, that symptoms of the intellectual impairment are not the only ones [4]. Motor functioning disturbances and symptoms of emotional blunting are also seen. Reduced libido and depressed mood are sometimes seen as early as the symptoms of intellectual impairment. From a pathogenetic point of view it can be accepted that disturbances of the ACh system may explain some of the intellectual symptoms seen in AD/SDAT. However, the parkinson-like symptoms common in AD [18] must be related to a disturbance in the DA metabolism. It is also logical to relate emotional and mood disturbances to defects in noradrenaline (NA) and 5-HT metabolism.

The main strategies in the treatment of dementias can be presented along five lines. The first line is pharmacologic substituting of defect neurotransmitter systems. By the use of precursors, enzyme inhibitors, and muscarinic cholinergic receptor agonists, the cholinergic system has been manipulated (for review see [19], [8]). In summary, the results of the investigations are disappointing. There seems to be some effect with physostigmine. Until recently physostigmine was available only for injections, but it can now be administered also orally. In total, however, the effect of cholinergic drugs has been rather disappointing and of no clinical utility.

The monoamine neurotransmitter systems can also be activated by drug treatment on the presynaptic, synaptic, and postsynaptic level. There are several studies in which attempts have been made to substitute or to activate the DA system. Some of the studies where L-dopa was used have reported a marginal clinical effect in patients with dementia, but many of the investigations have been negative.

Substitution of the disturbed serotoninergic system in AD and SDAT has also been discussed, especially in view of findings concerning tryptophan malabsorption, which according to some investigators [15] is a risk in these dementia patients. Treatment with precursors has not given impressive results, although only a few studies have been made [8]. Tricyclic antidepressants and MAO inhibitors may also be of interest. The few investigations made hitherto have, however, not given impressive results. Ergoloid mesylates have long been used in the treatment of symptoms of old age and dementia disorders. Originally it was claimed that these drugs increased the cerebral blood flow. However, ergoloid mesylates also seem to have an effect on neuronal metabolism. In terms of neurotransmitter activity, the ergoloid mesylates in use mainly block central alpha adrenergic and stimulate both DA and 5-HT receptor sites [17]. This effect of ergoloid mesylates may explain the clinical effect recorded with this drug.

The second line of treatment of dementias is to give patients neuropeptides. The theory for this is that some of the neuropeptides act as neurotransmitters or neurotransmitter modulators in the brain and at least some of them are reduced in AD. Vasopressin and parts of the ACTH molecule have been used in treatment studies. The effect of this treatment is marginal.

A third line in treatment of dementias is to give the patients nootropics. These are drugs that influence the metabolism of the neurons. Piracetam is such a drug. The result of treatment trials here are, however, inconclusive.

A fourth line in treatment of dementias, according to results about white matter would be to avoid blood pressure falls and hypoxia in old age. One important thing is, of course, to be careful with pharmacologic treatment in the elderly, as drugs may cause hypotension.

A fifth line in the treatment of dementias is nonpharmacologic treatment. Mental activation, psychotherapeutic support to the patient, and support to the family still are the treatment strategies that have given the best effect. According to an investigation by Karlsson et al. [14] it is shown that mental activation not only influences psychological but also biochemical factors. A group of patients with dementia, which was intensively treated with mental activation, not only had changes in psychological parameters but also in CSF markers; the somatostatin concentration increased and there was no decrease of HVA in CSF.

Acknowledgements. The study was supported by grants from the Swedish Medical Research Council, King Gustaf Vth and Queen Victoria Foundations, Fredrik and Ingrid Thuring Foundation, Greta and Einar Asker Foundation, and the Hjalmar Svensson Foundation.

References

1. Alzheimer A (1907) Über eine eigenartige Erkrankung der Hirnrinde. Cbl Nervenheilk Psychiat 18:177–179
2. Brun A (1983) An overview of light and electron microscopic changes. In: Reisberg B (ed) Alzheimer's disease. The standard reference. Free Press, New York, pp 37–47
3. Brun A, Gustafson L (1978) Limbic lobe involvement in presenile dementia. Arch Psychiatr Nervenkr 226:76–93
4. Bråne G, Gottfries CG (1985) Treatment with monoaminergic drugs in Alzheimer's disease and senile dementia. In: Gottfries CG (ed) Normal aging, Alzheimer's disease and senile dementia. Aspects on etiology, pathogenesis, diagnosis and treatment. Proceedings of two symposia, Collegium Internationale Neuro-Psychopharmacologicum 14th Congress, 22–23 June 1984, Florence, Italy. L'Université de Bruxelles, Brussels, pp 281–286
5. Carlsson A (1985) Neurotransmitters in old age and dementia. In: Häfner H, Sartorius N, Moschel G (eds) Mental health in the elderly: a review of the present state of research. Springer, Berlin Heidelberg New York Tokyo
6. Chia LS, Thompson JE, Moscarello MA (1984) X-ray diffraction evidence for myelin disorder in brain from humans with Alzheimer's disease. Biochim Biophys Acta 775:308–312
7. Gottfries CG (1983) Biochemical changes in blood and cerebrospinal fluid. In: Reisberg B (ed) Alzheimer's disease. The standard reference. Free Press, New York, pp 122–130
8. Gottfries CG (1983) Dementia. In: Hippius H, Winokur G (eds) Psychopharmacology 1, Part 2: Clinical psychopharmacology. Elsevier, Amsterdam
9. Gottfries CG, Kjällquist A, Ponten U, Roos BE, Sundbärg, G (1974) Cerebrospinal fluid PH and monoamine and glucolytic metabolites in Alzheimer's disease. Br J Psychiatry 124:280–287
10. Gottfries CG, Adolfsson R, Aquilonius SM, Carlsson A, Eckernäs SÅ, Nordberg A, Oreland L, Svennerholm L, Wiberg A, Winblad B (1983) Biochemical changes in dementia disorders of Alzheimer type (AD/SDAT). Neurobiol Aging 4:261–271

11. Gottfries CG, Karlssson I, Svennerholm L (1985) Senile dementia – a "white matter" disease. In: Gottfries CG (ed) Normal aging, Alzheimer's disease and senile dementia. Aspects on etiology, pathogenesis, diagnosis and treatment. Proceedings of two symposia, Collegium Internationale Neuro-Psychopharmacologicum 14th Congress, 22–23 June, 1984, Florence, Italy. L'Université de Bruxelles, Brussels, pp 111–118
12. Gottfries CG, Alafuzzof I, Carlsson A, Eckernäs SÅ, Karlsson I, Oreland L, Svennerholm L, Winblad B (1985). In preparation.
13. Hachinski VD, Lassen NA, Marshall J (1974) Multi-infarct dementia. A cause of mental deterioration in the elderly. Lancet 2:207–209
14. Karlsson I, Bråne G, Melin E, Nyth AL, Rybo E (1985) Mental activation – brain plasticity. In: Gottfries CG (ed) Normal aging, Alzheimer's disease and senile dementia. Aspects on etiology, pathogenesis, diagnosis and treatment. Proceedings of two symposia, Collegium Internationale Neuro-Psychopharmacologicum 14th Congress, 22–23 June, 1984, Florence, Italy, L'Université de Bruxelles, Brussels, pp 269–273
15. Lehmann J, Persson S, Wålinder J, Wallin L (1981) Tryptophan malabsorption in dementia improvement in certain cases after tryptophan therapy as indicated by mental behaviour and blood analysis. A pilot study. Acta Psychiat Scand 64:123
16. de Leon MJ, George AE, Ferris SH, Christman D, Gentes CI, Miller JD, Fowler J, Reisberg B, Wolf AP (1985) CT, PET and NMR brain imaging in aging and Alzheimer's disease. In: Gottfries CG (ed) Normal aging, Alzheimer's disease and senile dementia. Aspects on etiology, pathogenesis, diagnosis and treatment. Proceedings of two symposia, Collegium Internationale Neuro-Psychopharmacologicum 14th Congress, 22–23 June, 1984, Florence, Italy. L'Université de Bruxelles, Brusells, pp 199–202
17. Loew DM, van Deusen EB, Meier Ruge W (1978) Effects on the central nervous system. In: Berde B, Schild HO (eds) Ergot alkaloids and related compounds. Springer, Berlin Heidelberg New York, pp 421–532 (Handbook of experimental pharmacology, vol 49)
18. Pearce J (1974) Mental changes in Parkinsonism. Br Med J Lett 1:445
19. Reisberg B (1983) An overview of current concepts of Alzheimer's disease, senile dementia, and age-associated cognitive decline. In: Reisberg B (ed) Alzheimer's disease. Free Press, New York, pp 3–20
20. Reynolds CF, Kupfer DJ, Taska LS, Hoch CC, Sewitch DE, Spiker DG (1985) Sleep of healthy seniors: a revisit. Sleep 8:20–29
21. Sourander L, Polo O, Alihanka J (1985) Sleep apnea and hypoxia in patients with senile dementia. Paper presented at the Nordic Psychiatric Congress in Odense, May 29–June 1, 1985
22. Torack R (1971) In: Wells C (ed) Dementia. Davis, Philadelphia

Research Issues in Alzheimer's Disease

Analytic Epidemiology and Risk Factors in Alzheimer's Disease

L. AMADUCCI [1] and B. S. SCHOENBERG [2]

The study of the presence of associations between disease and host or environmental factors is the domain of analytic epidemiology [1]. During the course of their lives, different individuals are exposed to a variety of factors or conditions, some of which may play an important role in the occurrence of disease. Analytic epidemiology is aimed at identifying factors that are related to either a high or low risk of disease.

In the case-control investigation, one begins with a group of individuals who have the disease of interest (cases) and a group of individuals without the disease (controls) [2]. One then explores the present characteristics (in a cross-sectional study) or the history (in a retrospective study) of these two groups for the presence or absence of factors thought to be related to the occurrence of the disease. Obviously, one looks for factors that are distributed differentially in the group with the disease as compared to the group without the disease.

Case-control studies have a number of advantages that recommend such a strategy (Table 1). These studies can be carried out at low cost, and information can be

Table 1. Case-control studies

Advantages
Lower cost than prospective studies
Rapid answers
Possibility of examining multiple risk factors
No follow-up required
Low incidence diseases can be studied
Disadvantages
Problems with accuracy and completeness of retrospective inquiry
Problem with representativeness of sample cases and controls
Can only estimate relative risk
Presence of disease may influence factor being studied

[1] Department of Neurology, University of Florence, Viale Morgagni 85, Florence, Italy.
[2] Neuroepidemiology Branch, NINCDS-NIH, Room 804, Federal Building, 7550 Wisconsin Avenue, MD 20892, USA.

Neurology
Ed. by K. Poeck, H. J. Freund, and H. Gänshirt

obtained relatively quickly. Once suitable cases and control groups have been identified, a number of factors thought to be associated with the disease can be examined. Because one starts with identified patients and controls and determines past or current exposure to suspected risk factors, such studies do not require future follow-up of individuals. Finally, these studies can be used to investigate uncommon diseases, although a multicenter collaborative approach may be required to obtain a sufficient number of patients.

On the other hand, the case-control approach has its drawbacks (Table 1). To determine the past exposure of an individual with regard to a specific factor, one must rely on memory or medical records, the accuracy of which may be uncertain. Another major concern is the representativeness of cases and controls. With case-control studies, it is possible to provide only an estimate of relative risk. The relative risk is the ratio of the incidence rate of a disease in those with a given factor to the incidence rate of the same disease in those without the factor. Finally, the presence of the disease itself may influence the factor being studied.

Analytic epidemiologic investigations on dementia and Alzheimer's disease must deal with a number of methodological issues which pose special difficulties. Unless we want to restrict the study to patients with autopsy confirmation, we must rely on the accuracy of a clinical diagnosis. Since population-based studies are so difficult to carry out, it is usually necessary to search for cases among patients coming to a given hospital or clinic. This may lead to a selection bias, in that the patients receiving care at a particular institution may not be representative of all cases in the community. In obtaining required information about past exposure to putative etiologic factors, the epidemiologist frequently relies on data obtained by interview. With Alzheimer's disease, the cases, by virtue of their disease, generally cannot supply the required information. One must therefore identify an appropriate surrogate respondent and verify the reliability of data obtained in this manner [3]. As with most case-control studies, one must also be alert to the possibility of selective recall bias in which the family of a case may be motivated to remember past events possibly related to the occurrence of the disease of interest. Despite these problems, analytic epidemiologic studies of Alzheimer's disease have been successfully carried out.

There are several published studies aimed to identifying etiologic or pathogenetic factors in Alzheimer's disease [4–7], but only a few investigations meet the methodological requirements of case-control studies. The first well-organized comparative study on risk factors in dementia was published, in France, in 1838 by Esquirol, who compared cases from the Salpêtrière in Paris with those admitted to Charenton Asylum in Saint-Maurice [8]. He observed that the presenile forms of dementia were more frequent among the higher levels of French society. Hence he concluded that "the abuse of pleasures, the exaggeration of passions, and deviations from the normal life-style destroy human personality, disrupt the brain in early youth, predispose it to dementia and precipitate an early old age." The more recent and methodologically more complete studies are shown in the Table 2.

Heston et al. in 1981 published a study of the relatives of 125 probands who had dementia of the Alzheimer type as proved by autopsy [9]. When compared with a control group and general population figures, the relatives exhibited an excess of dementing illness consistent with genetic transmission. The relatives also had an excess of Down's syndrome, lymphoma, and immune diatheses.

Table 2. Case-control studies of Alzheimer's disease

	Cases	Controls	Data collection	Results
Heston et al. (1981) [9]	125	Population	Medical records next of kin interviews	Dementia in the relatives Down's syndrome in the relatives Lymphomas in the relatives Immune diatheses in the relatives
Whalley et al. (1982) [10]	74	Population	Medical records	Dementia in the relatives Increased parental age
Bharucha et al. (1983) [11]	53	Population	Medical records (Rochester)	(Herpes zoster infection)
Mortimer et al. (1983) [12]	78	Hospital population	Questionnaire to next of kin	Head trauma
Heyman et al. (1984) [15]	40	Population	Questionnaire to next of kin	Dementia in the relatives Thyroid disease Severe head trauma Down's syndrome in the relatives
Amaducci et al. (1985) [18]	116	Hospital population	Questionnaire to next of kin	Dementia in the relatives Head trauma

In 1982, Whalley et al. studied the families of 74 probands with autopsy proven Alzheimer's disease [10]. Whalley's findings did not support the hypothesis advanced by Heston. However the incidence of presenile dementia among first-degree relatives of probands was increased and was consistent with a simple polygenic model of inheritance.

Bharucha et al. in 1983, in a retrospective case-control study utilized clinical records for all 53 incidence cases of Alzheimer's disease occurring during a 5-year period in Rochester, Minnesota (in the north-central United States). Population controls were selected from the same community [11]. These investigators found only an association with herpes zoster infection, but this relationship was not statistically significant.

In the same year Mortimer and co-workers published the results of a case-control study based on 78 white males clinically diagnosed by a single examiner at the Veterans Administration Medical Center in Minneapolis (in the north-central United States) [12] and in 1985 French et al. presented a more extensive report of the same investigation [13]. Controls were obtained from the same hospital and a second set of controls were recruited from the same neighborhoods as the cases. There were some demographic differences between cases and controls: cases had more years of education and were more frequently Catholic than either hospital or neighborhood controls. Significantly more head trauma and depression were reported for cases than for hospital controls. The authors state however the possibility that the greater reporting of head trauma represented a recall bias.

In 1984 Heyman and collaborators published details of a case-control study (reported by Wilkinson in abstract form) [14] on 40 cases of clinically diagnosed Alzheimer's disease primarily from North Carolina (in the southeastern United States) Information was collected by means of a questionnaire administered to the next of kin [15]. There was a significantly higher frequency of prior thyroid disease in female patients than in female control subjects; in addition, a history of severe head injury was also obtained significantly more often among the patients than among controls. Finally, there was evidence of a possible genetic factor, manifested by an excess of dementia and mental retardation (including Down's syndrome) in families of patients with Alzheimer's disease.

As seen from the published studies, one particular problem is the question of sample size. We must therefore address the difficulty of having a large enough number of cases to reach statistical significance [16, 17]. Alzheimer's disease is still relatively uncommon in each individual center and the reported studies have dealt either with a small number of cases or with cases made up of special subgroups of patients (e.g., only males as in the Veterans Administration Study conducted by Mortimer) [12]. To deal with this problem, larger studies have adopted a multicenter collaborative approach. With a multicenter study of Alzheimer's disease one must exercise special care in standardizing: (a) diagnostic criteria; (b) the manner in which information is obtained; and (c) interviewing techniques and interviewers. To accomplish this, special forms and questionnaires must be prepared and all investigators must meet regularly to assure a uniform approach.

This is a problem that neurologists now involved in international collaborative studies are beginning to appreciate. A large number of issues must be carefully discussed. Investigators must decide what behavioral patterns are to be considered normal or abnormal in a specific population cohort and in a specific geographic region. Problems are magnified when collaborative studies involve populations living in different continents (even if these populations speak the same language). Difficulties were even encountered in a multicenter study on an Italian population from different regions of Italy (Table 3). However, in this Italian collaborative study these problems were compensated for by the larger number of cases included. The larger sample size yielded a higher statistical power, enabling us to compare the results with those reported previously.

Table 3. Multicenter Study on the Alzheimer's disease-senile dementia complex in the Italian population (SMICD)

Collaborative centers	Bari
	Florence
	Genoa
	L'Aquila
	Milan
	Padua
	Rome

Table 4. Major risk factors for Alzheimer's disease

Risk factors	Control group H = hospital; P = population	Odds ratio
Head trauma	H	3.50
	P	2.00
Mother's age at index delivery (>40)	H	2.50
	P	4.67 [b]
Any first- or second-degree relative with dementia	H	6.67 [a]
	P	3.44 [a]

[a] $P<0.001$; [b] $P<0.005$

Table 5. Presence of dementia in the family as a risk factor for clinically diagnosed Alzheimer's disease senile dementia

Dementia in	Control group H = hospital; P = population	Odds ratio
Any second-degree relative	H	11.00 [a]
	P	4.00 [b]
Any first-degree relative	H	5.00 [b]
	P	2.56 [c]
Siblings	H	11.00 [b]
	P	5.50 [c]
Mother	H	2.20
	P	3.33
Father	H	3.50
	P	1.00

[a] $P<0.001$; [b] $P<0.01$; [c] $P<0.05$

The most important findings of the Italian study recently reported in various international meetings [18, 19], are as follows (Table 4):

1. An increased relative risk for those with a history of head trauma (although this was not statistically significant).
2. A higher relative risk for people born to a mother aged 40 years or older.
3. An increased relative risk for people having a first or second-degree relative with dementia. This risk was greatest for siblings (Table 5).

Hence, from the data presented it appears that among the environmental factors, head trauma may be a possible risk factor [12, 13, 15, 18, 19]. In this regard, one must also consider the suggestions derived from cases of dementia pugilistica [20–22].

The most consistent results of these analytic studies indicate a familial association. This association can be interpreted again in terms of a microenvironmental influence, considering that in our cases, siblings rather than parents have the highest risk. However, this might be interpreted as possible recall bias. Nevertheless, the description of two large families affected by histologically proven Alzheimer's disease strongly suggests the possibility that a genetic factor may be important in the pathogenesis of the disease [23–24].

The association with Down's syndrome in one study [15] and the finding of a late maternal age in patients again point out some analogies between the two diseases [25–27]. The possibility that a gene defect either transmitted or modified during early life may be responsible at a later time for Alzheimer's disease appears consistent with the reported findings.

References

1. Lilienfeld AM, Lilienfeld DE (1980) Foundations of epidemiology. Oxford University Press, New York
2. Schoenberg BS (1977) Neuroepidemiology: incidents, incidence, and coincidence. Arch Neurol 34:261–265
3. Pickll LW, Brown LM, Blot WJ (1983) Information available from surrogate respondents in case-control interview studies. Am J Epidemiol 118:99–108
4. Hunter R, Dayan AD, Wilson J (1972) Alzheimer's disease in one monozygotic twin. J Neurol Neurosurg Psychiatry 35:707–710
5. Masters CL, Gajdusek DC, Gibbs CJ, Bernoulli C, Asher DM (1979) Familial Creutzfeldt-Jakob disease and other familial dementias: an inquiry into possible modes of transmission of virus-induced familial diseases. In: Prusiner SJ, Hadlow WJ (eds) Slow Transmissible Disease of nervous system. Academic press, New York
6. Nandy K (1981) Senile dementia: a possible immune hypothesis. In: Mortimer JA, Schuman LM (eds) Epidemiology of dementia. Oxford University Press, New York, pp 87–100
7. Perl DP, Brody AR (1980) Alzheimer's disease: X-ray spectrometric evidence of aluminium accumulation in neurofibrillary tangle-bearing neurons. Science 208:297–299
8. Esquirol JED (1838) Des maladies mentales considerées sous les rapports médicals, hygieéniques et medico-legales, vol. 2. Meline Lans, Bruxelles
9. Heston LL, Mastri AK, Anderson VE, White J (1981) Dementia of the Alzheimer type. Arch Gen Psychiatry 38:1085–1090
10. Whalley LJ, Carothers AD, Collyer S et al. (1982) A study of familial factors in Alzheimer's disease. Br J Psychiatry 140:249–256
11. Bharucha NE, Schoenberg BS, Kokmen E (1983) Dementia of Alzheimer's type: a case-control study of association with medical conditions and surgical procedures. Neurology 33 [Suppl 2] 85
12. Mortimer JA, French LR, Hutton JT, Schuman LM, Christians B, Boatman RA (1983) Reported head trauma in an epidemiologic study of Alzheimer's disease. Neurology 33 [Suppl 2] 85
13. French LR, Schuman LM, Mortimer JA, Hutton JT, Boatman RA, Christians B (1985) A case-control study of dementia of the Alzheimer type. Am J Epidemiol 121:414–421
14. Wilkinson WE, Heyman A, Sigmon A, Weinberg T (1982) Case-control study of possible environmental, infectious and genetic factors in Alzheimer's disease. Neurology 32 [part 2] A 228
15. Heyman A, Wilkinson WE, Stafford JA, Helms MJ, Sigmon AM, Weinberg T (1984) Alzheimer's disease: a study of the epidemiological aspects. Ann Neurol 15:335–341
16. Pasternack BS, Shore RE (1981) Sample sizes for group sequential cohort and case-control study designs. Am J Epidemiol 113:182–191
17. Schlesselman JJ (1974) Sample size requirements in cohort and case-control studies of disease. Am J Epidemiol 99:381–384
18. Amaducci LA, Fratiglioni L, Rocca WA et al. (1985) Risk factors for Alzheimer's disease (AD): a case-control study on an Italian population. Neurology 35 [Suppl 1] 277
19. Amaducci LA, Fratiglioni L, Rocca WA et al. (1985) Risk factors for clinically diagnosed Alzheimer's disease, a case-control study of an Italian population. Neurology (in press)

20. Corsellis JAN (1978) Posttraumatic dementia. In: Katzman R, Terry RD, Bick KL (eds) Alzheimer's disease: senile dementia and related disorders. Raven press, New York, pp 125–133
21. Corsellis JAN, Brierly JB (1959) Observation on the pathology of insidious dementia following head injury. J Ment Sci 105:714–720
22. Rudelli R, Strom JO, Welch PT et al. (1982) Posttraumatic premature Alzheimer's disease: neuropathologic findings and pathogenic considerations. Arch Neurol 39:570–575
23. Foncin JF, Salmon D, Supino-Viterbo V, Feldman RG, Macchi G, Mariotti P, Scoppetta C, Caruso G, Brumi AC (1985) Démence présénile d'Alzheimer transmise dans une famille étendue. Rev Neurol (Paris) 141 (3): 194–202
24. Nee LE, Polinsky RJ, Eldridge R, Weinartner H, Smallberg S, Ebert M (1983) A family with histologically confirmed Alzheimer's disease. Arch Neurol 40:203–208
25. Cohen D, Eisdorfer C, Leverenz J (1982) Alzheimer's disease and maternal age. J Am Geriatr Soc 30:656–659
26. Heyman A, Wilkinson WE, Hurwitz BJ et al. (1983) Alzheimer's disease: genetic aspects and associated clinical disorders. Ann Neurol 14:507–515
27. Ellis WG, McCulloch JR, Carley CL (1974) Presenile dementia in Down's syndrome. Neurology 24:101–106

Classical and Modern Neuropathological Approaches to Alzheimer's Disease

D. L. PRICE, R. G. STRUBLE, L. C. CORK, P. J. WHITEHOUSE, C. A. KITT, and J. C. TRONCOSO[1]

Introduction

Alzheimer's disease (AD), the most common type of adult-onset dementia [65], has been analyzed at several levels (Table 1; Fig. 1): regional distributions of disease; neuronal populations/systems at risk; abnormalities occurring in individual nerve cells; and molecular pathology of cellular constituents. These investigations have demonstrated that AD selectively involves specific parts of brain, certain transmitter systems, and components of the neuronal cytoskeleton. Dysfunction/death of at-risk populations of neurons in brainstem, basal forebrain, amygdala, hippocampus, and neocortex leads to impairments in memory, language, visual-spatial perceptions, etc. Human studies are complemented by investigations in animals that are essential for analyzing mechanisms, evolutions, and consequences of disorders in certain neuronal populations, for studying the cellular and molecular dynamics of disease processes, and for relating these processes to the clinical expressions of illness. This review discusses some new information derived from neuropathological and neurobiological studies of AD and of animal models sharing features with the human disease (Table 1; Fig. 1).

Regional and Systems Pathology

AD predominantly affects certain regions of the brain, including populations of nerve cells in the basal forebrain, brainstem, amygdala, hippocampus, and neocortex (Fig. 1).

Basal Forebrain Cholinergic System

Located within the medial septum, diagonal band of Broca (dbB), and nucleus basalis [27, 38], these nerve cells are the major source of cholinergic innervation to

[1] Neuropathology Laboratory, The Johns Hopkins University School of Medicine, Baltimore, MD 21205, USA.

Neurology
Ed. by K. Poeck, H. J. Freund, and H. Gänshirt

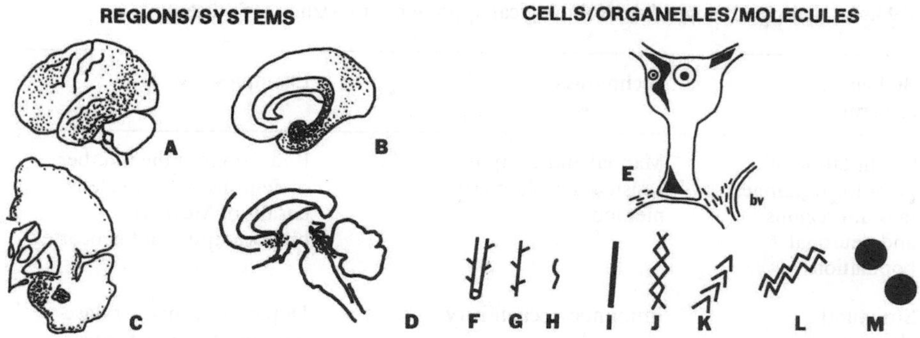

Fig. 1. This series of schematic drawings depicts the character and distributions of neuropathologic changes occurring in AD.
A and *B* are representations of lateral and medial aspects of hemispheres respectively; *stippling* indicates regions showing distributions of NFT, senile plaques, and loss of neurons (modified from Brun [11]
C and *D* are respectively a coronal section through the hemisphere and a midsagittal section through the lower forebrain, diencephalon, and brainstem. NFT and cell loss occur in the basal forebrain cholinergic system, amygdala, hippocampus, and neocortex (*C*). NFT and loss of nerve cells also occur in the basal forebrain cholinergic system, raphe complex, and locus coeruleus (*D*).
In *E*, a neuron synapses upon a target nerve cell; note blood vessel (*bv*). The neuron contains a normal nucleus, four types of inclusions (NFT *severe S-shape;* GVD *circular vacuoles with dark granule;* and Hirano body *dark rhomboid at base of dendrite),* and an accumulation of filaments in distal axon terminals (neurites) in plaque. The *short, dark lines* in the extracellular space around the enlarged neurite and the blood vessel indicate amyloid fibrils in the plaque and are associated with vessels (congophilic angiopathy).
F, G, and *H* depict normal microtubules, neurofilaments, and microfilaments, respectively.
I, J, and *K* illustrate 15-nm straight filaments, paired helical filaments, and paracrystalline arrays of actin, respectively.
L represents β-pleated amyloid fibrils, while *M* shows tubulin-immunoreactive granules

amygdala, hippocampus, and neocortex [61]. In AD, these neurons develop neurofibrillary tangles (NFT) [55, 71], and, by extrapolation from studies of aged macaques, their axons/terminals form neurites in senile plaques [34, 58, 59]. When these neurons degenerate [4, 55, 71], cholinergic markers, including presynaptic M2 muscarinic receptors, are reduced in amygdala, hippocampus, and neocortex [10, 37, 57]. Cholinergic denervation of these targets contributes to some of the behavioral, memory, and cognitive abnormalities occurring in AD [6, 17].

Brainstem Systems

NFT and neuronal loss may occur in the raphe complex [77]; reductions occur in levels of cortical 5-hydroxytryptamine (5-HT), uptake of 5-HT, and 5-HT metabolites [10]. Neurons in the locus coeruleus may also develop NFT and form neurites in plaques [80]; cell degeneration causes decreased noradrenergic cortical markers [9, 18, 66, 74, 78].

Impairments in arousal, mood, behavior, and memory may, in part, be related to lesions of these monoamine systems.

Table 1. Neuropathological-neurobiological approaches to Alzheimer's disease

Biological elements	Techniques	Examples
Quantitation of pathologic changes in brain regions and neuronal populations	Manual and computer-assisted morphometric methods	Reductions in the number of neurons in the nucleus basalis of Meynert, hippocampus, and neocortex
Structural changes in specific neurons	Immunocytochemistry	Dopamine β-hydroxylase-immunostained neurites in plaques; NFT in cholinergic and somatostatinergic neurons
Neuron shape and size	Golgi stains; computer-assisted morphometry	Abnormal dendritic arborizations; decreased size of neurons of the nucleus basalis
Transmitters and enzymes	Enzyme assays; radioimmunoassays	Reductions in cortical ChAT, somatostatin, and corticotropin-releasing factor
Receptors	Binding assays; in vitro autoradiography	Decreased M2 and somatostatin receptors; increase in corticotropin-releasing factor receptors
Components of abnormal organelles	Immunocytochemistry; electron microscopy; freeze-fracture/deep-etch	Decoration of PHF with anti-neurofilament antibody; actin microfilament lattices in Hirano bodies; tubulin in GVD
Abnormal constituents	Purification of constituents; analyses of proteins and other components; immunocytochemistry	Identification of amyloid protein in congophilic angiopathy; relative insolubility of PHF; sequencing of PHF proteins
Proteins and their modifications	Gels/Western blots; immunocytochemistry; in vitro incorporation of amino acids; protein purification/sequencing	Reduced protein synthesis; 200-kilodalton neurofilament protein phosphorylated in NFT-containing perikarya
Genes/RNAs	Southern and Northern blots; in situ hybridization; measurements of markers of RNA metabolism	Reduced cortical RNA; increased alkaline ribonuclease activity

Amygdala

NFT, senile plaques, and degeneration of neurons (somatostatinergic and perhaps other nerve cells) occur in the amygdala [31, 32]. Some of the emotional, motivational, and associative abnormalities occurring in patients with AD may be due to disease in the amygdala.

Hippocampus and Entorhinal Cortex

Hippocampal pyramidal neurons show NFT, dendritic pathology, granulovacuolar degeneration (GVD), Hirano bodies, and neuronal degeneration [5, 12, 23, 25, 28, 51, 64]. In the subiculum and entorhinal cortex, death of NFT-containing neurons of layers II and IV disconnects the hippocampal formation from association cortex [30]. In these regions, a variety of transmitter systems contribute neurites to plaques [62, 80]. Memory deficits occurring in AD have been attributed, in part, to a combination of deafferentation of hippocampus, intrinsic hippocampal pathology, and lesions in associated circuits, especially in entorhinal cortex.

Neocortex

NFT occur in cortex [72], particularly in temporal lobe and, to a lesser degree, in parietal and frontal association cortices [11]. Somatostatinergic cortical neurons develop NFT [53], form plaques [39, 60], and levels of somatostatin are reduced in neocortex [19, 54]. Levels of corticotropin-releasing factor, a peptide transmitter present in nerve cells intrinsic to cortex, are decreased, and corticotropin-releasing factor receptors are reciprocally increased [79]. A variety of other peptidergic systems appear to be relatively spared, but currently available neurochemical assays may not have detected some of the at-risk transmitter systems, including those using excitatory amino acids. Altered dendrites (arbors, receptor surfaces, etc.) failure to make/deliver/maintain receptors, and actual loss of neurons or their processes [12, 14, 40, 56] are pathologic conditions which may, in part, contribute to reductions in glutamate, somatostatin, serotonin S2, and nicotinic cholinergic binding sites in these regions [7, 26, 44, 70].

In AD, neocortical plaques are common [65], and studies in both aged macaques and humans with AD suggest that neurites in plaques may be derived from cholinergic, noradrenergic, serotonergic, γ-aminobutyric acid (GABA)ergic, and a variety of peptidergic systems [34, 35, 39, 60, 62, 63, 69, 80]. It is not yet known whether neurites in an individual plaque are homogeneous (i.e., only one transmitter marker in each plaque) or whether plaques show transmitter heterogeneity (i.e., more than one transmitter marker present in a single plaque) [50].

Cellular and Molecular Pathology

At-risk neurons in brainstem, basal forebrain, amygdala, hippocampus, and neocortex develop several types of structural pathology: NFT; enlarged neurites in senile plaques (associated with deposits of amyloid); GVD; and Hirano bodies. In addition, extracellular amyloid fibrils accumulate in the parenchyma (cores of plaques) and in proximity to blood vessels (congophilic angiopathy).

Neurofibrillary Tangles

NFT, which stain with antibodies directed against neurofilaments (including phosphorylated epitopes) as well as against microtubule-associated proteins (MAP2) and other novel antigens [3, 16, 21, 41], are intracytoplasmic fibrillary inclusions occurring in the perikarya/proximal dendrites of neurons. NFT are composed of accumulations of paired helical 10-nm filaments (PHF) [33], which are made up of insoluble protein polymers and are frequently associated with 10-nm neurofilaments and 15-nm straight filaments. These different types of filaments may be a "family" with differences resulting from compositional heterogeneity, modifications of component proteins, and/or stages in the evolution of filamentous pathology. Alternatively, elements of PHF could be derived either from noncytoskeletal host proteins (which are not normally assembled into filaments, but do form PHF in AD brain) or may be nonneuronal components (which gain access to neurons and assemble into filamentous forms). These issues will be clarified when sequences of normal and abnormal proteins can be compared [22, 24]. The formation of NFT is a stage in degeneration of neurons; when these cells die, their locations are marked by the presence of NFT-shaped accumulations of extracellular PHF [52, 55]. The presence of cortical NFT correlates with the presence of dementia [72] and with reductions in choline acetyltransferase (ChAT) activity in cortex [73].

Senile Plaques

These foci of enlarged axons/synaptic terminals/dendritic processes (neurites), associated with extracellular amyloid [51, 75], are most conspicuous within amygdala, hippocampus, and neocortex. Visualized using silver stains and antibodies directed against filament proteins, plaques represent sites of degenerating (possibly regenerating) axons/terminals derived from a variety of transmitter systems [34, 35, 39, 60, 62, 69]. The presence of plaques in AD correlates with reductions in cholinergic and somatostatinergic markers [45, 46]. These neurites are located in proximity to extracellular 7- to 10-nm amyloid fibrils composed of predominantly β-pleated sheet proteins. Sources of plaque amyloid are not yet clarified, but amyloid precursors could be derived from abnormal neuronal constituents, serum precursors, or other sources [24, 47, 49], which may be complexed with elements (including aluminum and silicon) [43]. Since plaques presumably represent sites of abnormal synaptic interactions, it is not surprising that, in both aged monkeys and humans with AD, the presence of neocortical plaques correlates with impaired performance on cognitive/memory tasks [36, 65].

Hirano Bodies

In AD, these rod-shaped cytoplasmic inclusions are common in the pyramidal cell layer of the hippocampus [23]. Transmission microscopy, immunocytochemistry, and freeze-fracture/deep-etch techniques have shown that Hirano bodies are made up of paracrystalline arrays of actin [25, 29] (J. Heuser and D. L. Price 1985, unpublished work).

Granulovacuolar Degeneration

GVD is frequently present in the cytoplasm of hippocampal pyramidal neurons in AD [5, 64]. Each granule lies within a vacuole, and granules contain tubulin-like immunoreactivity [81]. Newly available cDNA probes [13], which label tubulin mRNAs, should allow in situ hybridization analysis of specific tubulin mRNAs in GVD-containing and control neurons. Similar strategies can be used to examine mRNAs of other constituents of neurons [36] (P. N. Hoffman and D. L. Price 1985, unpublished work). The presence of GVD in these pyramidal neurons correlates with reductions in cell number [5], suggesting that the formation of GVD leads to cell death.

Animal Models

Animal models, which show AD-like abnormalities, are useful for combined behavioral, morphological, and chemical studies of mechanisms, evolutions, and consequences of molecular/cellular pathologic conditions involving specific systems. To illustrate investigations of pathology at the level of regions/systems and cells/organelles/molecules, we focus on three disorders: aluminium poliomyelopathy, a disorder useful for investigations of the pathogenesis of neurofibrillary perikaryal/axonal pathology; cholinergic deficiency in primate telencephalon, an experimental model in which behavioral changes can be correlated with transmitter deficits; and aged nonhuman primates in which age-associated behavioral abnormalities appear to be related to the presence of senile plaques.

Aluminum Poliomyelopathy

In AD, aluminum levels are increased in neurons containing NFT [42]. In experimental animals, intrathecal injections of aluminum chloride produce neurofibrillary pathology characterized by accumulations of neurofilaments (not PHF) in proximal axons, perikarya, and dendrites [68, 76]. It is possible that this neurofibrillary pathology could arise by increased synthesis of neurofilaments, a hypothesis that can be examined by visualizing in situ with cDNA probes levels of mRNA coding for the 68-kilodalton neurofilament protein [36]. However, it seems more likely that other mechanisms may be important in the pathogenesis of this type of neurofibrillary pathology. Recent studies have documented aberrant phosphorylation of the 200-kilodalton neurofilament protein in perikarya [67] associated with impaired axonal transport of neurofilament proteins [8, 67]. Similar posttranslational modifications may occur in the early stages of AD [16], leading to perikaryal accumulations of abnormal cytoskeletal proteins which may represent a nidus for the development of NFT.

Cholinergic Deficiency in Primate Telencephalon

To reproduce the forebrain cholinergic deficiency of AD, ibotenic acid has been microinjected into the substantia innominata of macaques, a procedure which destroys neurons in the basal forebrain cholinergic system [61]. Bilateral partial lesions of the nucleus basalis do not produce memory deficits, but task performance becomes sensitive to scopolamine [1]. Lesions involving medial septum, diagonal band, and nucleus basalis cause memory deficits [2], suggesting that cholinergic denervation of forebrain targets, particularly amygdala and hippocampus, is associated with impaired memory.

Aged Nonhuman Primates

To relate clinical findings to types of cortical pathology occurring in AD, we have begun to study aged macaques, which do not develop AD, but do exhibit a variety of cognitive/memory deficits [20] and develop senile plaques in cortex [48, 58, 60, 63]. Cross-sectional studies suggest that plaques evolve from neurite-rich to amyloid types, and immunocytochemical investigations indicate that neurites in plaques are derived from axons/terminals of cholinergic and a variety of other transmitter systems [34, 35, 50, 60, 69]. In individual animals, plaque densities tend to be better than chronological age as predictors of impaired cognitive function [63].

Conclusion

Classical and modern neuropathological approaches to AD have clarified aspects of the pathology occurring at several levels, including regions/systems and cells/organelles/molecules (Table 1; Fig. 1). With these approaches, investigators have begun to examine relationships of genes/RNAs, proteins and their modifications, organelles, transmitter markers (including enzymes and receptors), and evidence of involvement of specific neuronal populations. Moreover, some of these abnormalities can be reproduced in experimental models that are necessary for neurobiological studies of mechanisms, evolutions, and consequences of disease processes resembling those occurring in AD.

Acknowledgments. The authors gratefully acknowledge helpful discussions with Drs. John C. Hedreen, Paul N. Hoffman, John W. Griffin, Lary C. Walker, Douglas B. Murphy, Ludwig A. Sternberger, Nancy H. Sternberger, Thomas G. Aigner, Mortimer Mishkin, as well as Mr. Richard Altschuler and Ms. Sharon Presty. Mrs. Colleen Marine and Ms. Carla Jordon provided excellent secretarial assistance in the preparation of the manuscript.

This work was supported by funds from the U.S. Public Health Service (NIH AG 03359, NS 20471, AG 05146), The Commonwealth Fund, The McKnight Foundation, the Alfred P. Sloan Foundation, the American Health Assistance Foundation, and the Claster Family. Dr. Troncoso is the recipient of a Teacher-Investigator Development Award (NIH NS 00799).

References

1. Aigner T, Aggleton J, Mitchell SJ, Price D, DeLong M, Mishkin M (1983) Effects of scopolamine on recognition memory in monkeys after ibotenic acid injections into the nucleus basalis of Meynert. Soc Neurosci Abstr 9:826
2. Aigner T, Mitchell S, Aggleton J, DeLong M, Struble R, Wenk G, Price D, Mishkin M (1984) Recognition deficit in monkeys following neurotoxic lesions of the basal forebrain. Soc Neurosci Abstr 10:386

3. Anderton BH, Breinburg D, Downes MJ, Green PJ, Tomlinson BE, Ulrich J, Wood JN, Kahn J (1982) Monoclonal antibodies show that neurofibrillary tangles and neurofilaments share antigenic determinants. Nature 298:84–86
4. Arendt T, Bigl V, Arendt A, Tennstedt A (1983) Loss of neurons in the nucleus basalis of Meynert in Alzheimer's disease, paralysis agitans, and Korsakoff's disease. Acta Neuropathol (Berl) 61:101–108
5. Ball MJ (1977) Neuronal loss, neurofibrillary tangles and granulovacuolar degeneration in the hippocampus with ageing and dementia. A qualitative study. Acta Neuropathol (Berl) 37:111–118
6. Bartus RT, Dean RL III, Beer B, Lippa AS (1982) The cholinergic hypothesis of geriatric memory dysfunction. Science 217:408–417
7. Beal MF, Mazurek MF, Tran VT, Chattha G, Bird ED, Martin JB (1985) Reduced numbers of somatostatin receptors in the cerebral cortex in Alzheimer's disease. Science 229:289–291
8. Bizzi A, Crane RC, Autilio-Gambetti L, Gambetti P (1984) Aluminum effect on slow axonal transport: a novel impairment of neurofilament transport. J Neurosci 4:722–731
9. Bondareff W, Mountjoy CQ, Roth M (1982) Loss of neurons or origin of the adrenergic projection to cerebral cortex (nucleus locus ceruleus) in senile dementia. Neurology 32:164–168
10. Bowen DM (1983) Biochemical assessment of neurotransmitter and metabolic dysfunction and cerebral atrophy in Alzheimer's disease. Biological aspects of Alzheimer's Disease. Banbury Rep 15:219–231
11. Brun A (1983) An overview of light and electron microscopic changes. In: Reisberg B (ed) Alzheimer's disease. The Free Press, New York, pp 37–47
12. Buell SJ, Coleman PD (1981) Quantitative evidence for selective dendritic growth in normal human aging but not in senile dementia. Brain Res 214:23–41
13. Cleveland DW, Sullivan KF (1985) Molecular biology and genetics of tubulin. Annu Rev Biochem 54:331–365
14. Colon EJ (1973) The cerebral cortex in presenil dementia. A quantitative analysis. Acta Neuropathol (Berl) 23:281–290
15. Cork LC, Altschuler RJ, Struble RG, Casanova MF, Price DL, Sternberger N, Sternberger L (1985) Changes in the distribution of phosphorylated neurofilaments in Alzheimer's disease. J Neuropathol Exp Neurol 44:368
16. Cork LC, Sternberger NH, Sternberger LA, Casanova MF, Struble RG, Price DL (1986) Phosphorylated neurofilament antigens in neurofibrillary tangles in Alzheimer's disease. J Neuropathol Exp Neurol
17. Coyle JT, Price DL, DeLong MR (1983) Alzheimer's disease: a disorder of cortical cholinergic innervation. Science 219:1184–1190
18. Cross AJ, Crow TJ, Perry EK, Perry RH, Blessed G, Tomlinson BE (1981) Reduced dopamine-β-hydroxylase activity in Alzheimer's disease. Br Med J 282:93–94
19. Davies P, Katzman R, Terry RD (1980) Reduced somatostatin-like immunoreactivity in cerebral cortex from cases of Alzheimer disease and Alzheimer senile dementia. Nature 288:279–280
20. Davis RT (1978) Old monkey behavior. Exp Gerontol 13:237–250
21. Gambetti P, Shecket G, Ghetti B, Hirano A, Dahl D (1983) Neurofibrillary changes in human brain. An immunocytochemical study with a neurofilament antiserum. J Neuropathol Exp Neurol 42:69–79
22. Geisler N, Kaufmann E, Fischer S, Plessmann U, Weber K (1983) Neurofilament architecture combines structural principles of intermediate filaments with carboxy-terminal extensions increasing in size between triplet proteins. EMBO J 2:1295–1302
23. Gibson PH, Tomlinson BE (1977) Numbers of Hirano bodies in the hippocampus of normal and demented people with Alzheimer's disease. J Neurol Sci 33:199–206
24. Glenner GG, Wong CW (1984) Alzheimer's disease: initial report of the purification and characterization of a novel cerebrovascular amyloid protein. Biochem Biophys Res Commun 120:885–890
25. Goldman JE (1983) The association of actin with Hirano bodies. J Neuropathol Exp Neurol 42:146–152

26. Greenamyre JT, Penney JB, Young AB, D'Amato CJ, Hicks SP, Shoulson I (1985) Alterations in L-glutamate binding in Alzheimer's and Huntington's diseases. Science 227:1496–1499
27. Hedreen JC, Struble RG, Whitehouse PJ, Price DL (1984) Topography of the magnocellular basal forebrain system in human brain. J Neuropathol Exp Neurol 43:1–21
28. Hirano A, Zimmerman HM (1962) Alzheimer's neurofibrillary changes. A topographic study. Arch Neurol 7:227–242
29. Hirano A, Dembitzer HM, Kurland LT, Zimmerman HM (1968) The fine structure of some intraganglionic alterations. Neurofibrillary tangles, granulovacuolar bodies and "rod-like" structures as seen in amyotrophic lateral sclerosis and parkinsonism-dementia complex. J Neuropathol Exp Neurol 27:167–182
30. Hyman BT, Van Hoesen GW, Damasio AR, Barnes CL (1984) Alzheimer's disease: cell-specific pathology isolates the hippocampal formation. Science 225:1168–1170
31. Jamada M, Mehraein P (1968) Verteilungsmuster der senilen Veränderungen im Gehirn. Die Beteiligung des limbischen Systems bei hirnatrophischen Prozessen des Seniums und bei Morbus Alzheimer. Arch Psychiatr Z Neurol 211:308–324
32. Kemper TL (1983) Organization of the neuropathology of the amygdala in Alzheimer's disease. Biological aspects of Alzheimer's Disease. Banbury Rep 15:31–35
33. Kidd M (1963) Paired helical filaments in electron microscopy of Alzheimer's disease. Nature 197:192–193
34. Kitt CA, Price DL, Struble RG, Cork LC, Wainer BH, Becher MW, Mobley WC (1984) Evidence for cholinergic neurites in senile plaques. Science 226:1443–1445
35. Kitt CA, Struble RG, Cork LC, Mobley WC, Walker LC, Joh TH, Price DL (in press) Catecholaminergic neurites in senile plaques in prefrontal cortex of aged nonhuman primates. Neuroscience 16:691–699
36. Lewis SA, Cowan NJ (in press) Temporal expression of mouse GFAP mRNA studied by a rapid in situ hybridization procedure. J Neurochem
37. Mash DC, Flynn DD, Potter LT (1985) Loss of M2 muscarine receptors in the cerebral cortex in Alzheimer's disease and experimental cholinergic denervation. Science 228:1115–1117
38. Mesulam MM, Mufson EJ, Levey AI, Wainer BH (1983) Cholinergic innervation of cortex by the basal forebrain: cytochemistry and cortical connections of the septal area, diagonal band nuclei, nucleus basalis (substantia innominata), and hypothalamus in the rhesus monkey. J Comp Neurol 214:170–197
39. Morrison JH, Rogers J, Scherr S, Benoit R, Bloom FE (1985) Somatostatin immunoreactivity in neuritic plaques of Alzheimer's patients. Nature 314:90–94
40. Mountjoy CQ, Roth M, Evans NJR, Evans HM (1983) Cortical neuronal counts in normal elderly controls and demented patients. Neurobiol Aging 4:1–11
41. Nukina N, Ihara Y (1983) Immunocytochemical study on senile plaques in Alzheimer's disease. II. Abnormal dendrites in senile plaques as revealed by antimicrotubule-associated proteins (MAPs) immunostaining. Proc Jpn Acad 59:288–292
42. Perl DP, Brody AR (1980) Alzheimer's disease: X-ray spectrometric evidence of aluminum accumulation in neurofibrillary tangle-bearing neurons. Science 208:297–299
43. Perry EK, Perry RH (1985) New insights into the nature of senile (Alzheimer-type) plaques. Trends Neurosci 8:301–303
44. Perry EK, Perry RH, Candy JM, Fairbairn AF, Blessed G, Dick DJ, Tomlinson BE (1984) Cortical serotonin-S_2 receptor binding abnormalities in patients with Alzheimer's disease: comparisons with Parkinson's disease. Neurosci Lett 51:353–357
45. Perry EK, Tomlinson BE, Blessed G, Bergmann K, Gibson PH, Perry RH (1978) Correlation of cholinergic abnormalities with senile plaques and mental test scores in senile dementia. Br Med J 2:1457–1459
46. Perry RH, Candy JM, Perry EK (1983) Some observations and speculations concerning the cholinergic system and neuropeptides in Alzheimer's disease. Biological aspects of Alzheimer's Disease. Banbury Rep 15:351–361
47. Powers JM, Schlaepfer WW, Willingham MC, Hall BJ (1981) An immunoperoxidase study of senile cerebral amyloidosis with pathogenetic considerations. J Neuropathol Exp Neurol 40:592–612

48. Price DL, Cork LC, Stuble RG, Kitt CA, Price DL Jr, Lehmann J, Hedreen JC (1985) Neuropathological, neurochemical, and behavioral studies of the aging nonhuman primate. In: Davis RT, Leathers CW (eds) Behavior and pathology of aging in Rhesus monkeys. Alan R. Liss, New York
49. Price DL, Whitehouse PJ, Struble RG, Coyle JT, Clark AW, DeLong MR, Cork LC, Hedreen JC (1982) Alzheimer's disease and Down's syndrome. Ann NY Acad Sci 396:145–164
50. Price DL, Whitehouse PJ, Struble RG, Price DL Jr, Cork LC, Hedreen JC, Kitt CA (1983) Basal forebrain cholinergic neurons and neuritic plaques in primate brain. Biological Aspects of Alzheimer's Disease. Banbury Rep 15:65–77
51. Probst A, Basler V, Bron B, Ulrich J (1983) Neuritic plaques in senile dementia of Alzheimer type: a Golgi analysis in the hippocampal region. Brain Res 268:249–254
52. Probst A, Ulrich J, Heitz PU (1982) Senile dementia of Alzheimer type: astroglial reaction to extracellular neurofibrillary tangles in the hippocampus. Acta Neuropathol (Berl) 57:75–79
53. Roberts GW, Crow TJ, Polak JM (1985) Location of neuronal tangles in somatostatin neurones in Alzheimer's disease. Nature 314:92–94
54. Rossor MN, Emson PC, Mountjoy CQ, Roth M, Iversen LL (1980) Reduced amounts of immunoreactive somatostatin in the temporal cortex in senile dementia of Alzheimer type. Neurosci Lett 20:373–377
55. Saper CB, German DC, White CL III (1985) Neuronal pathology in the nucleus basalis and associated cell groups in senile dementia of the Alzheimer's type: possible role in cell loss. Neurology 35:1089–1095
56. Scheibel AB (1979) Dendritic changes in senile and presenile dementias. In: Katzman R (ed) Congenital and acquired cognitive disorders. Raven, New York, pp 107–124
57. Sims NR, Bowen DM, Allen SJ, Smith CCT, Neary D, Thomas DJ, Davison AN (1983) Presynaptic cholinergic dysfunction in patients with dementia. J Neurochem 40:503–509
58. Struble RG, Cork LC, Whitehouse PJ, Price DL (1982) Cholinergic innervation in neuritic plaques. Science 216:413–415
59. Struble RG, Hedreen JC, Cork LC, Price DL (1984) Acetylcholinesterase activity in senile plaques of aged macaques. Neurobiol Aging 5:191–198
60. Struble RG, Kitt CA, Walker LC, Cork LC, Price DL (1984) Somatostatinergic neurites in senile plaques of aged non-human primates. Brain Res 324:394–396
61. Struble RG, Lehmann J, Mitchell SJ, Cork LC, Coyle JT, Price DL, DeLong MR, Antuono PG (in press) Cortical cholinergic innervation: distribution and source in monkeys. In: Hanin I (ed) Dynamics of cholinergic function. Plenum, New York
62. Struble RG, Powers RE, Casanova MF, Kitt CA, O'Connor DT, Price DL (1985) Multiple transmitter-specific markers in senile plaques in Alzheimer's disease. J Neuropathol Exp Neurol 44:325
63. Struble RG, Price DL Jr, Cork LC, Price DL (1985) Senile plaques in cortex of aged normal monkeys. Brain Res 361:267–275
64. Tomlinson BE, Kitchener D (1972) Granulovacuolar degeneration of hippocampal pyramidal cells. J Pathol 106:165–185
65. Tomlinson BE, Blessed G, Roth M (1970) Observations on the brains of demented old people. J Neurol Sci 11:205–242
66. Tomlinson BE, Irving D, Blessed G (1981) Cell loss in the locus coeruleus in senile dementia of Alzheimer type. J Neurol Sci 49:419–428
67. Troncoso JC, Hoffman PN, Griffin JW, Hess-Kozlow KM, Price DL (1985) Aluminum intoxication: a disorder of neurofilament transport in motor neurons. Brain Res 342:172–175
68. Troncoso JC, Price DL, Griffin JW, Parhad IM (1982) Neurofibrillary axonal pathology in aluminum intoxication. Ann Neurol 12:278–283
69. Walker LC, Kitt CA, Struble RG, Schmechel DE, Oertel WH, Cork LC, Price DL (1985) Glutamic acid decarboxylase-like immunoreactivity in senile plaques. Neurosci Lett 59:165–169
70. Whitehouse PJ, Martino AM, Antuono PG, Coyle JT, Price DL, Kellar KJ (1985) Reductions in nicotinic receptors measured using [^{3}H] acetylcholine in Alzheimer's disease. Soc Neurosci Abstr 11:134

71. Whitehouse PJ, Price DL, Struble RG, Clark AW, Coyle JT, DeLong MR (1982) Alzheimer's disease and senile dementia: loss of neurons in the basal forebrain. Science 215:1237–1239
72. Wilcock GK, Esiri MM (1982) Plaques, tangles and dementia. A quantitative study. J Neurol Sci 56:343–356
73. Wilcock GK, Esiri MM, Bowen DM, Smith CCT (1982) Alzheimer's disease. Correlation of cortical choline acetyltransferase activity with the severity of dementia and histological abnormalities. J Neurol Sci 57:407–417
74. Winblad B, Adolfsson R, Carlsson A, Gottfries C-G (1982) Biogenic amines in brains of patients with Alzheimer's disease. In: Corkin S, Davis KL, Growdon JH, Usdin E, Wurtman RJ (eds) Alzheimer's disease: a report of progress in research. Raven, New York, pp 25–33 (Aging, vol 19)
75. Wisniewski HM, Terry RD (1973) Reexamination of the pathogenesis of the senile plaque. In: Zimmerman HM (ed) Progress in neuropathology, vol 2. Grune and Stratton, New York, pp 1–26
76. Wisniewski HM, Sturman JA, Shek JW (1980) Aluminum chloride induced neurofibrillary changes in the developing rabbit: a chronic animal model. Ann Neurol 8:479–490
77. Yamamoto T, Hirano A (1985) Nucleus raphe dorsalis in Alzheimer's disease: neurofibrillary tangles and loss of large neurons. Ann Neurol 17:573–577
78. Yates CM, Simpson J, Gordon A, Maloney AFJ, Allison Y, Ritchie IM, Urquhart A (1983) Catecholamines and cholinergic enzymes in pre-senile and senile Alzheimer-type dementia and Down's syndrome. Brain Res 280:119–126
79. DeSouza EB, Whitehouse PJ, Kuhar, MJ, Price DL, Vale WW (1986) Reciprocal changes in corticotropin-releasing factor (CRF)-like immunoreactivity and CRF receptors in cerebral cortex of Alzheimer's disease. Nature 319:593–595
80. Powers RE, Struble RG, Casanova MF, O'Connor DT, Kitt CA, Price DL (in press) Hippocampal anatomy and structural abnormalities of noradrenergic systems in aging and in Alzheimer's disease. Neuroscience
81. Price DL, Altschuler RJ, Struble RG, Casanova MF, Cork LC, Murphy DB (in press) Sequestration of tubulin in neurons in Alzheimer's disease. Brain Res

Structural Proteins in Alzheimer's Disease

D. SELKOE [1]

NFT	neuronal fibrillary tangle	AD	Alzheimer disease
PHF	paired helical filament	GFA	glial fibrillary acidic
SDS	sodium dodecyl sulfate	LF	lipofuscin
PHFP	paired helical filament protein	FACS	fluorescence activated cell sorting
βME	β-mercaptoethanol	SCN	thiocyanate
MW	molecular weight	CNBr	cyanogen bromide
EM	electron microscopy	HPLC	high performance liquid chromatography
NF	neurofilament		

Structural Changes in Alzheimer Neurons

Neuritic (senile) plaques and neurofibrillary tangles (NFT) represent the principal structural alterations of neurons in presenile and senile dementia of the Alzheimer type (Alzheimer's disease, AD). These two types of lesions are also found in much smaller numbers and in restricted topographical distribution in the brains of many neurologically normal individuals after the seventh decade. Tangles, plaques, and other structural changes found in Alzheimer brain tissue (granulovacuolar degeneration of neurons, amyloid angiopathy of small cerebral vessels, lipofuscin (LF) deposition in neurons and glia) are, therefore, qualitatively indistinguishable from the lesion that accompany normal brain aging, but are quantitatively much increased in AD. Neurofibrillary tangles are large, non-membrane-bound cytoplasmic masses of abnormal fibers found within the perikarya of neurons in hippocampus, amygdala, cerebral cortex, and certain deep gray nuclear structures. Numerous electron microscopic (EM) studies have concluded that the vast majority of fibers in these tangles have the appearance of tightly adherent pairs of helically wound, intermediate filaments, referred to as paired helical filaments (PHF) and having a maximum width of about 20 nm and a periodicity of roughly 80 nm [1–3]. It is also known that at least some of the abnormal neurites (dendrites and axonal terminals) making up the periphery of the senile plaque contain PHF [4]. Recently, a few laboratories have reported that bundles of straight (nonhelical) filaments of ap-

[1] Department of Neurology (Neuroscience), Harvard Medical School, and Center for Neurologic Diseases, Brigham and Women's Hospital, Boston, MA, USA.

Neurology
Ed. by K. Poeck, H. J. Freund, and H. Gänshirt

proximately 15 nm width may also be found in neurons in Alzheimer cortex and may coexist within perikarya containing PHF [5–8].

These observations as well as those in several other laboratories indicate that the fibrous cytopathology of neurons in AD is more complex and hetereogeneous than generally stated and includes the accumulation of straight cytoplasmic fibers with a spectrum of diameters from 10 to 20 nm as well as PHF. Molecular models for the reorganization of the fibrous neuronal cytoskeleton in AD will need to take this complexity into account.

In addition to the aforementioned intracellular changes, AD brain tissue displays abundant extracellular deposits of abnormal filaments that are found in the central "cores" of senile plaques, in random distribution in the cortical neuropil and in the walls of certain leptomeningeal and parenchymal vessels. Like the NFT, these fibrous extracellular deposits show characteristic green birefringence under polarized light after staining with the dye Congo red and are thus classified as amyloid deposits. EM demonstrates that the filaments comprising these deposits are generally in the range 5–10 nm in diameter. Their fine structure is distinct from that of the intraneuronal PHF and straight filaments. The protein chemical relationship of the intraneuronal and extracellular fibers that accumulate in AD is currently under investigation.

The accumulation of PHF-containing neuronal processes and cell bodies in Alzheimer brain tissue has been statistically correlated with several parameters of the disease, including degree of dementia [9–12], extent of neuronal loss in hippocampus [10], and degree of deficiency of cortical cholinergic function [12]. The marked loss of cholinergic perikarya recently reported in the nucleus basalis of Meynert and the septal nuclei in Alzheimer brains is associated with the presence of NFT in some of the remaining neurons in these nuclei [13, 14]. Thus, in contrast to Huntington's disease, in which striatal neuronal loss is unaccompanied by any characteristic ultrastructural change in adjacent neurons that have not yet died, neuronal attrition in Alzheimer brain is associated with marked structural changes in many remaining cells. In view of these observations, it seems important to identify the molecular nature of the PHF and ultimately the abnormal neuronal biochemical process or processes responsible for their progressive accumulation.

The principal objective of current work in several laboratories is to characterize the molecular mechanism of PHF and amyloid fiber formation and to establish what role this process may play in accelerated death of neurons during normal aging and in AD. In setting this goal, we are aware that neurofibrillary degeneration (PHF formation) is presumably a late and somewhat nonspecific event in the course of degeneration of certain human neuronal populations. However, understanding the basis for what is turning out to be an unusual, apparently irreversible and dramatic change in the neuron's internal organization may well provide important clues to abnormal molecular biologic events that precede PHF formation in neurons destined to die prematurely.

Immunocytochemical Studies of Neurofibrillary Degeneration

The identity and origin of the constituent proteins of the PHF has become a matter of considerable interest. The first reported protein chemical studies of cortical fractions containing NFT or partially purified PHF found enrichment of a polypeptide of molecular weight 50000 in such fractions [15]. This protein was felt to be a constituent of the PHF and was referred to as the paired helical filament protein (PHFP) [15, 16]. Immunocytochemical studies using polyclonal antisera raised against gel-purified PHFP [17] and against a partially purified human brain microtubule preparation [18] showed staining of Alzheimer NFT in tissue sections. These and other immunochemical studies by Wisniewski and Iqbal led to the conclusion that antigens other than tubulin, present in microtubule fractions from normal young brain, are shared with PHF [16]. More recently, Iqbal et al. achieved a much greater purification of PHF and reported that several polypeptides of approximate molecular weight 45–70000 were constituents of the PHF [19].

Studies by Yen and co-workers [20] have confirmed that polyclonal antisera to crude human microtubule preparations stain ~ 40% of neurofibrillary tangles in Alzheimer cortex as well as the neurites of the senile plaque. These authors as well as Eng et al. [21] find that antibodies to tubulin itself do not stain the tangles, and conclude that it is not tubulin in the microtubule preparations that is the shared antigen with PHF. Ihara and colleagues [22] have found staining of Alzheimer tangles and of some neurites in senile plaques with a rabbit antiserum to gel-purified neurofilament (NF) protein of molecular weight 200000. Gambetti et al. [23] and Dahl et al. [24] have reported immunostaining of in situ tangles with a polyclonal antiserum against a denatured chicken brain neurofilament preparation; this antiserum cross-reacts strongly with normal neurofilament proteins both by immunohistochemistry and by direct immunostaining of proteins in gels, but shows very little or no reaction with tubulin or glial filament protein. Anderton and co-workers [25] have produced monoclonal antibodies that react both with normal neurofilament proteins (polypeptides of molecular weight 150000 and 200000) and Alzheimer tangles and plaque neurites in tissue sections.

These various immunochemical studies are difficult to compare since the groups used different antisera or antibodies raised against a variety of partially purified, heterogeneous immunogens. More importantly, all of the studies described employed staining of in situ NFT in sections of Alzheimer cortex. It has subsequently been determined that some antibodies to normal cytoskeletal fibers (e.g., the monoclonals reported by Anderton et al.) label NFT weakly or not at all following their extraction from Alzheimer cortex in reagents (e.g., sodium dodecyl sulfate, SDS) that dissolve normal fibers [26, 27].

Biochemical Studies of the Neurofibrillary Tangle

Initial biochemical analysis of NFT and their constituent PHF used extraction with the nonionic detergent Triton X-100 and subcellular fractionation, as conventionally employed in cytoskeletal studies, to derive partially enriched PHF fractions from AD cortex [15, 28]. In the author's laboratory, one- and two-dimensional gel electrophoresis failed to demonstrate any consistently increased or unique neuronal polypeptides in PHF-enriched fractions compared with similar fractions from control brain [28]. After repeatedly finding no change in identifiable neuronal cytoskeletal proteins in PHF-enriched fractions compared with controls, we postulated that PHF might consist of insoluble proteins that did not enter gels after heating in sample buffer containing SDS and reagents that reduce disulfide bonds (e.g., β-mercaptoethanol, βME). EM of the SDS/βME-insoluble residue of the PHF preparation excluded at the top of the stacking gel demonstrated abundant PHF which retained their 80 nm periodicity, but were slightly thinner (~ 16–20 nm) in diameter than in situ PHF [28]. A method was developed for isolating whole NFT and many, though not all, NFT appeared to remain intact and retained their characteristic Congo red birefringence after heating in SDS/βME buffer. Further analyses showed that PHF remained insoluble and recognizable by EM after treatment with several strong denaturants, including 9.5 *M* urea, 6 *M* guanidine hydrochloride, and phenol [28, 29]. Since no quantitative assay for PHF in intact cortex or aqueous samples was available, we could not estimate the percentage recovery of PHF after SDS/βME extraction. It is possible, perhaps likely, that a portion of the PHF fiber is solubilized by harsh solvent extraction [19]. However, the marked enrichment of PHF after SDS/βME treatment, the preservation of their characteristic helical periodicity [28, 30], the fact that actual manual counts of NFT from most AD cases before and after treatment indicate no quantitative loss [28], and the absence of major polypeptides released into SDS acrylamide gels all suggest that most of the PHF fiber is stable in SDS/βME. The straight ~ 15 nm filaments found in degenerating neurons in some cases of AD can also be recovered, at least in part, in the SDS/βME-insoluble fraction of cortex.

Digestion of partially purified PHF fractions using specific or nonspecific proteases; e.g., trypsin or proteinase K, either with or without sonication of the fibers, has been attempted [29]. No soluble peptide fragments could be detected by SDS-polyacrylamide gel electrophoresis after such treatments and PHF could still be visualized by EM. We hypothesize that the rigid insoluble PHF polymers do not bind effectively to the active sites of proteolytic enzymes.

The discovery of the high degree of inertness of the abnormal fibers comprising NFT led to two general conclusions: (a) their relative insolubility enables the use of denaturant extraction to purify PHF to a greater extent than previously possible; (b) the insolubility of PHF in reagents such as SDS, urea, and βME suggests that covalent cross-links (other than disulfides) might be involved in part in assembling the subunits of PHF into their large polymeric forms. The shared properties of PHF fibers and known cross-linked protein polymers led us to hypothesize that covalent intermolecular cross-linking might be involved in PHF formation. A number of mammalian intracellular proteins have been shown to be cross-linked by glutamine-lysine bonds formed by the calcium-activated enzyme, transglutaminase. We have demonstrated that NF and other endogenous CNS proteins can serve as substrates for brain transglutaminase in vitro [31]. However, it has not been possible to demonstrate directly the presence of such cross-links in PHF since their identification requires the sequential degradation of the protein by proteolytic enzymes and subsequent isolation of the dipeptide cross-links, a technique which cannot yet be carried out on the highly inert PHF. Although the possibility of covalently cross-linking by ε-(γ-Glu)Lys bonds or some other intermolecular covalent cross link remains, no data are yet available to support this hypothesis. Alternative mechanisms for explaining the insolubility of PHF, such as the presence of extensive β-pleated sheet conformation, may be more likely.

The fact that PHF as well as extracellular amyloid deposits (senile plaque cores) share structural and tinctorial properties with amyloid proteins led to X-ray diffraction analyses of PHF and plaque amyloid [32]. Using considerably enriched, but not fully purified PHF preparations, characteristic 4.76 Å and 10.6 Å reflections consistent with a macromolecule containing cross-β-pleated sheet conformation were observed. This finding is consistent with the long-held hypothesis that, like other amyloids, the PHF and core fibers in AD contain β-pleated sheet structure. The apparent cross-β-pleated sheet conformation of PHF could explain, at least in part, their high degree of insolubility. However, the lack of quantitative solubilization of PHF and amyloid cores by concentrated guanidine hydrochloride differs from the behavior of non-CNS human amyloid proteins and suggests an even greater degree of insolubility.

Although considerable enrichment of PHF has resulted from the use of detergents during purification [19, 33], other SDS/βME-insoluble constituents of AD cortex (e.g., LF granules, amyloid fibers, denatured mitochondria, and unidentified granular material) still copurify with PHF. Because of their unusual nature, it has not been possible to obtain PHF that are at or close to structural homogeneity using biochemical purfication methods alone. Consequently, PHF-specific polyclonal antibodies [33, 34] and monoclonal antibodies (Mabs) [35–37] have been raised for characterizing PHF and for use as specific ligands for the further purification of the fibers. Characterization of our polyclonal PHF antibodies [33] demonstrated that they reacted at high dilution with both in situ and SDS-extracted NFT and senile plaque neurites but, unexpectedly, they labeled no structures in normal human or animal brain, other than the occasional senile plaque neurites and rare NFT found in normal aged human cortex. These PHF antibodies also failed to react with normal brain proteins (e.g., NF, tubulin, actin, glial fibrillary acidic protein) by Western blotting, a highly sensitive technique for the immunochemical detection of proteins. The specificity of our polyclonal antibodies for PHF contrasts with the fact that certain antibodies to normal NF cross-react with NFT (see, e.g., [25] and [38]). Several laboratories have characterized polyclonal or monoclonal NF antibodies on AD brain sections and have noted that the majority of antibodies to NF proteins do not label NFT, but a few do. In collaborative studies with Drs. Brian Anderton, Jacob Kahn and associates at St. George's Hospital Medical School, London, we observed that certain Mabs to the NF subunit proteins of molecular weight 200000 or 160000 labeled in situ NFT in identical fashion to our polyclonal PHF antibodies. However, after extensive SDS extraction, most NFT reacted very weakly or not at all with the NF Mabs [26]. We subsequently observed that following prolonged incubation of SDS-extracted NFT at room temperature under denaturing conditions, considerable immunoreactivity with the NF Mabs could be restored [39]. The results suggest that selected NF antigens may be incorporated into the SDS-insoluble fibers of NFT, but that under some conditions, such epitopes may not be readily detectable by immunocytochemistry. These observations underscore the difficulty of determining the protein composition of PHF by immunochemical methods and point to the need for a full protein chemical analysis of the purified fibers.

Several Mabs recently raised in our laboratory against SDS-extracted PHF show cross-reactivities with certain other brain structural proteins [37]. One of our Mabs reacts with SDS-isolated PHF as well as NF polypeptides and the glial filament subunit protein. Two Mabs react with glial filament protein alone and another reacts with determinants on myelin basic protein. Variability in the cross-reactivities of Mabs produced against PHF has been previously reported by other laboratories [35, 36].

Further evidence of the antigenic complexity of NFT is provided by studies by Kosik et al. [27] using Mabs to microtubule-associated protein 2 (MAP2). One of the MAP2 Mabs immunolabels NFT in sections of AD brain while two others do not. Following extraction of NFT in the presence of SDS, the MAP2 Mab no longer stains tangles. Thus, a portion of the MAP2 molecule, which has been postulated to have some role in the linking of microtubules to NF and other organelles in the neuron, may be closely associated with the abnormal fibers that accumulate in the NFT.

We are currently using PHF antibodies in an effort to purify PHF fibers fully. However, during initial attempts to devise a new method of immunopurification of these structures, we realized that the extracellular amyloid cores of senile plaques presented a more attractive candidate for immunopurification than the NFT because of the dense, spherical form of the cores, which retain their structure after isolation from brain tissue.

Purification and Partial Solubilization of Senile Plaque Amyloid: Comparison with PHF

In order to separate senile plaque amyloid from all other constituents of AD cortex, we used a novel strategy, namely the use of fluorescence-activated cell sorting (FACS) to isolate intact amyloid cores in an aqueous suspension [40]. The discrete, roughly spherical nature of the cores and the fact that their size (6–20 μm maximal diameter) is similar to blood cells that are routinely separated by flow cytometry led us to try this technique. Initial core fractions were prepared by centrifuging SDS-extracted homogenates of AD cortex at low speed (300 *g*), allowing quantitative pelleting of the cores while many LF granules, NFT, and small particles remained in the supernatant. The suspension was then sieved and separated on sucrose density gradients. Gradient interfaces that were particularly enriched in cores were subjected to FACS. On the basis of fluorescence and light-scattering (size) discriminants, unlabeled cores were separated from most autofluorescent LF granules by an initial FACS sort. The cores were then rhodamine labeled with a rat antiserum raised against partially purified amyloid cores and were separated from remaining contaminants by a second FACS sort. Bright-field, fluorescence, and polarization microscopy of the final fraction revealed highly purified, intact amyloid cores. EM shows that the cores are virtually free of contaminants except for occasional aggregates of LF. By particle counting, the final fraction consists of $\geqq 90\%$ amyloid cores.

We have subsequently carried out amino acid analyses of the purified cores [40, 41]. Each core contains approximately 60–120 pg protein. The amino acid composition shows an abundance of nonpolar residues with glycine being the most common residue ($\sim 18\%$). There is a small amount of methionine and no proline. The analyses show considerable similarity to the amino acid composition of partially purified PHF prepared by our biochemical method.

The solubility characteristics of purified amyloid cores are also similar to those of NFT. The cores are not quantitatively depolymerized in guanidine hydrochloride (6 *M*), urea or lithium bromide (7 *M*). However, following treatment in saturated guanidine thiocyanate (7 *M*), we no longer see any green birefringent cores after Congo red staining; they are replaced by amorphous congophilic aggregates. The guanidine SCN treatment clarifies the core fraction, but a small amount of particulate material can still be recovered by pelleting at 10000 *g*. Very similar effects are observed when the purified cores are treated with ~ 80% formic acid at room temperature for 1–2 h [41]. Formic acid was chosen because we had previously observed [42] that attempted CNBr cleavage of partially purified PHF in 70% formic acid caused a marked decrease in gel-excluded protein in the preparation and the appearance of a low molecular weight band migrating with the dye front in 10% acrylamide gels. Heating in SDS sample buffer and electrophoresis of such formic acid or guanidine thiocyanate-treated cores on urea/acrylamide gels (Coomassie Blue staining) reveals: (a) a diffuse smear of Coomassie-positive material throughout the entire running gel; (b) accentuation of this smear at the lower end of the gel, forming two broad bands at approximate molecular weight 5–7000 and 11–15000; and (c) some excluded insoluble material remaining at the top of the running and stacking gels. We have subsequently treated highly enriched PHF fractions with either 80% formic acid of 7 *M* guanidine thiocyanate followed by treatment with 1% SDS and have observed similar low molecular weight broad bands in urea gels which comigrate with the bands released from the cores [41]. These bands are not present in control brain fractions free of PHF or cores. By both dot blot immunoassays and Western blotting, these low molecular weight proteins (which can be separated and quantitatively prepared using size exclusion high performance liquid chromatography) react with amyloid antibodies but not PHF antibodies.

In summary, our present data suggest that the PHF fractions and the extracellular amyloid core fibers share some characteristics: (a) similar amino acid compositions; (b) similar solubility properties; (c) low molecular weight proteins released by formic acid/SDS or guanidine thiocyanate SDS which appear to derive from amyloid filaments, not PHF; and (e) apparent β-pleated sheet conformation.

Conclusion

Studies to date provide a complex picture of PHF composition with some data indicating a relationship to normal neurofilament and microtubule proteins, but several lines of evidence indicating unusual biochemical and antigenic properties that are distinct from those of normal intermediate filaments. The fact that a number of different antibodies produced in several laboratories react both with NFT and normal NF indicates that certain NF epitopes are either strongly associated with the PHF or actually incorporated into the PHF polymer. On the other hand, the fact that our PHF antibodies do not react with NF or other proteins in normal adult brain indicates that there are unique determinants on the PHF subunit proteins.

Further analysis of the PHF and amyloid core proteins released by formic acid or guanidine thiocyanate may clarify the relationship of these proteins to native fibrous proteins of the neuron. Our data are consistent with the hypothesis that PHF and the extracellular amyloid fibers in AD brain share properties but are chemically distinct. If this turns out to be the case, it may be that the amyloid fibers in the center of neuritic plaques precede the gradual degeneration of neurites and formation of PHF and straight filaments.

The central issue that remains is whether the unusual intra- and extracellular proteins that accumulate during normal aging and in AD derive from normal proteins by specific enzymatic or spontaneous posttranslational processing e.g., posttranslational modification of certain residues, or actually represent newly genetically expressed proteins. The latter possibility raises the question of a change in a regulatory or structural gene in the neuron and/or in non-neuronal cells.

References

1. Kidd M (1963) Paired helical filaments in electron microscopy of Alzheimer's disease. Nature 197:192
2. Terry RD, Gonatas NF, Weiss M (1964) Ultrastructural studies in Alzheimer's presenile dementia. Am J Pathol 44:269
3. Wisniewski HM, Narang HK, Terry RD (1976) Neurofibrillary tangles of paired helical filaments. J Neurol Sci 27:173
4. Gonatas NK, Anderson W, Evangelista I (1967) The contribution of altered synapses in the senile plaque: an electron microscopic study in Alzheimer's dementia. J Neuropathol Exp Neurol 26:25
5. Shiboyama H, Kitoh J (1978) Electron microscopic structure of the Alzheimer's neurofibrillary changes in case of atypical senile dementia. Acta Neuropathol (Berl) 41:229
6. Yagishita S, Itoh Y, Nan W, Amano N (1981) Reappraisal of the fine structure of Alzheimer's neurofibrillary tangles. Acta Neuropathol 54:239
7. Metuzals J, Monpetit V, Clapin DF (1981) Organization of the neurofilamentous network. Cell Tissue Res 214:455
8. Rudelli R, Strom JO, Welch PT, Ambler MW (1982) Posttraumatic premature Alzheimer's disease: neuropathologic findings and pathogenetic considerations. Arch Neurol 39:570
9. Tomlinson BE, Blessed G, Roth M (1970) Observations of the brains of demented old people. J Neurol Sci 11:205
10. Ball JJ (1976) Neurofibrillary tangles and the pathogenesis of dementia: a quantitative time study. Neuropathol Appl Neurobiol 2:394
11. Wilcock GK, Esiri MM (1982) Plaques, tangles and dementia. J Neurol Sci 56:343
12. Perry EK, Tomlinson BE, Blessed G et al. (1978) Correlation of cholinergic abnormalities with senile plaques and mental test scores in senile dementia. Br Med J 2:1457
13. Whitehouse PJ, Price DL, Struble RG, Clark AW, Coyle JT, DeLong MR (1982) Alzheimer's disease and senile dementia: loss of neurons in the basal forebrain. Science 215:1237
14. Nakano I, Hirano A (1982) J Neuropathol Exp Neurol 41:341 (Abstract)
15. Iqbal K, Wisniewski HM, Shelanksi ML et al. (1974) Protein changes in senile dementia. Brain Res 77:337
16. Wisniewski HM, Iqbal K (1980) Ageing of the brain and dementia. Trends Neurosci 3:226
17. Grundke-Iqbal I, Johnson AB, Terry RD, Wisniewski HM, Iqbal K (1979) Alzheimer neurofibrillary tangles: antiserum and immunohistological staining. Ann Neurol 6:532
18. Grundke-Iqbal I, Johnson AB, Wisniewski HM et al. (1979) Evidence that Alzheimer neurofibrillary tangles originate from neurotubules. Lancet 1:578

19. Iqbal K, Zaidi T, Thompson CH, Merz PA, Wisniewski HM (1984) Alzheimer paired helical filaments: bulk isolation, solubility, and protein composition. Acta Neuropathol (Berl) 62:167
20. Yen SH, Gaskin F, Terry RD (1981) Immunocytochemical studies of neurofibrillary tangles. Am J Pathol 104:77
21. Eng LF, Forno LS, Bigbee JW, Forno KI (1980) Immunohistochemical localization of glial fibrillary acidic protein and tubulin in Alzheimer's disease brain biopsy material. In: Amaducci L, Davison AN, Antuono P (eds) Aging of the brain and dementia. Raven, New York, p 49
22. Ihara Y, Nukina N, Sugita H, Toyokura Y (1981) Staining of Alzheimer's neurofibrillary tangles with antiserum against 200 K component of neurofilaments. Proc Jpn Acad 57:152
23. Gambetti P, Velasco ME, Dahl D, Bignami A, Roessmann V, Sindely SD (1980) In: Amaducci L, Davison AN, Antuono P (eds) Aging of the brain and dementia. Raven, New York, p 55
24. Dahl D, Selkoe DJ, Pero TR, Bignami A (1982) Immunostaining of neurofibrillary tangles in Alzheimer's senile dementia with neurofilament antiserum. J Neurosci 2:113
25. Anderton BH, Breinburg D, Downes MJ, Green PJ, Tomlinson BE, Ulrich J, Wood JN, Kahn J (1982) Monoclonal antibodies show that neurofibrillary tangles and neurofilaments share antigenic determinants. Nature 298:84
26. Rasool CG, Abraham C, Anderton BH, Haugh MC, Kahn J, Selkoe DJ (1984) Alzheimer's disease: immunoreactivity of neurofibrillary tangles with anti-neurofilament and anti-paired helical filament antibodies. Brain Research 310:249–260
27. Kosik KS, Duffy LK, Dowling MM, Abraham C, McCluskey A, Selkoe DJ (1984) Microtubule-associated protein 2: Monoclonal antibodies demonstrate the selective incorporation of certain epitopes into Alzheimer neurofibrillary tangles. Proc Natl Acad Sci USA 81:7941
28. Selkoe DJ, Ihara Y, Salazar FJ (1982) Alzheimer's disease: insolubility of partially purified paired helical filaments in sodium dodecyl sulfate and urea. Science 215:1243
29. Selkoe DJ, Ihara Y, Abraham C, Rasool CG, McCluskey AH (1983) Biochemical and immunocytochemical studies of Alzheimer paired helical filaments. In: Katzman R (ed) Biological aspects of Alzheimer's disease. Cold Spring Harbor Laboratory, New York, p 125 (Banbury Report no 15)
30. Yen SH, Kress Y (1983) The effect of chemical reagents or proteases on the ultrastructure of paired helical filaments. In: Katzman R (ed) Biological aspects of Alzheimer's disease. Cold Spring Harbor Laboratory, New York, p 155 (Banbury Report no 15)
31. Selkoe DJ, Abraham C, Ihara Y (1982) Brain transglutaminase: In vitro crosslinking of human neurofilament proteins into insoluble polymers. Proc Natl Acad Sci USA 79:6070
32. Kirschner DA, Abraham C, Selkoe DJ (1986) X-ray diffraction from intraneuronal paired helical filaments and extraneuronal amyloid fibers in Alzheimer disease indicates cross-β conformation. Proc Natl Acad Sci, USA, 83:503–507
33. Ihara Y, Abraham C, Selkoe DJ (1983) Antibodies to paired helical filaments in Alzheimer's disease do not recognize normal brain proteins. Nature 304:727
34. Brion JP, Couck AM, Passareiro E, Flament-Durand J (1985) Neurofibrillary tangles of Alzheimer's disease: an immunohistochemical study. J Submicrosc Cytol 17:89
35. Wang GP, Grundke-Iqbal I, Kascsak RJ, Iqbal K, Wisniewski (1984) Alzheimer neurofibrillary tangles: Monoclonal antibodies to inherent antigens. Acta Neuropathol 62:268
36. Yen SH, Gaskin F, Fu SM (1983) Neurofibrillary tangles in senile dementia of the Alzheimer type share an antigenic determinant with intermediate filaments of the vimentin class. Am J Pathol 113:373
37. Selkoe DJ, Abraham C, Rasool CG, McCluskey A, Duffy LK (1985) Production and characterization of monoclonal antibodies to Alzheimer paired helical filaments. In: E. Wang et al. (eds) Intermediate Filaments. Ann NY Acad Sci 455:774–778
38. Autiolio-Gambetti L, Gambetti P, Crane RC (1983) Paired helical filaments: relatedness to neurofilaments shown by silver staining and reactivity with monoclonal antibodies. In: Katzman R (ed) Biological aspects of Alzheimer's disease. Cold Spring Harbor Laboratory, New York, p 117 (Banburg Report no 15)

39. Rasool CG, Selkoe DJ (1984) Alzheimer's disease: Exposure of neurofilament immunoreactivity in SDS-insoluble paired helical filaments. Brain Res 322: 194
40. Selkoe DJ, Abraham C, Rasool CG (1984) Biochemical and structural studies of paired helical filaments and senile plaque amyloid in Alzheimer's disease. In: Glenner G (ed) Proceedings IV international symposium on amyloidosis. Plenum, New York (in press)
41. Selkoe DJ, Abraham CR, Duffy LK (1985) Purification by flow cytometry of amyloid fibers in Alzheimer disease. Abstract. American Society of Neurochemistry, March 1985
42. Selkoe DJ, Abraham C, Rasool CG, McCluskey A, Kosik KS, Duffy LK (1985) Paired helical filaments in human neurons: relationship to neurofilaments. Ann NY Acad Sci (in press)

Energy Metabolism and Neurotransmitters in Alzheimer's Disease

A. N. DAVISON [1]

Cerebral Blood Flow in the Ageing Brain

With the reduction in numbers of nerve cells and such structural changes as accumulation of lipofuscin and formation of neuritic plaques, it may be anticipated that there would be reduction in energy metabolism with advancing age. This is of especial importance because although the brain only accounts for some 2% of body weight, it consumes about 20% of the blood glucose and oxygen supply. However, there is little indication of reduction in cerebral blood flow (CBF) in ageing healthy human subjects in whom vascular disease is absent. Dastur and colleagues [9] found that the CBF of 62.1 ± 2.9 ml/100 g/min in young subjects with an average age of 21 years was relatively little reduced in normal old subjects with an average age of 71 years (57.9 ± 2.1 ml/100 g/min). The reduction in CBF reported by some other investigators could be due to subclinical atherosclerosis. There is also little to show that CBF alters with age in other species. Well-controlled in vitro studies on animal brain indicate changes in regional oxygen and glucose consumption with age. Peng, Peng and Chen [21] found that oxygen consumption in rat cortex falls between the ages of 4 and 24 months from 5.51 to 4.82 μl/mg dry tissue/h, with a 21% decrease in the hippocampus and a 24% decrease in the hypothalamus. As pointed out by these authors, the various decreases in oxygen consumption depend on the functional state of the individual neurons. They do not attribute changes to reduced hormonal control or to reduction in total neuronal number. However, it should be remembered that there is a continuous increase in the wet weight of rat brain during development, particularly in the first 6 months. This augmentation in brain weight tapers off by 1 year of age. The presence of considerable amounts of relatively inert myelin in the white matter of 2-year-old rats may account for the decreased oxygen consumption in comparison to young rats. The same explanation may apply to the findings of Frolkis and Bezrukov [14], who reported significant reductions with age in oxygen consumption in the hemispheres, the cerebellum and particularly in the brain stem. However, it has been found [2] that the rate of axonal flow decreases

[1] Department of Neurochemistry, Institute of Neurology, National Hospital, Queen Square, London WC1N 3BG, Great Britain.

Neurology
Ed. by K. Poeck, H. J. Freund, and H. Gänshirt

with age in the rat hippocampus, and this may be a key factor in controlling neurotransmitter synthetic enzyme activity in the nerve terminals.

Regional Glucose Metabolism in the Ageing Brain

Experimental studies on regional utilisation of glucose (using the Sokoloff deoxyglucose method) in rat brain show reductions of about 20% in glucose consumption of 26- and 36-month-old brains compared to that of 4- to 6-month-old animals [28]. Reductions were greatest in structures associated with visual and auditory function. There seems, therefore, to be a small decline in overall metabolic activity within certain sensory regions of maturing animals, but this difference does not continue to progress in the very old. With increasing age, reductions are seen in the oxidation of glucose and 3-hydroxybutyrate by rat brain slices. Changes have been found in synaptic and non-synaptic mitochondrial oxidation of pyruvate and hydroxybutyrate. There seems to be an age-related decrease in activity of tricarboxylic acid cycle and glycolytic enzymes in many brain regions, which may relate to the regional changes in glucose utilisation. It would be anticipated that as hearing and vision are impaired in the elderly human subject there would be a related decline in cerebral metabolism [8]. However, no significant change in oxygen consumption or the respiratory coefficient has been claimed. Using fluorodeoxyglucose uptake and positron emission tomography, no significant change was found in regional cerebral glucose utilisation as a function of age [8, 10]. In our study of utilisation of radioactive glucose by fresh human cortical tissue prisms [24] no significant reduction was found in production of labelled CO_2. The tissue prisms contain synaptic terminals and neurites severed from the cell body, so that even though some nerve cell loss may have occurred with age, reactive synaptogenesis with increased dendritic arborisation would compensate for such loss. The unaltered utilisation of glucose by the crude synaptosomal preparation may relate to dendritic metabolism rather than metabolism of cell bodies. Tricarboxylic acid cycle enzyme and cytochrome oxidase activities are particularly prevalent in the neuropil, while these enzymes can barely be detected in the perikarya. Lactic dehydrogenase, glycolytic and pentose phosphate shunt enzyme activities are relatively high in the cell body [13]. Thus the reduction in phosphofructokinase activity seen with increasing age in the human cortex may relate to loss of the perikarya of large pyramidal neurons of the fifth cortical layer, for they have a higher oxygen consumption than the surrounding neuropil.

Cerebral Blood Flow and Cerebral Metabolism in Alzheimer's Disease

In contrast to normal ageing there is a significant decline in CBF and mean oxygen utilisation in dementia. This decline correlates with increasing severity of cognitive loss in both degenerative and vascular cases [12]. Using positron emission tomography following administration of ^{18}F-deoxyglucose, decreased utilisation of glucose is seen in the cortex. In contrast, there is increased production of $^{14}CO_2$ from labelled glucose incubated with tissue prisms from the neocortex of Alzheimer patients [26]. Moreover, adenylate energy charge is unaltered in the tissue, although there is a reduction in the nucleotide pool, possibly related to loss of presynaptic terminals. The increased CO_2 production could be due to increased glycolysis. It is of interest that increased utilisation of glucose has been reported in fibroblasts from Alzheimer patients and glucose uptake is increased in peripheral blood B cells [16].

At an early stage in dementia the frontal cortex is relatively spared, yet reductions of glucose metabolism are seen [11]. These changes may be attributed to the loss of large neurons and the reduced dendritic arborisation which is a feature of Alzheimer's disease. Using monoclonal antibody to neurofilament protein, Rasool et al. [24] showed a 20%–30% deficit in perikaryal and neurite density in the inferior temporal and superior frontal gyrus of Alzheimer brain. Morphometric analysis shows a loss of about 40% of large neurons (those larger than 90 μm^2) from the midfrontal and superior temporal regions [29].

Cortical Neuronal Changes in Alzheimer's Disease

Other work points to the dysfunction or loss of cortical neurons and the correlation of a tangle formation to cognitive defect [31]. In Alzheimer's disease there is an unexplained reduction in the amount of deep gray matter, including the area containing the caudate nucleus, which is innervated by neocortical nerve cells from all lobes of the brain (see [7]). Some studies relate certain "cortical" cognitive symptoms to a probable dysfunction of the corticostriatal pathway, which is thought to use L-glutamate as its neurotransmitter. Unfortunately, the techniques used for studying excitatory amino acid-releasing nerve terminals in animals are difficult to apply to the subcortex of human brain. Thus, the binding of ^3H-L-glutamate to postsynaptic receptor sites on membranes prepared from the caudate nucleus has been examined [19]. Whereas the Alzheimer brains with high tangle counts had remarkable increases in specific binding of ^3H-L-glutamate at both concentrations of ligand tested, those with lower counts showed smaller increases in binding. This provides some evidence of a change in excitatory amino acid neurotransmission in Alzheimer's disease, for hemidecortication of rats also results in an elevated binding of ^3H-L-glutamate to striatal membranes. This may indicate a supersensitisation response to glutamate receptors in Alzheimer's disease, secondary to dysfunction of descending excitatory amino acid-releasing pathways from neurons in the neocortex [7].

Subcortical Neuronal Changes in Alzheimer's Disease

In 1981 Rossor proposed that Alzheimer's disease and Parkinson's disease were examples of conditions in which there was loss or dysfunction of nerve cells of the isodendritic core. He pointed out that cells from the locus coeruleus, substantia nigra, substantia innominata and septal nuclei share a non-specialised isodendritic pattern corresponding to the reticular formation. Loss of other cell groups could be due to trans-synaptic degeneration after the loss of ascending inputs. The dominant change in neurotransmitter metabolism is in markers of presynaptic cholinergic neuronal activity [3]. With the exception of the putamen, this loss occurs widely in the brain, especially in the hippocampus, amygdala and neocortex. In this respect the hippocampus [1] and the amygdala may turn out to be particularly critical brain regions. This points to a need to know more about septal-hippocampal pathways, as well as about the distribution of descending projections from large cortical neurons. Loss of activity of the acetylcholine-synthesising enzyme choline acetyltransferase (ChAT) is accompanied by an increase in the density of neuritic plaques in the neocortex, although the relationship is not linear [22]. Subjects with early-onset Alzheimer's disease are particularly severely affected histologically, and ChAT activity is proportionately lower than in elderly patients [4]. There is good evidence that loss [30] or shrinkage [20] of neurons from the nuclei of the basal forebrain is associated with neuritic plaque formation (somatostatin immunoreactivity has been detected in neuritic plaques [18]). The cholinergic system is particularly affected, since ascending projections from the nucleus basalis utilise acetylcholine as neurotransmitter. However, not all plaques are thought to be derived from degenerating cholinergic neurites. Muscarinic cholinergic receptor concentration does not alter, except possibly in down-regulation of presynaptic M2 receptors in the frontal cortex [17]. Since ChAT activity is not rate-limiting in acetylcholine synthesis, it was necessary to show that formation and stimulated release of the amine were impaired in Alzheimer's disease. Fresh surgical tissue samples were cut into prisms to produce crude synaptosomes, and these were incubated with ^{14}C-glucose [27]. Significant reduction was observed in acetylcholine synthesis under resting and stimulated conditions in Alzheimer patients with histological evidence of the disease [6]. Choline uptake into biopsy samples was similarly reduced [26]. However, despite the clinical appearance of Alzheimer's disease, examination of biopsy tissue in some presenile patients showed unexpectedly low plaque and tangle counts with no significant impairment of acetylcholine synthesis [5, 26]. Recent work [23] shows that loss of Meynert nucleus neurons and cortical ChAT activity can occur in mentally impaired patients with Parkinson's disease in the absence of Alzheimer-type neuropathology. Thus, although the cholinergic system is clearly affected in dementia, the neuropathological interpretation is not as straightforward as it once appeared.

The effect on other neurotransmitters in Alzheimer's disease may also be due to loss of neurons from discrete nuclei. The concentrations of serotonin and its receptors appear to be reduced in the temporal cortex [6], and this may relate to loss and damage of cells in the raphe nucleus [15]. Somatostatin concentration has been found to be reduced in the cortex.

Conclusion

There is current speculation concerning the possibility of a primary metabolic abnormality in the cortex of Alzheimer's patients which could explain the pathophysiology of the disease. Further research on energy metabolism and the anatomical and pathological changes in the neocortex with relation to neurotransmitter function must be made a major objective of further research.

References

1. Ball MJ, Fisman M, Hackinski V, Blume W, Fox A, Kral VA, Kirschen AJ, Fox H, Merskey H (1985) A new definition of Alzheimer's disease: a hippocampal dementia. Lancet 1:14–16
2. Bondareff W (1978) Effects of age-related changes in extracellular space and axoplasmic flow on neuronal aging. In: Kalzman R, Terry RD, Blick KL (eds) Alzheimer's disease: senile dementia and related disorders (Aging, vol 7). Raven, New York, pp 383–395
3. Bowen DM (1981) Alzheimer's disease. In: Davison AN, Thompson RHS (eds) The molecular basis of neuropathology. Arnold, London, p 649
4. Bowen DM, White P, Spillane JA, Goodhardt MJ, Curzon G, Iwangoff P, Meier-Ruge W, Davison AN (1979) Accelerated ageing or selective neuronal loss as an important cause of dementia? Lancet 1:11–14
5. Bowen DM, Benton JS, Spillane JA, Smith CCT, Allen SJ (1982) Choline acetyltransferase activity and histopathology of frontal neocortex from biopsies of demented patients. J Neurol Sci 57:191–202
6. Bowen DM, Allen SJ, Benton JS, Goodhardt MJ, Haan EA, Palmer AM, Sims NR, Smith CCT, Spillane JA, Esiri MM, Neary D, Snowdon JS, Wilcock GK, Davison AN (1983) Biochemical assessment of serotonergic and cholinergic dysfunction and cerebral atrophy in Alzheimer's disease. J Neurochem 41:266–272
7. Bowen DM, Davison AN, Francis PT, Palmer A, Pearce BR (1984) Neurotransmitter and metabolic dysfunction in Alzheimer's dementia: relationship to histopathological features. In: Rose FC (ed) Research progress in dementia. Karger, Basel (in press)
8. Creasey H, Rapoport SI (1985) Neurological progress – The aging human brain. Ann Neurol 17:2–10
9. Dastur DK, Lane MH, Hansen DB, Kety SS, Butler RN, Perlin S, Sokoloff L (1963) Effects of aging on cerebral circulation and metabolism in man. In: Birren JE, Butler RN, Greenhouse SW, Sokoloff L, Yarrow MR (eds) Human aging. A biological and behavioural study. US Government Printing Office, Washington DC, pp 59–78
10. Duara R, Grady C, Haxby J, Ingvar D, Sokoloff L, Margolin RA, Manning RG, Cutler NR, Rapoport SI (1984) Human brain glucose utilization and cognitive function in relation to age. Ann Neurol 16:702–713
11. Foster NL, Chase TN, Mansi L, Brooks R, Fedio P, Patronas NJ, De Chiro G (1984) Cortical abnormalities in Alzheimer's disease. Ann Neurol 16:649–655
12. Frackowiak RSH, Pozzilli C, Legg NJ, DuBoulay GH, Marshall J, Lenzi GL, Jones T (1981) Regional cerebral oxygen supply and utilization in dementia – a clinical and physiological study with oxygen-15 and positron tomography. Brain 104:753–778
13. Friede RL (1966) Topographic brain chemistry. Academic, New York, pp 50–51
14. Frolkis VV (1979) Blood supply and energy metabolism in the brain. In: Frolkis VV, Bezrukov VV (eds) Aging of the central nervous system. Karger, Basel, pp 16–24
15. Ishii T (1966) Distribution of Alzheimer's neurofibrillary changes in the brain stem and hypothalamus of senile dementia. Acta Neuropathol (Berl) 6:181–187
16. Khansari N, Whitten HD, Chou YK, Fudenberg HH (1985) Immunological dysfunction in Alzheimer's disease. J Neuroimmunol 7:279–287
17. Mash DC, Sevush S, Flynn DD, Norenberg MD, Potter LT (1984) Loss of M2-receptors in Alzheimer's disease. Neurology 34:120
18. Morrison JH, Rogers J, Scherr S, Benoit R, Bloom FE (1985) Somatostatin immunoreactivity in neuritic plaques of Alzheimer patients. Nature 314:90–92
19. Pearce BR, Palmer AM, Bowen DM, Wilcock GK, Esiri MM, Davison AN (1984) Neurotransmitter dysfunction and atrophy of the caudate nucleus in Alzheimer's disease. Neurochem Pathol 2:221–233
20. Pearson RCA, Sofroniew MV, Cuello AC, Powell TPS, Eckenstein F, Esiri MM, Wilcock GK (1983) Persistence of cholinergic neurons in the basal nucleus in a brain with senile dementia of the Alzheimer's type demonstrated by immunohistochemical staining for choline acetyltransferase. Brain Res 289:375–379

21. Peng MT, Peng YI, Chen FN (1977) Age-dependent changes in the oxygen consumption of the cerebral cortex, hypothalamus, hippocampus and amygdaloid in rats. J Gerontol 32:517–522
22. Perry EK, Tomlinson BE, Blessed Y, Bergmann K, Gibson PH, Perry RH (1978) Correlation of cholinergic abnormalities with senile plaques and mental test scores in senile dementia. Br Med J 2:1457–1459
23. Perry EK, Curtis M, Dick DJ, Candy JM, Atack JR, Bloxham CA, Blessed G, Fairbairn A, Tomlinson BE, Perry RH (1985) Cholinergic correlates of cognitive impairment in Parkinson's disease: comparison with Alzheimer's disease. J Neurol Neurosurg Psychiat 48:413–421
24. Rasool CG, Rogers SJ, Drachman DA (1984) Neuron and neurite loss in Alzheimer's disease. Soc Neurosci 10:273 (Abstracts) Rossor MN (1981) Parkinson's disease and Alzheimer's disease as disorders of the isodendritic core. Br Med J 283:1588–1590
25. Sims NR, Bowen DM, Davison AN (1981) [^{14}C]-acetylcholine synthesis and ^{14}C-carbon dioxide production from U-[^{14}C]-glucose by tissue prisms from human neocortex. J Biochem 196:867–876
26. Sims NR, Bowen DM, Allen SJ, Smith CCT, Neary D, Thomas DJ, Davison AN (1983a) Presynaptic cholinergic dysfunction in patients with dementia. J Neurochem 40:503–509
27. Sims NR, Bowen DM, Neary D, Davison AN (1983b) Metabolic processes in Alzheimer's disease, adenine nucleotide content and production of $^{14}CO_2$ from [U-^{14}C]glucose in vitro in human neocortex. J Neurochem 41:1329–1335
28. Smith CB, Goochee C, Rapoport SI, Sokoloff L (1980) Effects of ageing on local rates of cerebral glucose utilization in the rat. Brain 103:351–365
29. Terry RD, Peck A, DeTeresa R, Schechter R, Horopian DS (1981) Some morphometric aspects of the brain in senile dementia of the Alzheimer's type. Ann Neurol 10:184–192
30. Whitehouse PJ, Price DL, Struble RG, Clark AW, Coyle JT, Delong MR (1982) Alzheimer's disease and senile dementia; loss of neurons in the basal forebrain. Science 215:1237–1239
31. Wilcock GK, Esiri MM, Bowen DM, Smith CCT (1982) Alzheimer's disease. Correlation of cortical choline acetyltransferase activity with the severity of dementia and histological abnormalities. J Neurol Sci 57:407–417

Differential Cell Loss in (Peptide) Neurons in the Anterior Hypothalamus with Aging and Alzheimer's Disease: Lack of Changes in Cell Density

D. F. Swaab, E. Fliers, and E. Goudsmit [1]

Introduction

Cell loss is one of the characteristic symptoms of aging of the central nervous system. In addition, it is one of the neuropathological features in Alzheimer's disease (AD) and is commonly believed to underly the impairment of brain function found under these circumstances. Cell loss does not occur in a homogeneous way throughout the central nervous system [1] and it has often been proposed that ontogenetically and phylogenetically new structures would be affected more severely by cell loss in senescence and AD than would older structures [2]. However, few reliable data are available on this topic, while – to make things worse – cell loss in the human brain has generally been estimated by neuropathologists on the basis of the cell density in just a few microscopic sections.

A different approach towards categorizing changes in aging and AD is to observe the neurotransmitter content of those systems that show the most obvious changes. In addition to acetylcholine, the biogenic amines, amino acids and neuropeptides have been receiving increased attention lately. The neuropeptides will be discussed in the present paper. For historical reasons, this group of neuroactive compounds can be subdivided into the following groups: (a) peptides which were first known as hypothalamic hormones (i.e. vasopressin, oxytocin, LHRH, somatostatin and TRH); (b) peptides which were first known as pituitary hormones, but which are also produced by the nervous system (such as the opiomelanocortin family, e.g. α-, β- and γ-MSH, ACTH, β- and γ-LPH, α-, β- and γ-endorphin, and Met/Leu-enkephalin); (c) peptides which were not primarily known as hormones (e.g. substance P, angiotensin II, neurotensin, VIP, DSIP, CCK family, glucagon, carnosine and bradykinin); and (d) peptides that were first found in lower animals, but now appear to be present also in the human brain (e.g. bombesin, hydra head activator peptide, and FMRF-amide). All these peptides are produced by neurons and act in the brain as neurotransmitters or "modulators" (for details see [28]).

[1] Netherlands Institute for Brain Research, Meibergdreef 33, 1105 AZ Amsterdam (ZO), The Netherlands.

Neurology
Ed. by K. Poeck, H. J. Freund, and H. Gänshirt

Many neuropeptides show changes in concentration with aging and Alzheimer's disease [5, 8, 10, 28]. However, neurotransmitter concentration only reflects the net balance between the rates of synthesis, transport, release and degradation, and therefore does not reflect the functional state of a transmitter system (e.g. whether a system is degenerating or is activated). For this reason we have combined morphometric techniques, which reveal the direction of a change in neuronal activity (i.e. activation or inhibition) with immunocytochemical techniques, which can define the chemical nature of a given neuron.

With special reference to the two points mentioned in the first paragraph, we have studied four nuclei within a single structure, the anterior hypothalamus of the human brain. Three of the nuclei chosen are certain to contain peptide-producing neurons: the supraoptic nucleus (SON) and the paraventricular (PVN) nucleus, containing both vasopressin (VP-) and oxytocin (OX)-producing neurons [11], the suprachiasmatic nucleus (SCN), containing, among other things, VP and vasoactive intestinal peptide (VIP)-producing neurons. The chemical nature of the sexually dimorphic nucleus of the preoptic area (SDN) neurons is unknown at present. The four nuclei were studied morphometrically in a single series of formalin-fixed hypothalami, including five cases of neuropathologically confirmed AD. The measurements were often performed in the same sections. As will be documented below, considerable differences in cell loss were found among these four hypothalamic nuclei, while cell density measurements failed to elicit such changes.

The Supraoptic and Paraventricular Nuclei: a Stable Cell Population in Aging and in Alzheimer's Disease

The classical neurosecretory cells are found in the SON and PVN. Cells in these nuclei produce VP or OX. In order to see if the decreased production of VP, which was reported in the literature to take place in senescence and dementia [7, 18, 20, 21, 34, 37], entailed degeneration in these nuclei, we have measured cell and nucleolar sizes of immunocytochemically identified VP and OX cells in the SON and PVN as a parameter for peptide production by these neurons [11, 15, 24]. In addition, total cell counts were made for the SON and PVN.

The size of VP cell profiles in the dorsolateral SON and the PVN showed no statistically significant changes from childhood until 80 years of age. After this age a significant increase was observed in the size of VP cell profiles. In brains from patients with AD this morphometric parameter was within the range of the corresponding control age group [11, 30]. In contrast, OX cell size did not change, either with age or in Alzheimer patients. Nucleolar measurements showed similar results, viz. an increased number of VP cells in the SON and PVN in the oldest age group (80–100 years) and no change in the size of the OX cell nucleoli [15]. In view of the well- documented relationship in neurosecretory cells between cellular and nucleolar size, on the one hand, and peptide synthesizing activity on the other (for references see [11, 15]), the observed overall increase in VP cell and nucleolus size after 80 years of age implies an increased neurosecretory activity of these cells. This activation of VP cells appears to be reflected in augmented peripheral plasma levels of this peptide after the age of 70 [13, 17]. Similarly, Legros et al. [21] reported a secondary increase in immunoreactive blood levels of neurophysins – part of the VP and OX precursor – after the age of 70.

In a recent study (E. Goudsmit, E. Fliers, D. F. Swaab, 1986, Unaltered cell numbers in the human supraoptic and paraventricular nucleus with aging and senile dementia, in preparation), we have been able to show that the rise in activity of neurosecretory cells in the SON and PVN which accompanies normal aging is not a compensatory mechanism for cell loss in these nuclei. Total cell counts in the SON and PVN were the same in all age groups. In the PVN similar cell numbers were found in patients with AD and in controls, while the slightly lower SON cell counts in AD were not significantly different from the controls. Cell density in the SON and PVN did not show any significant change with aging. The SON of Alzheimer patients showed a significantly lower cell density as compared with the controls, but this was not the case with the PVN.

An activation of VP cells without cell loss was also found in aged Wistar rats [9]. A possible explanation of this phenomenon is suggested by recent immunocytochemical studies of VP binding sites in the kidney of the aged rat. Since VP staining was strongly diminished in comparison with young animals, the activation of VP cells in the brain of the aged rat is likely to be a functional compensation for decreased VP receptor affinity or receptor number in both the distal convoluted and the collecting ducts of the kidney (R. Ravid, E. Fliers, D. F. Swaab, 1986, Age-related changes in kidney vasopressin binding scores and urinary excretion in the rat, and [32]). The high neurophysin levels found after the age of 60 had in fact already been proposed to be based upon "an unrecognized renal tubulopathy" [19].

As mentioned already, in the 1950s the CNS was supposed to become less active in old age [12]. On the basis of this supposition as well as animal experiments apparently yielding beneficial effects of VP on cognitive functions, administration of this peptide was tried in patients with memory disturbances. The results of such attempts were inconsistent [16].

From the measurements of cell size and nucleolar size in the human SON and PVN, one cannot but conclude that VP "substitution therapy" in elderly people and perhaps also in some Alzheimer patients has probably been given to patients in whom neurophyophyseal function was not deficient at all – quite the opposite; it may have been activated, so as to compensate for a decreased renal sensitivity for VP. This consideration would at least partially explain the inconsistent results obtained with this therapy [16]. As reviewed in that paper, improvement of attention and memory following administration of VP analogues such as LVP or dDAVP to patients with AD were originally claimed, but subsequent, carefully controlled studies failed to confirm the effects. Nevertheless, "nonspecific activating effects" were reported to take place in these latter studies. The impression was that certain patients – especially those with relatively mild cognitive dysfunctions – had more energy and were less depressed than before treatment. One might, of course, wonder whether such effects are due to a central action of the peptide or, rather, to actions at the level of the kidney or peripheral blood vessels [22].

The Suprachiasmatic Nucleus: Cell Loss from the Age of 80 and in Alzheimer's Disease

The suprachiasmatic nucleus (SCN) is considered to be an endogenous "clock" of the mammalian brain, which coordinates hormonal and behavioral circadian rhythms. Age-related changes in biological circadian rhythms have been reported in humans as well as in other species. The increase in time spent both in wakefulness during the night and in daytime naps can be characterized as a disruption of circadian sleep/wake rhythms in senescence. Since this phenomenon is more prominent in patients with AD than in age-matched controls [26], the study of the SCN in relation to age and SDAT seemed of particular interest. However, the very existence of this nucleus in the human brain was questioned until recently, because of difficulties in visualizing it by conventional histological staining techniques [23]. Immunocytochemical staining with antibodies against VP has turned out to be an excellent marker for the human SCN [6], similar to what had been found earlier in the rat [33]. In the human SCN, ± 16% of the cells could be stained with anti-VP, irrespective of age, sex or the presence of AD. VP cells and fibres were visible throughout the nucleus [31], enabling us to apply morphometric techniques in order to follow age-related changes in volume and cell number.

A marked decrease in SCN volume, VP cell number and total SCN cell number was found in 80- to 100-year-old patients as compared with the younger age groups [30, 31]. Corresponding SCN changes in patients with AD were even more pronounced than those observed during normal aging. Neither VP cell density nor total cell density, as determined following staining with thionin, showed any significant changes with aging. In addition, no difference in VP cell density or total cell density was observed between Alzheimer patients and their age- and sex-matched controls.

Partial lesions in the SCN of the rat make it clear that the size of the SCN is crucial for expression of its pacemaker properties [25, 35]. The observed decrease in SCN volume and cell number in senescence and, even more pronounced in AD, therefore suggests a causal relationship between these changes in the SCN and disturbances of circadian rhythmicity, such as sleep/wake patterns. Abnormal temporal organization of sleep in combination with quantitative changes in various sleep parameters, in particular a reduction in the percentage of REM sleep, has also been found in aged Wistar and in Brown-Norway (BN/BiRij) rats [36]. This animal "model" may therefore enable us experimentally to analyse factors underlying age-related sleep changes.

The changes observed in VP cells and other cells in the SCN in senescence and, even more pronounced in AD, at first glance suggest that strong changes of neuronal systems in aging and dementia are not limited to the cholinergic system. On the other hand, one should keep in mind that data concerning a possible cholinergic innervation of the SCN are lacking, so that these observations do not necessarily argue against strong cholinergic involvement in AD [3].

The Sexually Dimorphic Nucleus of the Preoptic Area: Cell Loss from the Age of 40 Onwards

Since Raisman and Flied [27] reported sex differences in the synaptic organization of the preoptic area in the rat, reports pertaining to gender-linked differences in many brain components throughout the animal kingdom have increased (for review see De Vries et al. [4]). The most conspicuous of these sex differences was described by Gorski et al. [14], viz. in the preoptic area of the rat brain. One particular cell group within this area revealed such a clear cytoarchitectonic sex difference that it could be seen even with the naked eye in Nissl-stained sections. We have recently found an analogue of this sexually dimorphic nucleus (SDN) in the human brain [29]. Morphometric analysis demonstrated that the SDN was 2.5 ± 0.6 times (mean $\pm$ SEM) as large in men as in women and contained 2.2 ± 0.5 times as many cells in all age groups. From the age of 40 onwards the nucleus decreases gradually in volume and cell number in both sexes. The values for the Alzheimer patients were commensurate with their ages. No changes in cell density were observed, neither with aging, nor in AD. Although a function has yet to be established for this nucleus, it is located within an area that is essential for gonadotropin release and sexual behavior in other mammals.

Summary and Conclusions

In conclusion, VP neurons both in the supraoptic (SON) and in the paraventricular nucleus (PVN) become activated from the age of 80 during the course of normal aging and, to a similar extent, in Alzheimer patients. This activation is most probably induced by a decrease in VP receptor affinity or number in the kidney. Cell counts remain unaltered in the SON and PVN throughout life and so does cell density, apart from a decrease in the SON of Alzheimer patients. In contrast, VP neurons in the suprachiasmatic nucleus (SCN) show a marked reduction in number with senescence, while an even stronger numerical decrease was found in Alzheimer patients. Nucleoli measurements need to be performed in this brain area, in order to see if these changes are accompanied by a decrease in cell metabolism. Neither VP cell density nor total cell density change with age or in Alzheimer patients. Finally, a gradual decline in cell number is seen from the age of 40 onwards in the sexually dimorphic nucleus (SDN). However, no change in cell density could be observed either in aging or in Alzheimer's disease.

Consequently, cell loss with aging within a restricted region in the brain, viz. the anterior part of the hypothalamus, can range from no change at all until the age of 90 or beyond in the SON and PVN, to a strong and continuous cell loss starting at the age of 40 in the SDN.

The most obvious alterations took place in the volume of the hypothalamic nuclei, leaving cell density relatively intact. This means that important alterations in aging and dementia in the human brain may have been missed owing to the way neuropathologists have so far mainly depended on cell density changes.

Acknowledgments. This work was supported by the Foundation for Medical Research (FUNGO: project 13-51-30). We are grateful to O. Pach and P. J. van Nieuwkoop for their secretarial help. The material was obtained from the Brain Bank in the Netherlands Institute for Brain Research, Amsterdam.

References

1. Brody H (1973) Aging of the vertebrate brain. In: Rockstein M (ed) Development and aging in the nervous system. Academic, London, pp 121–133
2. Brody H, Vijayashanker N (1977) Cell loss with aging. In: Nandy K, Sherwin I (eds) The aging brain and senile dementia. Plenum, New York, pp 15–21
3. Coyle JT, Price DL, De Long MR (1983) Alzheimer's disease: A disorder of cortical cholinergic innervation. Science 219:1184–1190
4. De Vries GJ et al. (eds) (1984) Progress in brain research, vol 61. Elsevier Science, Amsterdam
5. De Wied D, Van Ree JM (1984) Neuropeptides, mental performance and aging. Life Sci 31:1691–1697
6. Dierickx K, Vandesande F (1977) Immunocytochemical localization of the vasopressinergic and the oxytocinergic neurons in the human hypothalamus. Cell Tissue Res 184:15–27
7. Durso R, Fedio P, Brouwers P, Cox C, Martin AJ, Ruggieri SA, Tamminga CA, Chase TN (1982) Lysine vasopressin in Alzheimer disease. Neurology 32:674–677
8. Faccinetti F, Nappi G, Petraglia F, Martignoni E, Sinforiani E, Genazzani AR (1984) Central ACTH deficit in degenerative and vascular dementia. Life Sci 35:1691–1697
9. Fliers E, Swaab DF (1983) Activation of vasopressinergic and oxytocinergic neurons during aging in the Wistar rat. Peptides 4:165–170
10. Fliers E, Swaab DF (1986) Neuropeptide changes in aging and Alzheimer's disease. In: Aging of the Brain and Alzheimer Disease. Prog Brain Res (in press)
11. Fliers E, Swaab DF, Pool ChrW, Verwer RWH (1985) The vasopressin and oxytocin neurons in the human supraoptic and paraventricular nucleus; changes with aging and senile dementia. Brain Res 342:45–53
12. Friedman SM, Friedman CL (1957) Salt and water balance in ageing rats. Gerontology 1:107–121
13. Frolkis VV, Golovchenko SF, Medved VI, Frolkis RA (1982) Vasopressin and cardiovascular system in aging. Gerontology 28:290–302
14. Gorski RA, Gordon JH, Shryne JE, Southam AM (1978) Evidence for a morphological sex difference within the medial preoptic area of the rat brain. Brain Res 148:333–346
15. Hoogendijk JE, Fliers E, Swaab DF, Verwer RWH (1985) Activation of vasopressin neurons in the human supraoptic and paraventricular nucleus in senescence and dementia. J Neurol Sci 69:291–299
16. Jolles J (1983) Vasopressin-like peptides and the treatment of memory disorders in man. In: Cross BA, Leng G (eds) The neurohypophysis: Structure function and control progress in brain research, vol 60. Elsevier, Amsterdam, pp 169–182
17. Kirkland J, Lye M, Goddard C, Vargas E, Davies I (1984) Plasma arginine vasopressin in dehydrated elderly patients. Clin Endocrinol 20:451–456
18. Legros JJ (1975) The radioimmunoassay of human neurophysins: contribution to the understanding of the physiopathology of neurohypophyseal function. Ann NY Acad Sci 248:281–303
19. Legros JJ (1979) The neurohypophyseal peptides: biosynthesis, biological role, and prospects of use in neuropsychiatric therapy. Triangle 18:17–30
20. Legros JJ, Gilot P, Seron X, Claessens J, Adam A, Moegen JM, Audibert A, Berchier P (1978) Influence of vasopressin on learning and memory. Lancet i:41–42
21. Legros JJ, Gilot P, Schmitz S, Bruwier M, Mantanus H, Timsit-Berthier M (1980) Neurohypophyseal peptides and cognitive function: a clinical approach. In: Brambilla F, Racagni G, de Wied D (eds) Progress in psychoneuroendocrinology. Elsevier/North Holland Biomedical, Amsterdam, pp 325–337
22. Le Moal M, Dantzer R, Mormède P, Baduel A, Lebrun C, Ettenberg A, Van der Kooy D, Wenger J, Deyo S, Koob GF, Bloom FE (1984) Behavioral effects of peripheral administration of arginine vasopressin: A review of our search for a mode of action and a hypothesis. Psychoneuroendocrinology 9:319–341
23. Lydic R, Schoene WC, Czeisler CA, Moore-Ede MC (1980) Suprachiasmatic region of the human hypothalamus: homolog to the primate circadian pacemaker? Sleep 2:355–361

24. Mann DMA, Yates PO, Marcynicek B (1985) Some morphometric observations on the cerebral cortex and hippocampus in presenile Alzheimer's disease, senile dementia of Alzheimer's type and Down's syndrome in middle age. J Neurol Sci 69: 139–159
25. Pickard GE, Turek FW (1983) The suprachiasmatic nuclei: two circadian clocks? Brain Res 268:201–210
26. Prinz PN, Vitaliano PP, Vitiello MV, Bokan J, Raskind M, Perskind E, Gerber C (1982) Sleep EEG and mental function changes in senile dementia of the Alzheimer's type. Neurobiol Aging 3:361–370
27. Raisman G, Field PM (1971) Sexual dimorphism in the preoptic area of the rat. Science 173:731–733
28. Swaab DF (1982) Neuropeptides, their distribution and function in the brain. Brain Res 55:97–123
29. Swaab DF, Fliers E (1985) A sexually dimorphic nucleus in the human brain. Science 228:1112–1115
30. Swaab DF, Fliers E, Fisser B (1984) The vasopressin containing neuron in the human brain. Changes during aging and senile dementia In: Knook DL, Galderini G, Amaducci L (eds) Aging of the brain and senile dementia: The inventory of EEC potentialities, pp 71–78
31. Swaab DF, Fliers E, Partiman TS (1985) The suprachiasmatic nucleus of the human brain in relation to sex age and senile dementia. Brain Res 342:37–44
32. Swaab DF, Fliers E, Ravid R (1986) The vasopressin neuron in the aging human and rat brain Suny-meeting (USA). Handbook of comparative opioid and related neuropeptide mechanisms, vol II. CRC, Boca Raton (FL) (in press)
33. Swaab DF, Pool CW, Nijvelt F (1975) Immunofluorescence of vasopressin and oxytocin in the rat hypothalamo-neurohypophyseal system. J Neural Transm 36: 195–215
34. Tinklenberg JR, Pigade R, Pfefferbaum A, Berger PA (1982) Vasopressin peptides and dementia. In: Corkin S, Davis KL, Growdon JH, Usdin E, Wurtman RL (eds) Alzheimer's disease: A report of progress in research. Raven, New York, pp 461–466
35. Van den Pol AN, Powley T (1979) A fine-grained anatomical analysis of the role of the rat suprachiasmatic nucleus in circadian rhythms of feeding and drinking. Brain Res 160: 307–326
26. Van Gool WA, Mirmiran M (1983) Age-related changes in the sleep pattern of male adult rats. Brain Res 279: 394–398
37. Weingartner N, Kaye W, Gold Ph, Smallberg S, Peterson R, Gillin JC, Ebert M (1981) Vasopressin treatment of cognitive dysfunction in progressive dementia. Life Sci 29:2721–2726

The Dementias: A View to the Future

K. L. Bick[1]

Today we have had the opportunity to consider the broad array of current approaches to the dementias with especial concern for the commonest form of dementia, Alzheimer's disease. As we look ahead to the next steps in our search for understanding, it is appropriate not only to look at where we are and where we have been, but also to take on that most dangerous of professions, that of the prophet. This discussion will focus on neurogenetic research strategies in Alzheimer's disease.

Why should research strategies targeted on the "new genetics" be considered relevant to Alzheimer's disease? Since the 1950s, there has been speculation that some percentage, ranging from 10% to over 50% in recent reports, of Alzheimer's disease cases fitted a pattern consistent with autosomal dominant inheritance, in which penetrance or expression of the gene is influenced by age, with expressivity reaching 40% or more in the tenth decade of life [1, 5, 13]. However, most studies have reported familial aggregations or clusters of Alzheimer's disease and rarely has it been possible to carry out the vertical transgenerational studies needed to document heritability. Professor Amaducci and his colleagues (this volume) report that the most significant risk factor for Alzheimer's disease in their Italian multicenter study was the presence of disease in first-degree relatives. This and other reports provide reason enough to consider whether the methodologically powerful approaches of recombinant DNA technology and molecular neurobiology can be useful in our attempt to understand Alzheimer's disease.

We must be careful to distinguish between a genetic component as contrasted with a genetic cause for human disease. If the presence of the mutant gene is not sufficient in itself to produce disease, then untangling the genetics will be a complex task. This appears to be the situation for some tumours and may be the case for the majority of patients with Alzheimer's disease. If, as may be true in neurofibromatosis, new pathological mutations occur in somatic cells in each generation, the question of heritability may be a moot one. And we must also remember that whether the genetic component produces frank disease often depends upon the environment in which that gene operates; as is true for symptoms of the porphyrias to be manifested.

[1] Nat. Inst. of Neurol. and Communicative Disorders and Strokes, National Institutes of Health, Bethesda, MD 20205, USA.

Neurology
Ed. by K. Poeck, H. J. Freund, and H. Gänshirt

Two approaches to the genetics of human disease have been exploited; one when the missing or defective gene product is known, as in enzyme deficiency diseases such as Gaucher's disease; the other when there is no clue to the nature of the mutant gene or its product.

As examples of the first approach, DNA segments have been isolated which contain genes of clinical neurological significance, e.g. phenylalanine hydroxylase (phenylketonuria), β-galactosidase (Gaucher's disease), hypoxanthine guanine phosphoribosyl transferase (Lesch-Nyhan disease). With a copy of the gene, it is often possible to demonstrate directly an abnormality in the DNA of individuals who carry the mutant gene. Attempts to use this candidate gene strategy [14] in Alzheimer's disease have focused on reported neurochemical differences between patients and those free of the disease. If one is convinced that neuropeptides and other neurotrophic proteins, such as nerve growth factor (NGF), are involved in the dystrophic response seen in the Alzheimer's disease brain [9], then chromosome 1, where a NGF gene has been localized by Francke [3], may be worth investigation. Further "candidate genes" for Alzheimer's disease might be considered from reports of anomalies in glucose metabolism, specifically in the pyruvate dehydrogenase complex [12], in looking at both synthetic and degradative pathways for neurotransmitters implicated in Alzheimer's disease, such as acetylcholine and the catecholamines, or considering the families of genes responsible for the production of the many neuropeptide modulators (somatostatin, for example) and trophic factors which play as yet unclear roles in this disease.

When there is no known or postulated gene product to use as a probe, genetic markers known as polymorphisms which travel with the disease in informative families may be used. It is important to remember that the polymorphisms are not the result of the lesion that caused the disease, but simply a pre-existing variation in the population which can be exploited to point the way to the unknown gene with its unknown role in the aetiology of Alzheimer's disease. As illustrated by the now well-known success in Huntington's disease, recombinant DNA technology provides the tools to obtain the requisite number of new genetic markers (polymorphisms) because it allows us to follow the heritable differences in the sequence of genomic DNA, markers known as restriction fragment length polymorphisms (RFLPs). RFLPs are detected as differences in the sizes of pieces of DNA broken up by restriction endonucleases. Unlike classical expressed markers, DNA polymorphisms can be found whether or not a given DNA sequence encodes a protein. Thus, the probes detecting RFLPs can be derived from known gene loci or from anonymous DNA segments. Fortunately, RFLPs appear to be present in all regions of the genome, thus making it feasible to construct a detailed human genetic linkage map to localize disease genes. Some 200 RFLPs are known today, and it is projected that sufficient markers to blanket the whole human genome will be available in the next 5 years.

For either of these genetic approaches to be used, clinical assessment of large families with informative individuals – those with the disease, unaffected, and at risk, who can be identified with reasonable certainty as belonging to one or other of these groups – is essential. This meshing of the clinician investigator with the skills of the molecular neurogeneticist is critical to any resolution of the role played by the genome in Alzheimer's disease. Given this interdependent collaborative unit, and access to sufficient numbers of families with multiple affected members (and more of these are being identified every year), it should be possible to tease out the details of the genetic aspects of Alzheimer's disease.

Efforts to look at the DNA directly in cases of Alzheimer's disease and other dementias have been fragmentary to date and not unexpectedly have led to controversial results. The story of defective DNA repair in response to ionizing radiation or alkylating agents in Alzheimer's disease lymphocyte-derived cell lines is still unclear, but enough evidence is now available to encourage further study of possible abnormalities in DNA repair. Robbins et al. [10] hypothesize that the death of neurons during the disease may be due to accumulation of unrepaired neuronal DNA damaged by radiomimetic agents, such as peroxides, originating in metabolism.

Two earlier reports of chromosome anomalies in Alzheimer's disease lymphocytes were not substantiated in further studies, with a recent report by Buckton et al. [2] indicating only changes similar to those seen in aged nondemented controls. McLachlan and co-workers [7] have reported altered chromatin structural conformations in Alzheimer's disease neocortex and have proposed that this may be a marker for Alzheimer's disease. Advances in our basic understanding of chromosomal organization and the cellular control of gene transcription are essential to clarify these approaches.

The putative mutant gene (or genes) in Alzheimer's disease might be recognized by the faulty protein they produce. The earlier thesis of molecular biology that the DNA sequence is transcribed into messenger RNA and translated into the linear array of amino acids which make up the primary structure of the protein must now be modified to take account of the phenomenon of reverse transcription and of the nuclear processing of primary transcript messenger to yield functional messenger RNA which translates the DNA message to the amino acid sequence in the cytoplasm. The extent of post-transcription processing in neurons is just beginning to be appreciated and greatly broadens the definition of possible mutational events.

The search for messenger RNAs in Alzheimer's disease brains and comparison of their amount and activity with that seen in control brains exemplifies another genetic strategy. In one kind of experiment, reverse transcriptases use the presumably mutant messenger as a template to make complementary DNA molecules which can be used as probes to search the genome directly for their mutant partners. In an appropriate translation system, messenger RNAs can direct the synthesis of the proteins they encode and thereby provide a lead to the nature of the mutant product.

Sajdel-Sulkowska and Marotta [11] have reported that protein synthesis directed by Alzheimer's disease brain messenger RNA is decreased as compared with that seen in controls. In dissecting out which facet of protein synthesis was affected, they provided evidence for a reduction in total cellular RNA and in active messenger RNA in Alzheimer's disease brains. This was associated with an increase in alkaline ribonuclease activity. They recently reported [6] that not only did messenger RNA derived from Alzheimer's disease brains translated in the reticulocyte lysate system produce less protein than controls, but also that a new species of protein of molecular weight 53000 is found. On the other hand, with another methodological approach, Morrison and co-workers [8] found only minor decreases of specific messenger RNAs in Alzheimer's disease cortex with no significant differences in translation into protein between control and Alzheimer's disease brains. Clarification of such discrepancies is essential.

The pathognomic lesions in the Alzheimer brain include plaques and tangles whose fibrous protein nature has long been the subject of much biochemical investigation. Increasingly, evidence is mounting that these abnormal fibrous elements are chemically related and share at least some immunological determinants. Could it be that these abnormal neurofilaments are the primary lesion or the primary cellular expression of the genetic lesion seen in Alzheimer's disease? Selkoe's elegant overview (this volume) of this active area of dementia research has already provided us with some intriguing insights into these questions. Gajdusek's provocative hypothesis [4], that interference with axonal transport of neurofilament proteins is induced by infection with atypical filamentous viruses, poses "a framework of thought" which must be subjected to rigorous investigation and analysis.

In their simplest form, the questions we seek to answer in research on Alzheimer's disease are as follows. Why do specific large neurons in the cortex and subcortical nuclei die? Are they genetically programmed to die or do they die because they lose their ability to respond to or transport trophic factors, or because the trophic factors are no longer produced? Are they killed by a noxious agent, either chemical or biological, produced endogeously or appearing from outside? I have focused on strategies to tease out the genetic contribution, if any, to this cell death. While today the panoply of ideas and data seems much too complex to be coherent, the confusion is an indication of life and vigour in our science. The answers to these questions will no doubt lead to new and more challenging questions about the cause and perhaps cure of this fascinating puzzle and dire dilemma of dementia.

References

1. Breitner JCS, Folstein M (1984) Familial nature of Alzheimer's disease. N Engl J Med 311:192
2. Buckton KE, Whalley LJ, Lee M, Christie JE (1983) Chromosomic changes in Alzheimer's presenile dementia. J Med Genet 20:46–51
3. Franke U, de Martinville B, Coussens L, Ullrich A (1983) The human gene for the β subunit of nerve growth factor is located on the proximal short arm of chromosome 1. Science 222:1248–1251
4. Gajdusek DC (1985) Hypothesis: interference with axonal transport of neurofilament as a common pathogenetic mechanism in certain diseases of the central nervous system. N Engl J Med 312:714–719
5. Heston LL, Mastri AR, Anderson VE, White J (1981) Dementia of the Alzheimer type: clinical genetics, natural history and associated conditions. Arch Gen Psychiatry 38:1085–1090
6. Marotta CA, Sajdel-Sulkowska EM (1985) Factors affecting brain protein synthesis in Alzheimer's disease. J Neurochem 44:S191
7. McLachlan-Crapper DR, Lewis PN, Lukiw WJ, Sima A, Bergeron C, deBoni U (1984) Chromatin structure in dementia. Ann Neurol 15:329–334
8. Morrison MR, Jamison S, Ojeda S, Pardue S, Griffin WST (1984) RNA isolation from Alzheimer's brain. Soc Neurosci Abstr 10(2):1062
9. Ojika K, Appel SH (1983) Neurotrophic factors and Alzheimer's disease. In: Biological aspects of Alzheimer's disease. Banbury Report 15:285–295
10. Robbins JH, Otsuka F, Tarone RE, Polinsky RJ, Brumback RA, Moshell AN, Nee LE, Ganges MB, Cayeux SJ (1983) Radiosensitivity in Alzheimer's disease and Parkinson's disease. Lancet i, 468–469

11. Sajdel-Sulkowska EM, Marotta CA (1984) Alzheimer's disease brain: alterations in RNA levels and in a ribonuclease-inhibitor complex. Science 225:947–949
12. Sheu K-FR, Kim Y-T, Blass JP, Weksler ME (1985), An immunochemical study of the pyruvate dehydrogenase deficit in Alzheimer's disease brain. Ann Neurol 17:444–449
13. Terry RD (1976) Dementia: a brief and selective review. Arch Neurol 33:1–4
14. White RL (1984) Human genetics. Lancet ii 1257–1262

The Dementias: A View to the Future

B. E. TOMLINSON [1]

Information on many aspects of Alzheimer's disease has enormously increased over the past 25 years, but there remain many areas of total ignorance in all investigational fields. This paper will mention only some fields where continuing work is crucial.

New Measuring Techniques: Their Value in Collaborative Studies

The availability of brain computerised tomography, PET scanning and NMR imaging provide the opportunity, along with other innovative techniques, for the elucidation of particular aspects of the disease and the correlation of these with clinical, and in some instances, neuropathological features. Much progress would be made in understanding the disease and its development if these techniques could be used in longitudinal studies. We know virtually nothing of the speed of development of brain atrophy, sulcal widening and ventricular dilatation in Alzheimer's disease nor the stage of the disease at which it actually develops. Limited personal experience suggests that neuropathological change is advanced when the patient first presents, but this is frequently many months, or even a year or more after relatives have first noted some change in cerebral function. We now have the opportunity to discover whether or not cerebral atrophy and ventricular dilatation are present early in the clinical presentation of the disorder or whether individual cases differ widely in this clearly fundamental feature. Similarly, it will shortly be possible to trace the development and localisation of metabolic abnormalities within the brain in life. Here again is the opportunity, through longitudinal studies, to trace the sequence of events with the strong possibility that this would lead to quite fundamental changes in our understanding of the disorder.

The Diagnosis of Early Cases

Quite clearly the use of new techniques in tracing cerebral changes which accompany the development of the disease would be much more certain if we had a

[1] Department of Pathology, Newcastle General Hospital, Newcastle Upon Tyne, NE4 6BE, Great Britain.

Neurology
Ed. by K. Poeck, H. J. Freund, and H. Gänshirt

reliable marker or procedure for early but certain diagnosis. In the absence of the former which is likely to come from biochemical or genetic developments, the production of more sophisticated psychometric tests which enable the confident detection of the earliest stages of the disease to be made would be a great step forward. The ability to differentiate the earliest stages of Alzheimer's disease from the non-progressive or more benign forms of memory and personality change which are relatively common in old age is clearly of great importance and failing the development of a reliable marker, patterns of change in batteries of psychometric tests may well be a method of investigation which, along with the various new procedures for examing in life the structure and function of the brain could lead (admittedly by arduous techniques) to the confident detection of the earliest cases showing minimal symptomatology.

The detection of such early cases and their thorough investigation in life by all possible means is of vital importance not only for our understanding of the disorder, but for the use of such cases in clinical trials of therapeutic agents and other forms of justifiable therapy. At this time we have to assume that the neuropathological changes which distinguish the later stages of the disorder, and which include nerve cell loss in the cerebral cortex and in a number of deep nuclei, are permanent and that detection of the earliest stages of the disorder only makes it possible to halt the neuropathological processes rather than reverse them. It seems absolutely certain that if we cannot influence or slow down the progress of the disease in its early, formative stages then there is no likelihood of affecting the great majority of patients who at this time are inevitably seen late in the development of the disorder.

Autopsy Study of the Earliest Cases: Contribution to Fundamental Knowledge of Pathology and Chemistry

The detection of the earliest stages of the disorder is not only of great importance clinically, but the investigation of such cases neuropathologically and biochemically, should they come to post mortem, could yield information which not only is totally defective now, but which might lead us to a reevaluation of our present concepts of the development of the disorder. The obtaining of even a small number of brains from people with the earliest symptomatology who die accidentally or from coincidental causes would give the opportunity to judge the significance of the present known neurochemical and neuropathological changes in the production of symptomatology. Detailed examination of the brain from individuals with minor symptoms could be most valuable. Such cases should be dissected and preserved in a way which enables all the necessary quantitative assessments of neuropathological change to be recorded, neuronal counts performed on precisely located cortical and deep nuclear structures and the widest range of neurochemical parameters determined on similar precisely identified samples. From such studies we might gain vital information about the sequence of involvement of the cortical and deep nuclear structures in pathological and chemical change. At the moment there is considerable argument and doubt about whether cortical or deep nuclear changes develop first or whether they progress together, and knowledge of the neuropathological and neurochemical changes which accompany early symptomatology or may occur without any apparent clinical abnormality is nonexistent. The detailed study of even a handful of very early cases could settle some of these important questions. Through the development of the new techniques which allow the earliest detection of both anatomical and biochemical change, and the study of occasional cases dying extremely early in the disease, we have the possibility of making fundamental advances in our knowledge of the natural history of the disease.

Need for Collaboration to Obtain the Most Information from Early Cases

Early cases coming to autopsy are too important to be retained by a single laboratory and the WFN would play a valuable role if, through its research groups, it enabled material obtained to be shared in a way which would produce the most information from the smallest number of cases. Naturally, to make significant progress there would need to be an agreement on the features which would establish the diagnosis for it is just possible that in the earliest stages of the disease neuropathological changes, particularly in the cerebral cortex, are minimal. If that were so it would indeed be a finding which would produce some optimism about possible therapy, but it seems much more likely that cortical changes, particularly in the presenile disease, would be sufficiently advanced in terms of plaque and tangle formation in the neocortex for the diagnosis to be made with confidence. Nevertheless, such agreement would be of fundamental importance for lack of uniformity in the use of diagnostic criteria for neuropathological diagnosis still produces unsatisfactory publications about Alzheimer's disease. World-wide agreement on the neuropathological changes which are necessary even in the late stage of the disorder to make a firm diagnosis is still needed and again the WFN could play a major role in setting these minimal criteria. All too often, even now, reliance is placed on examination of the hippocampus, and here, unless the most detailed and carefully controlled quantitative estimation of plaques and tangles are made, the diagnosis has to remain in some doubt since, as has been established in many studies in the past 20 years, all the cortical neuropathological stigmata of the disease tend to be more accentuated in the hippocampus and are, in occasional nondemented subjects, well developed and not readily distinguishable from demented cases without time-consuming quantitative procedures.

One Possible Source of Cases with Early Symptomatology

Acquiring confident contact with the earlier stages of the disorder may prove difficult. Physicians with knowledge of families in which an exceptionally high degree of Alzheimer's disease occurs have a unique possibility of seeing such early cases and subjecting them, through collaboration with other groups, to modern sophisticated investigations whereby the earliest symptomatology and its accompanying neuropathological and neurochemical changes may be defined. It could well be that the patterns of clinical development in cases with the familial form of the disease will differ from that of the more common nonfamilial cases of Alzheimer's disease, but even so, familial cases would present the possibilities of describing the very earliest changes and investigating all the features which accompany such early changes.

The Search for Subgroups

The delineation of what would appear to be subgroups of Alzheimer's disease or conditions of close similarity requires continuing further investigation. Patients with dyspraxia and further evidence of parietal lobe symptomatology have long been considered to have a shorter clinical course, and a group with dysphasia of slow progression associated with mild memory and personality disturbance has been delineated, the latter said to show an exceptional widening of the sylvian fissure on CT scanning. Are these "subgroups" distinguished by differences in neuropathological and neurochemical detail? Considerable effort continues to be put, quite rightly, into the investigation of the disease in the oldest affected groups, where beyond 80 years a number of investigators are convinced that the disorder is neuropathologically and possibly neurochemically and clinically of a modified kind. Particularly important for further investigation is the examination of the possibility that in old age, many cases which are clinically and perhaps biochemically indistinguishable from typical senile dementia of Alzheimer type (SDAT) occur in which senile plaques only are present in the neocortex either in the total absence of neurofibrillary tangles or in the presence of very few such changes. Considerable numbers of such cases have been reported in some series, but they are uncommon in the experience of many investigators. The detailed cerebral chemistry of such cases and the findings in the deep nuclei in both neuropathological and neurochemical terms is clearly of importance.

Do patients who are demented and with many senile plaques in the neocortex in the relative absence of neocortical tangles have the same changes in the deep nuclear structures as the typical case? Do they develop neurofibrillary tangles in the nucleus of Meynert, the locus coeruleus and the raphe nuclei of the brain stem? Is the biochemistry of these cases the same? If we can be certain that such cases exist in any number and that their symptomatology is indeed indistinguishable from that of the typical SDAT case and that no other disorder exists in these people which may contribute to their dementing syndrome then we would have to reassess the functional significance of neurofibrillary tangle formation in the disease process.

Further detailed analysis of cases above 80 years of age for comparison with younger Alzheimer disease subjects is also necessary to confirm that differences exist between the younger and old cases which are not merely those of degree. Great importance in pursuing this particular problem and indeed of the other variations which may occur, undoubtedly lies in the publication of authentic details of those cases which do not fit the standard recognised description of the pathology of presenile Alzheimer's disease. Editors and referees of papers published in reputable journals would do a great service if they insisted on the recording of the clinical, neuropathological and neurochemical details of such cases or refused their publication, as at present, with overwhelming interest world-wide in Alzheimer's disease there is much danger of confusion in the literature arising from the publication of articles in which some fundamental features are omitted in the final papers and possibly even from the initial protocols.

The Need for Investigation into the Neurochemistry of Dementia of Ischaemic Origin and its Influence on the Neurochemistry of Alzheimer's Disease

Intense interest in Alzheimer's disease has to some extent reduced the interest of many investigators into dementia resulting from ischaemic lesions; the latter are combined with the lesions of Alzheimer's disease in around 20% of cases developing in old age. Our knowledge of the influence of ischaemic destruction within the white matter or basal ganglia or stem on the neurochemistry of the cortex and the other deep nuclear structures is almost entirely defective at this time and yet such lesions present models for studying the effects on neurochemistry in anatomically related areas of lesions which can be precisely located within the brain. One of the sources of variation in neurochemical findings in cases of Alzheimer's disease lies in the methodology of examination of the brain in many laboratories since this may prevent the presence and anatomical location of ischaemic lesions being recorded. Tissue for neurochemistry should be obtained from precisely identified anatomical sites. This clearly requires skill and experience in anatomical dissection. Further, if the effects of ischaemic lesions on the neurochemistry of related brain areas is to be determined, or errors from ignoring ischaemic lesions are to be avoided, dissection and sampling of brain must be performed by someone with knowledge and experience of the recognition and anatomical location of ischaemic lesions. The prevailing habit of dividing the brain longitudinally through the midline with one hemisphere being made available for neurochemistry and the other for neuropathology carries with it the disadvantage that lesions in the two hemispheres may not be identical. If either of the hemispheres is examined by people unskilled in neuroanatomical dissection or the detection of other types of lesion there is the possibility that results will be misleading and the sources of error unrecognised. Obviously, in all studies of Alzheimer's disease careful note should be kept of the concomitant occurrence of other diseases and the neuropathological examination should be sufficient to eliminate other disorders, or if they are present, to define their severity and nature.

Alzheimer's Disease and Lewy Body Parkinson's Disease

The possible association between Alzheimer's disease and idiopathic or Lewy body Parkinson's disease needs detailed prospective studies which should involve both clinical, neuropathological and neurochemical investigation. The possible increased frequency of these two disorders occurring together raises important pathogenic and aetiological considerations. Our present knowledge of the association of these disorders is based on retrospective studies which have inevitable disadvantages, and this possible association requires careful reevaluation by prospective longitudinal studies at a number of centres throughout the world. Our present attitude towards Alzheimer's disease and SDAT is based on the presumption that it is a single disorder with uniform neuropathological and neurochemical characteristics, albeit with some possible subgroups, and that it has a common, single aetiology. Although this may well prove to be so there are many aspects of the disorder which need to be approached with the possibility in mind that aetiological factors may be multiple, that the disorder may differ in some fundamental respects in different parts of the world, and that genetic influences may, at least partially, determine these differences. The association of the disorder with idiopathic parkinsonism may also vary in different locations and it is not sufficient to accept the findings in a small number of centres as necessarily applying overall to the rest of the world.

Does the Disease Differ in Different Parts of the World?

The possibility that major variations exist within a framework of a basic neuropathological and neurochemical picture requires much further work. Variations in reported neuropathology, particularly in the cases in old age, illustrate this fact, but variations in molecular biological detail emphasise it more fundamentally. A significant illustration of the possibility of unidentified variations involves the study of amyloid in the brain in this condition and of neurofibrillary tangles. Different findings over the detailed investigation of both these important elements of the disease may not be simply the result of methodological differences. Is it necessary to assume that neurofibrillary tangles, because of their ultrastructural similarity from case to case, are necessarily biochemically the same in all cases or in all parts of the brain and that the factors which precipitate them are necessarily the same? Is it not possible that amyloid deposited in some brains and satisfying the ultrastructural definitions of that substance, may differ according to the aetiological mechanism which causes its deposition and which may not necessarily be the same from case to case and may indeed be varied by the genetic capability of the individual to produce biochemical sequences which may differ from that of other individuals. Our present techniques for isolating plaque amyloid and neurofibrillary tangles, although greatly advanced in the last decade, may nevertheless be insufficient at this time for settling many of the important problems which involve investigation of these structures. The elimination of contaminants is obviously of great importance and in relation to amyloid the separation of plaque amyloid from vascular amyloid, which is present in the majority of cases of Alzheimer's disease, is clearly of importance. Histological techniques allow such separation with exactitude, but limit the form of investigations which may be carried out.

Environmental Factors

The search for precipitating environmental factors is clearly vital. The influence of genetic factors in this disorder has become of even greater importance from recent studies of risk factors. We should nevertheless continue to pursue all avenues of research into other precipitating factors. It does not appear to be satisfactorily established that aluminium has no part to play. Here again we are in danger of assuming that because some investigations have produced negative results then those which have produced evidence of aluminium as a factor in the disease must necessarily be wrong. It seems unlikely that both are correct, but the possibility that there are cases in which aluminium has a role should not be eliminated because of carefully conducted studies which show no evidence of its involvement in another group of cases. Our thinking about Alzheimer's disease is too restricted if we assume that chemical and neuropathological findings and aetiology have to be identical and consistent from case to case. We had a simplified view of the development and aetiological factors of glomerulonephritic disorders 30 years ago and every year establishes the complex nature of the processes which may result in a terminal condition which on clinical and light microscopic grounds and without extremely sophisticated techniques, may appear to be a uniform end-stage disease. We must not ignore the possibility that in Alzheimer's disease we may be looking at the end-stage of a disorder to which there may be several different paths. The latter seems unlikely at this time and the obtaining of very early cases may well help settle the issue, but our thinking should not be restricted by assumptions on the uniformity of the disorder. Clearly, the search for a possible replicating agent has to be followed and in this respect the complicated relationship and influence of agent strain and the genetic constitution of the host (as illustrated by the scrapie model) may be of value in searching for the origins of the disorder.

Is All the Central Nervous System Involved?

A further important possibility needs to be established by detailed neuropathology and neurochemistry and that is whether all the central nervous system is involved in Alzheimer's disease. Many parts of the nervous system, particularly those affected by plaque and tangle formation, are subject to intense investigation, but structures apparently not affected by the disorder merit similar attention. The suggestion has been repeatedly made that neuronal RNA and nucleolar size are diminished in areas of the brain (cerebellum and brain stem nuclei) which are not apparently affected by any of the other characteristic changes of the disease. This raises the possibility that all the central nervous system may be involved in this disorder and that our present investigations and techniques are insufficient to detect the changes. It is necessary, therefore, to apply all available techniques to the investigation of those parts of the central nervous system not so far fully examined and which are not apparently or grossly affected in the disease. The publication of evidence of the normality of other areas of the brain is of equal importance to the publication of evidence of abnormality since widespread abnormality within the clinical nervous system has serious implications for therapeutic success and would strengthen the view that fundamental neuropathological and neurochemical changes throughout the whole nervous system are being produced by changes in genetic material.

2 Brain and Behavior

Mechanisms of Attention and Attentional Disorders. Session in Honor of the Late Dr. Norman Geschwind

The Impact of Dr. Geschwind's Work on Neuropsychology

K. Poeck [1]

This session is devoted to the memory of Dr. Norman Geschwind, who was one of the three organizers of the main topic of brain and behavior. He had just completed his part of the program, which was this session on mechanisms of attention and attentional disorders, when he was struck by a massive myocardial infarction. In fact, I learned the sad news one Monday morning, and in the afternoon I received a letter from him giving the final version of the program for this session.

In attempting to acknowledge the impact of Dr. Geschwind's work on present-day neurology and neuropsychology I am not going to describe his brilliant academic career with which you are all familiar. Rather, I shall try to highlight some fields where he was, and still is, in my view most influential. The first area is, of course, the reinstatement of neuroanatomy in behavioral neurology. In particular, Geschwind shifted the view from cortical centers that had been the sole preoccupation of localizationist researchers to the pathways connecting these centers. He elaborated on the notion that also those signals that underlie human behavior travel across the brain along certain fiber tracts from one distinct area to another. Symptoms and syndromes, consequently, were ascribed by him to disconnection of specified cortical areas, and this disconnection could be brought about either by subcortical damage to certain pathways or by damage to the cortical areas where those pathways originate or terminate. This held true for intrahemispheric as well as interhemispheric connections [3, 4].

The disconnection theory was inspired by Geschwind's acquaintance with eminent neuroanatomists, like Paul Yakovlev, by his knowledge of animal experimentation on the role of the corpus callosum, and by his avid reading and reinterpretation of the classical papers by Dejerine [1], Wernicke [2], and Liepmann [5]. Certainly, his close connection with Dr. Quadfasel gave him a familiarity with the older literature which surpassed that of any other living researcher. His interpretation of behavioral disturbances as disconnection phenomena was first received with admiration and enthusiasm. As with any theory that attempts to establish one basic

[1] Medizinische Fakultät der Technischen Hochschule Aachen, Abteilung Neurologie, Pauwelsstraße, 5100 Aachen, Federal Republic of Germany.

Neurology
Ed. by K. Poeck, H. J. Freund, and H. Gänshirt

explanatory model, it was later challenged under various aspects. Incidentally, this never offended him. Geschwind believed in the heuristic function of continuous discussion. Today most of us will agree that there are very many phenomena and groups of phenomena in behavioral neurology that simply cannot be explained otherwise. A field where his theory has proved most fruitful is that of the agnosias. Reading the classical papers, e.g., by Stauffenberg [10] in the light of Geschwind's interpretation makes one wonder why the classical authors did not explain the phenomena that were so brilliantly described by them on the basis of a disconnection mechanism.

The second aspect is the inauguration of studies on left–right asymmetries in the anatomic structure of the brain. Researchers had for decades looked in vain for asymmetries that simply had to be there, given the functional asymmetry of so many psychological performances. Geschwind's finding with Levitsky [9] on hemispheric differences in the size of the planum temporale was a revolutionary discovery that stimulated research in various directions. Wada was able to demonstrate the presence of these asymmetries as early as the middle of embryonic development. Other researchers, e.g., Galaburda or LeMay, described other aspects of asymmetry and, most important, there emerged an abundance of functional studies along this line. It is true that some of these studies have somehow simplified the principles of brain organization by treating the left and right hemispheres as if they represented the seat of unitary functions. This would not have been Geschwind's way of reasoning; he laid great stress on the differential intrahemispheric organization of functions. Shortly before his death he had just begun to summarize, together with Galaburda, his latest research on cerebral lateralization: biologic mechanisms, associations, and pathology [6–8]. Geschwind had conducted studies on the relationship between cerebral dominance and the human endocrinologic system. He recognized that certain immune disorders occur with especially high frequency in persons with anomalous cerebral dominance. The major three-part paper that has just appeared contains in the first line a hypothesis and a program for research. Whatever the final outcome of the wealth of pathophysiologic mechanisms suggested in these three papers, it is most impressive to consider the broad range of interest, covering virtually every part of medicine. At an age when many researchers are satisfied to work in one or two fields where they have gained international stature Geschwind embarked toward completely new areas. It is quite characteristic of him that he was driven to do so by one single pathogenetic concept, and it is equally characteristic that he began by posing a broad range of questions which he hoped to answer in future years of research.

As a clinician, Geschwind was equally outstanding. His rounds were legendary for their shrewd observation of patients and fascinating interpretation of findings. His lectures were didactic masterpieces. As a person, his most remarkable trait was an insatiable curiosity that led him to keep asking provocative questions. He was a multifaceted man. He certainly considered himself as one of the most influential neurologists of his time. Yet, he took critical comments in good spirit and enjoyed controversial discussions provided his partner had mastered the subject. He exhibited a rare blend of pride and modesty, and his appearance was enriched by a disarming generosity both in the field of science and in personal life. He was always fair, eager to inspire students, and to support junior researchers.

Geschwind was a great individualist. He was not in the strict sense of the word the founder of a school. Yet, his influence on contemporary behavioral neurology and on neurology in general is enormous, and there are few colleagues, even colleagues of his age, who have not been strongly influenced by his teaching. I think all of us who have had the pleasure of knowing him more closely were continuously stimulated, often instructed, sometimes irritated, but always attracted by his eminent scholarship. Personally, I have not known a man equally open-minded, curious, generous, and warmhearted. He has left his mark on contemporary neurology, and this will be true for a long time to come.

References

1. Geschwind N (1962) The anatomy of acquired disorders of reading. In: Money J (ed) Reading disability. Johns Hopkins Press, Baltimore, pp 115–129
2. Geschwind N (1963) Carl Wernicke, the Breslau School and the history of aphasia. In: Carterette EC (ed) Brain function, vol III: Speech, language and communication. University of California Press, Berkeley, pp 1–16
3. Geschwind N (1965) Disconnexion syndromes in animals and man. Brain 88:237–294
4. Geschwind N (1965) Disconnexion syndromes in animals and man. Brain 88:585–644
5. Geschwind N (1967) The apraxias. In: Straus EW, Griffith RM (ed) Phenomenology of will and action. Duquesne University Press, Pittsburgh, pp 91–102
6. Geschwind N, Galaburda AM (1985) Cerebral lateralization: Biological mechanisms, associations, and pathology: I. A hypothesis and a program for research. Arch Neurol 42:428–459
7. Geschwind N, Galaburda AM (1985) Cerebral lateralization: Biological mechanisms, associations, and pathology. II. A hypothesis and a program for research. Arch Neurol 42:521–552
8. Geschwind N, Galaburda AM (1985) Cerebral lateralization: Biological mechanisms, association, and pathology. III. A hypothesis and a program for research. Arch Neurol 42:634–654
9. Geschwind N, Levitsky W (1968) Human brain: Left–right asymmetries in temporal speech region. Science 161:186–187
10. von Stauffenberg W (1914) Über Seelenblindheit. Arb Hirnanat Inst, Zürich, H. 8

Anatomical Basis of Spatial Attention

G. Rizzolatti[1]

Attention is a term which derives from the common experience that physically identical stimuli may be perceived at different moments with different degrees of subjective clearness. Attention includes intensive phenomena, such as arousal, alertness, or attentiveness and selective phenomena. To the group of selective phenomena belongs the capacity to orient attention to different sectors of space: spatial attention. Deficits of this capacity are frequently encountered in patients in the form usually described as hemineglect. These patients, in the absence of primary sensory or motor deficits that may justify the symptoms, have difficulties in noticing events in the space contralateral to the lesion and to explore this space actively [see 1, 3].

One finding that clearly emerges from the literature on clinical and experimental neglect is that this syndrome may result following lesion of a large variety of cortical areas and subcortical centers [3, 10]. Among cortical areas the inferior parietal lobule, the frontal eye field (FEF), and the gyrus cinguli appear to play crucial roles; subcortical centers whose lesion produces neglect are the superior colliculus, the lateral hypothalamus, the substantia nigra, and parts of the striatum. Furthermore, some evidence exists that damage to intralaminar thalamic nuclei and to some parts of the brain stem reticular formation may also produce neglect [3, 10].

It is obvious that any theory of neglect must explain why attentional deficits are obtained with lesions of so many centers. The simplest way is to postulate that this occurs because the various centers and areas whose lesion produces neglect are part of a single attentional circuit. This type of explanation of neglect has been proposed, for example, by Heilman and his co-workers [3] and, in another form, by Mesulam [10]. Although this idea is appealing, an anatomic circuit including all the above mentioned centers appears to be extremely unlikely. The connections between some parts of it are very indirect and what is more important it does not appear that connections between centers forming the circuit are more direct or richer than those between the same centers and others not involved in attention.

In this paper I shall propose that neglect can occur following lesion of several circuits, each of them being to a large extent independent of the others. Each circuit has primarily a sensorimotor function. It extracts information from the environment and, in the presence of adequate stimuli, programs motor acts directed toward a specific part of space. When one of these circuits is internally activated it facilitates

[1] Istituto di Fisiologia Umana, Università di Parma, Via Gramsci 14, 43100 Parma, Italy.

Neurology
Ed. by K. Poeck, H. J. Freund, and H. Gänshirt

its afferent part [see 21], thus rendering it more sensitive to particular sectors of the environment, and simultaneously it inhibits other sensorimotor circuits, acting in this way as a filter for concurrent sensorimotor activities [15].

The strongest evidence in favor of this hypothesis comes from cases that I shall refer to as cases of atypical neglect, that is from syndromes in which the neglect is present and yet the attentional deficits are different from those classically observed in right parietal patients.

One type of atypical neglect can be demonstrated in cats after a sagittal section of the tectal commissures [9]. Animals with this lesion show motor and attentional deficits. Motor deficits consist in a marked reduction or even absence of vertical eye movements and in an abnormal posture of the head, which is held slightly ventro-flexed. At variance with normal cats, commissurotomized animals never look up and explore the space above their head. There is a clear deficit in their capacity to orient to visual stimuli abruptly presented in the upper visual space. The capacity to follow objects vertically is also impaired. When a piece of food is moved in an upward direction, starting in the lower field, the animal follows it until it reaches approximately the head midplane. Then the head movement stops and the cat appears to ignore where the food is. When the food is moved downward the animal has a startling reaction when the food reaches the lower visual space; until this moment the animal appears to be completely unaware of the stimulus. Formal testing of the upper and lower visual space carried out in our laboratory confirmed the upper space deficit. Animals with a complete lesion show a very slow recovery. Those with partial sections recover in less than 2 weeks.

In animals in which the lesion is anteriorly located and comprises the posterior commissure and the rostralmost part of the intertectal commissure, the deficits are different from those in which the intertectal commissures are severed [9]. There is no ventro-flexion of the head and no tendency to explore the lower space. In contrast, there is a slight head dorsiflexion and a preference to explore the upper space. Downward tracking head movements are slow and less accurate than upward movements. When two pieces of food held together in front of the animal are moved suddenly apart, one upward, the other downward, the animals constantly follow that moving upward. Similarly, if a piece of food is first moved downward and is then left in the lower visual space, the animal appears to be disoriented and is able to find it only after some time.

These data clearly indicate that in the cat the interruption of the midbrain commissures produces a vertical neglect. The attentional deficit is spatially correlated with postural and movement deficits. When the lesion is centered upon the posterior commissure the neglect involves the lower visual space and the head is dorsiflexed; when the lesion interrupts the intertectal commissures the neglect involves the upper visual fields and the head is ventriflexed.

Vertical attentional deficits similar to those experimentally obtained in the cat have also been observed in humans. Patients affected by progressive supranuclear palsy often show, beside other deficits, partial or total incapacity to move the eyes vertically and a slight dorsiflexion of the head [20]. These motor symptoms are accompanied by difficulties of orienting toward stimuli in the lower visual space [14]. For example, when eating they may stare straight ahead, fumbling with their meal, although they are quite able to look down on command, or they may stumble over objects in their path in the absence of motor deficits that may explain this behavior. The presence of attentional deficits in the vertical plane has been demonstrated in these patients by Posner et al. [13] in a series of elegant experiments. Recently, Camarda (personal communication) observed a patient with progressive supranuclear palsy who showed head dorsiflexion, paresis of downward directed eye movements, and marked attentional deficit in the lower visual space. CT scan showed a zone of hypodensity corresponding to the rostral pole of the superior colliculi, especially at the level of their midline. The analogy of the human syndrome with that experimentally obtained in animals is certainly compelling.

Another case of atypical neglect can be demonstrated in monkeys after lesion of lateral area 6 (areas FCBm and FBA of Von Bonin and Bailey) [17]. Prompted by some neurophysiologic data on the neuron properties of this region [18], we tested the animals by presenting stimuli outside their reach (far space), within the reach of their arm (distant peripersonal space), and around their mouth (pericutaneous buccal space). The testing was done by moving a piece of food held by a pair of forceps at different distances or by using two pieces of food. In this case the two pieces were initially kept close one to another, then, when the animal fixated them, one was moved while the other remained still in front of it; alternatively, both pieces were moved. Finally, frightening stimuli were presented far from or close to the monkey.

After lateral area 6 lesion, the animals did not show any visual deficit for stimuli presented in the far space and in distant peripersonal space. In contrast, striking disturbances were observed in the pericutaneous space around the mouth. When the animal was fixating a central stimulus, the introduction of a piece of food ipsilateral to the lesion produced, as in normal animals, an immediate mouth grasping response; the same stimulus shown contralaterally was ignored. When a stimulus was moved slowly from a central position near the mouth to the neglected side, the animal often appeared to be aware of the stimulus and tended to follow it, but had great difficulty in organizing the appropriate head and mouth movement necessary for grasping it. Most commonly the animal slowly opened its mouth and followed the stimulus with the mouth open, but without trying to take the object. With a simultaneous presentation of two stimuli, the monkey always tended to reach for the one ipsilateral to the lesion. Blinking in response to threatening stimuli moved toward the contralateral hemiface was absent. In contrast, facial movements were easily elicited by emotional stimuli presented far from the animal.

Deficits similar to those demonstrated with visual stimuli were present when the hemiface contralateral to the lesion was stimulated with tactile stimuli. Stimulation of the lips with food or other stimuli produced either no response or opening of the mouth not accompanied by any attempt to bite. Licking movements could not be elicited by wetting the contralateral lip with water or juice. Beside tactile and visual stimuli the animal showed a marked preference in using the hand ipsilateral to the lesion. Only when this hand was blocked did the animal, albeit reluctantly, employ the contralateral hand. There was no misreaching, but the movement was somewhat slower than with the normal arm.

There was a marked and rather fast recovery with time. The only residual deficits 60 days after the operation were the preference in using the hand ipsilateral to the lesion and a constant turning, in the test with two peribuccal stimuli, toward that ipsilateral to the lesion.

If the symptoms subsequent to a lateral area 6 lesion are compared with those of typical neglect, as for example that occurring in the monkey after a lesion of the FEF, the differences are remarkable. In the former case the attentional deficit is related to the peripersonal space, in the second it concerns essentially the far space. This last point has been well demonstrated by Gentilucci et al. [2] in conditioned monkeys by measuring the latency of saccadic eye movements to ipsilateral and contralateral visual stimuli presented far from and near the animal. A significantly greater latency increase was found after a FEF lesion for far stimuli than for those in the peripersonal space. A second remarkable difference between the two types of neglect concerns the types of motor deficits. After FEF lesion there is a decrease in saccadic eye movement and, more generally, a decrease of exploratory movements toward the contralateral field. These findings fit well with the electrophysiologic data showing that FEF play a central role in the generation of saccadic eye movements. In contrast, after a lateral area 6 lesion, the deficits affect the mouth–head movement and in lesser degree the arm movements. Thus, the attentional deficits concern different sectors of space and again, as in the case of midbrain lesions, they are congruent with the motor defect.

In recent years several studies have been devoted to the cortical areas presumably involved in spatial attention. In particular the corticocortical connections of parietal and frontal areas have been well established. The prediction of a single attentional circuit theory is that areas involved in neglect are either directly interconnected [10] or that they send axons to a unilateral "arousing" system whose activity is essential for rendering attentive the hemisphere where these areas are located [see 3]. This second possibility can easily be dismissed. If a lesion of a cortical area, let us say FEF, depresses the arousing system of an entire hemisphere, one would expect that all the attentional capacities of this hemisphere would be altered. The data show that this does not occur. In the case of an FEF lesion the animal can still direct attention to its personal and peripersonal space [6, 17]. This type of dissociation cannot be accounted for by an arousal interpretation. One may attempt to escape this conclusion by postulating the existence of arousing circuits limited to restricted regions of each hemisphere. However, although this proposal may save the arousing idea, it contradicts the main point of the arousing theory, that of a single attentional circuit.

The single circuit theory in its corticocortical version [10] is not supported by anatomic evidence. Broadly speaking there are at least three main pathways in the monkey that convey information from the association areas of parietal lobe to the frontal lobe [see 12]. The first connects the superior parietal lobule (area 5 or PE) with the dorsal parts of areas 4 and 6 and with the supplementary motor area. The second leaves the rostral part of the inferior parietal lobule (area PF or 7b) and terminates in the lateral area 6, in area 46 below the principal sulcus, and in the frontal and pericentral opercular cortex. The third connects the caudal part of the inferior parietal lobule (area PG or 7a) with area 8, 46, the anteriormost dorsal area 6, and the gyrus cinguli.

The first of these circuits conveys essentially proprioceptive information [11] and, as far as we know, is not related to attention. The third circuit is mostly, although not exclusively, involved in visually guided oculomotor behavior [5, 7]. The second circuit is formed by polysensory neurons that respond to somatosensory stimuli and to visual stimuli located in the animal's peripersonal space [5, 18]. A lesion of these last two circuits produces the classical "exploratory–oculomotor neglect" and "reaching–peripersonal space" neglect, respectively.

No connections appear to exist between areas belonging to these circuits in the intermediate part of the frontal lobe (areas 6 and 8) [8], and similarly there is no connection between areas PE on one side and PF and PG on the other [19]. However, reciprocal pathways link the rostral part of the inferior parietal lobule (area PF) to the caudal part of it (PE) [19]. These data may suggest that the inferior parietal lobule is a kind of master center of attention, controlling the two parietofrontal circuits involved in it. If this were so one would expect that: (a) this region were not parcellated, as it is, in anatomically distinct zones; and (b) that lesions of any part of it produced a global attentional deficit. Experiments performed by Rizzolatti et al. [16] showed that after lesion of area PF the consequent attentional disturbances are very similar to those following the lesion of lateral area 6. Conversely, lesion of area PE produces attentional deficits of the type observed after FEF lesion [5, 7]. Thus, the idea that the inferior parietal lobule is the master center for directing attention in space is not confirmed by empirical evidence.

The idea of a distributed system for attention, similar to that postulated for the organization of actions, may also explain the vertical subcortical neglect. Although anatomic and functional data on the brain stem mechanisms responsible for head movements are much less rich than those concerning the parietal and frontal lobes, the classical data of Hess and his co-workers [4] clearly support our proposal. On the basis of their lesion and stimulation studies they suggested that there are two brain stem systems involved in vertical head movements. The first, controlling head elevation, has its center corresponding to the rostral part of the nucleus interstitialis of Cajal and comprises the system of fibers descending from it and the reticular neurons located along their course. Electrical stimulation of this system elicits raising of the head, while its destruction causes ventro-flexion of the head. The second midbrain system controlling head movement includes the nucleus of the posterior commissure and its ascending and descending projections, most of which pass through the posterior commissure. Stimulation of the nuclei of the posterior commissure elicits lowering of the head and foretrunk, whereas its destruction causes dorsiflexion of the head and a peculiar goose-like gait. There is an obvious analogy between these data and those we obtained after midbrain lesions [9]. The novelty of our findings is that lesion of these premotor systems also produces neglect, the aspect of which depends upon the motor properties of the circuit that has been damaged. Thus, lesions of the midbrain circuits have consequences in attentional terms similar to those of cortical circuits, although their anatomic connections with the latter are rather indirect.

In conclusion, the available evidence appears to be incompatible with the notion that a single circuit is responsible for directing spatial attention. Spatial attention appears to be strictly linked with the organization of motor activity in space, and all those circuits that have this function, regardless of the effectors they control, also have attentional properties. This formulation of the spatial attention problem provides an explanation of the puzzling fact that so many centers and cortical areas appear to be involved in spatial attention and allows one to explain the atypical cases of neglect.

A weakness of the distributed theory of spatial attention is that it does not specify how the various attentional circuits interact or are controlled in order to give coherence to the behavior of the individual. It is indeed very plausible that some central system may exist and that, according to the motivational state, previous experience, and the environmental context, it may facilitate or inhibit the various sensorimotor circuits forming the distributed attentional system. It is important to note however that a lesion of this hypothetical control system should not necessarily produce spatial inattention. A lesion of it should produce an impairment in the choice of the appropriate sensorimotor circuit, that is of that circuit that more adequately responds to internal necessities and to the environmental challenges. Behaviorally, this will result in interference between various motor programs, perseveration, and confusion. It would be premature and beyond the scope of this paper to discuss where this hypothetical system is located, but I think it is important to keep in mind that the unity of our behavior does not necessarily imply a "center" whose lesion produces neglect.

References

1. De Renzi E (1982) Disorders of space exploration and cognition. Wiley, London
2. Gentilucci M, Gentilini M, Porro CA, Matelli M, Rizzolatti G (1986) Effects of unilateral frontal eye field lesions on saccadic eye movements to near and far targets (in preparation)
3. Heilman KM, Watson RT (1977) Mechanisms underlying the unilateral neglect syndrome. Adv Neurol 18:93–105
4. Hess WR, Bürgi S, Bucher V (1946) Motorische Funktion des Tektal- und Tegmentalgebietes. Monatsschr Psychiatr Neurol 112:1–52
5. Hyvärinen J (1982) The parietal cortex of monkey and man. Springer, Berlin Heidelberg New York, pp 202 (Studies of brain function, vol 8)
6. Latto R, Cowey A (1971) Visual field defects after frontal-eye-field lesions in monkeys. Brain Res 30:1–24
7. Lynch JL (1980) The functional organization of posterior parietal association cortex. Behav Brain Sci 3:485–499
8. Matelli M, Camarda R, Glickstein M, Rizzolatti G (1984) Interconnections within the postarcuate cortex (area 6) of the macaque monkey. Brain Res 310:388–392
9. Matelli M, Olivieri MF, Saccani A, Rizzolatti G (1983) Upper visual space neglect and motor deficits after section of the midbrain commissures in the cat. Behav Brain Res 10:263–285
10. Mesulam MM (1981) A cortical network for directed attention and unilateral neglect. Ann Neurol 10:309–325
11. Mountcastle VB, Lynch JL, Georgopoulos A, Sakata H, Acuna C (1975) Posterior parietal association cortex of the monkey: command functions for operations within extrapersonal space. J Neurophysiol 38:871–908
12. Petrides M, Pandya DN (1984) Projections to the frontal cortex from the posterior parietal region in the rhesus monkey. J Comp Neurol 228:105–116
13. Posner MI, Walker JA, Friedrich FJ, Rafal RD (1984) Effects of parietal injury on covert orienting of visual attention. J Neurosci 4:1863–1877
14. Rafal RD, Grimm RJ (1981) Progressive supranuclear palsy: functional analysis of the response to metysergide and anti-Parkinson agents. Neurology 31:1507–1518
15. Rizzolatti G (1983) Mechanisms of selective attention in mammals. In: Ewert JP, Capranica RR, Ingle DJ (eds) Advances in vertebrate neuroethology. Plenum, London, pp 261–297
16. Rizzolatti G, Gentilucci M, Matelli M (1985) Selective spatial attention: one center, one circuit or many circuits? In: Posner MI, Marin O (eds) Attention and performance XI. Erlbaum, Hillsdale, New Jersey, pp 251–265

17. Rizzolatti G, Matelli M, Pavesi G (1983) Deficits in attention and movement following the removal of postarcuate (area 6) and prearcuate (area 8) cortex in macaque monkeys. Brain 106:655–673
18. Rizzolatti G, Scandolara C, Matelli M, Gentilucci M (1981) Afferent properties of periarcuate neurons in macaque monkeys. II. Visual responses. Behav Brain Res 2:147–163
19. Seltzer B, Pandya DN (1980) Converging visual and somatic sensory input to intraparietal sulcus of the rhesus monkey. Brain Res 192:339–351
20. Steele JC, Richardson JC, Olszewski J (1964) Progressive supranuclear palsy. Arch Neurol 10:333–359
21. Wurtz RH, Goldberg ME, Robinson DL (1980) Behavioral modulation of visual responses in the monkey: stimulus selection for attention and movement. In: Sprague JM, Epstein AN (eds) Progress in psychobiology and physiological psychology, vol 9. Academic, New York, pp 43–83

The Contribution of Electrophysiology to the Study of Attention

M. E. GOLDBERG[1]

Introduction

One of the most difficult tasks that the central nervous system must perform is the filtering of the great mass of sensory data constantly impinging upon the organism. We live in a world of rich detail, only a small fraction of which can we use as data for behavior. We ignore most of the welter of sights, sounds, smells, and touches, responding only to those significant for our own lives. Attention is the selection process by which the brain filters out extraneous sensory information in order to concentrate on certain aspects of the environment. In the nineteenth century William James [8] wrote:

> Everyone knows what attention is. It is the taking possession of the mind, in clear and vivid form, of one out of what seem several simultaneous possible objects or trains of thought. Focalization, concentration of consciousness are of its essence. It implies withdrawal from some things in order to deal effectively with others.

A century later it is still appropriate to use James' concept as the starting point for a physiologic analysis of attention: the process by which the nervous system handles some stimuli at the expense of others [12].

In the primate the structure of the retina greatly facilitates the process of visual attention. Rather than acting as a homogeneous sheet of film, the retina concentrates most of its analytic power into a small portion of the center of the visual field, the fovea. Visual images falling on the fovea are analyzed in great detail. When a human or a monkey attends to an object it will most likely look at that object in order to analyze it with the greater power of the fovea. It is therefore possible to analyze what a subject is attending to by analyzing where it is looking [18]. In order to facilitate rapid shifts of attention by rapid shifts of eye position, the oculomotor system has developed the capacity to control eye position with great accuracy and speed, rapidly effecting changes of foveal position from one object of interest to another. The rapid change of foveal position is the saccade, a rapid conjugate eye movement with a reaction time of roughly 0.25 s, and a peak velocity of

[1] Laboratory of Sensorimotor Research, National Eye Institute, Building 10, Room 10B09, Bethesda, MD 20892, USA.

Neurology
Ed. by K. Poeck, H. J. Freund, and H. Gänshirt

close to 900°/s for a 20° eye movement. Much information about the physiology of attention has, perforce, come from the study of the neural mechanisms associated with saccadic eye movements.

Recently, several areas of the primate brain, including the superior colliculus [6], the frontal eye fields [5, 11], and the posterior parietal cortex [2, 10, 13], have been implicated in attentional processes, as a result of studies of the physiologic properties of single neurons studied in monkeys capable of making saccadic eye movements.

Methods for the Physiologic Study of Attention

In order to study the properties of neurons which might be related to attentional or oculomotor processes, it is necessary to record from single neurons in awake, behaving animals rather than the anesthetized, paralyzed preparation that has been the mainstay of neurophysiology since the nineteenth century. Combining techniques developed for studying the skeletal motor system [3] with techniques for conditioning eye movements, Wurtz [15] developed a method of studying visual and oculomotor properties of single neurons in awake monkeys. In this technique a monkey is trained to perform a series of visual tasks. The easiest task is to look at a spot of light and release a lever when the spot dims. A more complicated task is to look at the original light and make a saccadic eye movement if the light should disappear and another spot appear elsewhere on the screen. The first of these tasks is called the fixation task. Since the animal looks at the small spot (the fixation point), it does not break fixation to look at any other spots of light that may appear on the tangent screen. These stimuli are called passive or behaviorally irrelevant stimuli because the animal is not required to react in any way toward them. In the second task, called the saccade task, the stimulus is not behaviorally irrelevant. Instead of evoking no response, the stimulus becomes the target for an eye movement. In this latter case the animal has clearly attended to the stimulus. In the fixation case it is tempting to argue that the animal does not attend to the stimulus. It is, of course, impossible to know when an animal does not attend to a stimulus. All we can say is that the animal does not respond to the stimulus. However, there is some significant circumstantial evidence that in the fixation case the animal does indeed not attend to the passive stimulus, as will be discussed later.

After the animal has learned these two tasks it is prepared surgically for neurophysiologic recording. Under anesthesia, cylinders are placed stereotactically in the animal's skull with the underlying bone removed. After the animal recovers, microelectrodes can be passed through the intact dura and into the brain, and the activity of single neurons recorded while the animal is performing a task.

Behavioral Enhancement of Neuronal Visual Responses

The first step in analyzing a cell is to present a series of passive visual stimuli and find out where on the screen a light can evoke a response in the neuron. Figure 1*A* shows the visual response of a single neuron in the monkey frontal eye field. The illustration shows that in trial after trial the neuron discharges reliably after the onset of the visual stimulus. This neuron is therefore visually responsive. The superior colliculus, posterior parietal cortex, and frontal eye fields all have visually responsive neurons [17]. The receptive fields of these neurons lie generally (but not exclusively) in the contralateral visual field, and the neurons can be driven easily by spots of light without regard to stimulus orientation, color, or in most cases, direction of movement. Half of the neurons in these areas have a unique property: when the animal uses the stimulus in the receptive field as the target for an eye movement, the discharge of the neuron to the stimulus is markedly enhanced. Figure 1 *C* shows an example of this phenomenon in the frontal eye fields. The visual stimulus evoking the response is the same in Fig. 1*A* and 1*C*. However, in Fig. 1*A* the monkey is continuing to look at the fixation point, and is ignoring (not responding) to the stimulus in the receptive field. In the trials in Fig. 1*C*, the animal is making an eye movement to the stimulus in the receptive field. Note that the intensity of the discharge is increased, in this case by a factor of 3.4. The response to the stimulus is truncated by the animal's moving its eyes, and thus removing the stimulus from the receptive field. However, it is clear that as long as the stimulus is in the receptive field of the neuron, the discharge it evokes is markedly enhanced.

This presaccadic enhancement could be due to many factors. For example, there may be a pupillary dilatation preceding an eye movement, and the enhancement may be due to the increased luminous flux on the retina. Alternatively, the central fixation disappears when the saccade target appears, and the neuron might be responding to the release of the central fixation point. Another possibility is that the

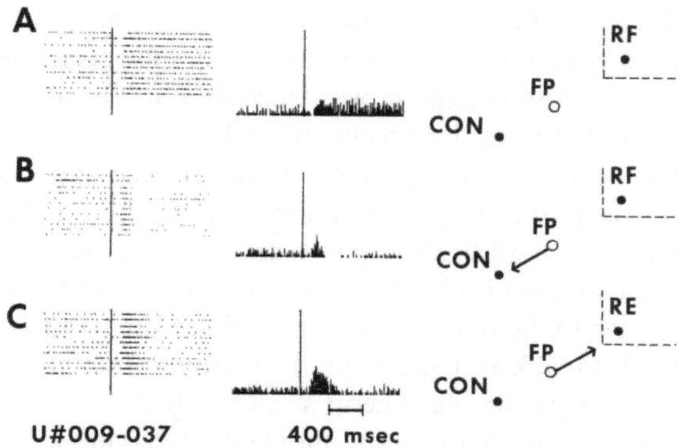

Fig. 1A–C. Presaccadic enhancement in a frontal eye field neuron. In this illustration the diagram on the left is a dot raster. Each *dot* corresponds to a neuronal action potential. Each *line* corresponds to a behavioral trial. The neuronal discharges in successive trials are synchronized on the onset of the passive visual stimulus, which is delineated by the *vertical line.* To the right of each raster the discharges are summed as a histogram. The *vertical trigger line* corresponds to a frequency of 152 Hz. **A** shows the discharge of the neuron to the onset of two stimuli; one (*CON*) outside the receptive field and one (*RF*) inside it. The approximate borders of the receptive field are shown by the *dotted line.* **B** shows the response of the same neuron when the animal makes a saccade to the control stimulus, even though the receptive field stimulus comes on. **C** shows the response of the same neurons when the animal makes a saccade to the receptive field stimulus. The *vertical trigger line* represents the onset of the stimulus in each display. Reproduced with permission from the *Journal of Neurophysiology* [5]

animal's level of arousal may be different when it performs the saccade task from when it performs the fixation task. This different level of arousal could result in an increase of excitability of all visual neurons, not only those in which the receptive field stimulus will be the target for an eye movement. Finally, the presaccadic enhancement could be spatially specific: the enhancement would only occur when a stimulus in the receptive field is the target for the eye movement. Figure 1 *B* shows that in the frontal eye fields the presaccadic enhancement is indeed spatially specific. In this experiment the animal is presented with two spots, one in the receptive field of the neuron (the receptive field spot, *RF*) and one far from the receptive field (the control spot, *CON*). Although both spots appear when the fixation point disappears, the animal is rewarded only when it makes an eye movement to the control spot, and not when it makes an eye movement to the spot in the receptive field. In this case the response is not significantly enhanced when compared with the fixation case. Thus, in the frontal eye fields the visual response of neurons can be enhanced only when the animal makes an eye movement to the stimulus in the receptive field, and not when the animal makes an eye movement elsewhere. This result can have two possible interpretations: the enhancement could be related to the eye movement itself, or it could be related to the shift of attention that precedes and accompanies the eye movement. Similar spatially specific presaccadic enhancement is found in the posterior parietal cortex and the superior colliculus.

The Dissociation of Eye Movement and Attention in the Posterior Parietal Cortex

The enhancement of visual response before a saccade seemed to be a good model for a central mechanism of attention. However, since eye movements and attention can be dissociated, it was necessary to see if the enhancement effect could be separated from the process of making saccades. A modification of the fixation task has been used to separate eye movements and attention in the monkey [2, 16]. In this task, the peripheral attention task, the monkey is presented with two stimuli. One is a small fixation point, and the other is a large peripheral stimulus. Either of the two stimuli can dim, and the monkey is rewarded for releasing the bar in response to the dimming of either. Since the fixation point is quite small, the monkey tends to look at it and to use its peripheral retina to perceive the much more obvious dimming of the peripheral stimulus. If the monkey does indeed break fixation, the computer monitoring the monkey's behavior will abort the trial. The result of this behavioral manipulation is that the monkey must attend to a stimulus to which it may not be able to make an eye movement.

In the superior colliculus [16] and the frontal eye fields [5] a stimulus which is the subject of a peripheral attention task will not evoke an enhanced response from a visual neuron, whether or not the neuron yields an enhanced response to a saccade target. In the posterior parietal cortex, however, enhancement of the visual response occurs in those neurons which do not yield an evoked response to saccade targets. Figure 2 compares the activity of neurons in the posterior parietal cortex and the frontal eye fields in the fixation, saccade, and peripheral attention tasks. Both neurons show presaccadic enhancement, and the parietal neuron also displays sac-

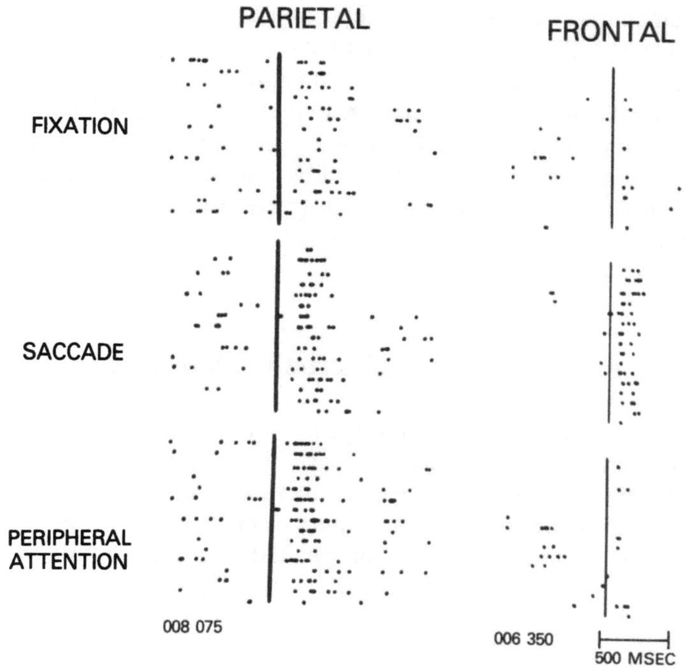

Fig. 2. Comparison of enhancement of visual response in parietal and frontal eye field neurons for fixation, saccade, and peripheral attention tasks. Each column shows the response of a neuron in the parietal cortex (*left column*) or frontal cortex (*right column*) to the onset of the visual stimulus in the fixation task, saccade task, or peripheral attention task. Note that although both neurons show presaccadic enhancement, only the parietal neuron shows enhancement in the peripheral attention task. Reproduced with permission from *Vision Research* [4]

cade-independent enhancement. This neuron has a rather weak visual response in the fixation task when the animal may ignore the stimulus, and gives a brisker response when the animal must make a saccade to the simulus or respond to it in the peripheral attention task. Peripheral attention enhancement is spatially specific in the posterior parietal cortex: when the animal attends to a stimulus outside the receptive field the response to the stimulus in the receptive field is not enhanced [2]. This experiment also provides circumstantial evidence that the animal does in fact not attend to a passively presented visual stimulus that has been presented for many consecutive trials. If the animal had been attending to the stimulus during the passive trials one would have expected the level of discharge to be the same as those in the peripheral attention task, because in the latter the animal is presumably attending to the stimulus. This is not the case, so the implication is that the animal is actually ignoring the stimulus during a series of passive trials.

The enhancement of visual responsiveness which occurs in the posterior parietal cortex is an excellent candidate for a neural mechanism for visual attention. Attended stimuli evoke more discharges than unattended ones. If we assume that the amount of effect that a stimulus has on the brain is a quantitative function of the number of discharges evoked by that stimulus, then an attended stimulus will have a greater effect than an unattended one. In the posterior parietal cortex, activity is dependent not only on the physical nature of the stimulus, but also on the behavioral significance of the stimulus. Activity in the posterior parietal cortex is subject to a gain control by an attentional factor, and only attended stimuli will have high rates of discharge in parietal neurons subject to behavioral enhancement. Since this gain control is independent of the strategy with which the animal will react to a stimulus, it must be related to the attentional factors which presumably accompany any response to a stimulus.

The Frontal Eye Fields and Attentive Movement

In the superior colliculus and the frontal eye fields, enhancement only occurs when the animal is going to make an eye movement to the stimulus, and not when the animal attends to it in some way that does not involve an eye movement. In these areas the quantitative enhancement of the effect of a stimulus is not involved in a general attentional mechanism, but rather in transmitting the enhanced visual re-

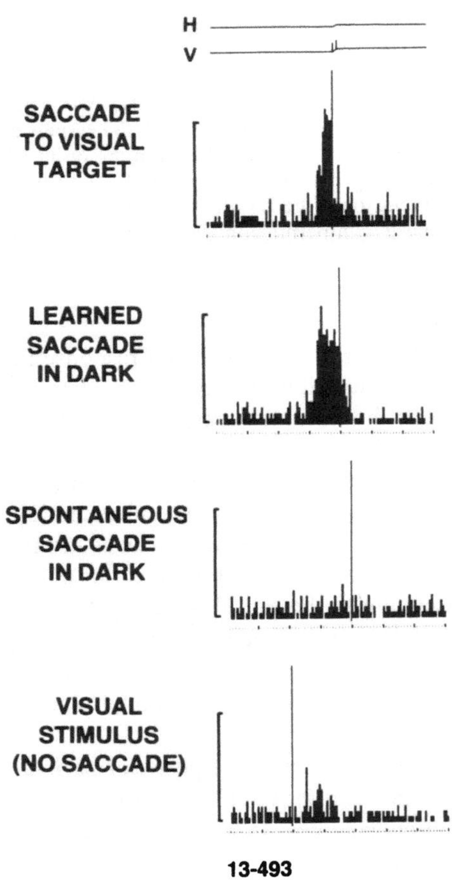

Fig. 3. Comparison of activity of a frontal eye field neuron before saccades of different motivation. The top histogram shows the activity before visually guided saccades, the second before learned saccades to a remembered point in total darkness, the third in association with spontaneous saccades, and the fourth in response to the same visual stimulus in a fixation task. Each histogram *calibration line* represents a discharge rate of 100 Hz. The *vertical line* in each histogram represents the alignment event, the beginning of the eye movement in the first three and the appearance of the stimulus in the receptive field in the fourth. Reproduced with permission from the *Journal of Neurophysiology* [1]

sponse to the oculomotor system. The frontal eye fields, however, are not unrelated to attentional mechanisms. The frontal eye fields contain a class of presaccadic movement neurons that discharge not only before visually guided saccades, but also before purposive saccades that are made to remembered targets for which there are no retinal stimuli [1]. These cells discharge much less, if at all, before spontaneous saccades made in total darkness.

Figure 3 gives an example of the dissociation in the frontal eye fields of discharge before two kinds of attentive movement and discharge before spontaneous saccades in darkness. Note the brisk discharge before visually guided and learned saccades, and the absent discharge before equivalent spontaneous saccades. It is not surprising that frontal movement neurons do not discharge before all saccades, since not all eye movements need be related to active visual attention. Monkeys make spontaneous eye movements in total darkness, and humans can make spontaneous saccades when they perform nonvisual tasks such as mental arithmetic. In these cases the eye movements are not a part of visual attentive behavior, and in these cases the frontal eye fields do not discharge before eye movements. This contrasts with movement-related neurons in the intermediate layer of the superior colliculus [17] which discharge before all saccades, even spontaneous saccades in total darkness and the quick phases of nystagmus. Thus, the presaccadic mechanism in the frontal eye fields can be considered to provide the motor signal for attentive exploration of the environment. The absence of such an attentive mechanism might explain the short-lived neglect associated with frontal lesions in humans [7] and monkeys [14]. Such patients have a less efficient method of making specific attentive eye movements because they lack the frontal eye fields, and in the early stages of recovery this deficit may be manifest as a more global neglect.

References

1. Bruce CJ, Goldberg ME (1985) Primate frontal eye fields. I: Single neurons discharging before saccades. J Neurophysiol 53:603–635
2. Bushnell MC, Goldberg ME, Robinson DL (1981) Behavioral enhancement of visual responses in monkey cerebral cortex. I. Modulation in posterior parietal cortex related to selective visual attention. J Neurophysiol 46:755–772
3. Evarts EV (1966) Methods for recording activity of individual neurons in moving animals. Methods Med Res 11:241–250
4. Goldberg ME, Bruce CJ (1985) Cerebral cortical activity associated with the orientation of visual attention in the Rhesus monkey. Vision Res 25:472–482
5. Goldberg ME, Bushnell MC (1981) Behavioral enhancement of visual responses in monkey cerebral cortex. II. Modulation in frontal eye fields specifically related to saccades. J Neurophysiol 46:773–787
6. Goldberg ME, Wurtz RH (1972) Activity of superior colliculus in behaving monkey. II. Effect of attention on neuronal responses. J Neurophysiol 35:560–574
7. Heilman KM, Valenstein E (1972) Frontal lobe neglect in man. Neurology 22:660–664
8. James W (1890) The principles of psychology. Holt, New York
9. Lynch JC (1981) The functional organization of posterior parietal association cortex. Behav Brain Sci 4:485–534
10. Lynch JC, Mountcastle VB, Talbot WH, Yin TCT (1977) Parietal lobe mechanisms for directed visual attention. J Neurophysiol 40:362–389
11. Mohler CW, Goldberg ME, Wurtz RH (1973) Visual receptive fields of frontal eye field neurons. Brain Res. 61:385–389

12. Posner MI (1980) Orienting of attention. Q J Exp Psychol 32:3–24
13. Robinson DL, Goldberg ME, Stanton GB (1978) Parietal association cortex in the primate: sensory mechanisms and behavioral modulations. J Neurophysiol 41:910–932
14. Welch K, Stuteville P (1958) Experimental production of unilateral neglect in monkeys. Brain 81:341–347
15. Wurtz RH (1969) Visual receptive fields of striate cortex neurons in awake monkeys. J Neurophysiol 32:727–742
16. Wurtz RH, Mohler CW (1976) Organization of monkey superior colliculus: enhanced visual response of superficial layer cells. J Neurophysiol 39:745–765
17. Wurtz RH, Goldberg ME, Robinson DL (1980) Behavioral modulation of visual response in the monkey: stimulus selection for attention and movement. In: Sprague JM, Epstein AN (eds) Progress in psychobiology and physiological psychology, vol 9. Academic, New York, pp 43–83
18. Yarbus AL (1967) Eye movements and vision. Plenum, New York

Representational Impairment as a Factor in Neglect

E. Bisiach[1] and A. Berti[1]

Unilateral neglect (UN) has become one of the major topics of modern behavioral neurology. The reason for this is evident: investigation of UN may provide substantial understanding of the mechanisms involved in spatial behavior of complex organisms. In particular, UN challenges current concepts of attention, representation, awareness, and control, insofar as these concepts relate to spatial behavior.

What we would like to do in this paper, is to argue that recent knowledge about UN forces a radical shift in our view of spatial attention and gives crucial support for the hypothesis that space representation in the brain should be construed as an analog of extrapersonal space. Further, we would like to present for discussion a more comprehensive view of UN, which implies a shift in emphasis from attentional to representational factors in the interpretation of the phenomenon.

The idea that UN is a representational disorder is far from new. It was clearly stated by the Austrian neurologist Zingerle in 1913 [8] (that is, before the identification of the syndrome had become an established fact in clinical neurology) that:

> The loss of sensory information may be placed alongside the impossibility of reproduction of earlier memories (from all sensory modalities) in the framework of a *disordered awareness of the laterality of one's own body* ... It is particularly important, not only that the manifest recall cannot be awakened by corresponding sensory information, but also that the defect cannot be amended through sight and touch and *the patient does not recognize the left half of his body, he does not see it as his property* ... In his consciousness, the body's representation is apparently confined to the right half...

Although Zingerle's paper focused on personal space, his intuition may also be applied to extrapersonal space, where it has recently received experimental support.

We [4] have indeed found that right-brain-damaged patients with neglect of the left half of space tend to omit details of the left side when asked to describe well-known views (such as the cathedral square in Milan) from a given vantage point from memory. If a description of the same view from the opposite vantage point is subsequently requested, the previously forgotten left-sided details – now on the right side – are reported, whereas details which the patient was able to report from the right half of the remembered perspective a moment before, now being located on the left, are thus subject to neglect. Dr. Messerli has recently sent us material from his files demonstrating that quite similar results, although unpublished, had al-

[1] Istituto di Clinica Neurologica, Università di Milano, Via F. Sforza 35, 20122 Milan, Italy.

Neurology
Ed. by K. Poeck, H. J. Freund, and H. Gänshirt

ready been obtained by his colleagues and himself by asking patients with neglect to give a mental description of the Place Neuve in Geneva. A parallel, though much more amazing phenomenon has more recently been described by Baxter and Warrington [2]. These authors had the opportunity to examine a patient with left neglect who misspelled the left half of words, both forward and backward, as if reading letter by letter from an imaginary display, of which the left half was invisible to the mind's eye. The same anomaly was observed by Gazzaniga and Barbut some months ago in another patient at Cornell University (personal communication).

Obviously, these patients are able to make adequate same-different judgments between visual patterns only if the difference in shape relates to the unimpaired half of space, whereas they make erroneous judgments if the difference relates to the neglected field. However, we [3] have found the same outcome in a condition in which patterns were moved to and fro behind a stationary vertical slit in the center of the visual field, so that all parts of the patterns could be attended to and perceived, but the apprehension of their whole shape required a process of representational reconstruction. These data have recently been replicated by Ogden, at Auckland University, with slightly different patterns [7].

The moral to be drawn from these findings seems to be clear-cut. UN is not to be explained in terms of sensory loss contralateral to the lesion or of defective movement (either exploratory or responsive) toward the impaired hemispace. On the other hand, its explanation in terms of spatial attention requires an unprecedented qualification: spatial attributes of attention should not only relate to external coordinates, but also to an inner representational frame. Concerning the structure of this frame, the data collected in patients with neglect provide the first unequivocal support for the claim that space representation has *analog* (as opposed to *propositional*) properties. Indeed, damage to a spatially circumscribed area of the brain may result not only in the topographically defined sensory loss which reflects the analog structure of early sensory processes, such as those taking place in the retina or in primary visual cortex, but also in a spatially circumscribed representational scotoma, which cannot be explained away as due to patients' tacit knowledge of the consequences of their sensory loss (such that they might mentally represent a complex object as they would *see* it, given their hemianopia): indeed, patients with neglect are as a rule totally unaware of their sensory disorders.

The evidence so far reviewed seems compatible with two different views about the neural mechanisms responsible for spatial behavior in complex organisms. According to both views, information relative to the environment must be laid down in an isomorphic *temporary* structure corresponding to Baddeley and Lieberman's [1] "scratch pad" metaphor for spatial working memory. However, from one point of view, this is an exquisitely active structure, the *intrinsic changes* of which directly precede overt behavior such as the description of mental images or the exploration of the environment – notably, that portion of the latter which falls outside the momentary compass of the senses. The other view maintains that it is a passive structure – much like an actual picture in the head – the exploitation of which requires a further component: namely an attentional mechanism operating as a scanning device, the nature of whose independent principles has never been specified. In the first view – let us term it *representational* – UN is simply the consequence of a local failure of the structure implementing space representation; in the second, which it seems more appropriate to call *attentional*, UN might result from selective failure in scanning an undamaged inner image of the environment.

Even in the absence of any empirical grounds for the choice, we would favor the first concept for a number of reasons: it is more parsimonious; it is less likely to cause distress to psychologists and philosophers afraid of "inner images"; it has no homuncular overtones; it does not require cumbersome models of neural activity and complex hypotheses about the processes which initiate and direct the activity of the putative scanning device. However, I am going to suggest that clinical neurology can indeed afford to argue for the representational hypothesis of UN from an empirical standpoint.

I will start by submitting that, shortly after the very first treatments of the subject, UN has become conceptually more and more segregated within a syndrome of which it constitutes the most frequent, but by no means the sole or even the necessary feature. This segregation might be arbitrary and misleading, since behavioral changes following lesions which ordinarily involve or approach the parietotemporo-occipital junction of the right hemisphere do not always render the contralateral hemispace void. Pathologic completion of patterns of which only the right half is correctly perceived constitutes the commonest instance of misrepresentation of the left side. Less frequent, but well known, is the intermixture of neglect phenomena with false (and often utterly fantastic) beliefs about the left side of the body and of the environment, which persist even when overt attention is occasionally directed to the abnormal side. Neurologists, indeed, are aware of the fact that denial of left hemiplegia and somatoparaphrenic phenomena may sometimes occur in the absence of neglect and even in patients whose attention is pathologically and inexorably drawn to the left side.

The hypothesis that the association of defective and productive hemispatial disorders is fortuitous cannot be argued from the frequent instances of double dissociation, since puzzling instances of this can also be found between different behavioral indicators of neglect. However, since the hypothesis, no matter how implausible, apparently cannot be dismissed altogether, it seems more fruitful to show how both defective and productive phenomena might be accommodated by a single, admittedly oversimplified neural model, given relatively subtle changes in basic dysfunction (Fig. 1).

In what follows, we will refer to the visual modality, although the model may fit any sensory channel. The diagram shows a sensory processor intervening between sensory transducer and the domain of nervous activities loosely conceived as thought processes. The processor is held to provide a spatially ordered organization of information coming from without the system (perception) as well as of information coming from within the system itself (representation).

The first layer shows the neural message carried by the sensory transducer from an elongated pattern *MN*. The second layer shows cell subassemblies which may be recruited by single portions of the pattern as well as by active subassemblies at the same level. It may be noticed that this design allows for the normal process of perceptual completion of a partially occluded pattern. The third layer is composed of subassemblies which, although being recruited by subassemblies active at layer II, do not match actual portions of the stimulus. Cell assemblies in layer III may also be recruited by autochthonous nervous activity – through pathways omitted in the

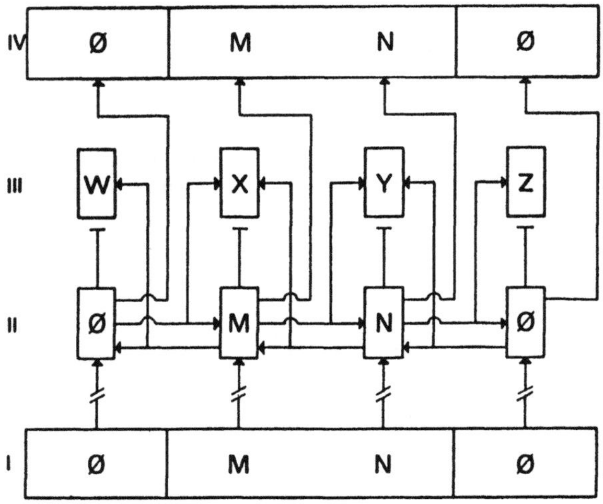

Fig. 1. Schematic model of the processing of a neural message (reproduced by permission from Bisiach et al. [5]

diagram – even in the absence of concurrent input from the sensory transducer. Subassemblies in layer II, besides allowing for perceptual completion of fragmentary patterns and for a reciprocal check of their actual correspondence to single portions of the sensory stimulus, inhibit spatially corresponding subassemblies in layer III. This inhibition prevents pathologic completion, so that the output of the sensory processor (layer IV) constitutes an adequate codification of the incoming stimulus. Complete inactivation of one half of the sensory processor would result in UN. If the inactivation is limited to one half of layer II, corresponding subassemblies in layer III would remain uninhibited, thus giving rise to pathologic representation (of the content of one hemispace) permeating thought processes unchecked by any hierarchically superordinate control unit.

The remarkable case of a patient which we presented at the Harvard University Meeting on Pattern Recognition and Concepts (Bisiach et al., [5]) however, suggests a more complex picture. This patient showed marked phenomena of hemineglect and of pathologic completion in reading words and readable non-words. The word *Carnagione* (complexion) and the non-word *Stomagione,* for instance, could either be read as *Ragione* (reason) or *Stagione* (season). On the contrary, when presented with unreadable non-words obtained by substituting the first half of words with a string of five consonants (for example, *Xrtmngione*) her performance was quite accurate and she would name all the consonants preceding the readable segment in perfect sequence.

This shows that under certain circumstances the sensory processor may work quite correctly in spite of the dysfunction provoking neglect and/or pathologic completion, and that this disorder relates to a level whose input is constituted by highly processed information. One might hypothesize that in our patient phenomena of neglect dyslexia do not indicate the absence of cell assemblies in one section of layer II, but their inability to inhibit layer III subassemblies, except in the case of additional activation dependent on an alerting mechanism triggered by the unexpectedness of unreadable strings of letters. It is worth noticing that this hypothetical mechanism, although entitled to be classed as attentional, implies a concept of attention referring to the *content* of information, not to its *location;* this is different from the concept of spatial attention which is at the heart of attentional explanations of unilateral neglect. Indeed, failure of this mechanism may cause misrepresentation of the content of one half of space, even when focal attention *is drawn* to that half.

Trying to bridge a gap between our speculative model and more factual neurophysiologic knowledge might seem rash. However, Crick [6] has recently suggested a hypothesis concerning the interplay of relay cells and reticular complex in the thalamus which, in spite of the metaphorical use of terms such as "internal attentional searchlight," might indeed realize the intrinsic modulation of a thalamocortical map in which perceptual and representational information is selectively processed relative to its content and location, as in the sensory processor of our model. Corticofugal input to the reticular complex of the thalamus might indeed constitute the determinative element of the recursive loop whereby stored knowledge relative to the symbolic value of sensory stimuli affects a gating mechanism, the inner vicissitudes of which might explain the apparently inattentive aspects of UN as well as the misrepresentation of the content of one side of space.

These two kinds of behavioral disorder were merged by Zingerle in a unitary syndrome which – borrowing the term from Jones – he named "dyschiria." Should the reunification of these symptoms prove well grounded, or at least heuristically helpful, reviving the term "dyschiria" would constitute an overdue tribute to the important, though badly neglected, contribution of Zingerle and should be welcome by those of us who appreciate our cultural heritage, as most certainly did Norman Geschwind, whose memory we are honoring in this session of the Congress.

References

1. Baddeley AD, Lieberman K (1980) Spatial working memory. In: Nickerson R (ed) Attention and performance VIII. Erlbaum, Hillsdale, NJ, pp 521–539
2. Baxter DM, Warrington EK (1983) Neglect dysgraphia. J Neurol Neurosurg Psychiatry 46:1073–1078
3. Bisiach E, Luzzatti C, Perani D (1979) Unilateral neglect, representational schema and consciousness. Brain 102:609–618
4. Bisiach E, Capitani E, Luzzatti C, Perani D (1981) Brain and conscious representation of outside reality. Neuropsychologia 19:543–551
5. Bisiach E, Meregalli S, Berti A (1985) Mechanisms of production-control and belief-fixation in human visuospatial processing. Clinical evidence from hemispatial neglect. Chapter for Commons ML, Herrnstein RJ, Kosslyn S (Eds.) Pattern recognition and concepts in animals, people, and machines. Eighth Symposium on Qualitative Analyses of Behavior, Harvard University, 1985 (in preparation)
6. Crick F (1984) Functions of the thalamic reticular complex: The searchlight hypothesis. Proc Natl Acad Sci USA 81:4586–4590
7. Ogden JA (1985) Contralesional neglect of constructed visual images in right and left brain-damaged patients. Neuropsychologia 23:273–277
8. Zingerle H (1913) Über Störungen der Wahrnehmung des eigenen Körpers bei organischen Gehirnerkrankungen. Monats Neurol 34:13–36

Disorders of Visual Perception and Recognition

Cortical and Subcortical Mechanisms of Visual Perception

G. Berlucchi [1]

Vision is the most important window of the human brain on the outside world. The predominance of vision over the other sense modalities is well expressed by two simple anatomical facts: in man, as in other primates, the three million fibers of the two optic nerves outnumber the sum total of the fibers in all other sensory nerves by a factor of about two, and probably more than one third of the entire neocortex is made up of areas that are exclusively visual in nature.

Contemporary science is making continuous progress in the study of vision using two approaches. On the one hand, the visual portions of the brain are directly explored at the systemic, cellular, and subcellular levels by traditional as well as recently developed anatomical, biochemical, and physiological methods. On the other hand, the new discipline of artificial intelligence considers vision as an information-processing task and utilizes computational techniques to tackle those problems that are solved naturally by the brain in the act of seeing. It should not be hard to convince an audience of clinical neurologists that these two approaches by no means supplant, but are complementary to, the old-fashioned studies which investigate the effects of pathological or experimental lesions of cortical and subcortical centers on visual performance. Analysis of visual deficits resulting from selective brain damage in man is essential not only for clinical purposes, but also as an indirect means for understanding the cerebral organization which subserves normal human vision. Similar analyses of the behavioral consequences of circumscribed experimental lesions in animals provide the opportunity for comparison with the human syndromes, as well as for direct correlation of specific visual disturbances with the findings of anatomy and physiology. A complete understanding of visual perception can be achieved only through such a multistage, multidisciplinary attack.

Changing Views of the Organization of the Visual System

In the last 20 years a major change has occurred in our concepts about the organization of the mammalian visual system. The traditional view was that the main sub-

[1] Istituto di Fisiologia Umana, Università di Verona, Strada Le Grazie, 37134 Verona, Italy.

Neurology
Ed. by K. Poeck, H. J. Freund, and H. Gänshirt

strate of visually guided behavior is a serially organized array of centers, from retina to lateral geniculate nucleus in the thalamus, from lateral geniculate nucleus to visuosensory cortex (striate cortex), from visuosensory to visuopsychic cortex (still modality-specific but of a higher order), from visuopsychic to polymodal association cortex, and from association cortex to the premotor and motor cortices for behavioral output. This traditional view assigned purely reflex functions – automatic oculomotor reactions, control of pupillary and ciliary muscles, and so on – to the pathway which goes from retina to pretectum and superior colliculus, and from these centers to premotor or motor neurons within the brain stem or the spinal cord.

Much of this view remains of course true, but parts of it have turned out to be wrong, and much further information has been added to the picture. The story of the birth and development of the newer concepts about the general organization of the visual system has been nicely recounted by Diamond [4] and by Diamond et al. [5], and I will present only a few crucial aspects of it.

1. There are many more than two visual areas in the cortex of most mammals (see, e.g., [19]). A visual cortical area is defined as a region of the cortex which has distinct cytoarchitectural and/or myeloarchitectural characteristics, receives projections from subcortical nuclei reached by the visual input and from other visual cortical areas, and can be shown by physiological methods to contain neurons which respond selectively to appropriate visual stimulation, often within a retinotopic organization. Much of what was known as polymodal, associational, or uncommitted cortex of the occipital, parietal, and temporal lobes is now believed to be constituted by visual cortical areas which overlap or adjoin the visuosensory and visuopsychic areas of classical neurology and are collectively named extrastriate visual cortex. Certainly more than ten such visual areas exist in the neocortex of cat and monkey, and there is reason to believe that in man the extrastriate visual areas are even more numerous. In fact, it could be argued that the expansion of the neocortex has occurred in evolution chiefly because of the increase in the number of areas selectively committed to visual functions. Although certain hierarchical aspects of the integration of the activities of the visual cortical areas have been convincingly emphasized (see, e.g. [9]), we shall see that other findings suggest that each visual area may constitute a separate functional unit and that the organization of these units may follow the principle of modularity (see, e.g. [2]).

2. Visual information can reach the extrastriate cortical areas not only through the classical route from lateral geniculate to striate cortex and from striate to extrastriate cortex, but also through other pathways, among which are direct projections from lateral geniculate to extrastriate cortex as well as conspicuous projections from the pulvinar thalami to several visual cortical areas. In turn, the pulvinar thalami receive visual inputs from the retina, the superior colliculus, and the pretectum, and at least in some species may project to striate as well as extrastriate areas [5].

3. There are thus multiple visual areas and multiple parallel pathways which convey information from retina to cortex. The attribute "parallel" is useful and correct insofar as it suggests that at least along portions of the visual pathways the anatomical organization is such as to allow the channeling of different retinal outputs into different visual stations. Thus the retinal outputs in the cat include at least three populations of fibers, corresponding to the X-, Y- and W-ganglion cell types. These

cells differ in size and consequently in conduction velocity, as well as in response properties. Among the large sized Y-cells and the medium-sized X-cells, the former show a better temporal resolution of the visual stimulus while the latter show a better spatial resolution. The small-sized W-cells form a heterogeneous population with poor contrast sensitivity, poor spatial and temporal resolution, and, at least in some cases, good motion sensitivity (for a review see [15]). At the lateral geniculate nucleus the three types of retinal afferents are kept segregated; further, lateral geniculate cells which receive an X-input project exclusively to area 17, or the striate cortex, whereas geniculate and extrageniculate (i.e., through tectum, pretectum, and pulvinar) projections conveying Y- and W-inputs to the cortex terminate in virtually all visual cortical areas, both striate and extrastriate. Thus the striate cortex is presumably indispensable for passing information transmitted along the X-retinal channel to other visual cortical areas, whereas the Y- and W-inputs can reach several cortical areas in addition to the striate area independently of the latter area (for reviews see [15, 18]).

A similar segregation of retinal afferents is manifest in the monkey, where small ganglion cells project exclusively to the four dorsal parvocellular layers of the lateral geniculate nucleus whereas larger ganglion cells project to the two ventral magnicellular layers of the lateral geniculate nucleus, to the superior colliculus, and to the pretectum. The small retinal ganglion cells of the monkey probably correspond to the X-cells of the cat; further, they are generally chromatically selective. At least one subpopulation of the large ganglion cells in the monkey retina is similar to the Y-cells of the cat retina, and shares their achromatic character (for a review see [2]). The corticopetal projection from the parvocellular and magnocellular layers of the lateral geniculate nucleus terminate in different layers of the striate cortex, and there is evidence that the segregation is maintained in the striate cortex itself as well as in other cortical areas (see, e.g., [8, 16]).

4. The strong evidence for the parallel arrangement of the multiple pathways projecting from retina to cortex should not mislead the observer into thinking that there are no serial connections within the visual system. On the contrary, serial connections are prominent in the visual system of both cat (see, e.g., [14]) and monkey (see, e.g., [20]), not only in the "orthodox" forward direction, i.e., from striate cortex onward, but also in a reciprocal "backward" direction. These feedback connections include descending projections from visual cortical areas to subcortical visual nuclei in the thalamus and the tectum.

Physiological Analysis of Single-Unit Activity in Visual Cortical Areas

After the initial discoveries of Hubel and Wiesel (see, e.g., [7]) it has become commonplace in contemporary visual physiology to make ample use of the somewhat anthropomorphic concept of single neurons specifically responsive to form, color, orientation, movement, and other parameters of the visual stimulus. Since neurons with similar response properties tend to be aggregated in visual cortical areas or subareas, the specific neuronal reactivity to visual stimulation has become a major means for the functional classification of cortical regions. On these physiological grounds and considerable anatomical evidence, Zeki [21] has suggested that in the monkey different classes of visual information such as color, form, motion, and depth are segregated in the striate cortex and distributed to different extrastriate areas for further processing. Mishkin et al. [10] also suggest that divergence of specific classes of information at the striate cortex is the premise for the constitution of the neural substrates of different visual perceptions, with an occipitotemporal pathway subserving object vision and an occipitoparietal pathway subserving spatial vision. The participation of the temporal cortex in object recognition is strongly suggested by the presence in this cortex of neurons which are selectively activated by extremely complex stimuli, such as hands or faces in different positions and seen from different angles [6, 12, 13].

The role of single neurons in the psychology of perception is of course a central issue in all theories of cerebral organization. Barlow [1] maintains that single neurons at high levels in the brain are capable of representing important events in the outside world and triggering the appropriate behavioral reactions to such events. Each perceptual event corresponds selectively to the firing of a large class of high-level neurons which are organized in parallel; any of these neurons can trigger the response by itself. In his words, "Whenever two stimuli can be distinguished, in normal life or in a psychophysical experiment, then proper analysis of the impulses occurring in *a single neuron* would enable them to be distinguished with equal or greater reliability." In the spirit of Barlow's hypothesis I would add to this claim the following corollary: Whenever the activity of a class of single neurons in the brain of an animal is correlated with the animal's discriminatory response to a given stimulus, the removal of that class of neurons should abolish the animal's ability to distinguish that stimulus. If a certain part of the brain contains neurons that are uniquely responsive to a certain stimulus, it is more than reasonable to assume that that part of the brain is indispensable for the recognition of that stimulus; however, the assumption must be substantiated by the suppression of the specific behavioral response following the removal of the part of the brain containing the specialized neurons. Experimental efforts along this line have not rarely been disappointing.

In the cat, for example, we have seen that area 17 (the striate area) of the cortex is the sole recipient of the information transmitted by the X-system of retinal ganglion cells, which possess the highest spatial resolution. Further receptive fields of neurons in area 17 and in the adjacent area 18 are finely tuned for orientation and the visuotopic map in area 17 is the most detailed and precise of all areas so far studied [18]. All these single-neuron characteristics point to area 17, alone or in combination with area 18, as the most likely substrate for the neural encoding of visual forms. However, cats trained on several form and pattern discriminations as normals could immediately recognize the discriminative stimuli a few days after bilateral removals of areas 17 and 18 [17]. The absence of area 17 and of the X-input to the cortex was obviously not incompatible with a good capacity for form vision, a fact which leads one to attribute this capacity to the remaining visual systems supplied with Y- and W-inputs from the retinas. That these extrastriate systems were indeed responsible for the good retention of destriated cats is shown by the presence of conspicuous retention deficits in cats trained and tested in the same way, but submitted to cortical lesions which extended outside areas 17 and 18 [17]. The response characteristics of neurons in these extrastriate areas would not suggest them as particularly important for the discrimination of simple geometric patterns.

A lesion experiment on the middle temporal (MT) visual area of the monkey was prompted by the response characteristics of neurons in this area. MT neurons are specifically sensitive to axis of motion and direction of motion of visual stimuli (see, e.g., [3]). Newsome et al. [11] found that chemical inactivation of MT in freely behaving monkeys reduced their ability to match the speed of pursuit eye movements to the speed of a moving target. However, the monkeys' ability to move the eyes in the appropriate direction of the stimulus movement was unimpaired. As stated by the authors, "this result is somewhat ironical since the cardinal characteristic of MT neurons has been their directional selectivity." The deficit in the speed of eye movements was of course compatible with the hypothesis of participation of the MT area in spatial analysis, but it was extremely short-lived, as it disappeared within a week of the operation. Newsome et al. [11] offer very reasonable interpretations of the incomplete match between the findings on single-neuron activity in MT and the effects of lesions of this area, but, as in the case of area 17 in the cat, it must be acknowledged that the expectations based on physiology are not totally fulfilled by the results of related lesion experiments.

Conclusions

The above comment should not sound too pessimistic. That selective lesions within the visual system produce different deficits depending on their location is a fact which has been demonstrated by clinical neurologists first and foremost in man. It is also well established that similarly different effects can be obtained in animals with experimental lesions of different parts of their visual systems. Cowey [2] has discussed how the specific visual effects of localized brain damage in man and in animals can be meaningfully related to anatomical and physiological knowledge. While I entirely agree with him that the planning of lesion experiments, as well as the interpretation of the results, must be guided by the available evidence of the structure and physiology of the brain, I am also aware of the difficulty of this task. Oversimplifications and overgeneralizations are not likely to make it easier.

References

1. Barlow HB (1985) The role of single neurons in the psychology of perception. Q J Exp Psychol [A] 37A: 121–145
2. Cowey A (1985) Aspects of cortical organization related to selective attention and selective impairments of visual perception: tutorial review. In: Posner M, Marin OSM (eds) Attention and performance, vol 11. Erlbaum, Hillsdale, pp 41–62
3. Desimone R, Schein SJ, Albright TD (1985) Form, color and motion analysis in prestriate cortex of the macaque monkey. Pontif Acad Sci Scripta Varia 54: 165–178
4. Diamond IT (1982) Changing views of the organization and evolution of the visual pathways. In: Morrison AR, Strick PL (eds) Changing concepts of the nervous system. Academic, New York, pp 201–233
5. Diamond IT, Fitzpatrick D, Sprague JM (1986) The extrastriate visual cortex: a historical approach to the relation between the "visuo-sensory" and "visuo-psychic" areas. In: Peters A, Jones EG (eds) Cerebral cortex, vol 4. Association and auditory cortices. Plenum, New York, pp 63–87

6. Gross CG, Desimone R, Albright TD, Schwartz EL (1985) Inferior temporal cortex and pattern recognition. Pontif Acad Sci Scripta Varia 54:179–201
7. Hubel DH, Wiesel TN (1977) Functional architecture of macaque monkey visual cortex. Proc R Soc Lond [Biol] 198:1–59
8. Livingstone MS, Hubel DH (1984) Anatomy and physiology of a color system in the primate visual cortex. J Neurosci 4:309–356
9. Maunsell JHR, Van Essen DC (1983) Hierarchical organization and functional streams in the visual cortex. Trends Neurosci 6:370–375
10. Mishkin M, Ungerleider LG, Macko KA (1983) Object vision and spatial vision: two cortical pathways. Trends Neurosci 6:414–417
11. Newsome WT, Wurtz RH, Dursteler MR, Mikami A (1985) Deficits in visual motion processing following ibotenic acid lesions of the middle temporal visual area of the macaque monkey. J Neurosci 5:825–840
12. Perret DI, Smith PAJ, Potter DD, Mistlin AJ, Head AS, Milner AD, Jeeves MA (1984) Neurones responsive to faces in the temporal cortex: studies of functional organization, sensitivity to identity and relation to perception. Hum Neurobiol 3:197–208
13. Rolls ET (1985) Neuronal activity in relation to the recognition of stimuli in the primate. Pontif Acad Sci Scripta Varia 54:203–213
14. Rosenquist AC (1984) Connections of visual cortical areas in the cat. In: Peters A, Jones EG (eds) Cerebral cortex, vol 3. Visual cortex. Plenum, New York pp 81–117
15. Sherman SM (1985) Functional organization of the W-, X-, and Y-cell pathways in the cat: a review and hypothesis. Prog Psychobiol Physiol Psychol 11:233–314
16. Shipp S, Zeki S (1985) Segregation of pathways leading from area V2 to areas V4 and V5 of macaque monkey cortex. Nature 315:322–325
17. Sprague JM, Berlucchi G, Antonini A (1985) Immediate postoperative retention of visual discriminations following selective cortical lesions in the cat. Behav Brain Res 17:145–162
18. Sprague JM, Hughes HC, Berlucchi G (1981) Cortical mechanisms in pattern and form perception. In: Pompeiano O, Ajmone-Marsan CA (eds) Brain mechanisms of perceptual awareness and purposeful behavior. Raven, New York, pp 107–132
19. Tusa RJ (1982) Visual cortex: multiple areas and multiple functions. In: Morrison AR, Strick PL (eds) Changing concepts of the nervous system. Academic, New York, pp 235–259
20. Ungerleider LG (1985) The corticocortical pathway for object recognition and spatial perception. Pontif Acad Sci Scripta Varia 54:21–33
21. Zeki S (1978) Functional specialization in the visual cortex of the rhesus monkey. Nature 274:423–428

Visual Agnosia for Objects

J. L. SIGNORET[1]

A 70-year-old patient who presented with an infarct in the distribution of the left posterior cerebral artery was asked to name a watch put before her; the patient answered that it was "something with which to see ... a pair of glasses." Is this an aphasic error or an error of recognition? The patient was asked again "with what object do you cut cloth?" she answered immediately "with scissors," thus confirming the absence of an anomia. The patient was then asked to mime how she would use a pair of scissors; she mimed how to wind up a watch. Her vision did not allow her to recognize the watch, if you consider the verbal response as the criterion of recognition. But the object "watch" was well known, as witnessed by her miming the rewinding of the watch, even if the miming did not occur at the appropriate moment.

Visual Agnosia for Objects is a Complex Syndrome, in Spite of a Definition Accepted by All

Visual agnosia for objects is a difficulty in recognizing objects presented visually. This difficulty can not be explained by mental deterioration, a disorder of attention, or a lack of familiarity with the object. Above all, two criteria are essential, but always disputed, because their significance is imprecise: (a) the absence of visual sensory difficulty necessary for adequate perception; (b) possible recognition of the object by another sensory modality. Visual agnosia for objects, confined by these two criteria risks becoming more or less an elementary sensory visual difficulty, or it might be considered as a reflection of a more generalized disorder concerning the "cognition" of objects.

Visual Agnosia for Objects is an Ambiguous Syndrome

The ambiguity of visual agnosia for objects is explained by its origins. A dog sees objects, but it does not recognize them after bioccipital lesions; this is the example

[1] Clinique des Maladies du Système Nerveux, Hôpital de la Salpêtrière, 47 Boulevard de l'Hôpital, 75013 Paris, France.

Neurology
Ed. by K. Poeck, H. J. Freund, and H. Gänshirt

that Munk [35] used to define psychic blindness. Lissauer [31] reported a human study and proposed a model for the recognition of objects: the visual perception of an object must first of all be pertinent, and must then be associated with anterior images left by the object in order to result in its recognition. Thus, psychic blindness is made up of two levels: one perceptive and the other associative. The same year as Lissauer's observation, Freund [21] posed the question whether certain types of psychic blindness were not in fact the result of an interruption of the association between normal visual perception and language which was also normal. Some cases of psychic blindness were then really optic aphasias. Freud [20], having read Freund, developed the concept of agnosia. Objects have a mental representation different from that of words. Agnosia is defined as the alteration of the mental representation of objects. It is important to emphasize that according to Freud, all sensory modalities originate as mental representations of objects. Psychic blindness is therefore a form of agnosia.

What is Recognizing an Object?

The recognition of an object cannot be reduced to a single response. An object is characterized by multiple associations. An object is first of all a form: we construct, by visual and tactile experience, an internal representation of this form, a sort of "template." An object also has a function; we know how to use it. An object has a name. An object is therefore associated with form, function, and name. Each is included in a sort of "thesaurus" where a relationship is established with other forms, other functions, and other names. Recognition is "the totality of all the associations aroused by any object" [22].

Using pictures which are more difficult to recognize than objects is often necessary in order to demonstrate the difficulty in recognition. Pictures allow one to explore all the forms that make up our visual world and to carry out a number of semantic matchings. On the other hand, using fragmented and incomplete pictures, or mixtures of pictures, tests perceptive competence rather than the recognition of objects.

Pathophysiology

It is important, regarding the interpretation of visual agnosia for objects, to remember its initial ambiguity. The interpretations stemming from the evolutionary model consider the disorder as testifying to a regression affecting the faculty of visual perception, while the interpretations stemming from the associationist model consider the disorder as resulting from functional ruptures, disconnections between the many and varied mental capacities; this associationist model relies on anatomic data. These two types of interpretation could seem opposite, indeed irreconcilable. In fact, different interpretations do not apply to the same disorder. In order to propose a pathophysiology of visual agnosia for objects, it is first important to recognize that visual agnosia for objects is not a single entity. In the same fashion, in order to propose a pathophysiology of aphasia, it is necessary to recognize several types of aphasia. Thus we are led to break down visual agnosia for objects into three types: (a) aperceptive agnosia; (b) associative agnosia; and (c) asemantic agnosia.

Aperceptive Visual Agnosia for Objects or Visual Form Agnosia

Patients can generally describe the parts of the object to be recognized. Morphological errors are frequent. Recognition is sometimes possible, but slow, and only after numerous hesitations. Patients are conscious that they see badly, and their behavior is reminiscent of that of a blind person. Recognition upon touching the object is immediate and correct [7, 9, 10]. It is generally admitted that these patients can not sketch the object to be recognized. Some sensory deficits are frequently seen in this type of agnosia, making it the most visual type of agnosia for objects. It must be noted that reading can be preserved, while prosopagnosia and memory deficits are as a rule present; the observations of Albert et al. [1] seem to correspond to an aperceptive agnosia. It is therefore understandable that this type of agnosia has in some ways served to repudiate the concept of agnosia [5, 11]. Most likely the patient reported by Goldstein and Gelb [23] represented this type of agnosia where one is justified in applying the Gestalt theory [9]: the patient can not extract from the object presented visually the "template" which permits recognition. It is important to remember that there is no obligatory relationship between these sensory deficits and the presence of an aperceptive agnosia [17]. Efron [15] was able to show in the patient reported by Benson and Greenberg [7] that discrimination between a square and a rectangle was defective despite perfect visual acuity. These data were confirmed by Warrington [45], who also pointed out the inability to detect a simple form fragmented and presented against a fragmented background; she felt that this difficulty should therefore be considered a pseudoagnosia. We believe that such a difficulty certainly belongs to the visual agnosias, because it is something more than the elementary sensory process which is involved in this case.

The lesions responsible for such an aperceptive agnosia are bilateral [2, 10]; they affect the lingual and fusiform gyri, and also the inferior longitudinal fasciculus. It seems reasonable to speculate that in humans there are functionally equivalent areas in the cortex to those of the inferior temporal cortex of monkeys; it is known that in monkeys these areas of cortex somehow reconstruct the form of a visual stimulus by starting with fragment analysis which takes place in the striate and prestriate cortex [43]. The lesion must be bilateral because otherwise interhemispheric transfer can take place, by the anterior commissure [40]. This lesion can also account for prosopagnosia which as a rule is due to a visual-limbic disconnection. As far as difficulty in recognition would allow, it would be interesting to know if these patients are able to identify their own personal possessions [12]. There remain two points to be discussed:

1. Is there a functional hemispheric prevalence for this perceptual activity? A number of works [e.g., 14] have suggested that, associated with right postrolandic hemispheric lesions, there are deficits in visual perception. It seems that the critical region responsible for this deficit must be the right parietal region [47], affecting visual attention and strategy rather than visual perceptual synthesis.
2. The existence of an aperceptive agnosia does not exclude the possibility of another coexistent visual agnosia for objects, in particular associative [8, 41].

It was probably just such a patient who led Alexander and Albert [3] to say that all visual agnosias are a result of bilateral occipital lesions, affecting the inferior longitudinal fasciculus which contributes to the visuoverbal connections; it does not seem legitimate, as these authors suggested, to consider isolated prosopagnosia as a minor form of agnosia, since it occurs as a result of an altogether different pathophysiology.

Associative Visual Agnosia for Objects or Agnosia by Disconnection

The behavior of these patients is not that of a blind person. Indeed when objects are presented visually, patients seem perplexed and lost; they give erroneous, even fantastic, verbal responses. Thus, for Lissauer's patient: candle = "pencil," glasses = "candlestick," handkerchief = "glasses," bottle = "candlestick," pen holder = "scissors to clean the light" [31]. There exists an ordered semantic rapport between the object presented and the erroneous verbal responses, such that morphological errors are rare; these responses are especially contaminated by previously presented objects, and by preceding verbal responses. Patients can verbally define an object from its name and find the name of the object from a definition; this attests to the absence of an anomia. If patients are asked to imitate the use of the object presented they frequently carry out the gesture corresponding to the erroneous verbal response, but this is not the rule; there is no apraxia on verbal command. Tactile recognition is exceptionally perfect, often better than visual recognition [19, 34]. Patients find it impossible to match objects which have categorical and semantic links. It is important to note the variability of the responses. Other disorders are constantly involved: right homonymous hemianopia generally without macular sparing, pure alexia, anomia-agnosia for colors. There is no prosopagnosia; indeed, pictures of famous people can give rise to erroneous verbal responses, but patients recognize their relatives and identify unfamiliar faces. Copying is generally satisfactory. The behavior of these patients is sometimes baffling; they are frequently elderly and could be considered demented. From the strict point of view of their behavior, however, a simple clinical examination should suggest the possibility of a visuoverbal, visuotactile, or visuogestural disconnection, since their visual sensory, tactile sensory, gestural, and verbal capacities are preserved. Looking at the anatomic lesions confirms this.

Lissauer's patient, when studied by Hahn [25], showed a unilateral left cortical lesion, affecting the two labia of the calcarine sulcus, the cuneus, the lingual gyrus, and a commissural lesion, affecting the white matter in the periventricular region (tapetum, posterior forceps) and the splenium of the corpus callosum. Nodet's patient had an identical lesion [38]. The most recent studies confirm that a unilateral left occipital or occipitoparietal lesion affecting the cortex and the commissural fibers could be the origin of an associative agnosia [4, 18, 26, 28, 28, 34]. So a left occipital lesion, causing a right homonymous hemianopia inhibits access of visual information to the left hemisphere. A lesion in the commissural fibers inhibits or disturbs the transfer of information from right to left hemisphere. This explains why the form of the object as perceived by the right hemisphere cannot be named by the left hemisphere; such an interpretation was proposed by Freund [21] in justification of the concept of an optic aphasia. But this interpretation does not account for the defect of tactile recognition and gesture. There must then be two other possibilities as proposed by Geschwind [22]: either the inability of the right hemisphere to arouse a tactile representation, or an anterior extension of the lesion in the corpus callosum. Instead of these two proposals which do not seem to correspond to the clinical and anatomic data, it seems legitimate to consider the angular gyrus (PG area) of the left hemisphere as the key area in explaining the associative agnosia, as Nielsen had suggested earlier [37]. This area is a multisensory convergence zone [33] which is more developed in humans on the left side [16]. It receives fibers from the ipsilateral and contralateral hemispheres [39]. Visual, tactile and other information converges on this area. The functional role of this area is supramodal: it associates information between them and orients this information according to the chosen response, either toward the parietal lobe for gestures, or toward the temporal lobe for language. A white matter lesion in the parieto-occipital region can, therefore, disrupt the interhemispheric connections and the intrahemispheric connections which conduct visual and tactile information to the PG area. Just as in pure alexia [24], right homonymous hemianopia is without doubt a necessary condition for the occurrence of an associative agnosia. The rarity of the associative agnosias as a result of an infarct in the left posterior cerebral artery territory is due to the fact that these connections are located in the watershed zone between the middle and posterior cerebral artery and they are rarely affected. The pathologic data show the anatomic proximity of the visual and tactile connections since the difficulty in tactile recognition is often associated with visual recognition difficulty. In some cases, however, where there is isolated visual recognition difficulty, visuoverbal and visuogestural disconnections are produced [4]. The tactile connections are situated in front of the visual connections as indicated by the fact that an anterior extension of the lesion causes both visual and tactile recognition disorders [34]. The independence of the visual and tactile connections is confirmed by other pathologic data: one can observe an optic aphasia or a visuoverbal disconnection, and also a bilateral tactile aphasia or a tactoverbal disconnection [6, 30]. These two syndromes show that the connections between area PG and the temporal and parietal areas are also independent. Auditory information likewise converges on area PG, accounting for their parietal position; but they are situated in front of the visual and tactile connections. Moreover, patients who present with associative agnosia are generally capable of recognizing the sounds characteristic of an object. This associative function of area PG also involves different elements of the same modality: classification of images and coloring of drawings [13]. Injury to area PG is without doubt responsible for the major comprehension disorder exceeding the verbal information in certain global aphasias.

Asemantic Visual Agnosia for Objects or Agnosia by Defect of the Cognition of Objects

In 1971 Taylor and Warrington [42] reported a case of visual agnosia which was called associative, but presented with three singular features: (a) a loss of the meaning of words (generally concrete terms); (b) the absence of any visual sensory abnormalities; (c) probable cerebral atrophy. In 1975 Warrington [44] reported three similar cases: visual and tactile difficulty in recognizing objects was accompanied by difficulty in recognizing the meaning of words (verbal agnosia). The difficulty thus affected the recognition of all the visual and verbal information which had meaning, justifying the term of "selective impairment of semantic memory." It could be argued whether or not this kind of difficulty should be included with the visual agnosias. Our experience is that these patients frequently present as if they had visual agnosia. It seems difficult to establish anatomic correlates for eventual pathophysiologic interpretation in a degenerative disease. However, it is important to point out that similar disorders have been described during herpes encephalitis [36]. The frontotemporolimbic connections seem to be involved since the prevalence of these lesions in Alzheimer's disease seems similar to that in herpes encephalitis. Finally, interest in this form of agnosia is twofold since it allows one: (a) to show the remarkable visual performances beside the disorder of meaning; [32]; (b) to analyze the organization of the semantic system of these patients [46].

One, Two or Three Visual Agnosias?

It seemed legitimate to distinguish three types of visual agnosia for objects, at least to try to avoid the lexical and pathophysiologic confusions. Between visual agnosia considered due to a problem of visual perception of forms and visual agnosia considered due to a problem of cognition of the meaning of objects, there probably exists only one "true" visual agnosia for objects. This rare but authentic syndrome is that which was described by Lissauer, the associative visual agnosia for objects or difficulty with visual connections.

Acknowledgement. We thank Dr. Robert O'Hara for his critical review of the English version of this paper.

References

1. Albert ML, Reches A, Silverberg R (1975) Associative visual agnosia without alexia. Neurology 25:322–326
2. Albert ML, Soffer D, Silverberg R, Reches A (1979) The anatomic basis of visual agnosia. Neurology 29:876–879
3. Alexander MP, Albert ML (1983) The anatomical basis of visual agnosia. In: Kertesz A (ed) Localization in neuropsychology. Academic, New York, pp 393–415
4. Assal G, Regli F (1980) Syndrome de disconnexion visuo-verbale et visuo-gestuelle. Aphasie optique et apraxie optique. Rev Neurol 136:365–376
5. Bay E (1953) Disturbances of visual perception and their examination. Brain 76:515–550
6. Beauvois MF, Saillant B, Meininger V, Lhermitte F (1978) Bilateral tactile aphasia: a tacto-verbal dysfunction. Brain 101:381–401
7. Benson DF, Greenberg JP (1969) Visual form agnosia. A specific defect in visual discrimination. Arch Neurol 20:82–89
8. Benson DF, Segarra J, Albert ML (1974) Visual agnosia – prosopagnosia. A clinico-pathologic correlation. Arch Neurol 30:307–310
9. Brain WR (1941) Visual object-agnosia with special reference to the Gestalt theory. Brain 64:43–62
10. Cambier J, Masson M, Elghozi D, Henin D, Viader F (1980) Agnosie visuelle sans hémianopsie droite chez un sujet droitier. Rev Neurol 136:727–740
11. Critchley M (1964) The problem of visual agnosia. J Neurol Sci 1:274–290

12. Damasio AR, Damasio H, Van Hoesen GW (1982) Prosopagnosia: anatomic basis and behavioral mechanisms. Neurology 32:331–341
13. De Renzi E, Faglioni P, Scotti G, Spinnler H (1972) Impairment in associating colour to form concomitant with aphasia. Brain 95:293–304
14. De Renzi E, Scotti G, Spinnler H (1969) Perceptual and associative disorders of visual recognition. Relationship to the side of cerebral lesion. Neurology 19:634–642
15. Efron R (1968) What is perception? Boston Studies in the Philosophy of Science 4:137–173
16. Eidelberg D, Galaburda AM (1984) Inferior parietal lobule. Divergent architectonic asymmetries in the human brain. Arch Neurol 41:843–852
17. Ettlinger G (1956) Sensory deficits in visual agnosia. J Neurol Neurosurg Psychiatry 19:297–307
18. Ferro JM, Santos ME (1984) Associative visual agnosia: a case study. Cortex 20:121–134
19. Frederiks JAM (1969) The agnosias. Disorders of perceptual recognition. In: Vinken PJ, Bruyn GW (eds) Handbook of clinical neurology, vol 4. North Holland, Amsterdam, pp 13–47
20. Freud S (1891) On aphasia. A critical study. Imago (1953), Londres
21. Freund DC (1889) Über optische Aphasie und Seelenblindheit. Arch Psychiatr Nervenkr 20:276–297, 371–416
22. Geschwind N (1965) Disconnexion syndromes in animals and man. Brain 88:237–294, 585–644
23. Goldstein K, Gelb A (1918) Psychologische Analysen hirnpathologischer Fälle aufgrund von Untersuchungen Hirnverletzter. Z Gesamte Neurol Psychiatr 41:1–142
24. Greenblatt SH (1973) Alexia without agoraphia or hemianopsia. Brain 96:307–316
25. Hahn E (1895) Pathologisch-anatomische Untersuchung des Lissauerschen Falles von Seelenblindheit. In: Arbeiten der Psychiatrischen Klinik, Breslau, H 2. Thieme, Leipzig
26. Hécaen H, de Ajuriaguerra H (1956) Agnosie visuelle pour les objets inanimés par lésion unilatérale gauche. Rev Neurol 94:222–233
27. Hécaen H, Angelergues R (1963) La cécité psychique. Masson, Paris
28. Hécaen H, Goldblum MC, Masure MC, Ramier AM (1974) Une nouvelle observation d'agnosie d'objet. Déficit de l'association ou de la catégorisation spécifique de la modalité visuelle? Neuropsychologia 12:447–464
29. Larrabee GJ, Levin HS, Huff FJ, Kay MC, Guinto FC Jr (1985) Visual agnosia contrasted with visual-verbal disconnection. Neuropsychologia 23:1–12
30. Lhermitte F, Beauvois MF (1973) A visual-speech disconnexion syndrome. Report of a case with optic aphasia, agnosic alexia and colour agnosia. Brain 96:695–714
31. Lissauer H (1889) Ein Fall von Seelenblindheit nebst einem Beitrage zur Theorie derselben. Arch Psychiatr Nervenkr 21:222–270
32. Marin OSM, Glenn CG, Rafal RD (1983) Visual problem solving in the absence of lexical semantics: evidence from dementia. Brain Cognition 2:285–311
33. Mesulam MM, Van Hoesen GW, Pandya DN, Geschwind N (1977) Limbic and sensory connections of the inferior parietal lobule (area PG) in the rhesus monkey: a study with a new method for horseradish peroxydase histochemistry. Brain Res 136:393–414
34. Morin P, Rivrain Y, Eustache F, Lambert J, Courtheoux P (1984) Agnosie visuelle et agnosie tactile. Rev Neurol 140:271–277
35. Munk H (1881) Über die Functionen der Großhirnrinde. Gesammelte Mittheilungen aus den Jahren 1877–1880. Hirschwald, Berlin
36. Newcombe F, Ratcliff G (1974) Agnosia: a disorder of object recognition. In: Michel F, Schott B (eds) Les syndromes de déconnexion calleuse chez l'homme. Lyon, pp 317–341
37. Nielsen JM (1937) Unilateral cerebral dominance as related to mind blindness. Minimal lesion capable of causing visual agnosia for objects. Arch Neurol Psychiatr 38:108–135
38. Nodet V (1899) Les agnoscies. La cécité psychique en particulier. Félix Alcan, Paris
39. Pandya DN, Karol EA, Heilbronn D (1971) The topographical distribution of interhemispheric projections in the corpus callosum of the rhesus monkey. Brain Res 32:31–43
40. Rocha Miranda CE, Bender DB, Gross CG, Mishkin M (1975) Visual activation of neurons in inferotemporal cortex depends in striate cortex and forebrain commissures. J Neurophysiol 38:475–491

41. Rubens AB, Benson DF (1971) Associative visual agnosia. Arch Neurol 24:305–316
42. Taylor A, Warrington EK (1971) Visual agnosia: a single case report. Cortex 7:152–161
43. Ungerleider LG, Mishkin M (1982) Two cortical visual systems. In: Ingle DJ, Goodale MA, Mansfield RJW (eds) Analysis of visual behavior. MIT Press, Cambridge, pp 549–566
44. Warrington EK (1975) The selective impairment of semantic memory. Q J Exp Psychol 27:635–657
45. Warrington EK (1985) Agnosia: the impairment of object recognition. In: Frederiks JAM (ed) Clinical neuropsychology. Elsevier, Amsterdam, pp 333–349 (Handbook of clinical neurology, vol 1, no 45)
46. Warrington EK, Shallice T (1984) Category-specific semantic impairments. Brain 107:829–853
47. Warrington EK, Taylor AM (1973) The contribution of the right parietal lobe to object recognition. Cortex 9:152–164

Disorders of Face Recognition

H. D. Ellis [1]

Introduction

It is with some surprise and not a little amusement that we learn that the prolific writer and composer of hymns, Sabine Baring-Gould, once lifted up a child, saying "And whose little girl are you, my dear?" She replied, sobbing "I'm yours, Daddy."

Face recognition is one of the skills that the majority of us daily display throughout most of our lives. Therefore, even allowing for the fact that Baring-Gould had 14 children, it seems odd to us that he failed to recognise one of them. Each of us carries around in our head a portrait gallery comprising at least a couple of thousand faces of people we know either personally or through public media [14]. When encountering one of the people we know the memory store corresponding to the person can be accessed almost instantaneously. Exceptions to this rule do occur, of course, as the above example shows – and I shall devote the main part of this paper to considering both everyday and pathological disturbances of face perception and face memory.

Models of Face Recognition

In recent years a number of cognitive models of face recognition have been proposed [13, 14, 16, 29]. In each case the process is assumed to involve a series of states leading from early structural processes to eventual identification. In between these stages information about the category of a face (e.g. male/female) and its familiarity is extracted at independent stages. In much simplified form the models envisage a process like that shown in Fig. 1.

Notice that analysis of facial expression does not appear as part of the main sequence of operations. Instead, there are grounds for thinking that expressions are handled by a parallel system [13]. The type and order of operations depicted in Fig. 1 will later be used to construct a taxonomy of prosopagnosic disorders.

[1] Department of Psychology, University of Aberdeen, Old Aberdeen, AB9 2UB, Great Britain.

Neurology
Ed. by K. Poeck, H. J. Freund, and H. Gänshirt

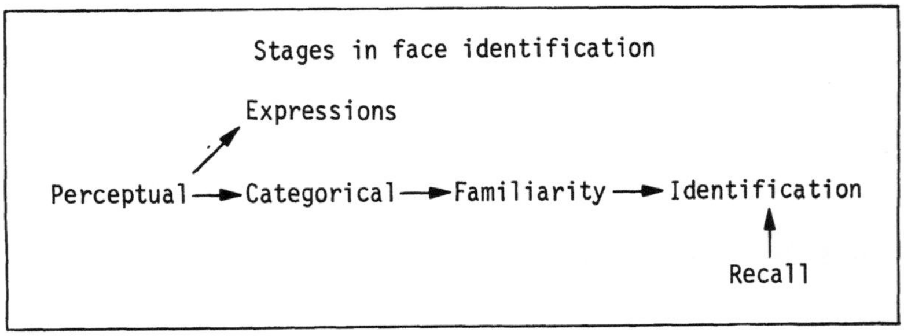

Fig. 1. Simplified outline of the hypothesised stages underlying face recognition

Disordered Face Recognition

Disorders of face recognition ability may take many forms, ranging from small impairments to profound inability to recognise previously familiar faces. Problems may also be transient or permanent – few of us can fail to have experienced some mild temporary failures of recognition, but comparatively few cases of complete inability to recognise others have been reported. In between, there are many neurological conditions producing moderate to severe problems in identifying others and/or interpreting their facial expressions, most of which can be explained within the model shown in Fig. 1.

According to Sergent [31] about 1% of brain-damaged patients show some impairment in recognising faces. However, only some 100 patients have ever been reported displaying prosopagnosia, the most extreme disorder in face perception [33].

By contrast everyday failures in face recognition are comparatively common. Young et al. [38] asked 22 people to keep diaries recording slips or errors in identifying people over a 7-week period. This exercise produced almost 1000 instances of the kinds of errors that people with intact brains can make when looking at other people. Young et al. have categorised these slips into the following types; most of them are from the first four categories:

1. Person unrecognised
2. Person misidentified
3. Person seemed familiar only
4. Difficulty in retrieving biographical details
5. Uncertain of recognition
6. Thought it was not someone it was
7. Wrong name retrieved

Brain Damage

Focal Injury

As Sergent [31] reminds us, the integrity of the whole brain and the joint participation of the two hemispheres are necessary for optimal functioning. Early research into brain damage and face perception concentrated on the particular association between right-sided injury and disorders in recognising people [11, 27, 37]. According to Yin [37] right hemisphere (RH) damage may lead to impaired memory for upright faces, but does not affect memory for inverted faces.

Sergent [31], however, argues that it is a mistake to concentrate exclusively on right hemisphere involvement in face recognition for it may be that the left hemisphere (LH) also possesses mechanisms suited to handling physiognomic patterns, but that it may be more severely affected by any sensory deficits accompanying the injury. That is, the LH is at a cognitive disadvantage compared with the RH which can more easily operate on degraded or distorted input. She continues by stating that the two cerebral hemispheres are sensitive to different bands of spatial frequency: the LH is responsive to high frequencies and the RH to the low frequencies that seem particularly important in face perception. Since it is the high frequency information that is most likely to be lost as a result of brain damage, Sergent insists that the apparent *cognitive* asymmetry in face recognition may be attributed instead to early perceptual factors. Asymmetries do exist, but they are qualitative rather than quantitative in character. The LH processes faces by concentrating largely on high frequency information (which requires good viewing conditions, including long presentation durations), while the RH predominantly makes use of low frequency input that is preserved under impoverished viewing conditions. Sergent's interesting theoretical analysis has yet to be supported by empirical evidence.

Diffuse Damage

A number of general neurological conditions have been examined in relation to their effects on face recognition. Moreover, Levin and Benton [23] have shown that a simple test of face matching skills, in which target faces have to be located among arrays of alternatives, can be reliably used to differentiate neurological cases from those with functional disorders.

Other tests of face processing skills have also been employed. In two related studies patients diagnosed as suffering "chronic organic brain syndrome" were examined on a test of memory for famous faces and a test of ability to identify facial expressions correctly [20, 21]. Interestingly, scores on the two tests were entirely unrelated: some patients were impaired on the memory test, but responded appropriately to the facial expressions; others were able to identify famous faces, but could not label expressions.

Recently, work by an interdisciplinary team at Aberdeen University has begun to explore, inter alia, face processing skills among different groups of dementing patients (Korsakoff, Alzheimer, multi-infarct, chronic alcoholic). Tests were designed to measure: (a) face matching (Benton test); (b) memory for stranger's faces (based on Milner [27]); (c) recognition of famous faces; and (d) ability to interpret facial expression. Patients' brains were examined using nuclear magnetic resonance and blood flow imaging techniques.

The results of this study shown in Table 1 are at present only preliminary, but already they look quite interesting. Korsakoff patients were impaired relative to controls on all four tests, including those that did not require a memory component. The Alzheimer group, while scoring significantly below controls on the first three tests, were normal on the expression test. Interestingly, the Alzheimer patients were

Table 1. Mean raw scores of four patient groups and controls on four face tests

	Famous faces	Facial memory (corrected)	Benton (corrected)	Affect recognition
Controls	19.11	8.67	51.08	14.25
Korsakoff psychosis	5.91	1.25	41.90	11.10
Alcoholic dementia	15.17	5.82	45.44	13.75
Dementia, Alzheimer type	5.78	2.00	40.86	12.86
Multi-infarct dementia	7.89	1.33	39.50	9.00

Table 2. Percentages of prosopagnosias arising from different aetiologies (derived from 74 cases reviewed by Mazzucchi and Biber [25])

Vascular	Neoplastic	Trauma	Infarct	Toxic	Lobectomy
74	9	7	4	3	3

superior to the multi-infarct dementia group on the expression test. With conventional psychometric tests patients suffering from these two conditions are often difficult to distinguish.

Prosopagnosia

By far the most striking disorder in ability to analyse facial images is prosopagnosia, which, as was mentioned earlier, is a fairly unusual syndrome in which patients fail to identify previously familiar faces, usually display difficulties in learning new faces, but sometimes are able to make simultaneous matches to faces [3, 5, 36]. As Table 2 indicates, most cases of prosopagnosia arise from vascular disorders.

At times claims for prosopagnosia following right hemisphere injury alone have been made [10, 18, 22]. As Damasio et al. [9] point out, however, none of these cases has received post-mortem analysis and even if unilateral damage were certain, the fact that the majority were bilateral would be of greater significance. The brain structures closely identified with prosopagnosia are the ventromedial aspects of the occipitotemporal gyri, usually involving bilateral disconnection of the inferior longitudinal fasciculus [19, 26]. However, subcortical structures, particularly the amygdala may also play a part and should not, therefore, be overlooked [30].

At this point it is worthwhile referring back to the earlier discussion of Sergent's [31] ideas concerning the dual nature of face perception. It is clearly predictable from her analysis that bilateral brain damage should be necessary for prosopagnosia to ensue, because unilateral RH damage could leave LH processing intact, allowing some face processing to occur, albeit limited. A similar conclusion may be drawn from a consideration of the work on patients with cerebral commissurotomy who appear able to "identify" faces using either hemisphere [32].

Hecaen [17], it should be noted, cautioned against the facile use of a single term to cover all cases of prosopagnosia. He distinguished perceptual from mnestic prosopagnosia. I believe that the prosopagnosias may usefully be further subdivided and that one way of doing so is to make use of the kind of information-processing model of face recognition that was presented earlier in Fig. 1. Table 3 summarises the argument.

My contention is that the prosopagnosias comprise four types of patients: (a) those who display gross perceptual difficulties; (b) those who cannot classify faces as belonging to certain simple categories (male/female, black/white, old/young); (c) those who can classify correctly, but fail to proceed beyond that point; and (d) those who can not only perceive and classify faces, but who are also aware of faces as being unfamiliar or familiar in some undefined way and yet can not fully identify people they encounter.

It is possible to subdivide prosopagnosics further into those who have additional problems in analysing facial expressions or revisualising faces. Equally a distinction may be made between those who retain some memory for familiar as opposed to famous faces, but the number of cases of prosopagnosia is too small either to warrant or to substantiate such a fine classification scheme. Recent work by Bauer [2] and Damasio et al. [9] has added further complication to the analysis of the prosopagnosias. In each of these studies patients have been reported who, while failing consciously to recognise name-face combinations or simply to identify previously familiar faces, nonetheless displayed evidence of autonomic "recognition".

I should like now to mention briefly a case of prosopagnosia that Andrew Young and I are studying, not because the work throws any theoretical light on the subject of disordered face perception, but because it has revealed a gap in the literature. As far as we can tell no one has reported any systematic attempt to help prosopagnosic patients overcome their visual difficulties. The reasons for this are obvious: the patients often have other, more important, problems; they can usually manage by using nonphysiognomic cues to person identification (voice, gait, etc.); and most patients are past middle age and, perhaps, therefore are beyond any socially crippling consequence of their disability. The following case is the first reported instance of prosopagnosia acquired in early life.

In the case of K. D., therefore, there are good reasons for wanting at least to try to provide remedial help in face perception. She is a 9-year-old girl who suffered meningitis when 14 months old, followed by hydrocephalus, and subsequent anaesthetic complications. She now has mild left-sided hemiparesis and is severely visually impaired with poor contrast sensitivity across a wide range of frequencies. When we first tested her she was of about average intelligence and had a reading age only slightly below chronological age. She is able to recognise people by voice and shows good object recognition.

K. D. cannot recognise anyone by face, however. This includes her family, classmates and teachers. When given photographs of herself mixed with photographs of other children she cannot pick out her own face. She can indicate parts of faces when asked, however, and displays a reasonable ability to perceive and interpret facial expressions. She achieved a score of 37 on the Benton test – but only by laboriously comparing faces feature by feature, which seems to be the way many prosopagnosic patients cope with this task [2]. K. D. does have other visuospatial problems, including poor copying skills and limited topographical memory, but her inability to recognise people's faces is the most pronounced disorder and is already

Table 3. Six-way classification of prosopagnosic deficits

	Perceptual	Categorical	Expression	Familiarity	Identification	Recall
Symptoms of disorders	Metamorphosia. Faces look "glob"-like. Faces seem cartoon-like. Eye region looks strange	Inability to discern: sex; race; age from faces. All faces appear similar	Inability to extract affective information from faces. (Most prosopagnosic patients are able to read facial expressions)	Inability to experience any vestige of familiarity from previously known faces that are not otherwise distorted, etc.	Ability to discern some familiarity, but inability to connect percept to semantic/contextual information about the person	Problems with "revisualising" or recalling facial features. (Many prosopagnosics can recall faces that they are unable to recognise)
Case examples	Shuttleworth et al. [33]	Bodamer [5]	Bauer [2]	Agnetti et al. (1978)	Bornstein [6]	Charcot (1883)
	Whitely and Warrington [35]	Pallis [28]	Bornstein [6]	Cohn et al. (1974)	Bruyer et al. [7]	Shuttleworth et al. [33]

beginning to be a social handicap which will no doubt become a bigger problem as she gets older.

Other Face Perception Disorders

In rare psychiatric cases there are disorders of face perception that usually involve the patient searching for dissimilarity (as opposed to the search for identity made by prosopagnosic patients). In Capgras syndrome patients identify a familiar face, but claim that it is an imposter. In the illusion of Fragoli the same person may appear to undergo transformations of face. Tzavaras et al. [34] have reported that such patients, with what they term delusional misidentification syndrome (DMS), are also likely to be impaired on tests of face matching and short-term face memory which may imply that the origins of DMS may not be so very different from those of prosopagnosia. A similar conclusion may be drawn from work associating bilateral frontal and right hemisphere lesion with Capgras syndrome [1]. This suggests that DMS may have an organic basis similar to that for other forms of reduplicative paramnesia.

Conclusions

Disorders in face perception range from the normal everyday slips in recognition to the profound disturbances in physiognomic analysis shown in rare neurological cases and the equally rare bizarre delusions of identity found in some psychiatric patients. Some of the disorders clearly involve early perceptual processes and may reflect a loss of contrast sensitivity at mid to low spatial frequencies. Other disorders, however, are more properly viewed as originating later in the system and mostly seem to result from problems of accessing stored information, either about general face properties (e.g. what features indicate a male face) or about the familiarity of an individual face, or about its identity. Normal subjects as well as prosopagnosics may display some of these latter disorders, albeit in a much reduced form, but they do not experience the severe perceptual distortions reported by some prosopagnosic/metamorphopic patients, who usually have bilateral posterior brain damage.

Acknowledgements. The interdisciplinary work on face processing is being carried out by Besson, Cherryman, Crawford, Ellis, Parker, Salzen and Smith, and is funded by the Scottish Home and Health Department. The joint work with Andrew Young is supported by a grant from the Economic and Social Research Council. Details of K. D.'s diagnosis and treatment were kindly supplied by Mr. J. F. Shaw, Consultant Neurosurgeon, Western General Hospital, Edinburgh.

References

1. Alexander MP, Stuss DT, Benson DF (1979) Capgras syndrome: a reduplicative phenomenon. Neurol 29:334–339
2. Bauer RM (1984) Autonomic recognition of names and faces in prosopagnosia: A neuropsychological application of the guilty knowledge test. Neuropsychologia 22:457–469

3. Benton AL (1980) The neuropsychology of face recognition. Am Psychol 35:176–186
4. Benton AL, Gordon MC (1971) Correlates of face recognition. Trans Am Neurol Assoc 96:146–150
5. Bodamer J (1947) Die Prosop-Agnosie. Arch Psychiatr Nervenkr 179:6–53
6. Bornstein B (1963) Prospagnosia. In: Halpern L (ed) Problems of dynamic neurology. Hadassah Medical Organization, Jerusalem
7. Bruyer R, Laterre C, Seron X, Feyereisen P, Strypstein E, Pierrand E, Rectem D (1983) A case of prosopagnosia with some preserved covert remembrance of familiar faces. Brain Cogn 2:257–284
8. Damasio AR, Damasio H, Van Hoesen GW (1982) Prosopagnosia: Anatomic basis and behavioral mechanisms. Neurology 32:331–341
9. Damasio AR, Damasio H, Tranel D (1985) Prosopagnosia: Anatomic and physiologic aspects. Paper presented at NATO ARW Aspects of Face Processing, Aberdeen
10. De Renzi E (1985) Prosopagnosia. Paper presented at NATO ARW Aspects of Face Processing, Aberdeen
11. De Renzi E, Spinnler LH (1966) Visual recognition in patients with unilateral brain disease. J Nerv Ment Dis 142:513–525
12. Ellinwood EH (1969) Perception of faces. Psychiatr Q 43:622–646
13. Ellis HD (1983) The role of the right hemisphere in face perception. In: Young AW (ed) Functions of the right cerebral hemisphere. Academic, London
14. Ellis HD (in press) Processes underlying face recognition. In: Bruyer R (ed) The neuropsychology of face perception and facial expression. Erlbaum, Hillsdale NJ
15. Fagan JF (1976) Infants' recognition of invarient features of faces. Child Dev 47:627–638
16. Hay DC, Young AW (1982) The human face. In: Ellis AW (ed) Normality and pathology in cognitive functions. Academic, London
17. Hecaen H (1981) The neuropsychology of face recognition. In: Davies GM, Ellis HD, Shepherd JW (eds) Perceiving and remembering faces. Academic, London
18. Hecaen H, Angelergues R (1962) Agnosia for faces. Arch Neurol 7:92–100
19. Jeeves MA (1985) The historical roots and recurring issues of neurobiological studies of face perception. Hum Neurobiol 3:191–196
20. Kurucz J, Feldmar G (1979) Prosopo-affective agnosia as a symptom of cerebral organic disease. J Am Geriatr Soc 27:225–230
21. Kurucz J, Feldmar G, Werner W (1979) Prosopo-affective agnosia associated with chronic brain syndrome. J Am Geriatr Soc 27:91–95
22. Landis T, Christen L, Cummings JL (1984) Prosopagnosia and associated symptoms in unilateral right posterior lesions: clinical and radiological findings in five patients. Poster presented at 2nd European Workshop on Cognitive Neuropsychology, Bressanone
23. Levin HS, Benton AL (1977) Facial recognition in "pseudo neurological" patients. J Nerv Ment Dis 164:135–138
24. McKellar TPH (1957) Imagination and thinking: a psychological analysis, Cohen and West, London
25. Mazzucchi A, Biber C (1983) Is prosopagnosia more frequent in males than females? Cortex 19:509–516
26. Meadows JC (1974) The anatomic basis of prosopagnosia. J Neurol Neurosurg Psychiatry 37:489–501
27. Milner B (1968) Visual recognition and recall after right temporal lobe excision in man. Neuropsychologia 6:191–209
28. Pallis CA (1955) Impaired identification of faces and places with agnosia for colour. J Neurol Neurosurg Psychiatry 18:218–224
29. Rhodes G (1985) Lateralized processes in face recognition. Br J Psychol 76:249–271
30. Sarter M, Markowitsch HJ (1985) The amygdala's role in human mnemonic processing. Cortex 21:7–24
31. Sergent J (1984) Inferences from unilateral brain damage about normal hemispheric functions in visual pattern recognition. Psychol Bull 96:99–115
32. Sperry RW, Zaidel D (1979) Self-recognition and social awareness in the deconnected minor hemisphere. Neuropsychologia 17:153–166

33. Shuttleworth EC, Syring V, Allen N (1982) Further observations on the nature of prosopagnosia. Brain Cogn 1:207–322
34. Tzavaras A, Luaute JP, Bidault E (1985) Face and psychopathology. Paper presented at NATO ARW Aspects of Face Processing, Aberdeen
35. Whiteley AM, Warrington EK (1977) Prosopagnosia: a clinical, psychological and anatomical study of three patients. J Neurol Neurosurg Psychiatry 40:395–403
36. Wilbrand H (1892) Ein Fall von Seelenblindheit und Hemianopsie mit Sectionsbefund. Dtsche Z Nervenheilk 2:361–387
37. Yin RK (1970) Face recognition by brain-injured patients: a dissociable ability? Neuropsychologia 8:395–402
38. Young AW, Hay DC, Ellis AW (in press) The faces that launched a thousand slips: everyday difficulties and errors in recognising people. Br J Psychol

Recovery of Visual Field in Patients with Postgeniculate Damage

J. ZIHL and D. VON CRAMON[1]

Introduction

Human neuropsychology usually centres on diagnostic assessment and definition of functional disturbances after brain damage in humans. Another aspect of equal relevance is the evaluation of changes of cerebral disorders over the course of time. Poppelreuter, in 1917 [6], and more recently Miller [4] stressed that human neuropsychology should deal with both of these aspects.

Changes in neuropsychological impairment can be expected either owing to recovery of disturbed functions or as a result of a patient's adaptation to his handicap by, for example, compensation. Regarding recovery, one has to distinguish between *spontaneous return* of function and *recovery following intervention*. In the case of spontaneous recovery, the essential question is to what extent function can be expected to return. Insufficient spontaneous recovery does not a priori mean, however, that a particular function cannot be restored in principle, for example, following intervention.

This paper addresses recovery of visual field from scotoma in patients suffering from unilateral postgeniculate damage. Visual field defects are undoubtedly the most frequent cerebral visual disorders, which have the particular advantage that they can be measured quantitatively using standardised stimulus and response parameters. They can serve, therefore, as a good model for the study of recovery of an elementary sensory brain function.

It is surprising that even though the different field defects and their underlying brain pathology were established at the beginning of this century (see, e.g., [8]), no systematic quantitative follow-up studies have been performed except for single cases or small patient groups. From the studies available we have learned, however, that visual field regions can recover spontaneously from scotoma within a relatively short time following brain damage [2, 3]. Even though complete or near complete recovery has been reported in single cases, spontaneous recovery was most often

[1] Max Planck Institute for Psychiatry, Department of Neuropsychology, Kraepelinstr. 10, 8000 München 40, Federal Republic of Germany.

Neurology
Ed. by K. Poeck, H. J. Freund, and H. Gänshirt

limited to the return of fairly small field portions, insufficient to significantly alter patients' levels of disability.

The main complaints of patients with homonymous field loss regard the problem of avoiding obstacles or persons appearing on the defective side, and difficulties with reading. Reading impairment can be observed mainly in cases with field defects reaching the fovea (hemianopia, paracentral scotoma), because the visual field remaining is too small to permit sufficient text to be simultaneously perceived – words disappear at the left or right side of the line, or appear cut off at the beginning or the end, depending on the side of the field defect. Wilbrand [7], who first described this disorder in 1907, called it hemianopic dyslexia. As Poppelreuter [6] pointed out, such patients are not usually in a position to improve their condition through compensatory strategies for themselves.

The objective of our study was to find out (a) how frequently, to what extent, and over what time period spontaneous recovery of visual field could be observed, and (b) whether it is possible to reduce the extent of the field defect by systematic intervention. The group of 111 patients (35 females, 76 males) participating in this study was an ad hoc sample, all of them suffering from unilateral postgeniculate damage. Clinical details are summarised in Table 1. Most patients (69%) had sustained infarction in the area of the posterior cerebral artery. Cases with right-sided brain damage predominated (62, or 56%), in that patients with aphasia were not accepted. Most of the patients (79%) showed homonymous hemianopia. The percentage of cases with upper and lower quadrantanopia were about equal (13% and 11%); six patients (5%) suffered a paracentral scotoma. Except for their visual field loss the patients did not demonstrate any neuropsychological deficit. Oculomotor performance was not disturbed and no obvious ophthalmological disorder was present in any case. All patients except those with closed head injury showed clear signs of a structural lesion as evidenced by hypodensity in the computed tomography (CT) scan.

Visual fields were mapped by standardised kinetic and static perimetry using a modified Tübingen perimeter, which allows fixation monitoring by means of an infrared camera and offers a spatial resolution of 0.25° visual angle up to 15° eccentricity, and 1° beyond.

Table 1. Clinical details of patients ($n = 111$)

Aetiology		PI[a]	IC[b]	CHT[c]	TU[d]
	n	76	8	18	9
	%	68.5	7.2	16.2	8.1
Age	Mean	50.2	53.3	33.9	36.4
	Range	27–76	33–61	15–51	13–46
Sex	Females	26 (34%)	1	4	4
	Males	50 (66%)	7	14	5
Side of damage	Left	28 (37%)	3	11	7
	Right	48 (63%)	5	7	2

[a] Posterior infarction, [b] Intracerebral haemorrhage, [c] Closed head trauma, [d] Tumour (operated)

Spontaneous Recovery

The visual field was determined several times at different intervals following brain damage. The majority of patients (97, or 88%) were examined for the first time within 6 weeks after brain damage. Spontaneous recovery was observed only in a small group of patients (13, or 12%) and occurred either in the central region (see Fig. 1a) or in the periphery of the visual field (Fig. 1b). The extent of spontaneous recovery in the central field region ranged from 2° to 5° ($n=6$; mean: 2.8°). In the periphery (i.e. beyond 5° eccentricity) it ranged from 3° to 8° ($n=7$; mean: 6.3°). With respect to the different aetiologies, 8 out of 76 patients with infarction, 3 out of 18 patients with closed head trauma and 2 out of 8 patients with intracerebral haemorrhage showed spontaneous recovery. Only in one patient who had suffered from intracerebral haemorrhage did we observe a nearly complete recovery from hemianopia within 4 weeks (Fig. 1c).

The percentage of patients showing spontaneous recovery is, therefore, rather small and the extent of recovery limited. It could be suspected, however, that in the early stages spontaneous recovery might be observed in a higher percentage of patients, but only a very few patients can be tested so early on.

We did not find any evidence for significant recovery after more than 6 weeks, although we conducted follow-up investigations in some cases as much as 2 years later (Table 2). It can be concluded that after 6 weeks no further recovery of visual field can be expected.

Visual field data taken at least 6 weeks after the occurrence of brain damage are shown in Table 2. Residual visual field did not exceed 3° visual angle in about 60% of patients. These patients exhibited marked reading disabilities because the field remaining was too small to allow normal reading [10, 11]. In addition, about 90% of the patients, all possessing a residual field smaller than 10°, complained of severe problems in avoiding obstacles or people on the affected side.

Hence one is left with the question whether visual field regions can be restored by systematic intervention. Since intervention techniques were not available in this area, our main effort was to find and develop a training procedure, leaving system-

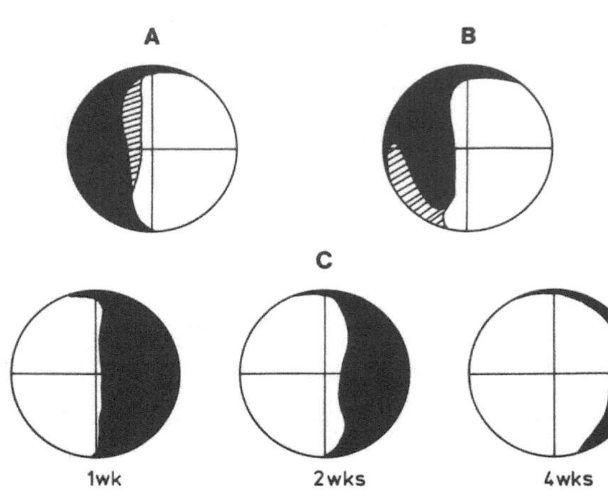

Fig. 1. A, B Partial spontaneous recovery of binocular visual field in two patients with cerebral infarction (**A** of the inner field; **B** in the periphery); **C** complete recovery in a patient with intracerebral haemorrhage. Field maps are shown up to 60° eccentricity

Table 2. Time since lesion, residual visual field before and field enlargement after treatment

Time since lesion (in months)	1	2	3
PI	10 (13%)	28 (37%)	38 (50%)
IH	0	4	4
CHT	0	4	4
TU	1	4	4
Total	11 (10%)	40 (36%)	60 (54%)

Residual visual field (°) before treatment[a]	<1.5	2–3	3.5–5	5.5–10	10
n	18	51	14	19	9
%	16.2	46.2	12.6	17.1	8.1

Visual field enlargement (°) after treatment[a]	<1.5	1.5–3	3.5–5	5.5–10	10
n	32	28	15	15	21
%	28.8	25.3	13.5	13.5	18.9
		35.0[b]	19.0	19.0	27.0

[a] Values refer to meridians along which training was performed
[b] Percentage of cases of the group benefiting from treatment ($n = 79$)

atic quantitative testing of behavioural effectiveness to come later. The objective of this study was, therefore, to find out whether parts of the visual field can be restored, and what factors influence intervention.

Recovery of Visual Field Following Systematic Intervention

The hypothesis that visual field can be restored after brain damage has been supported by experimental studies with primates after striate cortex lesions. Cowey [1] and Mohler and Wurtz [5] showed that detection and localisation of light spots can be restored by systematic training. The observed recovery from scotoma did not occur spontaneously, indicating that improvement resulted from specific intervention. Furthermore, recovery was mainly observed in the field portion subjected to training and was thus not a general effect in terms of a global increase in sensitivity.

On the basis of the training procedure used by Mohler and Wurtz [5] we developed a technique for the treatment of visual field defects in patients with postgeniculate brain damage, using the Tübingen perimeter. This technique has been described elsewhere [9] and will not be presented here in detail. In brief, the patient was asked to shift his gaze, at the onset of an acoustic signal, in one sweep from the fixation point in the centre of the perimeter towards the scotomatous side. Here light targets were presented for 1 s randomly at different positions along a particular meridian. The patients were informed along which meridian targets would appear so that they were able to direct their attention to the field region subjected to training. They were not, however, informed as to the positions of the target and the order of presentation. Usually training sessions were performed daily, and in any session

80–120 trials were conducted. Patients were never informed about the outcome of the sessions.

The visual field was mapped at the beginning of training and at regular intervals. Enlargement of the field of at least 1.5° visual angle was accepted as a significant increase. In a smaller group of patients (49, or 44%) we introduced intervals without treatment lasting 1–9 weeks, to rule out field enlargement independent of systematic intervention. The time between the first evidence of the field loss and the beginning of training varied between 1 and 28 months (see Table 2). In this time no significant change in field size was observed (*t* test: $p > 0.50$). After treatment was finished (i.e. when no further increase larger than 1.5° was observed), measurement of the visual field was continued for at least 4 months.

Amount and Quality of Recovered Field Region

The majority of patients (71%) benefited from treatment, showing a field enlargement which varied between 1.5° and 46°. In approximately half of the patients, field increase did not exceed 5° visual angle. Even this rather small increase was associated, however, with a significant reduction of reading disabilities in 94% of the patients showing this visual disorder before treatment. Difficulties in avoiding obstacles were reduced in about half (52%) of the patients complaining it before treatment.

Enlargement of visual field was restricted to particular field regions and was not obtained along the whole field border. In the restored field region, colour and form vision returned in most of the patients [10]. These patients reported that vision was qualitatively the same in this region as in the corresponding region in the intact hemifield. In some patients, however, colour and form vision did not return in the restored field region, and even light sensitivity remained reduced. This cerebral hemiamblyopia was mainly observed in patients who had suffered closed head trauma (9 out of 11 cases) and, less frequently, in patients with cerebral infarction (6 out of 63 patients).

Enlargement of visual field was linked to periods of treatment. In training-free intervals no significant change in visual field border was obtained ($n = 49$; *t* test: $p > 0.20$). Furthermore, field enlargement did not disappear after the end of the

Table 3. Recovery of visual field by systematic treatment: Pearson correlation coefficients for 7 variables. 1 Sex; 2 Age; 3 Aetiology; 4 Side of brain damage; 5 Time since lesion; 6 Residual field before treatment; 7 Field enlargement after treatment

	1	2	3	4	5	6	7
1	–	−0.08	0.06	0.15	−0.07	−0.15	−0.19
2		–	0.39 [a]	0.27	0.03	−0.06	0.02
3			–	−0.23	−0.05	−0.03	−0.01
4				–	0.01	−0.25	−0.05
5					–	0.09	−0.07
6						–	0.28

[a] $p < 0.001$.

training period. Follow-up measurements extending to about 4 years (range: 4–52 months) did not reveal any significant change in field size in any of the patients when compared with the field border immediately after the end of training (Wilcoxon test: $p > 0.20$).

An important aspect of this study was the identification of factors which may determine or influence recovery of visual field following systematic intervention. Surprisingly enough we could not find any significant correlation between the amount of field enlargement and age, sex, aetiology, side of brain damage, time since lesion and residual visual field (see Table 3). The significant correlation between age and aetiology is due to the fact that patients suffering from posterior cerebral infarction or intracerebral haemorrhage were on average much older than patients with closed head trauma or tumour (cf. Table 1).

Conclusions. The main conclusions which can be drawn from this study are as follows:

1. Spontaneous recovery of visual field from scotoma can be observed within about the first 2 months after brain damage. The percentage of cases showing spontaneous recovery is rather negligible.
2. Visual field restoration by systematic treatment is possible; the extent of enlargement is, however, limited.
3. Several factors, especially age at injury and time since brain damage, were not found significantly to influence recovery following systematic intervention.

What are the possible neural mechanisms underlying the observed recovery? One may hypothesise that the loss of visual field as initially plotted may have resulted from both irreversible and reversible damage to the optic radiation and/or the striate cortex. Recovery of visual field may be interpreted as the reappearance or increase of functional efficiency previously reduced by reversible damage. Recovery will not occur, therefore, following almost complete destruction of neuronal tissue. In fact, we did not find any significant recovery in patients with pseudocystic necrosis, showing hypodense areas with values below 15 HU in the CT scan. On the other hand, almost complete hemianopia was also present in patients with CT density values ranging between 20 and 30 HU. In these patients we observed field enlargement following treatment [10]. It seems reasonable, therefore, to assume that neuronal damage was incomplete in patients benefiting from treatment, so that residual neurons able to subserve visual functioning remained intact.

A final comment is required as to the behavioural significance of the effect of systematic intervention described in this paper. After treatment of the total group of 111 patients, 69 cases (62%) did not present a visual field larger than 10° eccentricity in the affected hemifield, either because patients did not benefit from treatment or because recovery was too small. Thus, these patients are still handicapped by their difficulty in seeing objects and persons on the affected side. For this group of patients we therefore have to identify other means of intervention leading to a successful adaptation to their handicap. One strategy which presents itself is compensation of the irreversibly lost visual field by eye and head movements. The majority of our patients did not compensate spontaneously for their field defect to a sufficient extent by such means. They showed a restricted field of search in the hemifield on the affected side, with an average extent of 9° along the horizontal axis (range: 3–28°). For comparison, in the intact hemifield the average extent of the field of search was 46° (range: 40–52°). If a patient's field of search can be improved by intervention, the degree of compensation for the lost hemifield may hopefully be improved and his visual disability thus be reduced. Using a specially developed training technique, we were able to improve patients' exploration, leading to a significant enlargement of the field of search (mean extent after treatment: 28°; range: 18–42°; t test: $p < 0.001$).

In conclusion, patients with homonymous field loss can be treated either by direct restoration of visual field or by the introduction of new search strategies. These alternatives are not mutually exclusive. With respect to rehabilitation, the main goal of intervention is the reduction of patient's impairment. The means of intervention, however, remain to be determined individually depending on the prognosis for recovery of function.

Acknowledgement. Part of this work has been supported by Deutsche Forschungsgemeinschaft.

References

1. Cowey A (1967) Perimetric study of field defects in monkeys after cortical and retinal ablations. Q J Exp Psychol 19:232–254
2. Gloning I, Gloning K, Tschabitscher H (1962) Die occipitale Blindheit auf vaskulärer Basis. Graefes Arch Clin Exp Ophthalmol 165:138–177
3. Haerer AF (1973) Visual field defects and the prognosis of stroke. Stroke 4:163–168
4. Miller E (1984) Recovery and management of neuropsychological impairment. John Wiley, Chichester New York
5. Mohler CW, Wurtz RH (1977) The role of striate cortex and superior colliculus in visual guidance of saccadic eye movements in monkeys. J Neurophysiol 40:74–94
6. Poppelreuter W (1917) Die psychischen Schädigungen durch Kopfschuß im Kriege 1914/16. Band I: Die Störungen der niederen und höheren Sehleistungen durch Verletzungen des Okzipitalhirns. Voss, Leipzig
7. Wilbrand H (1907) Über die makulär-hemianopische Lesestörung und die v. Monakowsche Projektion der Makula auf die Sehsphäre. Klin Mbl Augenheilk 45:1–39
8. Wilbrand H, Saenger A (1917) Die homonyme Hemianopsie nebst ihren Beziehungen zu anderen cerebralen Herderscheinungen. Bergmann, Wiesbaden
9. Zihl J (1980) Recovery of visual function in patients with cerebral blindness: effect of specific practice with saccadic localization. Exp Brain Res 44:159–169
10. Zihl J, von Cramon D (1985) Visual field recovery from scotoma in patients with postgeniculate damage. Brain 108:439–469
11. Zihl J, Krischer C, Meißen R (1984) Die hemianopische Lesestörung und ihre Behandlung. Nervenarzt 55:317–323

Memory and its Disorders

Is Vascular Thalamic Amnesia a Disconnection Syndrome?

D. von Cramon, N. Hebel, and U. Schuri [1]

"Is amnesia a disconnection syndrome?" This question, raised by Warrington and Weiskrantz in 1982 [23], will be reexamined in the context of circumscirbed vascular thalamic lesions followed by memory dysfunction. It is through the knowledge of vascularization patterns and angioarchitectonic features of the human thalamus that we hope to further the discussion on vascular thalamic amnesia. Over the last decade several cases of vascular thalamic lesions have been reported where by CCT evidence small hypodense lesions, representing selective thalamic infarctions, in the "polar" region of the thalamus have been held responsible for severe memory dysfunction [2, 5, 8, 9, 11, 17, 18, 24].

Regarding some of these papers a somewhat hazardous interpretation of the anatomical structures presumably involved in the thalamic amnesia may be noticed. Most authors hypothesize without further proof, that a lesion of the mediodorsal thalamic nucleus (MD) is crucial to memory dysfunction. Because MD lesions are said to cause amnesia in patients with thiamine deficiency [22] and because MD lesions actually lead to memory disorders in animals (cf. [10]) amnesia due to vascular thalamic lesions is also attributed to MD lesions. It is necessary to examine whether this analogy-based argument is not in fact circular.

It is the aim of this study to speculate on the anatomical implications of thalamic, not diencephalic, amnesia on the basis of 11 of our own patients with selective vascular thalamic lesions, 4 of them suffering from memory dysfuncion, the other 7 with no memory disorder. In addition we reevaluated 5 amnesic patients with vascular thalamic lesions reported in the literature. The central question concerns whether lesions of the thalamic grey or *white* matter play a decisive role in vascular thalamic amnesia.

Before entering into the anatomical discussion we need to establish whether there are clear-cut differences in test data on memory performance among the 11 patients with thalamic lesions whom we had the opportunity to examine repeatedly over a period between 8 months (patient 7) and 84 months (patient 3) after the event (see Table 1).

---

[1] Max Planck Institute for Psychiatry, Department of Neuropsychology, Kraepelinstrasse 10, 8000 Munich 40, Federal Republic of Germany.

Neurology
Ed. by K. Poeck, H. J. Freund, and H. Gänshirt

Table 1. Data on 11 patients with circumscribed vascular thalamic lesions

Patient	1	2	3	4	5	6	7	8	9	10	11
Age	67	42	44	58	61	66	46	60	64	19	14
Sex	M	F	F	F	F	F	M	M	M	F	F
Site of lesion	P/B	P/B	P/B	P/L	C/B	C/L	V/B	V/L	V/R	V/L	V/L
Time since lesion (months)	14	12	84	26	13	36	8	10	11	35	16
Chronic amnesia	Yes	Yes	Yes	Yes	No	No	No	No	No	No	No

C, central (paramedian); P, polar; V, ventrolateral; B, bilateral; L, left; R, right

Beginning with the short-term retention of verbal stimuli, the digit span was normal in all patients. If the amount of isolated verbal information exceeded the attention span considerably – as in a 15-item word list – the recall performance was impaired in only one patient (patient 1) with bilateral lesions in the polar region. The same patient revealed an increased rate of forgetting in a word list with delayed recall. The recall of sentences, however, was not impaired in any patient. Increasing the amount of semantically connected verbal information – as in a short story with 57 semantic units – only two patients (patients 1 and 2) with bilateral polar lesions showed a poor performance. The short-term retention of nonverbal stimuli such as block span or the recognition of Benton's figures, faces and odours was normal in all patients.

The long-term retention – over a period of 48 h – of complex verbal material (the short story) was disturbed in all patients with bilateral polar lesions (patients 1–3) whereas the recognition of faces was impaired in one patient only. We had expected the long-term retention of faces to be more severely afflicted in patients with significant lesions in the right thalamus (patients 1–3). It is likely that the recognition task (choosing one face out of four in a series of ten faces presented 48 h before) may have been too easy.

The three patients with bilateral and the patient with the left-sided polar lesion showed a very poor performance in verbal learning tasks. Comparing our own results with those reported in the literature, the verbal learning deficit may be considered a key symptom of vascular thalamic amnesia. The learning of nonverbal, i.e. complex figurate stimuli is not so consistently impaired. Nevertheless, three of four patients with polar lesions also showed poor performances in object paired associates learning. None of them obtained good results in a visual maze learning task. It is noteworthy also that the patient with the left-sided lesions was impaired in two nonverbal learning tasks. The question arises whether (a) there might be an additional right-sided lesion not visible in the CCT, or more likely (b) that the "nonverbal" learning tasks require verbal strategies as well. On the other hand we were surprised by the fact that patient 3, whose bilateral polar lesions had occurred 7 years before, showed a normal performance in object paired associates learning. One may speculate that in chronic thalamic amnesia the nonverbal learning capacity can be better compensated than the verbal one.

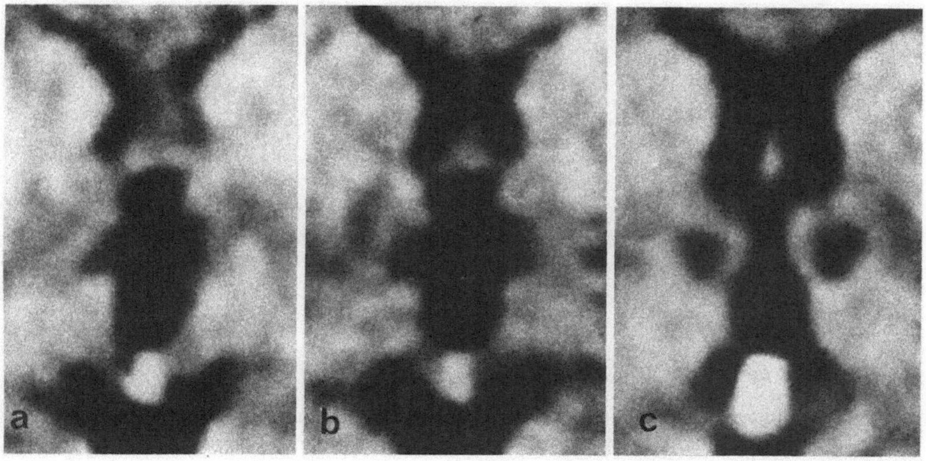

Fig. 1 a–c. Bilateral thalamic lesions in a 44-year-old female suffering from a long-lasting amnesia that had occurred 7 years before. The hypodense areas afflicting only the caudal and middle thalamic level (excluding the cranial thalamic level and presumably also the hypothalamic level) are located almost symmetrically in the polar region of both thalami. At the middle thalamic level (slice **c**) the hypodense lesions are separated from the third ventricle by a small normodense band, whereas at the caudal level the lesions come close to the third ventricle

Anterograde amnesia in vascular thalamic lesions is not necessarily associated with a retrograde amnesia. Patient 1 had a poor performance in a famous faces test and only two amnesic patients had difficulties in recalling the main events of their lives.

All amnesic patients had an unrealistic view of their memory deficits, considerably overestimating their performances. It is possible, in view of this lack of insight, that at least patients with bilateral polar lesions may to some extent appear as "happy amnesics". General intelligence, as tested with a short German version of the WAIS [6], was within the normal range in all 11 patients. Furthermore, amnesic and nonamnesic patients could not be distinguished by attentional deficits. There is obviously no doubt that the three patients with bilateral and the one with the left-sided lesion in the "polar" region of the thalamus showed the constitutive features of chronic amnesia (cf. [24]).

We would like to turn to the discussion of the pathoanatomical prerequisites of vascular thalamic amnesia with the presentation of the CCT scans of two patients (patients 3 and 4) which prove that we based our investigations on well-defined and selective thalamic lesions (Figs. 1 and 2).

Thalamic vascularization is complex; thus it is not surprising that there are divergent classifications reported in the literature. We follow the description of Buettner [3] and Percheron [13–15].

In 60%–70% of the cases reported in the literature the ventral thalamic region consists of two vascular subterritories, one supplied by the paramedian thalamic arteries and a more oral one supplied by a single polar artery (Fig. 3). If this latter vessel is absent the polar territory is irrigated by the paramedian thalamic arteries.

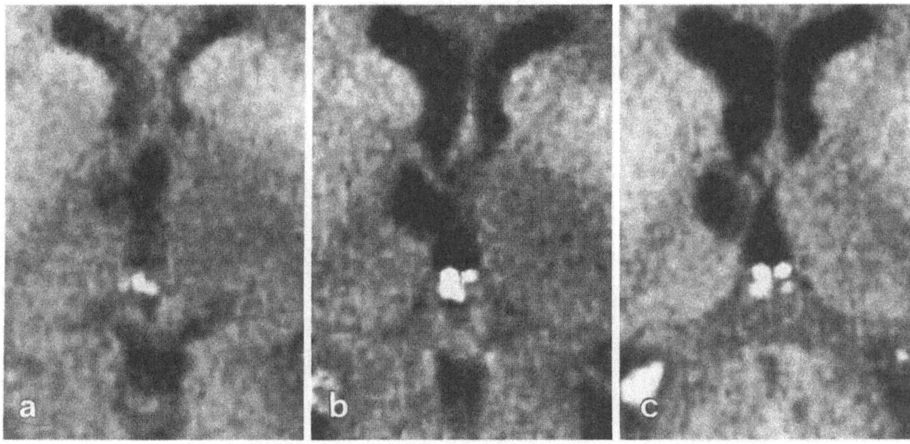

Fig. 2a–c. Unilateral thalamic lesion in a 58-year-old female suffering from chronic amnesia. The CCT was done 26 months after the "brain event". The anterior horn of the left ventricle is slightly enlarged; the polar region of the *left* thalamus shows a hypodense area restricted to the caudal and middle level of the thalamus. Again the large hypodense lesion reaches the third ventricle at the caudal thalamic level and is presumably separated from it at the middle thalamic level

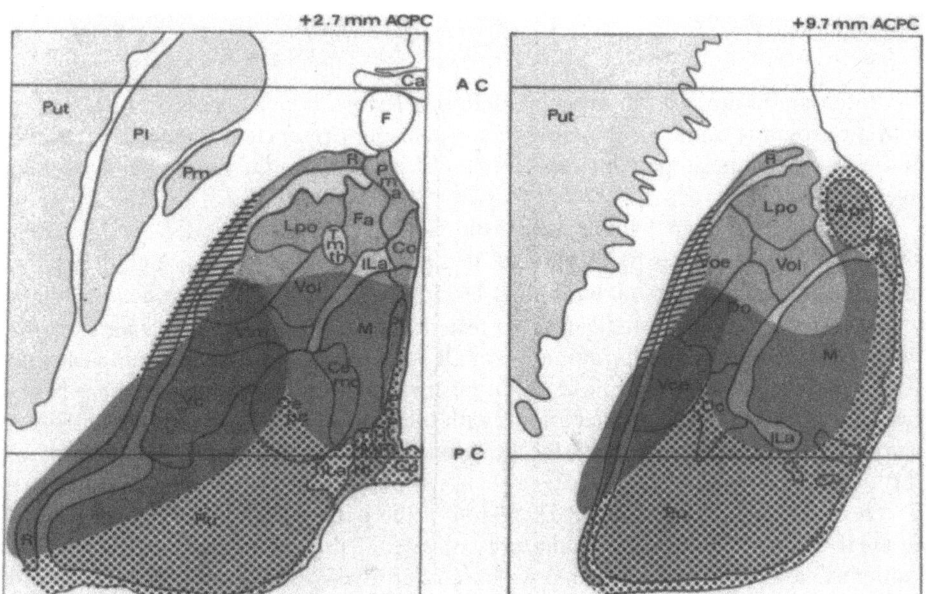

Fig. 3. The two vascular subterritories of the ventral thalamic region are shown in grey; the *light grey area* depicts the territory of the polar thalamic artery; the *medium grey area* that of the paramedian thalamic arteries. The irrigation areas are indicated for the caudal thalamic level (2.7 mm above ACPC line) and for the middle thalamic level (9.7 mm above ACPC line) on two horizontal sections of Van Buren and Borke's atlas [21]. The grey irrigation area reaches the third ventricle at the caudal thalamic level, but is separated from it at the middle thalamic level by a small band of tissue supplied by the medial branch of the posterior choroidal arteries (*stippled area*). The *dark grey area* represents the vascular subterritory of the geniculate arteries, the *diagonally hatched area* that of the anterior choroidal artery

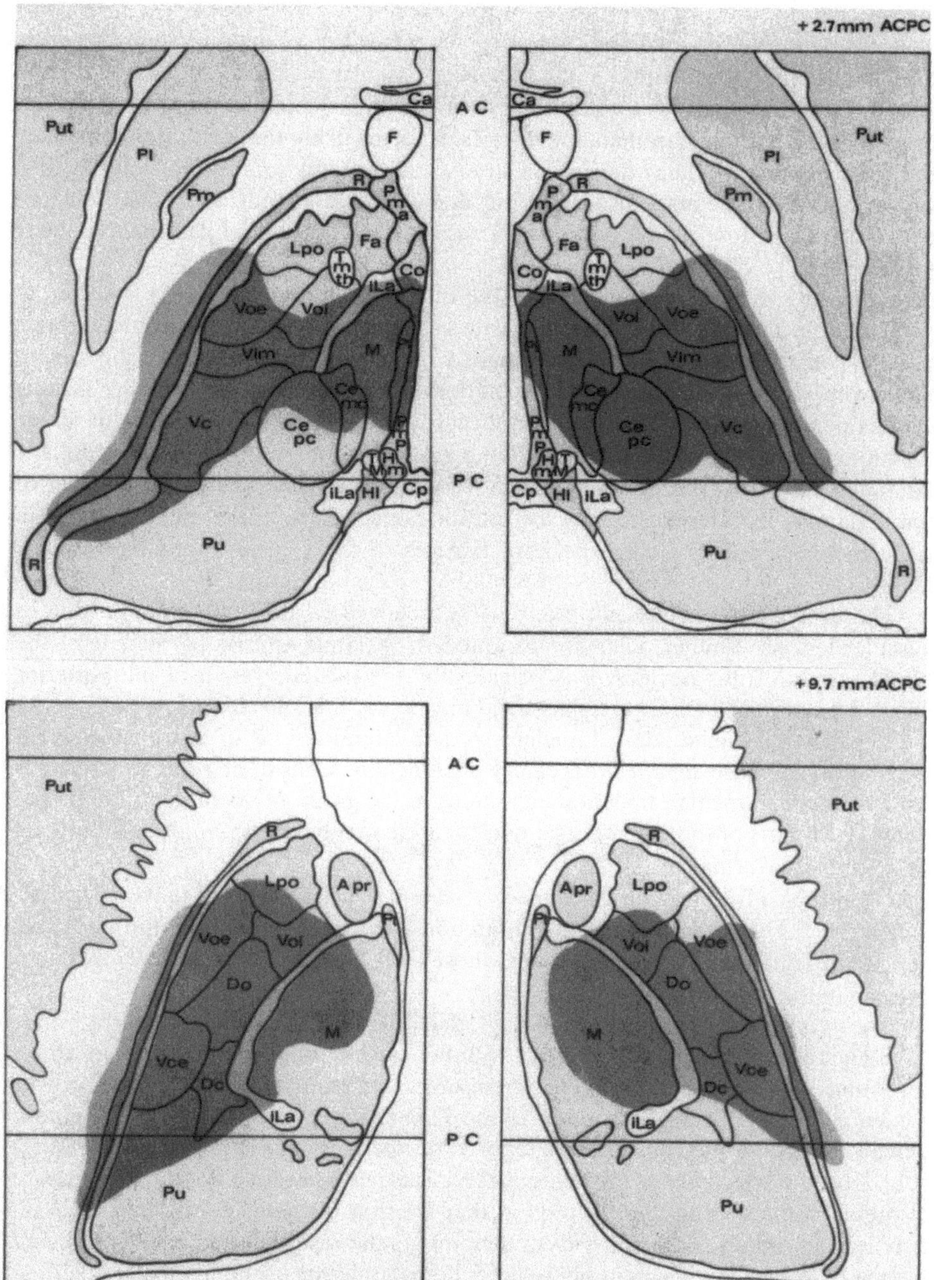

Fig. 4. The thalamic infarction areas (*dark grey*) of seven patients who did not reveal significant memory disorders at the caudal (upper diagrams) and the middle (lower diagrams) thalamic level. The vascular lesions included the territory of the geniculate and paramedian thalamic arteries. In two cases larger parts of the mediodorsal nucleus were affected, leaving, however, its ventromedial portion spared. There were no isolated infarctions in the territory of the posterior choroidal vessels; they are usually combined with an infarction of other branches of the posterior cerebral artery, afflicting memory-related brain structures, e.g. in the postcommissural hippocampus and posterior parahippocampal gyrus

Comparing the original CCT scans of our own cases of thalamic amnesia with those sufficiently documented in the literature, vascular thalamic amnesia obviously depends on infarctions in the subterritory of the polar thalamic artery or the polar branch of the paramedian thalamic arteries. It seems likely that central paramedian thalamic infarction when there is an artery sufficient to supply the polar region causes no severe memory disorder. This assumption is supported by two nonamnesic patients, whose infarct patterns are restricted to the central paramedian territory (Fig. 4).

Regarding the angioarchitecture of the human thalamus, we find a specific organization of the arterial vessels. The arteries and arterioles have a rectilinear and parallel course, their ramifications are mostly rectangular. As a characteristic feature larger vessels are located in the white matter of the thalamus; only smaller ramifications penetrate into the grey matter. Accordingly, a high concentration of larger thalamic vessels is found in the mamillothalamic tract and in the internal medullary lamina as well [16]. The polar thalamic artery ramifies at the ventrobasal border of the thalamus; its arterioles follow the intrathalamic course of the mamillothalamic tract and may also run with the fibre bundles of the ventral internal medullary lamina.

The anterior nuclei are not likely to be involved in thalamic amnesia due to vascular lesions. Neither polar nor paramedian thalamic arteries participate in the blood supply of this nucleus; it is irrigated by the medial branch of the posterior choroidal arteries which is rarely involved in vascular thalamic lesions.

Regarding the mediodorsal nucleus, even bilateral lesions of this nucleus seem insufficient to cause *significant* memory dysfunction. Considering the two patients with central paramedian thalamic infarctions in the group of seven nonamnesic patients large parts of the mediodorsal nucleus were involved with no relevant impact on memory performance.

We received fresh insight into memory-related structures crucial to vascular thalamic amnesia by superimposing the infarction areas of our own four amnesic cases and, additionally, of five amnesic cases whose CCT "lesions" were sufficiently documented in the literature (Fig. 5).

The overlap area encircles the mamillothalamic tract, a component of the Papez circuit connecting the mamillary body with the anterior thalamic nucleus, two structures that are obviously not afflicted themselves. There appears to be a vast body of evidence that a bilateral disruption of the Papez circuit alone may cause memory deficit. Regarding the clinical cases reported in the literature (e.g. the case of Sweet et al. [20]) the selectivity of the anatomical lesions seems at least doubtful. There are also data contradicting the assumption that a lesion restricted to the Papez circuit may lead to significant memory dysfunction (e.g. the case reported by Woolsey and Nelson [25]). The involvement of the mamillothalamic tract is highly likely in vascular thalamic lesions; this is corroborated by pathoanatomical findings [4, 7].

The other structure located within the overlap area is the ventral portion of the internal medullary lamina. Its possible role in memory processes has not been discussed so far. Fibres travelling within the anterior and the inferior thalamic peduncle reach the mediodorsal nucleus passing this part of the internal medullary lamina. The anterior thalamic peduncle contains bidirectional fibres connecting the prefrontal, orbitofrontal and anterior cingulate cortex with the mediodorsal nucleus.

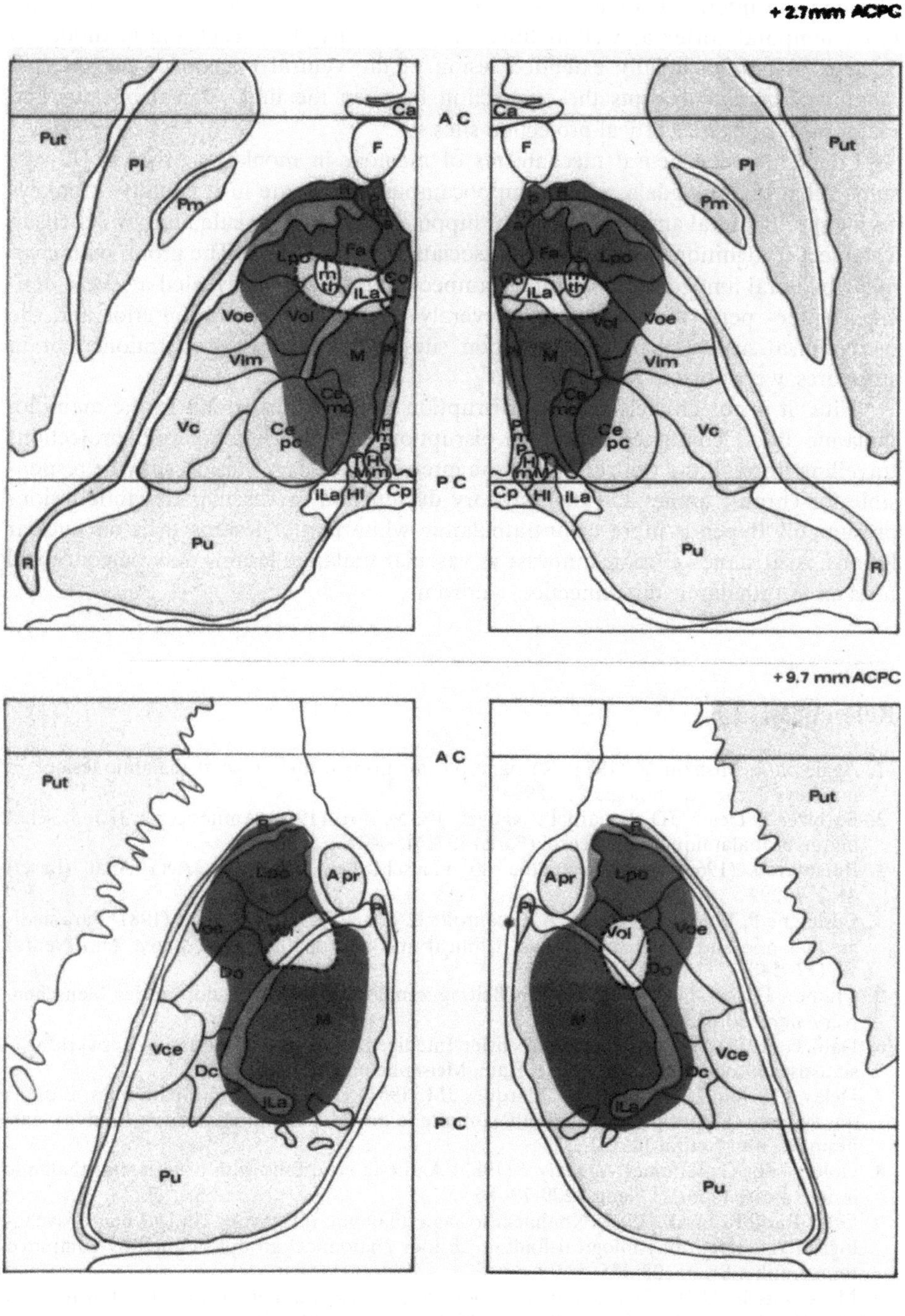

Fig. 5. Overlap areas of the thalamic lesions of four of our own and five other cases reported in the literature at the caudal (upper diagrams) and the middle (lower diagrams) thalamic level. The overlap areas encircle two fibre structures: the mamillothalamic tract and the ventral part of the internal medullary lamina. The *dark grey area* represents the vascular territory of the polar and paramedian arteries

Through the inferior thalamic peduncle fibres from the orbitofrontal, insular, anterior temporal cortex as well as fibres from the amygdala reach the mediodorsal nucleus. A craniocaudally extended lesion of the ventral portion of the internal medullary lamina disrupts the connection between the mediodorsal nucleus and major parts of its neocortical projection sites.

Concerning the neural mechanisms of memory in monkeys, Mishkin [12] assumed that the amygdala and the hippocampus participate in it equally. Monkeys with either bilateral amygdalectomy or hippocampectomy revealed minor deficits in an object recognition and also in an associative memory task. The group with *combined* bilateral amygdalectomy-hippocampectomy, however, revealed a severe deficit. Memory performance was also severely impaired when the anterior and the mediodorsal nuclei, thalamic projection sites of the previously mentioned brain structures, were ablated bilaterally [1].

Thus, it is not unlikely that the disruption of the Papez circuit in the mamillothalamic tract, combined with the disruption of amygdalothalamic projections travelling through the ventral part of the internal medullary lamina, may be responsible for chronic amnesia. Thus, memory dysfunction in vascular thalamic lesions presumably depends more on intrathalamic white matter lesions than on nuclear lesions. As it stands chronic amnesia in vascular thalamic lesions may be conceived of as an intrathalamic disconnection syndrome.

References

1. Aggleton J, Mishkin M (1983) Recognition impairment after medial thalamic lesions in monkeys. Neuropsychologia 21:189–197
2. Barbizet J, Degos JD, Louarn F, Nguyen JP, Mas JL (1981) Amnésie par lésion ischémique bi-thalamique. Rev Neurol (Paris) 137:415–424
3. Buettner J (1960) Die Blutgefäße im menschlichen Thalamus. Acta Anat (Basel) 41:279–299
4. Castaigne P, Lhermitte F, Buge A, Escourolle R, Hauw JJ, Lyon-Caen O (1981) Paramedian thalamic and midbrain infarcts: Clinical and neuropathological study. Ann Neurol 10:127–148
5. Cramon D von, Eilert P (1979) Ein Beitrag zum Amnestischen Syndrom des Menschen. Nervenarzt 50:643–648
6. Dahl G (1972) WIP reduzierter Wechsler Intelligenz Test – Anwendung – Auswertung – statistische Analysen – Normwerte. Hain, Meisenheim am Glan
7. Delay J, Brion S, Escourolle R, Marques JM (1961) Démences artériopathiques. Lésions du système hippocampo-mamillothalamique dans le déterminisme des troubles amnésiques. Rev Neurol 105:22–33
8. Goldenberg G, Wimmer A, Maly J (1983) Amnesic syndrome with a unilateral thalamic lesion: a case report. J Neurol 229:79–86
9. Graff-Radford et al. (1985) Nonhaemorrhagic thalamic infarction: clinical neuropsychological and electrophysiological findings in four anatomical groups defined by computed tomography. Brain 108:485–516
10. Markowitsch HJ (1982) Thalamic mediodorsal nucleus and memory: a critical evaluation of studies in animals and man. Neurosci Biobehav Rev 6:351–380
11. Michel D, Laurent B, Foyatier N, Blanc A, Portafaix M (1982) Infarctus thalamique paramedian gauche. Rev Neurol 138:533–550
12. Mishkin M (1982) A memory system in the monkey. Philos Trans R Soc Lond [Biol] 298:85–95

13. Percheron G (1966) Etude anatomique du thalamus de l'homme adulte et de sa vascularisation artérielle. Medical thesis, Paris
14. Percheron G (1976a) Les artères du thalamus humain. I. Artère et territoire thalamique polaires de l'artère communicante posterieure. Rev Neurol (Paris) 132:297–307
15. Percheron G (1976b) Les artères du thalamus humain. II. Artères et territoire thalamiques paramedians de l'artère basilaire communicante. Rev Neurol (Paris) 132:–309–324
16. Plets C, de Reuck J, van der Eecken H, van den Bergh R (1970) The vascularization of the human thalamus. Acta Neurol Belg 70:687–770
17. Schott B, Mauguire F, Laurent B, Serclerat O, Fischer C (1980) L'amnésie thalamique. Rev Neurol 136:117–130
18. Speedie LJ, Heilman KM (1982) Amnesic disturbance following infarction of the left dorsomedial nucleus of the thalamus. Neuropsychologia 20:597–604
19. Squire LR, Moore RY (1979) Dorsal thalamic lesion in a noted case of human memory dysfunction. Ann Neurol 6:503–506
20. Sweet WH, Talland GA, Ervin FR (1959) Loss of recent memory following section of fornix. Trans Am Neurol Assoc 84:76–82
21. Van Buren JM, Borke RC (1972) Variations and connections of the human thalamus. 2. Variations of the human diencephalon. Springer, Berlin Heidelberg New York
22. Victor M, Adams RD, Collins GH (1971) The Wernicke-Korsakoff syndrome. Blackwell Scientific, Oxford
23. Warrington EK, Weiskrantz L (1982) Amnesia: A disconnection syndrome? Neuropsychologia 20:233–248
24. Winocour G, Oxbury S, Roberts R, Agnetti V, Davis C (1984): Amnesia in a patient with bilateral lesions to the thalamus. Neuropsychologia 22:123–143
25. Woolsey RM, Nelson JS (1975): Asymptomatic destruction of the fornix in man. Arch Neurol 32:566–568

What Amnesics Can and Can Not Do

A. BADDELEY[1]

Human memory is not of course a unitary function, and there has over the last 10 or 20 years been considerable controversy as to how many kinds of memory should be assumed. While this is still an area of lively disagreement, at least some of this is probably more terminological than conceptual. There would probably be relatively broad agreement about a preliminary analysis of memory into at least three separate domains, namely sensory memory, working memory and long-term memory. The term sensory memory refers to the brief storage of information presented to the senses which forms part of the process of perception. It seems likely that brain damage will on occasion produce deficits in these systems, but they are likely to present as perceptual rather than memory problems, and as such are beyond the scope of the present review.

Information passes from the sensory systems into working memory, a system concerned with the temporary maintenance and manipulation of information that is required by a wide range of tasks ranging from the comprehension of spoken language to the performance of reasoning and arithmetic tasks. The concept of working memory developed from that of short-term memory (STM), but differs from it in a number of important respects. Within experimental psychology, the term STM implies a unitary store capable of holding small amounts of information over a matter of seconds. The terms is an unfortunate one, since it is used by the general public, and by some of the medical profession, in a much looser way to refer to remembering things that happened a matter of minutes, hours or days ago, as opposed to years, a distinction which does not in fact seem to map onto empirical results. In recent years it has become clear that the concept of a unitary STM is over-simplified, and consequently it has been replaced by the concept of working memory which refers to an alliance of interacting temporary storage systems, the subsystems themselves often being directly involved in other cognitive processes such as hearing, talking and seeing. In its current form the model assumes three main components: the central executive, a control system that is probably tied up with the processes of attention, which is supplemented by two slave systems; the visuospatial

[1] Medical Research Council, Applied Psychology Unit, Cambridge, Great Britain.

Neurology
Ed. by K. Poeck, H. J. Freund, and H. Gänshirt

sketchpad, a system responsible for maintaining and manipulating visual images; and the articulatory loop which stores and manipulates phonological information.

Long-Term Memory

Traditionally, long-term memory (LTM) has been regarded as a unitary system. In recent years however, its unity has been increasingly questioned, and it certainly has proved useful to make a number of conceptual distinctions, although whether these represent separate underlying neural systems, or are reflections of the same system operating under different circumstances, remains in dispute. One distinction that has been made is that between *semantic* and *episodic* memory. The term semantic memory essentially refers to our knowledge of the world, whether it comprises knowing the colour of a banana or the meaning of the French word *chat* or how many inches there are in a foot. This was distinguished, in an influential paper by Tulving [5], from episodic memory, which represents our memory for personally experienced events such as having breakfast this morning or meeting someone on holiday last year. There is no doubt that these two modes in which the memory system operates are different in many ways, although I would not regard the evidence as forcing one to assume separate underlying systems. For example, it may be the case that semantic memories are the residue of large numbers of episodes, each having something in common, the semantic component, which builds up and is much more durable than the recollection of the individual episodes on which the semantic information is based.

A third category of human learning does present a much stronger case for depending on a separate system. This is what has sometimes been termed procedural learning and it comprises essentially the acquisition of skills, whether perceptual, such as learning to scan an X-ray and detect a diseased lung; motor, as in learning to ride a bicycle; or intellectual, as in learning to solve puzzles such as the Tower of Hanoi. The evidence that this is a separate memory system comes primarily from studies of the amnesic syndrome, where this type of learning appears to be intact, despite the presence of dense and global amnesia. I shall return to this point later.

The study of human memory was for many years largely confined to the laboratory, where it is relatively easy to control the amount of learning, the retention interval and the conditions of retrieval. In recent years however there has been an increasing concern with the ecological validity of the techniques developed within the laboratory.

Broadly speaking the concepts developed within the laboratory are, I am happy to say, generally applicable outside. There are however two areas which have been neglected in laboratory research which are now starting to be investigated in more detail, namely autobiographical memory, the capacity of a subject to recollect events from earlier life, and prospective memory, remembering to do something at a particular time, for example to buy bread on the way back from the office. While these aspects of memory do not necessarily involve separate memory systems, they probably do involve different uses of these systems, and since they are more central to the lives of patients than learning lists of unrelated words, they are of very direct clinical relevance within neuropsychology.

Amnesia

Memory problems of a greater or lesser degree are characteristic of a very wide range of patients suffering from any form of brain damage, be it the result of head injury, stroke, presenile dementia or indeed normal ageing. The term amnesic syndrome however would typically be applied only to patients whose memory deficit is substantial, a deficit which may occur in a relatively pure form, unaccompanied by other signs of cognitive impairment. Such "pure" amnesics are of course comparatively rare, but are theoretically very important because of their implications for the existence of a specific system concerned with long-term memory. Subjects with pure amnesia offer a natural experiment which allows us to draw strong conclusions about the memory system involved, in contrast to patients who have multiple cognitive deficits, making interpretation of their remaining capacities extremely difficult. However, such patients are of course much more numerous than pure amnesics, and from a practical viewpoint if from no other, it is important that our theories are also applicable to them. Fortunately, in recent years there has been a considerable increase in work on such cognitively varied, but important groups as those suffering from closed head injury, stroke, senile dementia, and of course normal ageing.

There is however no doubt that neuropsychologists have been particularly interested in the study of pure amnesics. Since such cases are rare, in practice this has meant studying groups such as those suffering from Korsakoff syndrome, who are identified as being *relatively* cognitively intact. It has however become increasingly clear that many such patients do suffer from secondary deficits, as indeed one might expect, bearing in mind the very varied pattern of brain damage that is associated with virtually any given aetiology, including of course that of Korsakoff syndrome. However, after a period of controversy, largely generated by the problem of comparability of patients, there now appears to be considerable agreement as to what a relatively pure amnesic patient can and can not do. Since cases of comparatively pure amnesia have been reported in a wide range of patients, including alcoholics with Korsakoff syndrome, postencephalitics, CVA patients and patients suffering from anoxia or poisoning, the question obviously arises as to whether they show a common syndrome. While the detailed pattern of impairments may vary somewhat from patient to patient, I do not feel that there is as yet any conclusive evidence to suggest that the pattern varies with aetiology. This would certainly not be a universal view; Squire [3] for example has suggested that two types of amnesia exist, one reflecting damage to the temporal lobes, showing relatively rapid forgetting, and a second, associated with subcortical damage, showing normal forgetting rates. The evidence for such differences in forgetting rate appear to me to be at present very slim, with subsequent evidence seeming to suggest that rates of forgetting are remarkably normal across a wide range of patients. Hence, in the absence of evidence to the contrary I shall discuss the amnesic syndrome as if it were a unitary memory deficit. I shall illustrate the discussion with data from a single very pure amnesic patient, K.J., who became densely amnesic following an attack of meningitis and who was studied jointly by Dr. Barbara Wilson and myself. Though not highly educated he is of superior intelligence (verbal IQ 133, performance 131).

A classic amnesic patient will show impaired learning of new material, regardless of modality of presentation and regardless of whether it is based on language, meaning or spatial coding. In terms of performance on psychological tests, one would expect such patients to have great difficulty learning to associate pairs of words, to learn the names or faces of new people, or to recall passages of prose, stories or incidents after a brief delay. Recognition memory would similarly be impaired for verbal or visual material. The performance of K.J. on some standard long-term memory tasks is shown in Table 1, from which it will be clear that he has a substantial memory deficit.

Laboratory-based memory tests have been used for many years and found to be reliable and sensitive measures of memory deficit. They are however somewhat artificial, and a patient might well argue that he or she can cope very well without needing to commit to memory 40 unrelated words or 40 strange faces, and that the verbatim recall of news items is only marginally more important than the capacity to remember complicated but meaningless designs. In fact of course there is no doubt that in densely amnesic patients, abysmally poor performance on the tests described is associated with major everyday memory problems, which may well be sufficiently incapacitating to make it impossible for the patient to work, or live a normal life. A series of interview and questionnaire studies carried out on both closed head injury patients and the normal elderly suggested that everyday memory problems certainly do occur, but indicated that they are not necessarily well predicted by performance on standard clinical tests [4].

Table 1. Performance of a post-meningitic patient K. J. on a range of standard memory tests

Test	Score	
Digit span	14[a]	
Logical memory (prose)		
Immediate	12[a]	
Delayed	0[a]	
Visual memory (Rey)		
Copy	35/36	
Recall	0/36	
Warrington forced choice recognition		
Words	5[a]	
Faces	6[a]	
Rivermead behavioural memory test	0/12	
Semantic memory		
Silly sentences test	K. J.	Controls (sd)
Time/sentence (s)	2.03	1.98 (0.79)
Errors (%)	0.7	1.8
Category judgement		
Time/pair (s)	1.65	1.57 (0.30)
Errors (%)	2.1	4.8 (3.1)
Category generation		
30 s	10.0	8.6
60 s	12.5	14.3
Vocabulary		
WAIS (production)	16[a]	
Mill Hill (recognition) (percentile)	95	95

[a] Scaled score: mean normal performance = 10

In an attempt to provide an objective measure of such everyday memory problems, Barbara Wilson of the Rivermead Rehabilitation Centre in Oxford devised a behavioural memory test which comprises a total of ten subtests, each aimed at providing an objectively scorable measure of some everyday memory problem that is commonly reported by or observed in patients. The tasks include learning the name of a person portrayed, learning and recognising a series of objects and faces, learning a simple route, questions about orientation in time and space and a number of measures of prospective memory. For example on arrival the patient is asked for some small personal object such as a comb, which is then placed in a drawer and the patient is requested to ask for it at the end of the session. The test can be scored either in terms of the number of items passed, or on a more finely graded basis [7]. Normal adult subjects under the age of 65 pass all the subtests, and even brain-damaged patients typically fail on no more than one or two, provided they are rated as having no memory problems. A sample of 25 brain-damaged patients who were rated by the therapists treating them as having memory problems that were sufficient to have some bearing on their treatment passed a mean of 3.76 items. K. J. failed on all items, a result that would be typical of a dense global amnesic patient. This is consistent with everyday observation, which suggests that he has great difficulty in recalling what happened earlier in the day, learning his way around a new environment, learning to recognise new acquaintances and learning their names. There is no doubt that K. J., as is typical of amnesic patients, shows grossly impaired functioning of the system we previously referred to as episodic memory.

What is Spared in Amnesia?

Working Memory

A patient may be densely amnesic and yet have intact functioning of working memory as measured on the basis of a range of tests. For example the digit span test in which the subject is required to repeat back a string of numbers may be quite normal in amnesic patients. The recency effect, the tendency for the last few items encountered to be well recalled, is also typically intact, hence the patient presented with a list of 20 unrelated words would probably recall 2 or 3 of the last 4 presented, but very few earlier items. Another task that may be intact in amnesic patients is the short-term forgetting test devised by Peterson and Peterson in which the subject is presented with a short list of items, for example three unrelated words, and required to recall them after a brief interval ranging from 0 to perhaps 30 s during which rehearsal is prevented by having the patient perform a counting task. It seems likely that this task makes heavy demands on the central executive as well as the articulatory loop, and tends to be impaired in patients who have even relatively mild information processing deficits. There is however now general agreement that it can be unimpaired in the presence of dense amnesia (see [1] for a discussion).

A task that depends on spatial working memory is the Corsi blocks test. This comprises an array of nine blocks placed in front of the patient; the tester taps a number of blocks in sequence, and the patient attempts to imitate, the score being determined by the longest correct sequence. This again may be quite intact in densely amnesic patients.

Semantic Memory

The tasks so far developed to look at semantic memory are primarily language based. They include vocabulary tests, for example that included in the WAIS or the Mill Hill vocabulary test. These offer a relatively static measure of information that the patient has acquired about the meaning of words. A more dynamic measure is given by the "silly sentences" test which measures the speed with which the patient can judge whether simple sentences about the world are true (e.g. *Robins have red breasts* or *U. S. Presidents hold political office*), or are false sentences, made by combining the elements of two true sentences (e.g. *Robins hold political office* or *U. S. Presidents have red breasts*). A second test that measures speed of access to semantic memory is the fluency or item generation test in which the subject is required to produce as many words beginning with a particular letter, or items belonging to a particular semantic category, such as birds' or boys' names, as possible within a specified period. Tests of vocabulary tend to be very resistant to the effects of brain damage, while speed of sentence verification, and number of items generated are much more susceptible. However in the case of a pure amnesic such as K. J., performance on all these tests may be quite normal, as the data in Table 1 suggest.

Procedural Learning

It has been known for a number of years that amnesic patients can learn motor skills, but in recent years it has become clear that they are capable of learning relatively normally a very wide range of tasks ranging from classical conditioning to perceptual skills like reading words written in mirror writing where their performance shows excellent improvement with practice. Another task that reveals procedural learning is that of repeatedly solving the same jigsaw puzzle, where learning occurs and is well retained, and characterises that particular puzzle rather than simply a general improvement in solving skills. Amnesic patients can learn to solve complex puzzles like the Tower of Hanoi; they can also show excellent learning of words when cued in certain ways. Warrington and Weiskrantz [6] showed that if given a series of words (*stamp, frame*) and subsequently tested by being given the first few letters (*sta-*, *fra-*), then amnesic patients show excellent learning. It is characteristic of all these circumstances that the learning may occur with no conscious recollection of ever having encountered the task before. As would be expected, K. J.'s procedural learning was normal as measured by a range of tasks, the results of some of which are shown in Table 1.

What characterises those tasks which show procedural learning, and how are they different from the episodic memory tasks on which performance is so poor? The procedural tasks all appear to test learning by performance, with subjects not needing to know whether or not they have experienced the task before; they merely tackle the task, and learning is demonstrated by the fact that they can do it more efficiently. This contrasts with episodic memory tasks in which the patients are essentially recollecting some previous experience. Hence if they have been shown the word *stamp,* and are asked to recall it they need some form of direct access to that experience. Given the first few letters as a cue however, the task becomes one of solving a problem, namely producing a five-letter word beginning with *sta.* Having previously been presented with the word *stamp,* that item will have been primed in some aspect of the memory system, and hence will be readily available as an answer.

On this broad characterisation of the procedural learning effect, virtually everyone is agreed; there is however much less agreement on its appropriate theoretical interpretation. One interpretation suggests that there are two separate memory systems, one system is dependent on conscious awareness and is assumed to be defective in amnesic patients, while the other is said to be independent of conscious monitoring, and may be intact in amnesic patients. Another possibility is that episodic, semantic and procedural learning are all modes of operation of the same unitary learning system, with amnesic patients lacking one source of the feedback from this system. At present we do not have good experiments to differentiate between these two views, but it may be that work such as that described by Mishkin on the anatomical correlates of memory may throw light on this issue.

Autobiographical Memory

This is an area of considerable recent interest in both normal subjects and brain-damaged patients. Techniques for investigating it are still relatively primitive, but it is already clear that wide differences exist, with some amnesic patients such as K. J. having an apparently normal access to memories that occurred before the illness that produced the amnesia, while others who appear to be almost equally pure amnesics have a very clouded and uncertain access to information about their life, whether before or after the onset of amnesia. Finally, in the case of patients who have bilateral frontal damage, the request for autobiographical recollections may produce confabulation (for a more detailed discussion see [2]).

Other Memory Disorders

Having established a reasonably clear pattern of deficits in the case of the classic amnesic syndrome, there is now a good deal of interest in the extent to which a similar pattern is shown by patients whose memory deficit is less pure. It is still too soon to draw firm conclusions, but our own preliminary work on patients suffering from closed head injury and on the normal elderly suggests that both groups show impaired learning as measured by episodic memory tasks, while their performance on working memory tasks that do not place heavy demands on the central executive appears to be relatively spared. In the case of semantic memory, performance on vocabulary tests appears to hold up extremely well, but speed of performance on the silly sentences test and verbal fluency both show a decline. Perhaps the most interesting question concerns procedural learning, and here the data are still sparse. However, both groups showed poor performance on the reading of transformed script, while other evidence seems to suggest that the elderly perform poorly on learning the pursuit rotor, a motor task. This suggests that, unlike amnesic patients, the head injured and the elderly probably do not show normal procedural learning.

References

1. Baddeley AD (1982) Amnesia: a minimal model and an interpretation. In: Cermak LS (ed) Human memory and amnesia. Erlbaum, Hillsdale, pp 305–336
2. Baddeley AD, Wilson BA (to be published) Amnesia, autobiographical memory and confabulation. In: Rubin D (ed) Autobiographical memory. Cambridge University Press, London
3. Squire LR (1981) Two forms of amnesia: an analysis of forgetting. J Neurosci 1:630–635
4. Sunderland A, Harris JE, Baddeley AD (1983) Do laboratory tests predict everyday memory? A neuropsychological study. JVLVB 22:341–357
5. Tulving E (1972) Episodic and semantic memory. In: Tulving E, Donaldson W (eds), Organisation of memory. Academic, New York
6. Warrington EK, Weiskrantz L (1968) A new method of testing long-term retention with special reference to amnesic patients. Nature 217:972
7. Wilson BA, Cockburn J, Baddeley AD (1985) The Rivermead Behavioral Memory Test. Thames Valley Test Company, 22 Bulmershe Road, Reading, England

3 Neuroepidemiology and Clinical Trials

Neuroepidemiology

Neuroepidemiology as the Basis of Scientific Clinical Neurology

B. P. M. SCHULTE [1]

On the eve of the VIth World Congress of Neurology held in Brussels in 1957, Wilder Penfield opened an Anglo-American Symposium in London on the history and philosophy of the brain and its functions with a Hippocratic preamble. In this lecture Penfield [1] quoted a personal communication from Dr. Gordon Holmes as follows: "The claim of Hippocrates that knowledge comes only from direct observation, observation controlled by experiment, remains today the essential basis of our science."

This statement is applicable without restriction to neuroepidemiology. Neuroepidemiology begins with direct observation of neurologic disease in well-defined populations. Data from descriptive neuroepidemiologic studies often provide the necessary framework to formulate hypotheses concerning the etiology of neurologic diseases. With the techniques of analytic neuroepidemiology, such as case-control or prospective studies, these hypotheses can be formally tested. Hypotheses concerning treatment or prevention can be examined scientifically with the methods of controlled clinical trials [3]. Defined in this way neuroepidemiology – descriptive, analytic, and experimental – is strictly in concordance with the claim of Hippocrates.

Through the centuries the Hippocratic emphasis on prevention, prognosis, and natural history of disease (i.e., the scope of epidemiology) faded away and was overruled by an ever-expanding diagnostic technology [2]. But with the discovery of bacteria there was an abrupt change and epidemiology began to flourish [4]. Initial efforts were devoted to infectious diseases. The same techniques were later found useful in evaluating chronic, noninfectious disorders. Neuroepidemiology has become more established in recent decades. It is now being accepted as an essential basis for scientific clinical neurology. There are some obvious reasons for this development. Dissatisfaction with the unfavorable cost : benefit ratio of diagnostic procedures for individual patients is growing. The same applies to expensive therapeutic approaches that often lack a rational basis. While the socioeconomic burden of traditional medical care is criticized in developed countries, it is unacceptable for de-

[1] Institute of Neurology, Catholic University, Reinier Postlaan 4, 6500 HB Nijmegen, The Netherlands.

Neurology
Ed. by K. Poeck, H. J. Freund, and H. Gänshirt

veloping countries. Faster communication between nations and mutual influence promote interdependence in the solution of health care problems. Since neuroepidemiologic research yields better knowledge of the natural history of neurologic diseases and can identify risk factors for these disorders, rational programs of prevention and control can be designed. Therefore, neuroepidemiology is at the focus of world attention.

At the previous twelve World Congresses of Neurology since the first in Bern in 1931, neuroepidemiology has never been a main theme. Therefore, the XIIIth World Congress of Neurology in Hamburg is a landmark for neuroepidemiology and for scientific clinical neurology, as the papers in this session demonstrate.

References

1. Penfield W (1958) Hippocratic preamble: the brain and intelligence. In: Poynter FNL (ed) The history and philosophy of the brain and its functions. Blackwell Scientific, Oxford, p 3
2. Riese W (1959) A history of neurology. MD Publications, New York, p 171
3. Schoenberg BS (1982) Hypothesis testing in neuroepidemiology: experiments of nature and experiments of man. Neuroepidemiology 1:85–101
4. Tower DB (1978) Neurological epidemiology: an introductory perspective. Adv Neurol 19:1

Epidemiology of Cerebrovascular Disease: International Patterns

SHI-CHUO LI [1] and B. S. SCHOENBERG [2]

Investigations of the distribution of cerebrovascular disease in different parts of the world have provided important information useful in formulating etiologic hypotheses. In any epidemiologic investigation, it is essential to define the disease being studied. The various terms included in this category of cerebrovascular disease are outlined in Table 1, together with corresponding code numbers from the World Health Organizations's *International Classification of Diseases* [1]. In most epidemiologic studies the categories of cerebral thrombosis and cerebral embolism are combined into a single group referred to as cerebral infarction.

Cerebrovascular disease is one of the most common neurologic diseases, with a relatively high case fatality ratio and a substantial personal, familial, and social impact among the survivors. In a number of countries, cerebrovascular disease is one of the three leading causes of death. For example, data from Taiwan, 14 cities in the People's Republic of China, and Japan show that cerebrovascular disease was the leading cause of death. In the United States, Canada, Cuba, and Barbados, it is the third leading cause of death [2, 3].

Figure 1 shows the average annual mortality rates (age-adjusted to the 1950 United States population) for cerebrovascular disease in different countries. They are for various years between 1967 and 1973, except for data from the People's Republic of China, which are for 1982. The average mortality rate of cerebrovascular disease in the world is about 100 deaths per 100000 per year, and is generally higher for males [4, 5].

Geographic differences were found in the mortality rates for cerebrovascular disease both between countries and within countries. For instance, Japan has a mortality rate which is more than four times that for the Philippines or Poland. As for China, areas in the northeast report the highest rate for any area of the world where the disease has been studied.

In the United States, the southeastern region has the highest mortality, whereas in Japan and China, the northeast reports the highest mortality [4, 5]. Research on

[1] Beijing Neurosurgical Institute, Tiantan Xili, Beijing, People's Republic of China.
[2] Neuroepidemiology Branch, NINCDS-NIH, Room 804, Federal Building, 7550 Wisconsin Avenue, Bethesda, MD 20892, USA.

Neurology
Ed. by K. Poeck, H. J. Freund, and H. Gänshirt

Table 1. ICD code for cerebrovascular disease[a]

ICD code	Category of cerebrovascular disease
430	Subarachnoid hemorrhage
431	Cerebral hemorrhage
432	Occlusion of precerebral arteries
433	Cerebral thrombosis
434	Cerebral embolism
435	Transient cerebral ischemia
436	Acute but ill-defined cerebrovascular disease
437	Generalized ischemic cerebrovascular disease
438	Other and ill-defined cerebrovascular disease

[a] International Classification of Diseases, 8th revision [1]

Japanese migrants shows that cerebrovascular mortality rates are highest for Japanese in Japan, intermediate for Japanese residing in Hawaii, and lowest for Japanese living in California (on the west coast of the United States). This is in marked contrast to the mortality rates for coronary heart disease, which show a trend in the opposite direction [6]. This suggests that environmental factors play more important roles in the geographic variations than do racial or genetic factors.

With regard to the incidence rates of cerebrovascular disease, the worldwide average is about 200 new cases per 100000 per year [7]. There is considerable variation from country to country, as illustrated by tabulations for populations in the United States, Japan, and China (Table 2). The age-adjusted average annual inci-

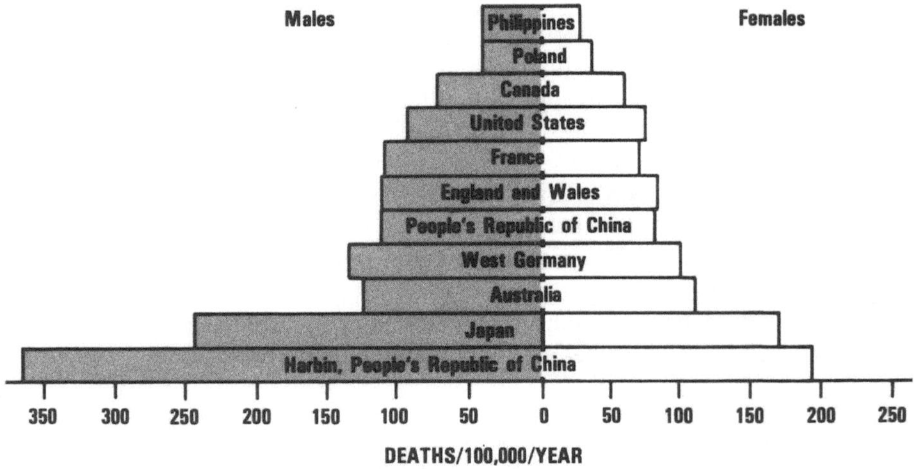

Fig. 1. Average annual age-adjusted mortality rates for cerebrovascular disease by sex, various countries, 1967–1973 (data from China are for 1982, age-adjusted to the 1950 United States population, using the direct method of age-adjustment)

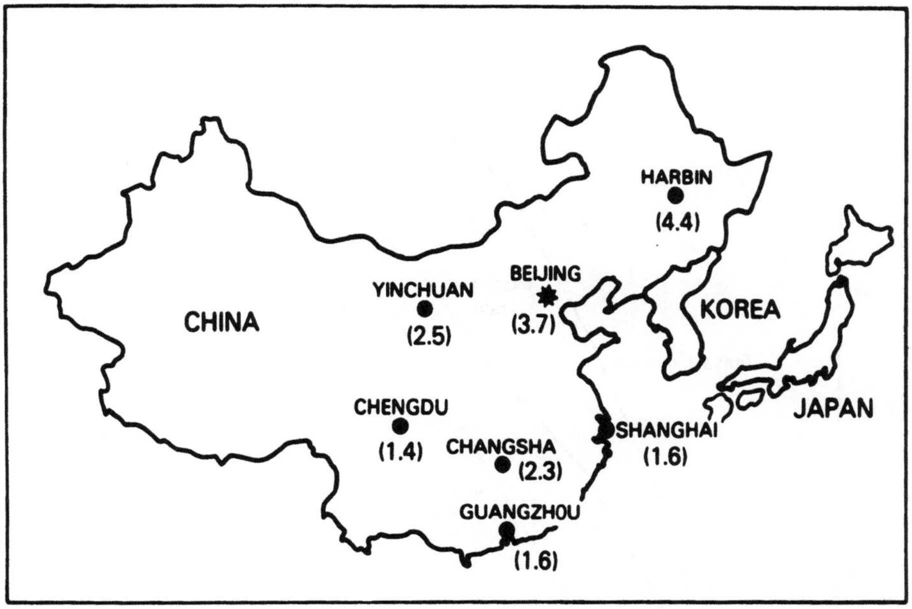

Fig. 2. Incidence rates (per 1000 per year) of completed stroke in different cities of the People's Republic of China [5]

Table 2. Crude and age-adjusted incidence rates of first completed stroke

Population	Years	Age groups	First stroke per 1000 per year	
			Crude	Age-adjusted[a]
Rochester MN, USA [8]	1955–1969	All	1.5	1.7
Hisayama, Japan [9]	1961–1963	All	2.3	2.9
Shibata, Japan [10]	1966–1978	20+years	2.6	2.7
6 cities, People's Republic of China (PRC) [5]	1982	All	1.8	2.2
		20+years	2.5	3.6
Harbin, PRC [5]	1982	All	3.1	4.4

[a] 1960 United States population as standard

dence rate for all ages from Hisayama, Japan is high (2.9 per 1000); from six cities of China, 2.2 per 1000; and from Rochester, Minnesota, 1.7 per 1000. The rates for those 20 years of age and older from six cities in China, however, are higher than that from Shibata, Japan [5, 8–10]. The rate from Harbin, in northeast China, is among the highest rates in the world.

Annual incidence rates for completed stroke in China show a south-to-north gradient (Fig. 2). The rates are highest from northeastern China (Harbin) and lowest in southern China (Chengdu and Guangzhou). This geographic difference is similar to the geographic distribution of cerebrovascular disease in Japan [4, 5, 11].

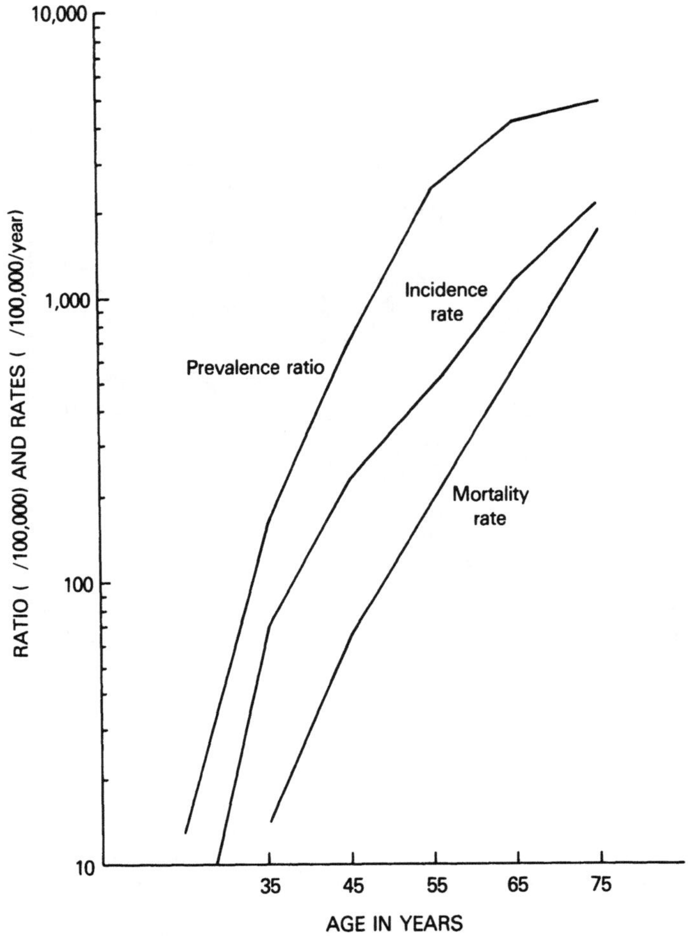

Fig. 3. Age-specific rates for completed stroke plotted on a logarithmic scale against age, 6 cities, People's Republic of China (prevalence ratio: 1 January 1983; incidence and mortality rates: 1 January–31 December 1982)

Table 3. Percentage distribution by type of first completed stroke

Type of stroke	Weighted average white population[a] [7] (%)	Shibata, Japan [10] (%)	6 cities, People's Republic of China [5] (%)
Subarachnoid hemorrhage	8	8	2
Intracerebral hemorrhage	12	23	44
Cerebral infarction	69	58	51
Ill-defined stroke	11	11	3

[a] These figures were compiled from studies before the routine use of computerized axial tomography to evaluate individuals with completed stroke

In cooperation with the United States National Institutes of Health, the World Health Organization has developed a protocol to measure the prevalence of major neurologic disorders, including cerebrovascular disease. Using this protocol, investigations have been carried out in the United States, Nigeria, and seven different cities in the People's Republic of China. Smaller pilot studies have been conducted in Chile, Colombia, Ecuador, India, Italy, Mexico, Peru, and Venezuela [12]. Generally speaking, the prevalence ratio for cerebrovascular disease throughout the world is about 500–700 per 100000 [13, 14]. The geographic differences in prevalence ratios are similar to the figures for mortality and incidence rates already mentioned.

Figure 3 is from a recent survey which was carried out in six cities in the People's Republic of China [5]. It can be seen that the morbidity and mortality rates increase dramatically with age. They appear as almost straight lines when a logarithmic scale is used for the magnitude of the rates; this corresponds to an exponential increase with age.

In terms of the specific types of cerebrovascular disease, data from the United States, Japan, and China are compared in Table 3 [5, 10, 13]. The percentage of different categories of completed stroke shown here are for incident cases of first completed stroke from different studies. Although cerebral infarction is responsible for the majority of completed strokes, the percentage of intracerebral hemorrhage is much higher for Chinese and Japanese populations than for white populations.

In conclusion, cerebrovascular disease represents one of the most common neurologic diseases and a serious health problem internationally. The descriptive epidemiologic investigations of cerebrovascular disease have explored its distribution by sex, age, race, and geography, suggesting the importance of environmental etiologic factors. Analytic epidemiologic studies to identify specific risk factors for cerebrovascular disease will hopefully lead to rational programs of prevention and control of this disorder.

References

1. World Health Organization (1969) International classification of diseases, 8th revision, Geneva
2. Li SC, Cheng XM (1982) Epidemiology of cerebrovascular disease, a general review. Chin J Nerv Ment Dis 8:50–55
3. Pan American Health Organization (1982) Health conditions in the Americas, 1977–1980. Washington, D.C., Scientific Publication 427
4. Schoenberg BS (1980) Epidemiology of cerebrovascular disease. South Med J 72:331–336
5. Li SC, Schoenberg BS, Wang CC et al. (1985) Cerebrovascular disease in the People's Republic of China: epidemiologic and clinical features. Neurology 35:1708–1713
6. Worth RM, Kato H, Rhoads GG et al. (1975) Epidemiologic studies of coronary heart disease and stroke in Japanese men living in Japan, Hawaii, and California: mortality. Am J Epidemiol 102:481–490
7. Kurtzke JF (1976) An introduction to the epidemiology of cerebrovascular disease. In: Scheinberg P (ed) Cerebrovascular disease, tenth Princeton conference. Raven, New York, pp 239–253
8. Matsumoto N, Whisnant JP, Kurland LT et al. (1973) Natural history of stroke in Rochester, Minn., 1955 through 1969: an extension of a previous study, 1945 through 1954. Stroke 4:20–29
9. Katsuki S, Hirota Y, Akazome T et al. (1964) Epidemiological studies in Hisayama, Kyushu Island, Japan. Jpn Heart J 5:12–36

10. Tanaka H, Heda Y, Date C et al. (1981) Incidence of stroke in Shibata, Japan: 1976–1978. Stroke 12:460–466
11. Wang CC, Cheng XM, Li SC et al. (1983) Epidemiology of cerebrovascular disease in an urban community of Beijing, People's Republic of China. Neuroepidemiology 2:121–134
12. Schoenberg BS (1983) Neuroepidemiologic generalizations: high tax on importing data, low tax on importing principles. Neuroepidemiology 2:117–120
13. Kurtzke JF (1980) Epidemiology of cerebrovascular disease. In: Siekert RG (ed) Cerebrovascular survey report for joint council subcommittee on cerebrovascular disease. Whiting, Rochester, Minn, pp 135–176
14. Kurtzke JF (1982) The current neurologic burden of illness and injury in the United States. Neurology 32:1207–1214

Cerebrovascular Risk Factors

V. C. HACHINSKI [1]

Introduction

Prevention offers the most efficacious management of cerebrovascular disease and the treatment of risk factors the most effective means of prevention. The 10% of people who sustain 50% of strokes can be identified through the presence of risk factors [10].

Age

While stroke can occur at any age, even prenatally, its incidence rises sharply after the age of 55 years [15]. Age is the single most powerful predictor of stroke. However, to paraphrase Mark Twain "everybody talks about getting older, but nobody does anything about it." Not yet.

Hypertension

The most important treatable risk factor for stroke is hypertension. The risk increases with increasing levels of systolic and diastolic blood pessure, beginning in the normal range [24]. Hypertension represents a risk for atherothrombotic, lacunar, and hemorrhagic stroke and for subarachnoid hemorrhage (Longstreath et al. 1985) in both sexes and all ages. Treatment of hypertension decreases the hazard of stroke substantially and promptly [19–21]. Cardiac disease, ischemic, hypertensive, and valvular heart disease, and arrhythmias pose significant and largely treatable risks for stroke (Table 1) [2, 23] (Hinton et al. 1977).

Diabetes Mellitus

The presence of glucose intolerance increases the risk for stroke two- to threefold [24]; moreover, hyperglycemics tend to suffer larger cerebral infarcts than normoglycemic patients [14]. Unfortunately, controlling blood glucose levels seems to have scant impact on the progression of the vascular complications.

[1] Department of Clinical Neurological Sciences, University Hospital, University of Western Ontario, London, Ontario, Canada.

Neurology
Ed. by K. Poeck, H. J. Freund, and H. Gänshirt

Table 1. Risk factors for stroke

1. Hypertension (diastolic and systolic)
2. Cardiac disease
    - Ischemic/hypertensive
        - Coronary heart disease
        - Myocardial infarction
            - Acute – endocardial damage → thrombi
            - Chronic – akinetic segments → thrombi
        - Congestive heart failure
        - Left ventricular hypertrophy
            - On ECG
            - On chest X-ray
    - Valvular
        - Rheumatic heart disease
        - Prolapsing mitral valve
        - Endocarditis
            - Infectious
            - Marantic
        - Aortic stenosis
        - Prosthetic heart valves
        - ? Calcified mitral annulus
    - Arrhythmias such as:
        - Atrial fibrillation
        - Sick sinus syndrome
3. Diabetes
4. Erythrocytosis
5. Cigarette smoking
6. Other
    - Physical inactivity
    - Hyperlipidemia
    - Heredity
    - Environmental factors

Erythrocytosis

The hematocrit value relates to stroke risk, beginning in the normal range, in part from associated hypertension [12] and in part from increased viscosity and perhaps other factors. Although decreasing the hematocrit ameliorates symptoms in polycythemics, it remains plausible, but uncertain, whether lowering the hematocrit also lowers the risk for stroke.

Cigarette Smoking

Although cigarette smoking represents a small risk factor for stroke, it is a powerful contributor to coronary artery disease [24] and as such deserves rigorous curbing.

Physical Inactivity

Physical inactivity may be a risk for stroke [7], but is not a well-studied one.

Hyperlipidemia

Elevated blood cholesterol poses a small risk for stroke, an effect that dissipates after the age of 55 years. According to the Framingham data, an inverse relationship between blood levels of LDL and the risk of stroke obtains, especially in women [24]. On the other hand, other studies have documented low HDL levels (Murai et al. 1981) in stroke patients and it has been recently shown that stroke itself affects serum lipid levels [13].

Heredity

Strokes occur more commonly among siblings of stroke patients than among the siblings of their spouses (Alter and Kluznich 1972) although it remains uncertain to what degree the raised risk reflects familial agglomerations of hypertension, diabetes, and other risk factors.

Environmental Factors

Hawaiians of Japanese descent have a lower incidence of stroke than Japanese from the same area of Japan as their ancestors. On the other hand, they have more heart attacks. The differences likely arise from differences in life-style and diet (Tillotson et al. 1973; Kagan et al. 1985).

Cerebrovascular Risk Factors in the Young

The young by this definition are adults aged 45 years or under. The etiology of stroke in this age range is broader with different entities predominating than at a later age [6]. The risk factors are also different (Table 2).

Cardiac Disease

Valvular heart disease is an important cause of stroke in the young. Rheumatic heart disease has dropped dramatically in North America in the past 25 years [18], but remains a menace in the developing world. Mitral stenosis, especially with associated atrial fibrillation is the commonest lesion leading to neurologic sequelae [2]. Mitral valve prolapse, although innocent and symptomless in the vast majority of subjects, has become a leading cause of stroke and transient ischemic attacks in the young [2]. Bicuspid aortic valves, idiopathic hypertrophic subaortic stenosis, infective and idiopathic cardiomyopathies, and atrial myxoma represent uncommon, but important causes of stroke in the young. Paradoxical emboli may occur when increased pressure in the right heart pushes a clot into the left heart through a patent foramen ovale [9]. Increased blood pressure as a result of hypertension is an important risk factor for hemorrhage and ischemic stroke, especially if untreated or combined with other risk factors such as diabetes or a hyperlipidemia.

Table 2. Risk factors for stroke in the young

1. Cardiac disease	4. Hyperlipidemia
Valvular heart disease, especially	5. Oral contraceptives
mitral valve prolapse	6. Cigarette smoking
Cardiomyopathies	7. Trauma
Atrial myxoma	8. Drug abuse
2. Hypertension	9. Alcohol
3. Migraine	10. Neurosyphilis

Migraine

Migraine is a common condition and hence it occurs coincidentally in patients with strokes due to other causes. It should be a diagnosis of exclusion unless the deficit follows a previous series of transient deficits of the same nature. There is also some evidence that migraine compounds the risk of stroke in women taking oral contraceptives [4].

Hyperlipidemia

A direct correlation between serum cholesterol levels and risk of stroke exists up to the age of 55 years, although the association is not powerful [24].

Oral Contraceptives

The best evidence for an association between oral contraceptives and the risk for stroke comes from the large prospective study being carried out by the Royal College of General Practitioners [16] which showed that the risk of cerebral thrombosis and cerebral embolism among users is 19 times that of nonusers, although the absolute risk remains small. The risks for stroke rise sharply with increases in the level of blood pressure and also with increasing age, heavy smoking, and migraine [4]. Pregnancy and the puerperium also increase the risk for stroke [1].

Cigarette Smoking

Cigarette smoking enhances the risk for stroke among oral conraceptive takers and represents a strong risk for coronary heart disease [24].

Trauma

Direct trauma to the cervical arteries or damage from chiropractic manipulation may lead to dissection or occlusion and stroke (Easton and Sherman 1977).

Drug Abuse

Oral or intravenous amphetamines and intravenous heroin can lead to arteritis and cerebral infarction or hemorrhages [3].

Alcohol

Alcoholic intoxication has been reported to be a significant prelude to stroke [8]. The mechanism has not been elicited and includes contraction of cerebral and systemic vessels, platelet activation, and unreported or forgotten trauma.

Neurosyphilis

Although neurosyphilis has declined considerably since the advent of penicillin, meningosyphilis accounts for a small, but significant proportion of strokes, especially among the young [17].

Aggregation and Interaction of Risk Factors

The Framingham data show that the presence of one risk factor may potentiate that of another [24]. Moreover, there is some evidence that siblings of stroke patients are more likely to have multiple risk factors than the relatives of their spouses [5]. An example of potentiation among the young is the augmentation of risk for stroke by oral contraceptives in the presence of hypertension and smoking [4].

The Need to Search for New Risk Factors

All the known risk factors only account for a fraction of the risk for stroke [24]. The search for genetic markers to identify patients at high risk may prove rewarding. Buck et al. in a prospective study (C. Buck, W.B. Chodirker, A.P. Donner, 1986, The C3F phenotype and the occurrence of stroke in hypertensives, unpublished data) found that among male hypertensives the possession of the C3F complement fragment carried a 9.1 greater likelihood of sustaining a stroke than if the trait was absent. New risk factors such as raised fibrinogen levels [22] are being delineated. Studies comparing the differing incidence of stroke and coronary heart disease among ethnically similar populations in Japan and Hawaii strongly suggest that life-style, diet, and environment play major roles (Tilloston et al. 1973; Kagan et al. 1985). The World Federation of Neurology is in an excellent position to foster comparative studies that may elicit new and treatable risk factors for stroke.

Conclusion

The acute stroke gets most of the attention, while the management of cerebrovascular risk factors gets most of the results. Treatment of hypertension and heart disease offer the most direct and effective means of preventing stroke. While many risk factors for cerebrovascular disease have been discovered, many more remain to be defined. Further advances are likely to come from genetic studies, changes in life-style, and the diligent management of known risk factors for cerebrovascular disease.

References

1. Amies AG (1970) Cerebral vascular disease in pregnancy I. Hemorrhage. J Obstet Gynaecol 77:100
2. Barnett HJM (1983) Heart in ischemic stroke – A changing emphasis. Neurol Clin North Am 1:291
3. Caplan LR, Hier DB, Banks G (1982) Stroke and drug abuse. Stroke 82:869
4. Collaborative Group for the Study of Stroke in Young Women (1975) Oral contraceptives and stroke in young women. JAMA 231:718
5. Diaz JF, Hachinski VC, Pederson L, Donald A (1985) Prevalence of risk factors for stroke in families of patients with cerebral infarct and transient ischemic attacks. Can J Neurol Sci 12:177
6. Hachinski VC, Norris JW (1985) The acute stroke. In: Plum F (ed) Contemporary neurology series, vol 27. FA Davis, Philadelphia

7. Herman B, et al. (1982) An evaluation of risk factors for stroke in a Dutch community. Stroke 13:334
8. Hillbom M, Kaste M, Rasi V (1983) Can ethanol intoxication affect hemocoagulation with increased risk of infarction in young adults? Neurology 33:381
9. Jones HR Jr, et al. (1983) Cerebral emboli of paradoxical origin. Ann Neurol 13:314
10. Kannel WB (1976) Epidemiology of cerebrovascular disease. In: Ross Russell RW (ed) Cerebral arterial disease. Churchill-Livingstone, Edinburgh, p 1
11. Kannel WB, Wolf PA, Verter J et al. (1970) Epidemiologic assessment of the role of blood pressure in stroke: The Framingham study. JAMA 214:301
12. Kannel WB, et al. (1972) Hemoglobin and the risk of cerebral infarction: The Framingham study. Stroke 3:409
13. Mendez I, Hachinski VC, Wolfe BM (1986) Serum lipids after stroke. Neurology (in press)
14. Plum F (1983) What causes infarction in ischemic brain? The Robert Wartenberg lecture. Neurology 33:222
15. Robins M, Baum HM (1981) National survey of stroke. Incidence. Stroke [Suppl 2] 12:1–45, 1–57
16. Royal College of General Practitioners (1983) Incidence of arterial disease among oral contraceptive users. J R Coll Gen Pract 33:75
17. Simon RP (1985) Neurosyphilis. Arch Neurol 42:606–613
18. Statistics Canada (1980) Statistics Canada: Causes of death 1978. Queen's Printer, Ottawa
19. Veterans Administration Cooperative Study in Antihypertensive Agents (1967) Effects of treatment on morbidity in hypertension: results in patients with diastolic blood pressures averaging 115 through 129 mm Hg. JAMA 202:1028–1034
20. Veterans Administration Cooperative Study in Antihypertensive Agents (1970) Effects of treatment on morbidity in hypertension – results in patients with diastolic blood pressure averaging 90–114 mm Hg. JAMA 213:1143–1152
21. Veterans Administration Cooperative Study in Antihypertensive Agents (1972) Effects of treatment on morbidity in hypertension III. Influence of age, diastolic pressure and prior cardiovascular disease; further analysis of side effects. Circulation 45:991–1004
22. Wilhelmsen L, Svardsudd K, Korsan-Bengtsen K, et al. (1984) Fibrinogen as a risk factor for stroke and myocardial infarction. N Engl J Med 311:501–511
23. Wolf PA, et al. (1978) Epidemiologic assessment of chronic atrial fibrillation of risk of stroke: The Framingham study. Neurology 28:973
24. Wolf PA, Kannel WB, Verter J (1983) Current status of risk factors for stroke. Neurol Clin North Am 1:317

Epidemiology of Epilepsy

M. E. CRUZ [1], P. BARBERIS [1,2], and B. S. SCHOENBERG [2]

Available data suggest that the disorders affecting the nervous system are important public health problems in developed [3, 60] as well as in developing countries [15–17, 47, 48]. Among such diseases *epilepsy* stands out not only because of its high prevalence but because of its particular individual, familial, and social implications. Epidemiologic studies of epilepsy are needed to broaden our knowledge and understanding of factors associated with an increased risk for this condition.

The unqualified term "epilepsy" has no more precision than others such as "headache." The definition of epilepsy in recent epidemiologic studies is based on the recurrent presentation of two or more afebrile seizures.

Single afebrile seizures, febrile convulsions, and seizures as acute manifestations of abnormal metabolic states are excluded. The diagnosis is primarily clinical since there is no laboratory test which can confirm the presence or absence of the condition. The electroencephalogram (EEG) can assist the clinician in reaching the diagnosis, but it is neither very sensitive nor very specific. On the other hand, the term epilepsy includes several types of seizures, each having a different age of onset, response to treatment, prognosis, EEG correlates, and, possibly, risk factors. It is clear that secondary epilepsy due to parasitic infestation of the brain is a totally different condition than genetically determined epilepsy. However, there is a need for an all-inclusive term useful for estimating the demand for services and for other public health purposes.

Descriptive epidemiologic studies providing incidence and prevalence data on the epilepsies have been conducted in numerous geographic areas. The comparability of their results, however, is limited by the lack of consistency in definitions and by major differences in methodology.

Specifically, there is a wide variation in case ascertainment: studies based on medical chart reviews, medical registries, or surveys conducted through questionnaires sent by mail are all reported, making it difficult to compare their results. Hospital and private practice based data usually underestimate by as much as one-third

---

[1] Dept. of Medical Statistics and Epidemiology, Mayo Clinic, 200 First St. SW, Rochester, MN 55905, USA.
[2] Center for Research and Training in Neurosciences, Quito, Ecuador, and Neuroepidemiology Branch, NINCDS, NIH, Bethesda, MD, USA.

Neurology
Ed. by K. Poeck, H. J. Freund, and H. Gänshirt

the prevalence of epilepsy at the community level [2]. Community-based surveys are the best way of accurately assessing disease magnitude and distribution.

Such surveys are influenced, however, by local customs or beliefs. If epilepsy is considered a social stigma, patients suffering from this condition are concealed from the researchers [60]. Despite multiple difficulties in implementing these studies, data have recently become available from a World Health Organization-sponsored international study suggesting that epilepsy is a public health problem, especially in rural areas of the most socioeconomically deprived parts of the world [15, 57].

Part of the information that follows stems from this program that has promoted epidemiologic studies of neurologic disorders in developing countries, using a standardized protocol applied by nondoctor personnel in door-to-door surveys. Countries in which this methodology has been applied are: Nigeria, (urban) Peoples Republic of China (PRC), (urban) Chile, (urban) Peru, and (rural areas of) Venezuela, Colombia, and Ecuador.

In the three last studies, accuracy of diagnosis was stressed through the use of standardized criteria applied by clinical neurologists. The definition of epilepsy used was: two or more afebrile seizures (clinically obvious episodes) not as a result of alcohol or drug withdrawal and unrelated to acute metabolic disorders. Only "active" cases were considered. These were defined as: (a) individuals who are not on anticonvulsant medication and had a seizure during the year prior to prevalence day, or (b) individuals on antiepileptic therapy with a seizure during the 5 years before prevalence day.

Mortality Data on Epilepsy

The available information on mortality rates from epilepsy is limited [68]. Information is lacking particularly from developing countries. Moreover, less than one-third of patients with epilepsy have this diagnosis mentioned on their death certificates [70, 71]. However, some general trends can be deduced from the available figures. The highest reported mortality rates are from Chile, Colombia, and Venezuela; and the lowest are from the USA, Japan, and England. Table 1 shows the temporal trends in the average annual (age-adjusted to 1950 US population) mortality rates per 100000 for epilepsy in various nations [44].

Mortality data for epilepsy should be interpreted cautiously as these may be a reflection of different case ascertainment and different management of cases [39].

Age-, sex-, and race-specific death rates for epilepsy are available only from the USA [2, 39]. In comparing the sexes, rates were consistently higher for both white and nonwhite males. Racial comparison showed higher rates in nonwhites than whites [8]. However, this racial variation has not been reflected in incidence studies [31]. Death rates for single individuals were higher than those for married and widowed. Rates were also higher in rural areas [31].

The life expectancy of persons with epilepsy is estimated to be shortened by about 6 years [68]. The cause of death in epileptics is directly related to seizures in only 27.5% of cases. Drowning, accidents, and suicide accounted for 19%, while 49% of the causes were unrelated to the epilepsy [68].

Table 1. Temporal trends in the average annual age-adjusted[a] mortality rates per 100000 for epilepsy in various nations [44]

Country	Years	Rate	Years	Rate
Australia	1954–1958	1.6	1967–1973	1.3
Austria	1953–1957	2.1	1967–1973	1.7
Belgium	1954–1958	1.9	1967–1972	1.3
Canada	1953–1957	1.6	1967–1973	1.1
Chile	1956, 1958	4.6	1967–1973	3.8
Colombia	1957	4.6	1967–1969, 1972	3.7
Czechoslovakia	1953–1957	1.5	1967–1973	1.7
Denmark	1953–1957	1.1	1967–1973	0.6
England and Wales	1953–1957	1.6	1967–1973	1.3
Finland	1954–1958	2.4	1967–1973	1.1
France	1953–1957	1.3	1967–1973	1.1
Greece	1956–1957	1.6	1967–1973	1.6
Iceland	1951–1955	1.6	1967–1973	1.8
Ireland	1954–1958	2.5	1967–1972	1.4
Israel (Jewish)	1956–1958	1.2	1967–1973	0.8
Italy	1953–1957	1.9	1967–1973	1.1
Japan	1953–1957	1.9	1967–1973	1.0
Luxembourg			1967–1973	1.6
Mauritius			1967–1973	3.9
Mexico	1956	3.6	1967–1973	2.9
Netherlands	1953–1957	1.4	1967–1973	1.1
New Zealand (excludes Maori population)	1952–1956	2.3	1967–1972	1.1
Northern Ireland	1951–1955	1.9	1967–1973	1.3
Norway	1953–1957	2.1	1967–1973	1.6
Philippines	1956–1957	1.3	1967–1973	1.7
Poland	1954–1957	1.1	1967–1973	1.6
Portugal	1955–1958	4.2	1967–1973	4.0
Scotland	1951–1955	2.2	1967–1973	1.3
Sweden	1953–1957	1.1	1967–1973	1.0
Switzerland	1953–1957	1.5	1967–1973	0.7
United States	1953–1957	1.3	1967–1973[b]	1.0
Uruguay	1955–1957	2.2	1967–1973	1.7
West Germany (Federal Republic of Germany)	1953–1957	1.8	1967–1973	1.4

[a] Adjusted to 1950 US population as a standard
[b] 1972 US rate is based on a 50% sample of death certificates
Reproduced with permission from reference 44.

Prevalence

Prevalence data for epilepsy are available from different geographic regions. Table 2 summarizes the information derived from community-based surveys.

In Africa, the prevalence ratio of epilepsy in the population of Igbo-Ora, Nigeria is 5.3 per 1000 [49], which is similar to the 4.6 per 1000 reported for Caucasians [39]. In rural Aiyete, Nigeria, the prevalence is 37 per 1000 [48], while it is from 29 to 49 per 1000 in Liberia [24, 27, 66]; 13 per 1000 in Lagos [18]; and 20 per 1000 in Tanzania [1]. The substantial differences encountered in the studies cited above within

Table 2. Prevalence ratios for epilepsy from community-based surveys (per 1000 population)

USA	6.6–9.1	Nigeria	5.3–37
England	3.3–6.2	Colombia	17–19.5
Poland	7.5	Ecuador	12.7
Guam	2.3–5.4	Venezuela	17.5
Tanganyika	15	China (PRC)	4.6
Liberia	26–49		

the same ethnic population are thought to represent differences of exposure to improved primary health care. This may explain the low prevalence in the population of Igbo-Ora [49]. The focus of endemic epilepsy in Liberia probably represents a particular disease entity and more research is needed to clarify this point.

In Asia, the reported prevalence ratio varies from 4.6 per 1000 in urban China (PRC) [42] to 9 per 1000 in India [34]. In Israel, a figure of 4.1 per 1000 was reported [39].

In Oceania, one study reports a prevalence figure of 7.5 per 1000 in Australia [5], and another cites the figure of 3 per 1000 in Guam [39].

In South America, an earlier study reported the high figure of 19.5 per 1000 in Colombia [25]. Recent studies using a uniform methodology confirmed this high prevalence ratio in rural South American populations. In Ecuador, the prevalence ratio was 12.7 per 1000 [16, 17], in Venezuela, 17.5 per 1000 [52], and in rural Colombia, 17 per 1000 [54].

Prevalence figures from English surveys vary from 3.5 per 1000 [43] to 6.2 per 1000 [53]. Other figures from European countries show: Norway, 3.5 per 1000; urban Poland, 4.9 per 1000; rural Poland, 2.9 per 1000 [46]; Warsaw, Poland, 7.8 per 1000 [70]; Italy, 6.2 per 1000 [29].

In the Rochester, Minnesota (USA) population, the prevalence ratio is 6.6 per 1000 [32]; in an American Indian population, it is reported to be 9.1 per 1000 (J.G. Levy and S. Ghachu, 1981, cited by Aird et al. [2]).

The prevalence of all types of epileptic seizures has been found to be 24.4 per 1000 in Denmark [35]. In England the lifetime prevalence of epilepsy was 17 per 1000 excluding single seizures [26].

The regional differences of epilepsy prevalence ratios presented here appear to reflect not only differences in methodology, but also geographic, ethnic, and socioeconomic factors. However, the exact role of each of these remains to be determined.

There is an overall tendency for rural deprived areas of the Third World to report higher figures for epilepsy prevalence.

In South America, the prevalence ratio of epilepsy rises with increasing age to a peak in the fourth decade and then declines (Table 3). In these populations, head trauma and CNS parasitosis probably constitute the majority of cases [14], although detailed case-control studies will better define this problem. It appears that biopsychosocial deprivation of both the inhabitants of the Andean and subtropical areas in South America and rural areas in Africa is associated with the high prevalence ratios for epilepsy in these populations [16, 17, 21, 47].

Table 3. Age- and sex-specific prevalence ratios for epilepsy for Venezuela, Colombia, and Ecuador, 1985 (cases/1,000)

Age group (years)	Males	Females	Total	95%	Confidence Interval
0– 9	10.30	11.75	11.02	7.64	15.43
10–19	13.02	20.38	16.80	12.85	21.50
20–39	14.72	18.18	18.84	12.61	22.06
40–59	12.03	24.75	19.31	13.03	27.61
60+	11.46	25.32	18.82	10.27	31.61
Total	12.42	18.62	15.79	13.67	18.23
Total age adjusted to 1960 US population			16.39	14.19	18.93

Most of the studies conducted with the use of the standard WHO protocol show lower prevalence ratios of epilepsy in the population older than 60 years of age, both because epileptics have a greater risk of dying than the general population and those with seizures due to cerebrovascular disease and brain tumors have a relatively poor survival [17]. Only in Rochester, Minnesota (USA) is there a continually increasing prevalence ratio with increasing age [32], probably representing careful follow-up of identified cases [60].

Epilepsy in Children

Seven studies of children are worth reviewing. Four of them used the same methodology: Oregon [45], Maryland [59], Chile [10], and Mexico [22]. Table 4 compares these data.

Another three studies from Kentucky, USA [6] and Italy [7, 67] are also very similar. Criticism has been made of somewhat different wording of the definition of epilepsy among these studies.

The higher figures reported from Chile and Mexico cannot be accounted for only by the fact that complicated febrile seizures were included. Data using the uniform protocol described from South America, China (PRC), and Nigeria on the point prevalence of "active" epilepsy in children 0–9 years of age are summarized in Table 5.

In Cuba, the prevalence ratio of epilepsy in children aged 0–14 years was found to be 7.5 per 1000. Thirty-nine percent of the cases had a first attack during the first

Table 4. Prevalence ratios for childhood epilepsy (per 1000 population)

USA	7.8–14.1
Mexico	18.3
Chile	21.1

Table 5. Prevalence ratios for childhood epilepsy from community-based surveys (per 1000 population, under 10 years)

China (PRC)	3.5
Venezuela	12.1
Ecuador	9.4
Colombia	13.5
Nigeria	5.8–26

year of life [50]. In Italy, the prevalence of epilepsy was about 3 per 1000 among 13000 children, aged 6–14 [51]. In northern Italy, another study found 6.1 per 1000 prevalence in children under 14 [29]. In Poland, the prevalence ratio of epilepsy in school children (7–15 years) was reported to be 6.7 per 1000 [37]. In 3-year-old children from Japan, the prevalence ratio for afebrile convulsions was 9 per 1000 [64].

In a clinical epidemiological study conducted in Moscow, USSR, one-third of all cases of epilepsy had their first seizure at under 3 years of age [56]. In a German city, two-thirds of epileptic children had their first seizure prior to the third birthday [19].

In Sudan, Africa, an unusually low prevalence ratio of 0.9 per 1000 was reported among the entire school population in Khartoum Province [69].

A detailed review of epidemiologic aspects of childhood epilepsy has been published [41].

Types of Epilepsy

It is difficult on clinical grounds alone to be certain of the type of epilepsy. Usually a more detailed investigation, including EEG, is needed for accurate classification.

The fact that generalized convulsive epilepsy constitutes the majority of the identified cases of epilepsy in China (PRC) and South America may reflect the obvious nature of tonic-clonic convulsions. Partial seizures with secondary generalization could have been erroneously classified as generalized tonic-clonic seizures on the basis of the information obtained from clinical history alone. In a study from South America [15], 23% of the seizures were classified as partial and 69% as generalized tonic-clonic. In the study from China (PRC) [42], 8% were partial and 81% generalized. In Nigeria, 55% were partial and 25% generalized [49].

On the contrary, in studies from industrialized countries, partial seizures, simple and complex, constitute between 43%–68% of all cases [23]. However, a study from India reported 20% of generalized epilepsies and 80% of partial seizures [34]. So, the differences among developed and developing countries with regard to seizure types may not be real and may represent only methodologic variations. Clinical field research surveys may tend to report generalized seizures more frequently than surveys based on hospital data, where sophisticated methods facilitated more accurate diagnosis.

Absence seizures have been reported in defined populations as follows: South America [15], 5%; China [42], 8%; Nigeria [49], 3%; Italy [29], 4%.

Incidence

Average annual age-specific incidence rates per 100000 population in Rochester, Minnesota (USA, 1935–1974) reveal a curious U-shaped curve with high rates for infants and the elderly. This marked increase in incidence rates at age 75 and over has not been found in other studies and may be due to better case ascertainment and medical care among the elderly in Rochester. Childhood incidence rates in developing countries should be higher, reflecting the additional effect of poorer peri-

Table 6. Incidence rates for epilepsy (per 100000/year)

USA	48	Norway	33
England	45	Japan	17
Italy	33	China (PRC)	25
Iceland	26		

natal medical care, infections, and parasitic brain lesions (both congenital, such as toxoplasmosis, and acquired, such as cysticercosis). At least one study done in Reunion [63] shows this to be the case, although more complete surveys are needed in this respect.

Incidence rates from some of the most important studies conducted are presented in Table 6 [30, 32, 42, 53].

Temporal trends for epilepsy incidence were investigated in the USA [32]. This study shows a decrease in incidence rates over time for subjects under age 20, reflecting better prenatal and perinatal care.

Cumulative incidence is the cumulative effect of age-specific incidence rates. It has also been defined as the proportion of an initially disease-free group developing the disease over a fixed time interval [40]. These data are useful for genetic counseling, prognostic information, and eventually therapeutic intervention. By age 20 years, 4.1% of the population will have had a single seizure and 1.1% recurrent seizures (epilepsy). At age 80, these figures are 8.6% and 3.2%, respectively [33].

Risk Factors

Most authors report retrospective studies. The most recent are two case-control studies conducted in China (PRC) and Nigeria. In China (PRC) [42], a carefully designed study found the following to be significant risk factors for idiopathic epilepsy: premature or difficult birth, maternal illness during pregnancy, previous febrile seizures, family history of epilepsy, and maternal age above 30 years. Putative causes of symptomatic epilepsy were head injury (47.5%), intracranial infection (24.6%), cerebrovascular disease (16.4%), intracranial tumors (3.3%), and other causes (8.2%).

In Nigeria putative risk factors for epilepsy were: febrile convulsions, malnutrition, alcohol intake, and lack of immunizations [49]. Other important factors in de-

Table 7. Etiology of epilepsy (%)

	USA	Europe	Asia	Africa
Idiopathic	76.7	40–45	79	60
Symptomatic	23.3	55–60	21	40
Head trauma	20.8	15–26	47.5	4–12
Cerebrovascular disease	22.5	–	16.4	6–20
Infection	12.5	13–15	24.6	10–20
Congenital	16.7	–	–	–
Tumor	1.5	4–2	3.3	3–10
Perinatal factors	7.5	12–27	–	1–2
Other	2.5	–	8.2	1–2

veloping countries include head trauma and cerebral parasitosis [14]. Table 7 compares these data with those reported from the USA and Europe [32, 36, 58].

In Italy 40% of the epileptic cases studied had antecedent perinatal brain injuries [29]. A study performed in a Danish county [20] revealed that 17% of mentally retarded persons had epilepsy. An increased prevalence ratio of epilepsy has also been reported in coeliac disease [9]. Quattrini et al. [55] report that 15% of drug abusers present with epilepsy as a neurological complication of drug dependence. The latency between the onset of drug abuse and occurrence of the seizures was 1–2 years. Partial complex seizures with secondary generalization were more frequent than generalized seizures. The prevalence of active epilepsy is significantly increased in the teen-age population exposed prenatally to thalidomide [61].

For all these reasons further analytic epidemiologic research is needed with the aim of identifying risk factors which may be different for the various geographic regions. Such investigations will lead the way for the implementation of effective programs to prevent epilepsy.

Simultaneously, treatment programs with community participation, within the context of primary health care delivery systems, should be initiated to dampen the socioeconomic burden of epilepsy for developing nations.

Acknowledgements. We thank Walter Rocca, Patricia Davis, and Vijay Chandra, from the Neuroepidemiology Branch, NINCDS, NIH, Bethesda, for their useful comments to the manuscript; as well as Mrs Sandi Chartier and Ms Linda Davis for secretarial assistance.

References

1. Aall-Jilek LM (1965) Epilepsy in the Wapagoro tribe in Tanganyika. Acta Psychiatr Neurol Scand 41:57–86
2. Aird RB, Masland RL, Woodbury DM (1984) The epilepsies: a critical review. Raven, New York, pp 99–116
3. Anderson DW, Bryan FA, Harris BSH, Lessler JT, Gagnon JP (1985) A survey approach for finding cases of epilepsy. Public Health Rep 100:386–393
4. Annegers JF, Hauser WA, Shirts SB (1984) Heart disease mortality and morbidity in patients with epilepsy. Epilepsia 25:699–704
5. Beran RG, Hall L, Pesch A, Ho P, Lam S, Leung PY, Cheung P, Fung M (1982) Population prevalence of epilepsy in Sydney, Australia. Neuroepidemiology 1:201–208
6. Baumann RJ, Marx MB, Leonidakis MG (1978) Epilepsy in rural Kentucky: Prevalence in a population of school age children. Epilepsia 19:75–80
7. Cavazzuti GB (1980) Epidemiology of different types of epilepsy in school age children of Modena, Italy. Epilepsia 21:57–62
8. Chandra V, Bharucha NE, Schoenberg BS (1983) Deaths related to epilepsy in the United States. Neuroepidemiology 2:148–155
9. Chapman RW, Laidlow JM, Colin-Jones D, Eade OE, Smith CL (1978) Increased prevalence of epilepsy in coeliac disease. Br Med J 2:250–251
10. Chiofalo N, Kirschbaum A, Fuentes A, Cordero ML, Madsen J (1979) Prevalence of epilepsy in children of Melipilla, Chile. Epilepsia 20:261–266
11. Crombie et al. (1960) A survey of the epilepsies in general practice. Br Med J 2:416–422
12. Cruz ME et al. (1977) Endemic neurological syndromes in the high Andean iodine deficiency region. Proceedings. XI World Congress of Neurology. Excerpta Medica, Amsterdam, pp 366–374
13. Cruz ME, Ramirez I (1981) Causas de dano cerebral congenito en el altiplano andino. In: Cruz ME, Espinoza E (eds) Nuevas perspectivas de la Paralisis Cerebral. Publitec, Quito, pp 45–54

14. Cruz ME, Utreras A, Canelos P, Malo L (1984) Guia de tomografia axial computarizada. Pub Med Quito, pp 85–124
15. Cruz ME, Ponce PL, Pradilla G, Barberis P, Gonzalez B (1985) Community based neuroepidemiologic studies in South America using a uniform protocol. Paper presented at the First Panamerican Congress of Neuroepidemiology, Bogota, April 24–27, 1985
16. Cruz ME, Schoenberg BS, Ruales R, Barberis P, Proano J, Bossano F, Sevilla F, Bolis CL (1985) Pilot study to detect neurologic disease in Ecuador among a population with a high prevalence of endemic goiter. Neuroepidemiology 4:108–116
17. Cruz ME, Tapia D, Enriquez J, Izurieta H, Barberis P, Schoenberg BS, Bolis CL (to be published) Prevalence of epilepsy in children of Ecuador, South America. Community Neurology (in press)
18. Dada TO (1968) Epilepsy in Nigeria: a study of the incidence, pathogenesis, clinical pattern and sociopsychological problems of epilepsy; MD thesis, University of Bristo
19. Doose H, Sitepu B (1983) Childhood epilepsy in a German city. Neuropediatrics 14: 220–224
20. Dyggve H, Kodahl T (1979) Disease pattern among 942 mentally retarded persons in a Danish county. Acta Psychiatr Scand 59:381–394
21. Fierro Benitez R, Cruz ME, Estrella E, Ramirez I, Stanbury JE (1978) Protein-calorie malnutrition and iodine deficiency. Effect on mental development, language and audition. In: American Medical Association (ed) Nutrition in transition. American Medical Association, Chicago, pp 254–263
22. Garcia-Pedroza F, Rubio-Donnadieu F, Garcia Ramos G, Escobedo-Rios F, Gonzalez Cortez A (1983) Prevalence of epilepsy in children: Tlalpan, Mexico City, Mexico. Neuroepidemiology 2:16–23
23. Gastaut H, Gastaut JL, Goncalvez e Silva GE, Fernandez Sanchez GR (1975) Relative frequency of different types of epilepsy: a study employing the classification of the International League Against Epilepsy. Epilepsia 16:457–467
24. Gerrits C (1983) A West African epilepsy focus. Lancet I: 358
25. Gomez JG, Arciniegas E, Torres J (1978) Prevalence of epilepsy in Bogota, Colombia. Neurology (Minneap) 28:90–94
26. Goodridge DM, Shorvon SD (1983) Epileptic seizures in a population of 6000. Br Med J (Clin Res) 287:641–644
27. Goudsmit J, van der Waals FW, Gajdusek DC (1983) Epilepsy in the Gbawein and Wroughbarh clan of Grand Bassa county. Liberia: The endemic occurrence of "see-ee" in the native population. Neuroepidemiology 2:24–34
28. Granieri E, Rosati G, Tola R, Pavoni M, Paolino E, Pinna L, Monetti VC (1983) A descriptive study of epilepsy in the district of Copparo, Italy, 1964–1978. Epilepsia 24: 502–514
29. Granieri E, Paolino E, Tola MR, Carreras R, Monetti VC, De Bastiani P, Pinna L, Merlin I, Altobelli A, Finotti L, et al. (1984) Epidemiology of epilepsy in the U.S.L. 34, Copparo, Emilia Romagna. Riv Neurol 54:245–264
30. Gudmundsson G (1966) Epilepsy in Iceland. Acta Neurol Scand [Suppl] 25/43:124
31. Hauser WA (1978) Epidemiology of epilepsy. Adv Neurol 19:313–339
32. Hauser WA, Kurland LT (1975) The epidemiology of epilepsy in Rochester, Minnesota, 1935 through 1967. Epilepsia 16:1–66
33. Hauser WA, Annegers J, Anderson N (1981) Epidemiology and the genetics of epilepsy. Arch Neurol 38:735
34. Joshi V, Katiyar BC, Mohan PK, Misra S, Shukla GD (1977) Profile of epilepsy in a developing country: a study of 1000 patients based on the international classification. Epilepsia 18:549–554
35. Juul-Jensen P, Foldspang A (1983) Natural history of epileptic seizures. Epilepsia 24:297–312
36. Krohn W (1961) Study of epilepsy in northern Norway, its frequency and character. Acta psychiatr Scand [Suppl] 150/36:215–227
37. Kuran W (1975) Epidemiology of epilepsy in school children at Pruszkow and Ursus. Neurol Neurochir Pol 9:57–63

38. Kurland LT (1959/60) The incidence and prevalence of convulsive disorders in a small urban community. Epilepsia (Amst) 1:143–161
39. Kurtzke JF, Kurland LT (1984) The epidemiology of neurologic disease. In: Baker and Baker (eds) Clinical neurology, Chapter 66. Harper and Row, Philadelphia, pp 27–42
40. Last JM (1983) Dictionary of epidemiology. Oxford University Press, New York
41. Leviton A, Cowan LD (1982) Epidemiology of seizure disorders in children. Neuroepidemiology I:40–83
42. Li SC, Schoenberg BS, Wang CC, Cheng XM, Zhou SS, Bolis CL (1985) Epidemiology of epilepsy in the urban population of the People's Republic of China. Epilepsia 26:391–394
43. Logan WPD, Cushion FA (1958) Studies on medical and population subjects, no. 14. Morbidity statistics from general practice, vol I. His Majesty's Stationery Office, London, England
44. Massey EW, Schoenberg BS (1985) Mortality from epilepsy: international patterns and changes over time. Neuroepidemiology 4:65–70
45. Meighan SS, Queener L, Weitman M (1976) Prevalence of epilepsy in children of Multnomah county, Oregon. Epilepsia 17:245–256
46. Nowak S (1972) Epidemiology and socio-medical problems of epilepsy in urban and rural populations. Neurol Neurochir Pol 23:373–374
47. Osuntokun BO (1980) Neuroepidemiology in Africa. In: Rose FC (ed) Clinical neuroepidemiology. Pitman Med, Kent, pp 57–86
48. Osuntokun BO, Schoenberg BS, Nottidge VA, Adeuja A, Kale O, Adeyefa A, Bademosi O, Olumide A, Oyediran ABO, Pearson CA, Bolis CL (1982) Research protocol for measuring the prevalence of neurologic disorders in developing countries. Neuroepidemiology I:143–153
49. Osuntokun BO, Adeuja AOG, Schoenberg BS, Bademosi O, Nottidge VA, Olumide AO, Ige O, Yaria F, Bolis CL (to be published) Prevalence of neurological disorders in a Nigerian suburban community. Proceedings of the XIII World Congress of Neurology
50. Pascual Lopez MA, Pascual Gispert J, Rodriguez Rivera L, Rojas Ochoa F, Tejeiros A (1980) Epilepsy: Epidemiological study in a child population. Bol Med Hosp Infant Mex 37:811–821
51. Pazzaglia P, Frank-Pazzaglia L (1976) Record in grade school of pupils with epilepsy: an epidemiological study. Epilepsia 17:361–366
52. Ponce Ducharne PL et al. (1985) Estudios neuroepidemiologicos en Venezuela. Ministerio de Sanidad
53. Pond DA, Bidwell BH, Stein L (1960) A survey of epilepsy in fourteen general practices. I. Demographic and medical data. Psychiatr Neurol Neurochir 63:217–236
54. Pradilla-Ardila G, Puentes F, Rivera R, Ballesteros G, Flantamsky H, Benavides MC, Vargas P, Rey N (1984) Estudio Neuroepidemiologico en Giron Santander. UIS
55. Quattrini A et al. (1982) Neurological complications in drug dependence with special reference to the development of epileptic syndromes. Riv Patol Nerv Ment 103:262–270
56. Remezova ES, Airapetova ES, Andreeva LA, Gorlina IS (1984) Clinical picture and treatment of epilepsy and epileptic syndromes in children. Zh Nevropatol Psikhiatr 84:882–885
57. Robinson N (1982) The epidemiology of epilepsy. Nursing Times 78:1717–1722
58. Roger J (1970) Epidemiology of epilepsy in European and American populations: a review. Afr J med Sci 1:237–245
59. Rose SW, Penry JK, Markush RE, Radloff LA, Putnam PL (1973) Prevalence of epilepsy in children. Epilepsia (Amst) 14:133–152
60. Schoenberg BS (1985) Epidemiology of Epilepsy. In: Porter and Morselli (eds.) Epilepsies. Butterworth, Kent, pp 94–105
61. Stephenson JB (1976) Epilepsy: Neurological complication of thalidomide embryopathy. Dev Med Child Neurol 18:189–197
62. Subianto DB, Tumada LR, Margono SS (1978) Burns and epileptic fits associated with cysticercosis in mountain people of Irian Jaya. Trop Geogr Med 30:275–278
63. Soulayol R, Yoyer-Vidil N (1974) L'Epilepsie dans la Reunion. Doin, Paris
64. Tsuboi T (1984) Epidemiology of febrile and afebrile convulsions in children in Japan. Neurology (Cleveland) 34:175–181
65. Ueki K, Sato S (1963) An epidemiological study of epilepsy in infancy and childhood in Niigata city. Psychiatr Neurol Pediatr (Japan) 3:3–13

66. van der Waals FW, Goudsmit J, Gajdusek DC (1983) See-ee: clinical characteristics of highly prevalent seizure disorders in the Gbawein and Wroughbarh clan region of Grand Bassa county, Liberia. Neuroepidemiology 2:35–44
67. Violante F, Serena M, Taroni G (1979) Epidemiological investigation on epilepsy in children of school age. Riv Patol Nerv Ment 99:255–266
68. Woodbury L (1978) Epidemiological characteristics. In: Plan for nationwide action on epilepsy. Report of the commission for the control of epilepsy and its consequences, vol. IV, USDHEW publ no. (NIH) 78-279, Washington, D.C., pp 1–114
69. Younis YO (1983) Epidemiology of epilepsy among school populations in Khartoum Province, Sudan. J Trop Med Hyg 86:213–216
70. Zielinski JJ (1974) Epilepsy and mortality rate and cause of death. Epilepsia 15:191–201
71. Zielinski JJ (1974) Epileptics not in treatment. Epilepsia 15:203–210

Epidemiology of Head Injury

B. JENNETT[1]

Accidents now account for more deaths than any other condition under the age of 45 in developed countries. Even in Africa accidents more commonly cause death between the ages 5 and 45 years than any WHO listed disease. In more than 70% of accidental deaths head injury is the major component. Serious persisting disability after trauma is much more commonly due to head injury than to any other kind of trauma. There is no ICD code for this condition; instead there are some 10 rubrics which do not reflect either severity or complications as recognised by clinicians; moreover there is such overlap between different codes that coding practices probably account for many of the discrepancies between different places or different time periods. Good data therefore depend on planned collection and even then there are difficulties.

There have now been a number of surveys on head injuries in Britain, Australia and the United States in the last decade [1–6]. These make it possible to make comparisons between certain clearly defined categories in different places, in particular for deaths and for patients admitted to hospital. Many trivial injuries never reach hospital, but it is difficult to ascertain these by questioning sample populations or doctors and nurses employed in places of work or providing primary care in the community.

Mortality statistics may omit deaths at the scene of the accident which account for two-thirds of fatalities in the United States and Australia and rather less than half in Britain. Studies based on hospital admissions omit the 5–10 times greater number of patients who attend emergency rooms and are sent home. These mild injuries consume considerable resources and are a source of appreciable anxiety because a small number of mild injuries develop serious complications; moreover, many patients have symptoms for at least 2–3 weeks after mild head injury, accounting for a considerable aggregate morbidity on account of their very large numbers.

Studies of *hospital admissions* pose problems because head-injured patients are often dispersed through several different specialties within a hospital. The proportion that reach a neurosurgeon varies considerably according to the availability of neurosurgical services in different places. Most acute American hospitals have a

[1] Department of Neurosurgery, Institute of Neurological Sciences, Glasgow, G51 4TF, Scotland.

Neurology
Ed. by K. Poeck, H. J. Freund, and H. Gänshirt

neurosurgeon whereas in Europe and Australia neurosurgery is a regionalised specialty; with only one unit for 1 million population or more, only severe or complicated injuries may be accepted. In Britain only about 5% of head injuries admitted to hospital are referred to neurosurgeons, but the proportion varies between 0.5% and 50%. Yet most detailed clinical reports of hospitalised cases are limited to this small subset of head-injured patients that reach neurosurgeons.

The most complete data are those available for Scotland where the provision of national statistics on deaths and on all hospital discharges coded by diagnosis makes ascertainment relatively reliable [2]. However, it has needed a special study to discover the number of patients who attend emergency departments and are sent home [7]. In Scotland, about 20% of attenders are admitted whereas in parts of the United States only 10% of attenders come into hospital. In Britain, guidelines have been published [8] based on estimating the risk of complications – especially intracranial haematoma [9]. These indicate that patients who have recovered from brief unconsciousness and have no fracture on skull X-ray can safely be sent home provided that there is a caring relative available. Such cases account for more than 90% of attenders and 70% of admissions in Britain. Places adopting these guidelines report marked reduction in admission rates since doing so, although admission rates for mild injuries had been rising in the country as a whole [10]. Incidence rates based on admissions will therefore vary according to local policies for dealing with attenders.

Death rates from head injuries per unit of population vary considerably between different countries. These reflect published differences in death rates due to accidents in general as well as from road accidents [11]. In Britain there are only 9 head injury deaths per 100000 population per year compared with 25–28 in the United States and in Australia.

In the United States there are considerable variations in both death rates and admission rates between urban and rural areas, between white and black races and between sexes. In the age group 10–25 years head injuries account for some 15% of all deaths in Britain and for over 20% in Australia and the United States. Death rates are slowly falling in all three countries.

Admission rates per 100000 population are about 200 in the United States, 300 in Britain and almost 400 in Australia. That there are fewer admissions and more deaths in the United States may reflect a greater proportion of severe injuries, but the lower rate of admission of mild injuries who come to hospital also contributes. Many injuries admitted in Britain are mild and leave hospital within 24–48 h. One American survey was limited to injuries associated with "significant damage to the brain" but such vague descriptions are not easy to apply [12]. However, the use of the Glasgow Coma Scale now makes it possible to compare injuries of similar severity in different places and better data are emerging as this severity scale is increasingly used throughout the world [5]. Other measures of severity are the presence of a skull fracture, the duration of stay in hospital and whether or not the patient is referred to a neurosurgeon. Length of stay may be prolonged owing to major extracranial injuries which occur in one-third of patients admitted to hospital after head injury.

It is commonly assumed that *road accidents* are the most frequent cause of head injuries. In fact they account for only about half the fatal cases in the United States, but for two-thirds in Australia, where about 20% of fatal injuries are due to falls and rather more than 10% to assault. The more detailed data available for Scotland show marked differences in the distribution of causes according to the severity of injury. Road accidents account for 56% of *fatal* head injuries, but for only 13% of head injuries who are *sent home* from accident departments; for admissions the proportion is intermediate (38%). Among road accidents pedestrians form a significant proportion in Britain and these unprotected road users often suffer more severe injuries than vehicle occupants. Alcohol is an important contributing cause for road accidents, falls and assaults. In some parts of Britain the drunken pedestrian is particularly at risk. Causes also vary with age, falls being more common in the elderly. Children and the elderly are frequent pedestrian victims.

Epidemiology should also take account of the prevalence of disabled survivors in the population. As well as the large number of mildly injured people suffering temporary disability there is an accumulating number with major, persistent disability. The average age of survivors after severe injury is 27 years and these victims face 40 years of disability and their numbers in Britain are similar to those for disability after stroke. In most countries severe head injuries are 2–3 times as common as in Britain, making it likely that their population of disabled people is also greater.

The purpose of head injury management should be to reduce avoidable mortality and morbidity. It is therefore sensible to ask the question "of deaths that occur after head injury, which could have been prevented." Most avoidable deaths are due to mismanagement in hospital, not lack of care at the roadside or delays in getting to the first hospital. The commonest avoidable factors are delay in dealing with remediable complications such as acute intracranial haematoma or hypotension and hypoxia due to extracranial injuries that cause secondary brain damage. It is estimated that about half of all deaths in hospital could have been avoided with better management and some avoidable mismanagement is a feature of about 50% of those who survive with serious disability.

For this reason improvement in the organisation and delivery of health care to all head-injured patients within a community can reduce mortality and morbidity significantly. Indeed this is more effective than increasingly aggressive means of treating the small minority of patients who are severely injured. Adequate services can be planned only if there are good data about how many injuries occur, and about where and when they happen. For example we have calculated a need for seven neurosurgical beds per million population in Britain for cases of serious injury or at risk from complications [13]. The epidemiology of head injury is therefore far from being an academic enterprise, for its practical applications could yield significant benefits in improved health care.

Prevention should apply at several levels – trying to prevent the original accident and once an accident has occurred to minimise the degree of brain damage at impact. It should aim to organise medical care in the community as a whole so that the risks of a second insult to the brain by avoidable mismanagement are minimised. It is fair to ask when conducting continuing audit of head injury care in a community what proportion of deaths and disabilities are associated with avoidable factors – in the way that has been done for 25 years in Britain in looking at maternal and more recently perinatal mortality. Measures directed to prevention in this broad sense are both political and medical. But neither political nor medical measures can be proposed, organised or audited unless there is an epidemiological base.

References

1. Jennett B, Murray A, MacMillan R, Macfarlane J, Bentley C, Hawthorne V (1977) Head injuries in Scottish hospitals. Lancet 2:696–698
2. Jennett B, MacMillan R (1981) Epidemiology of head injury. Br Med J 282:101–104
3. Simpson D, Antonio JD, North JB et al. (1981) Fatal injuries of the head and spine. Epidemiological studies in New South Wales and South Australia. Med J Aust 2:660–664
4. Frankowski RF, Klauber MR, Trabbador K et al. (1984) Head injury mortality: a comparison of three metropolitan counties. Am J Public Health (in press)
5. Jagger J, Levine JI, Jane JA et al. (1984) Epidemiologic features of head injury in a predominantly rural population. J Trauma 24:40–44
6. Kraus JF, Black MA, Hessol N et al. (1984) The incidence of acute brain injury and serious impairment in a defined population. Am J Epidemiol 119:185–201
7. Swann IG, MacMillan R, Strang I (1980) Head injuries at an inner city accident and emergency department. Injury 12:274–278
8. A Group of Neurosurgeons (1984) Guidelines for initial management after head injury in adults. Br Med J 288:983–985
9. Mendelow AD, Teasdale G, Jennett B, Bryden J, Hessett C, Murray G (1983) Risks of intracranial haematoma in head injured adults. Br Med J 287:1173–1176
10. Miller JD, Jones PA (1985) The work of a referral head injury service. Lancet 1:1141–1144
11. Jennett B, Teasdale G (1981) Management of head injuries. FA Davis, Philadelphia
12. Annegers JF, Grabow JD, Kurland LT, Laws ER (1980) The incidence, causes and secular trends of head trauma in Olmsted Country, Minnesota, 1935–1974. Neurology 30:912–919
13. Bryden JS, Jennett B (1983) Neurosurgical resources and transfer policies for head injuries. Br Med J 286:1791–1793

Discussion

Environmental vs. Genetic Factors in Ischemic Cerebrovascular Disease

W. S. FIELDS [1]

Specific patterns of atherosclerotic lesions in patients with ischemic cerebrovascular disease have emerged from analysis of arteriograms in approximately 7500 patients in three large-scale multicentered clinical trials, for which I have had the privilege of being the coordinator. In each of these trials aortocranial arteriography was a requisite for entry. The first of these was the Joint Study of Extracranial Arterial Occlusion, which included 23 institutions in the United States and the Institute of Neurology in Montevideo, Uruguay. The primary objective of this study was to determine the role of reconstructive arterial surgery in the prevention of stroke. It soon became apparent that among whites in North America the predominant lesion was atherosclerotic stenosis situated at the extracranial bifurcation of the common carotid artery. Lesions at this location were deemed appropriate and readily accessible for carotid endarterectomy. Among persons of similar European background, living in Uruguay, Argentina, and Southern Brazil, cerebral ischemic symptoms occurred in approximately 35% as a consequence of dilatation, elongation, and kinking of the extracranial arteries. Kinking was considered an indication for reconstructive arterial surgery. Among North American blacks admitted to the Joint Study, it was noted that the offending lesions were more often found in the carotid siphon, at the origin of the middle cerebral artery, or at both locations. Lesions of this nature are virtually unknown among West Africans of the same ethnic origin.

As already pointed out by Professor Shi-chuo Li, Japanese and Chinese living in the Orient have different patterns of cerebrovascular disease than do those of the same ethnic origin living in Hawaii and North America. The anatomical patterns of cerebral atherosclerotic lesions in these two populations also differ, with intracranial arterial lesions being more frequently associated with cerebral symptoms in those persons living in the Far East, while in North America the patterns of atherosclerotic lesions tend to conform to the pattern seen among whites in the same geographic region. Differences of this nature have also been apparent in the three parts of the recently completed Extracranial-Intracranial Bypass Study conducted in North America, Europe, and the Far East about which you will hear more from Professor Barnett.

[1] University of Texas, The M. D. Anderson Hospital and Tumor Institute at Houston, Houston, TX 77030, USA.

Neurology
Ed. by K. Poeck, H. J. Freund, and H. Gänshirt

I hasten to point out that the foregoing statements are general conclusions and that one can find exceptions to the rule in each of the aforementioned populations. All of this evidence, however, when considered together, tends to confirm the observations of Professor Li that patterns of cerebrovascular disease appear to relate more closely to environmental than to genetic factors. One must, therefore, take these differences into consideration before making the assumption that the conclusions drawn from a clinical treatment trial conducted in one geographic location are equally applicable to the population in another region, even though the subjects may have a common genetic background. Geographic factors must be considered in attempting to determine the weight to be given to any one or a group of risk factors for cerebrovascular disease. Data of this nature should be of great interest to physicians in clinical practice who must base treatment decisions on the best available information about the characteristics of the population from which their patients are drawn. Information of this nature is not readily available at the present time to the average primary physician or for that matter to the specialist in neurological diseases. These differences in the patterns of lesions in persons with ischemic cerebrovascular disease must also be considered in the future by those planning multicentered clinical trials.

Case-Control Study of Focal Cerebral Ischemia in Young Adults

C. FIESCHI [1]

This paper is a preliminary report of the "CNR cross-sectional case-control study of focal cerebral ischemia in young adults" (CNR PFMPR SP4 OB. 38) [1]. Eight neurological departments are participating in this study: four in northern Italy (Genoa, Milan, Padua, Parma), three in central Italy (Florence, L'Aquila, Rome) and one in southern Italy (Messina). The final sample will consist of 350 patients of ages between 15 and 44 years, and 700 controls.

This discussion reports data from 235 patients recruited until 30 June 1985; 125 patients (53%) were males and 117 (47%) females. The frequency distribution of patients recruited increases linearly with age. Males outnumber females in the older age groups (35–39 and 40–44) respectively, while females are more numerous in the age group 20–34 years (Fig. 1).

Among the 235 patients recruited, 134 (57.5%) had reversible cerebral ischemic attacks and the remaining 101 (42.5%) had strokes (Table 1). Carotid attacks included 76.6% of all the cases; 17.4% of patients had vertebral basilar attacks while a definite diagnosis of arterial territory was not reached in 6.0% of all included cases.

All patients had brain CT scan while angiography has been performed in 156 patients (66.3%) (Table 2). Congruous angiographic lesions have been detected in 12 of 85 RIA patients (14%) and in 44 of 71 stroke patients (61.9%). Globally, 56 patients had congruous lesions: 31 (55.3%) in extracranial vessels and 25 (44.7%) in intracranial vessels. Associated risk factors and concomitant diseases are variably distributed among the patients recruited (Table 3).

At present, the main characteristics of these young Italian adults with focal cerebral ischemia are the following:

1. A strong female prevalence in the age group 20–34 years, possibly indicating different clusterings of ethopathogenic mechanisms in the young.
2. 20% of angiographically documented cases have congruous extracranial lesions, indicating that atherosclerotic disease is already active in our young population. Besides, 16% of patients have congruous intracranial lesions suggesting an embolic mechanism, the source of which is not always detectable.

---

[1] On behalf of the CNR Study Group on Stroke, III Cattedra di Clinica Neurologica, Dipartimento di Scienze Neurologiche, Università degli Studi di Roma "La Sapienza", 00185 Rome, Italy.

Neurology
Ed. by K. Poeck, H. J. Freund, and H. Gänshirt

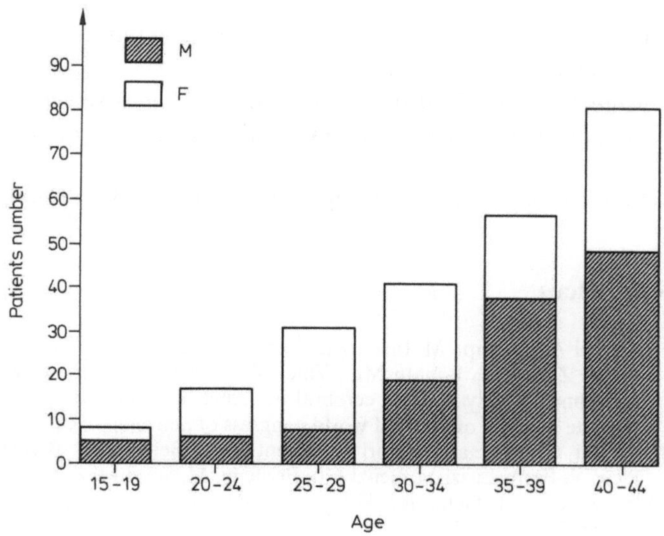

Fig. 1. Age groups and male:female ratio in 235 young adults with focal cerebral ischemia

Table 1. Clinical diagnosis and arterial territories

	Patients No.	Carotid No. (%)	Vertebral basilar No. (%)	Undetermined No. (%)
TIA	82	61 (74.5)	14 (17.0)	7 (8.5)
P-TIA	29	20 (68.9)	7 (24.2)	2 (6.9)
TIA-IR	23	20 (86.9)	3 (13.1)	
Stroke	101	79 (78.3)	17 (16.8)	5 (4.9)
Total	235	180 (76.6)	41 (17.4)	14 (6.0)

Table 2. Clinical diagnosis and congruous angiographic lesions

	Patients	Carotid	Vertebral basilar	Congruous	Angiographic (%)
TIA	49	7		7	(14.2)
P-TIA	20	1	1	2	(10.0)
TIA-IR	16	3		3	(18.7)
Stroke	71	33	11	44	(61.9)
Total	156	44	12	56	(35.9)

Table 3. Risk factors and associated diseases

Cardiac diseases	16.5%	Smoking	51.2%
Mitral valve prolapse	NA	Alcohol	12.2%
Hypertension	12.7%	Oral contraceptives	18.9%
Diabetes mellitus	5.1%	Vascular migraine	16.8%
Dyslipidemia	17.7%	Associated diseases	5.9%

3. 17% of young adults with focal cerebral ischemia did not show any apparent risk factor or associated disease. However, data on mitral valve prolapse [2] are not yet available for this analysis.
4. More than one-third of patients, with proven associated risk factors (hypertension, diabetes mellitus, and cardiac disease) ignored their associated disease.

Acknowledgement. This work is supported by CNR grant 84.02328.56.

References

1. Carolei A, Prencipe M, Inzitari D, Landi G, Gandolfo C, Tomasello F, Parma M, Frontoni M, De Zanche L, Bonatti ML., Vinci M, Loeb CW, Fieschi C (1985) CNR Cross-sectional case-control study in focal cerebral ischemia in young adults. Acute brain ischemia 1985. Satellite meeting of the XIII world congress of neurology. Raven, New York (in press)
2. Fieschi C, Francia A, Allori L, Argentino C, Bernardi S, Bertazzoni G, Carpinteri F, Di Piero V, Ferro Luzzi M, Lenzi GL, Prencipe M, Servi M, Zanette E (1983) Mitral valve prolapse as a risk factor for TIA. A study with echocardiography and dynamic ECG. Eur Neurol 22:233–239

Guillain-Barré Syndrome Following (A/New Jersey/76) Influenza (Swine Flu) Vaccine: Epidemic or Artifact?

L. T. KURLAND [1], W. C. WIEDERHOLT, E. BEGHI, J. W. KIRKPATRICK, H. G. POTTER, and F. P. ARMSTRONG

Physicians in the United States have generally accepted as fact that the (A/New Jersey/76) swine flu vaccine administered to nearly 45 million people from October through December 1976 was responsible for an increase in Guillain-Barré syndrome (GBS). However, the only substantive evidence for that association is a single study based on data collected by health officers during the highly publicized swine flu program and the moratorium on the immunizations which was declared on 16 December 1976.

The foundation for the thousands of claims against the U.S. government for compensation for GBS and other disorders is the report by Schonberger et al. [1] which describes the epidemiologic features of the 1098 cases reported to Centers for Disease Control (CDC) as GBS by the state and territorial health officers. The authors show the epidemiologic curve for the 532 vaccinated and 543 unvaccinated cases. For the 532 cases reported among vaccine recipients, the epidemic curve showed a marked increase of cases in the first 6 weeks after vaccination, with a peak during the 3rd week. Within the first 6 weeks, the attributable risk of vaccine-related GBS in the adult population was estimated at nearly 1 case per 100000 vaccinations, which corresponds to an attributable risk ratio of 8.8 if one accepts as baseline the incidence rate for GBS in the unvaccinated population as estimated by CDC. If one uses, instead, the baseline rate for Olmsted County, Minnesota, the relative risk is much lower and the "epidemic" terminates at 6 weeks [2, 3]. The attack rates reported by CDC were similar for the monovalent and bivalent vaccines and for whole and split product vaccines by different manufacturers. Studies of subgroups (Ohio and Michigan) [4, 5] and a reanalysis of the CDC computerized summary data appeared to confirm the general conclusions reached by CDC [6].

This remarkable association of swine flu vaccine and GBS is contrary to past experience in the United States, where some 300 million doses of influenza vaccines have been administered since 1945 without evidence of an increase in neurologic

[1] L. T. Kurland, Department of Medical Statistics and Epidemiology, Mayo Clinic and Mayo Foundation, Rochester, MN 55905, USA.

Neurology
Ed. by K. Poeck, H. J. Freund, and H. Gänshirt

disorders. Killed swine flu virus was a component of many of these vaccines, particularly during the period 1955–1969. Furthermore, studies of other influenza vaccines from 1978 through 1981 have shown no significant increase in GBS.

The high relative risk and temporal association noted in the CDC report on the swine flu vaccine must be regarded as strong epidemiologic evidence of a causal relationship. Yet it is remarkable that no other independent population-based study has been published which supports that position. The only large-scale independent study suggested that the number of cases of GBS among personnel in the U.S. Army was appreciably less than anticipated from the CDC report [7]. The study in Olmsted County, Minnesota, where some 40000 adults received the vaccine showed no case among the vaccinees, although this might be expected if the risk were 1 in 100000 as reported by CDC. The completeness of case ascertainment in Olmsted County led us to examine this question on the assumption that the attack rate might be greater. Under these circumstances, the lack of cases in Olmsted County, although of interest, does not contribute to the question of the true relative risk of the vaccine [3].

Since the Army study [7] had a number of methodological faults, the lists for GBS diagnosed from 1974 through 1978 were requested from among active duty military personnel in the U.S. Army, Navy, and Air Force. The results have provided impressive evidence that GBS was not a complication of the swine flu vaccination program in the military services. Between 1 October and 16 December 1976, more than 80% of the 2.1 million active duty personnel in the armed forces received 400 CCA units of killed whole virus vaccine – double the dose used in the civilian

Table 1. Guillain-Barré syndrome in active duty Army personnel by month of admission, 1974–1978

	1974	1975	1976	1977	1978
January	3	4	2	2	2
February	3	5	4	0	3
March	1	2	0	1	3
April	4	1	1	0	3
May	0	2	0	2	3
June	1	0	1	2	3
July	0	0	3	2	2
August	1	2	1	0	0
September	3	2	1	0	2
October	0	2	1	2	0
November	2	2	1	1	0
December	1	1	1	3	1
Total	19	23	16	15	22
Strength	780000	779000	775000	779000	777000
Rate/10^5	2.44	2.95	2.06	1.93	2.83
Mean rate for 1974–1978	2.44				

Incidence includes all diagnoses reported for a case (both principal and secondary).
ICDA-8 diagnosis code 3540 was used for 1974–1978.

Table 2. Guillain-Barré syndrome in active duty Navy/Marine Corps personnel by month of admission, 1975–1978

	1975	1976	1977	1978
January	0	3	2	1
February	0	1	3	1
March	2	3	1	4
April	2	2	2	2
May	0	3	1	1
June	0	6	2	2
July	1	2	0	1
August	0	2	2	1
September	2	1	2	1
October	1	2	1	1
November	2	2	2	0
December	1	0	2	0
Total	11	27	20	15
Strength	732000	719000	717000	717000
Rate/10^5	1.50	3.76	2.79	2.09
Mean rate for 1975–1978	2.53			

Incidence includes all diagnoses reported for a case (both principal and secondary).
ICDA-8 diagnosis code 3540 was used for 1975–1978.

Table 3. Guillain-Barré syndrome in active duty Air Force personnel by month of admission, 1975–1979

	1975	1976	1977	1978	1979
January	4	2	0	2	0
February	0	2	3	1	2
March	0	2	1	1	0
April	0	0	0	1	1
May	1	1	1	0	2
June	0	3	0	2	0
July	3	0	1	0	3
August	0	1	0	0	2
September	2	2	0	1	3
October	2	0	2	1	3
November	2	1	3	1	1
December	2	1	0	0	0
Total	16	15	11	10	15
Strength	612000	584000	571000	570800	563000
Rate/10^5	2.61	2.56	1.93	1.75	2.66
Mean rate for 1975–1979	2.31				

Incidence includes all diagnoses reported for a case (both principal and secondary).
ICDA-8 diagnosis code 3540 was used for 1975–1979.

Table 4. Guillain-Barré syndrome in active duty personnel

Service	Years	Average strength	Number of GBS cases	Average annual rate/ 100000	Percentage vaccinated	Number vaccinated 1976
Army	1974–1978	778000	95	2.44	88	682000
Navy/Marines	1975–1978	721000	73	2.53	68	490300
Air Force	1975–1979	595462	67	2.31	90	525600
Total		2094462	235	2.40	80.5	1697900

Table 5. Guillain-Barré syndrome in active duty personnel[a]

	Average annual number of GBS cases	Average number of cases in any 4 months	Number observed 1 October 1976– 31 January 1977	Number expected from civilian swine flu vaccine (RR 3.96)	*P*
Army	19	6.3	5	11.94	0.021
Navy/Marines	18.3	6.1	6	10.26	0.115
Air Force	13.4	4.7	2	8.41	0.01
Total	50.7	17.1	13	30.61	0.0003

[a] Olmsted County, Minnesota. Average annual rate aged 18 and over, 1935–1980 = $2.23/10^5$ (approximately 1.5 million patient years).

population. Since virtually all cases in the military services suspected of having GBS would be hospitalized, but only those fulfilling reasonable diagnostic criteria would have a discharge diagnosis of GBS, the evaluation was based on those discharge diagnoses (Tables 1–5). The results show no excess of cases during the 4-month critical period for the vaccine (October 1976 through January 1977) compared with other similar periods between 1974 and 1978.

Because of the ongoing litigation, CDC did not release its raw data to anyone outside CDC until required to do so by a Federal court order in November 1981. The CDC then made available the computer line listings on all of the cases included in its report published in 1979. This proved to be an opportunity for those of us who were now concerned about the validity of the CDC study, but had also been denied access to their data because of all the pending litigation. The Department of Justice then commissioned a panel of experts in neurology and epidemiology to analyze the computer printouts on these 1098 cases which had formed the basis for the CDC report; again, we emphasize that the hospital records were not made available for review. The analysis of the 1098 data summary sheets by the panel led to a detailed report, referred to as the Langmuir panel report, released in the June 1984 issue of the *American Journal of Epidemiology* which provided several important items of information [6]:

1. In 122 of the CDC data sheets, the information was so incomplete or contradictory that the case could not be adequately classified.

2. The epidemic curve for cases classified as having extensive motor involvement fitted a log-normal distribution with a peak at 3 weeks and a return to baseline at 6 weeks.
3. Using Olmsted County, Minnesota, rates as baseline, there was now an excess of only 211 cases among the vaccinees to account for the "epidemic."

In other words, if 211 cases reported as GBS in the vaccinees were found not to be GBS, the epidemic could evaporate.

It was not until mid-1983 that the actual CDC report forms (questionnaires) were made available to us for examination, again as a result of a Federal court order. A review of the questionnaires completed by the health officers, the computer line listings, as well as interviews with several of the health officers (or the paramedical assistants who collected the data that went to the CDC) provided serious and disquieting results. The material now available showed that:

1. The CDC did not establish diagnostic criteria for GBS that could guide health officers and their nonphysician assistants in case ascertainment.
2. Records were abstracted in the field and no copies of clinical records for subsequent review were retained.
3. No systematic follow-up of cases had occurred – and this for a disease which requires outcome information to provide high assurance of a correct diagnosis.
4. No neurologic assessment of the clinical records was ever carried out.

We also became aware that CDC had continued to count as cases those which had subsequently been shown not to be GBS, and that there may have been greater efforts to recruit the vaccinated over the nonvaccinated cases which could further have biased the results. In view of the tremendous repercussions of the CDC report in terms of litigation and the question of the general safety of vaccines as perceived by the public, a most serious issue was the failure of the CDC to obtain confirmation of the diagnoses and evaluation of the epidemic pattern from some independent source. We have now seen that the data from such an independent source, namely, the three military services, showed no increase whatsoever in GBS incidence rates in spite of substantial exposure to swine flu vaccine.

Further review of the CDC abstracts revealed a number of other curious findings pertaining to diagnosis. In 10% of cases accepted by the CDC as GBS there was no evidence of progression, in 13% weakness was not bilateral, 22% were reported as having had no evidence of lower motor neuron involvement. Since the CDC report was not published until 2½ years after the immunization program, another curious fact which emerged is that 80% of patients accepted as GBS were listed as not recovered – this, in spite of the well-known fact that the majority of patients with GBS make an excellent recovery within several months. It is also of interest that the rate of GBS cases reported to CDC dropped precipitously in both the vaccinated and nonvaccinated cases in January 1977, suggesting that proximity to the time of greatest publicity may have had an effect on case ascertainment. Another curious observation is that of 532 vaccinated individuals accepted by the CDC as GBS, nearly 100 did not file administrative claims for compensation against the U.S. government and another 100 did not bring their claims for compensation to trial. Were these 200 cases extremely mild, or did they occur in nonlitigious persons, or were they not cases of GBS? Additional studies of the influenza vaccine in the years after 1976 have shown no significant association with GBS [8–11].

On the basis of these observations, we have advised the Director of the Centers for Disease Control of our concern over quality control and our reservations about the accuracy of diagnosis of the cases which were accepted as GBS. We have recommended that a panel of neurologists, with expertise in the diagnosis of GBS, review the actual medical records of each of the 1098 cases and classify them on the basis of reasonable diagnostic criteria. The identification and vaccination status would be masked on each case prior to review.

We are pleased to report that the Director of CDC has approved such a reappraisal of the cases in Minnesota and Michigan and by the end of 1985 we expect to know if our concern is reasonable with respect to the accuracy of diagnosis and reporting bias.

References

1. Schonberger LB, Bregman DJ, Sulliban-Bolyai JZ, Keenlyside RA, Ziegler DW, Retailliau H, Eddins DI, Bryan JA (1979) Guillain-Barre syndrome following vaccination in the National Influenza Immunization program, United States, 1976–1977. Am J Epidemiol 110(2):105–123
2. Kennedy RH, Danielson MA, Mulder DW, Kurland LT (1978) Guillain-Barre syndrome: a 42-year epidemiologic and clinical study. Mayo Clin Proc 53:93–99
3. Beghi E, Kurland LT, Mulder DW, Wiederholt WC (1985) Guillain-Barre syndrome: clinicoepidemiologic features and effect of influenza vaccine. Arch Neurol 42:1053–1057
4. Marks JS, Halpin TJ (1980) Guillain-Barre syndrome in recipients of A/New Jersey influenza vaccine. JAMA 243(24):2490–2494
5. Breman JG, Hayner NS (1984) Guillain-Barre syndrome and its relationship to swine influenza vaccination in Michigan, 1976–1977. Am J Epidemiol 119:880–889
6. Langmuir AD, Bregman DJ, Kurland LT, Nathanson N, Victor M (1984) An epidemiologic and clinical evaluation of Guillain-Barre syndrome reported in association with the administration of swine influenza vaccines. Am J Epidemiol 119:841–879
7. Johnson DE (1982) Guillain-Barre Syndrome in the United States Army. Arch Neurol 39:21–24
8. Schonberger LB, Hurwitz ES, Katona P, Holman RC, Bregman DJ (1981) Guillain-Barre syndrome: its epidemiology and associations with influenza vaccination. Ann Neurol 9 [Suppl]:31–38
9. Kaplan JE, Schonberger LB, Hurwitz ES, Katona P (1983) Guillain-Barre syndrome in the United States, 1978–1981: additional observations from the national surveillance system. Neurology 33:633–637
10. Hurwitz ES, Holman RC, Nelson DB, Schonberger LB (1983) National surveillance for Guillain-Barre syndrome: January 1978–March 1979. Neurology 33:150–157
11. Hurwitz ES, Schonberger LB, Nelson DB, Holman RC (1981) Guillain-Barre syndrome and the 1978–1979 influenza vaccine. N Eng J Med 304:1557–1561

Co-authors

W. C. Wiederholt, Department of Neurosciences, University of California, San Diego.
E. Beghi, Mario Negri Institute, Milan, Italy.
J. W. Kirkpatrick, Office of the Surgeon General, U. S. Army.
H. G. Potter, U. S. Navy Environmental Health Center, Naval Station, Norfolk.
F. P. Armstrong, U. S. Air Force School of Aerospace Medicine, Brooks Air Force Base.

The views expressed by the participants in the military services represent their own opinions and should not be construed as an official position of the Department of Defense.

Epidemiology of Head Injury: Future Perspective

M. GOLDSTEIN [1]

Professor Jennett, a world authority on both the clinical care of the head injured and on the epidemiology of head injury, once again challenges us; this time, to address the sparse information available on the incidence, morbidity, and mortality associated with head injury. In many of the developed and newly developing nations of the world, plans are under way to improve health care services. However, the data necessary to develop realistic and efficient plans in the area of head injury are at best minimal, and too often could be inadequate.

Professor Jennett has reviewed for us the epidemiologic data available. He points out that there are important similarities and differences in the information available among studies done in different parts of the world and that there is a critical need for an international endeavor for the collection of comparable epidemiologic data on head injury. Similar problems have been addressed in the past by WHO in areas such as stroke, diabetes, and schizophrenia. I would hope that the WFN Research Committee would develop the protocol necessary for the collection of such data and work with WHO to initiate an international research effort. Only with such data can meaningful and efficient programs of health care be initiated.

We now have a substantial body of information about the pathogenesis of cerebral damage due to head injury, including focal and diffuse vascular lesions and more recently, further elucidation of diffuse axonal injury due to the shearing effect of physical forces, particularly when they occur in the lateral plane [1]. The pathogenesis of coma as a result of individual and combined pathologies is now much clearer; hence, more specific diagnostic and therapeutic approaches offering improved outcomes are in sight. Thus, there is every probability in the near future for improved therapies with important reductions in morbidity and mortality.

However, these improved clinical interventions may still be quite inadequate to meet our goals since such a very large proportion of head injury deaths occur before the patient is admitted to hospital. As you recall, even in the 1980s only one-third of head-injured patients survive long enough to undergo significant medical-surgical therapy. Even if we reduced in-hospital head injury deaths by 50%, this would result in a 16% reduction in total head injury deaths. On the other hand, if we could re-

[1] Director, National Institute of Neurological and Communicative Disorders and Stroke, National Institutes of Health, Bethesda, MD 20892, USA.

Neurology
Ed. by K. Poeck, H. J. Freund, and H. Gänshirt

duce all head injury deaths by 15%, there would be an 18% reduction in total head injury mortality [2].

A 15% reduction in total head injury deaths is not an unrealistic goal. This achievement is probably more attainable than the 50% reduction of in-hospital deaths required to obtain comparable results.

The keys to obtaining these results are the continuing improvement of the in-hospital armamentarium of medical-surgical procedures *combined* with the initiation of community-based programs. Community programs need to include measures to prevent and minimize the occurrence of head injury, provide for emergency on-site treatment and establish systems for rapid transportation to centers prepared to provide the clinical skills required for proper care of the head injured. Prevention and improved immediate care are the essential ingredients of community-based programs.

Head injury has the dubious distinction of being among the leading causes of death and disability in every environment in which it has been studied. It seriously threatens our teenage and young adult populations. There are now demonstrated models of community intervention that must be considered if we are to address this epidemic of modern times adequately. Professor Jennett's plea for the necessary data should not go unheeded.

References

1. Becker DP, Povlishock JT (eds) Central nervous system trauma status report, 1985. NINCDS-NIH, Bethesda, Md
2. Frankowski RF (1985) Head injury mortality in urban populations and its relation to the injured child. In: Brooks BF (ed) The injured child. University of Texas Press, Austin, p 28

Epidemiology of Peripheral Neuropathies

B. O. OSUNTOKUN [1]

Introduction

Although the peripheral neuropathies (PN) occur world-wide, there are few community-based studies. For valid epidemiological studies, subjects must be representative of the community and the diagnosis must be accurate. Most studies of PN have been done in hospital populations and diagnostic criteria have varied among investigators, making comparison difficult.

PN may involve various topographical sites, with bilateral symmetrical, focal and multifocal disturbance of function, either in isolation or as part of widespread multisystem disease. The possible causes are numerous and may be multiple in the same patient: e.g. the alcoholic diabetic patient who is also susceptible to pressure palsies. The pathological process may affect neurones (neuronopathy), distally directed, centrally directed or both centrally and distally directed axons (axonopathy), Schwann cells, interstitial supporting tissues and vascular supply; the derangement may be mediated from without (trauma, compression, inflammation etc.); and combinations of these may occur. Because of the heterogeneity of PN, classification into aetiological subtypes is important for epidemiological studies. The problems inherent in the epidemiological studies of peripheral nerves have been highlighted by Schoenberg [104]. Perhaps because of these, less is known about the epidemiology of PN compared with common diseases of the nervous system such as stroke and epilepsy. This communication presents a distillation of the epidemiology of PN as seen world-wide.

Usefulness of Epidemiology in Peripheral Neuropathies

Epidemiological studies have been valuable in indicating the causes of clusters and outbreaks of PN. Examples include the following:

1. Organic mercury intoxication (Minamata disease) first recognised in 1953 among the residents of fishing villages surrounding Minamata Bay in Japan [65] and also described in Iraq [24], Pakistan [46, 55], Guatemala [87] and Ghana [28].

[1] Neurology Unit, Department of Medicine, University of Ibadan, Ibadan, Nigeria.

Neurology
Ed. by K. Poeck, H. J. Freund, and H. Gänshirt

2. Intoxication with triorthocresyl phosphate (TOCP) which contaminated cooking oil and has been reported from South Africa [116], Morocco [109], India [123], United States of America [80] and Sri Lanka [105].
3. The tracing of the gene which determines variegate porphyria in white South Africans, among whom the prevalence is 3 per 1000, to a seventeenth century Dutch emigrant couple.
4. The identification of a tick-borne (*ixodes dammini*) spirochaete as the cause of Lyme disease, a multisystem disorder which affects the skin, joints, heart and the nervous system, including the peripheral nerves, first described in the Lyme district of Connecticut, and found in at least 14 of the United States, as well as in Scandinavia (where a mosquito vector may be involved) and Australia [76, 113].
5. The classification of the hereditary neuropathies that present clinically as Charcot-Marie-Tooth disease [47].
6. Others include the identification of the cause of PN in humans with exposure to *n*-hexane, acrylamide, methyl-*n*-butyl-ketone, dimethylaminopropionitrile, chlordecone and clioquinol; increased incidence of Guillain-Barré syndrome (GBS) following swine influenza immunization in the United States in 1976; and an outbreak of beriberi among schoolboys in southern Japan due to thiamine deficiency [31]. Epidemiological studies provide data on efficacy, effectiveness of treatment and on prognosis

Some General Epidemiological Considerations

Prevalence

There are few studies to determine prevalence ratios of *all* types of PN. In the last 5 years, the World Health Organization- (WHO-)sponsored community-based neuroepidemiological studies have made some data available. Excluding isolated cranial nerve disease such as Bell's palsy, prevalence ratios of PN per 100000 vary from 300 to 1100 in Nigeria [93, 94], 113 in urban China [68], 1498, 1172, and 129 in Colombia, Ecuador and Venezuela, respectively [22].

Age and Sex Distribution

PN (especially acquired ones) commonly occur in adults and the elderly, although GBS may afflict children. Poliomyelitis, a scourge in many developing countries, is essentially a disease of young children under the age of 5 years, after which almost 100% of the population have acquired immunity. The onset of many hereditary PN is in childhood and adolescence.

There is no sex bias; however in nutritional PN, the onset may be precipitated by pregnancy and lactation. Females suffer more from diseases such as systemic lupus erythematosus (SLE) and sarcoidosis in which PN are common. Males are more affected by PN of chronic renal failure.

A decade ago many cases of PN could be assigned no identifiable cause – 40% or more. With increasing sophistication in investigation, epidemiological and family studies, the percentage of cryptogenic PN was 24% of 205 patients at the Mayo

Clinic, in the United States [32], 10% of 519 patients in Australia [75], 20% of 114 patients in India [61] and 26% of 358 patients in Nigeria [7].

In developed countries, the commonest causes of PN are, in descending order, trauma, diabetes, acquired demyelinating disorders, nutritional deficiencies and toxins, while in the developing countries, leprosy, acquired demyelinating disorders, nutritional deficiencies, diabetes and toxins are the commonest. Traumatic PN predominantly afflict working class males. World-wide GBS seems to be the most common acute areflexic PN [4, 7, 61].

Nutritional neuropathies occur in circumstances which differ from one part of the world to the other. In developing countries shortage of or inadequate dietary intake due to poverty and lack of food compounded by factors such as ignorance, unbalanced and vegetarian diets, drought, flood, famine and wars are the main causes. Alcoholism unfortunately is increasing in the developing countries. Infections, pregnancy and prolonged lactation may constitute precipitating factors. By contrast, in the developed countries, the common primary nutritional causes of PN are chronic alcoholism, food faddism, neglect and ignorance. In all parts of the world, secondary nutritional neuropathies are due to malabsorption, excessive vomiting from pregnancy and disease, chronic illnesses from neoplasms, psychoses, dementia and depression. Apart from specific nutritional deficiencies of thiamine, folate, vitamin B_{12}, pyridoxine, panthothenic acid, biotin, vitamin E, which may cause PN, protein-energy malnutrition (PEM), which in varying severity may afflict 4%–40% of the population in developing countries may cause mild and reversible PN [25, 85, 86]. Subclinical malnutrition may explain the high frequency (20% or more) of absent ankle jerk in apparently normal Africans aged 20–45 years, as found in Nigeria and Tanzania [90] in contrast to retention of ankle jerk in 94% of 200 elderly white people [54]. Of 898 former prisoners of war in the Far East, 36 years after exposure to malnutrition, 5.5% still had evidence of neuropathy [38]. It is doubtful if deficiencies of riboflavin and nicotinic acid cause PN. Vitamin B_{12} deficiency as addisonian pernicious anemia is very rare in Africa and India, where it is usually due to malabsorption.

Toxic PN are frequent in developed countries owing to industrial exposure. Genetic predisposition is important in PN caused by drugs such as isoniazid (liver acetylation phenotype). Two-thirds of black Africans are fast acetylators [101].

Peripheral neuropathies associated with infections are common in developing countries. Leprosy afflicts 12 million people (4 million in India and 1 million in Africa). Herpes zoster is universal. In rabies, endemic in Africa, Asia and South America, segmental demyelination with or without wallerian degeneration of axons occurs [20, 119]. South American trypanosomiasis is a major cause of autonomic PN. Schistosomiasis which afflicts about 400 million people infrequently causes PN [70, 96]. A syndrome caused by the bite of tick (*Ixodes*), due to botulinum-like intoxication from the female tick's salivary fluid, may simulate GBS although sensory signs are absent and the cerebrospinal fluid is persistently normal [100]. Tick-transmitted spirochaetal infection is the cause of Lyme disease or Bannwarth's syndrome, a meningoencephalomyeloradiculopathy, in which PN occur in 10%–20% of patients, associated with increased CSF protein and pleocytosis [113, 131]. Malaria, endemic in areas of the world inhabited by 1 million people, is said to cause PN, but the evidence is dubious. Reversible PN has been associated with infection by *Giardia lamblia* [9].

Hereditary PN is rare or under-reported in many developing countries [1] with few exceptions such as Tunisia [10, 11] and India [124, 125]. Vasculitis as a cause of PN is uncommon in some regional group such as black Africans among whom diseases such as SLE, polyarteritis nodosa, rheumatoid arthritis and even the microangiopathy of diabetes mellitus occur at a much lower prevalence compared with other races and black Americans.

Some Epidemiological Features of the Common and Specific Peripheral Neuropathies

Leprosy

As an entity, leprosy is the commonest cause of PN in the world. Leprosy spreads between humans with no alternate host, and transmission requires prolonged contact. The incubation period is long, 5–15 years or more. All leprosy is neural leprosy [37] since in *all* cases, the peripheral nerves are involved: 4.3% of 11000 patients had PN without any cutaneous manifestations [29]. Types of leprosy depend on the levels of immunity. The range of immunity is from the "immunocompetent" tuberculoid leprosy in which the cutaneous infiltrates contain well-organised epithelioid and giant cell granulomas, predominant helper/inducer T-cell subset and scanty bacilli or remnants of them, through borderline and indeterminate leprosy to the "immunodeficient" lepromatous type in which the cutaneous infiltrates consist of macrophages heavily parasitised with bacilli, and predominant suppressor/cytotoxic T-cell subset [122]. Sensorimotor or sensory PN, mononeuritis multiplex and simplex are the usual presentations. The prevalence ratio of leprosy in India is 2–6 per 1000 [125].

Recent advances in sequencing, isolating and cloning the approximately 5000 genes of *Mycobacterium leprae* [133] open enormous opportunities for accurate epidemiological surveillance, early diagnosis, treatment and evolution of a potent vaccine. Advances in chemotherapy using once-monthly rifampicin and clofazimine and daily dapsone with or without ethionamide and prothionamide and other drug regimens [66, 128] have considerably improved the cure rate. A vaccine is currently undergoing trial. Immunisation with BCG vaccine offers some protection.

Acquired Demyelinating Polyneuropathy

Both cell and humorally mediated autoimmune factors are involved. It may be acute or chronic.

Acquired Acute Demyelinating Polyneuropathy (GBS). The prevalence ratios per 100000 in urban China were 9.5 (16.0 in males and 3.0 in females) [68]. In many countries crude incidence rates per 100000 per year ranged from 0.5 to 1.9 [8, 50, 60, 111]. In the United States the incidence rate was highest in persons aged 50–74 with another high but lesser peak in persons aged 15–34 [60]: the findings in Denmark were similar [8]. In most reports, there is no sex bias: excess of males were reported in Denmark [8] and China [68].

Risk factors include antecedent acute upper respiratory infection in about two-thirds, viral infections including acute exanthemata, infectious mononucleosis, cytomegalovirus infection, acute diarrhoeal diseases, receipt of biological materials (stings, vaccinations) and rarely surgery [100]. About 90% of infections occurred within 30 days of onset of neurological illness. There was a specific association of the severe disease with vaccination against swine influenza/New Jersey A in the United States in 1976: but this may not apply to other strains of influenza vaccine.

The prognosis of the disease is often good with or without steroid treatment: steroid therapy may be harmful [53]. The mortality rate is about 5%–8%: of those who recovered, 15% showed considerable residual morbidity. Clinical trials of plasma exchange showed acceleration of recovery [40, 43, 88]. The major factors which adversely affect prognosis are severe maximum deficit requiring ventilation, failure to improve within 3 weeks of reaching the peak of neurological deficit and within 1 month of onset [130].

Acquired Chronic Demyelinating Polyneuropathy (ACDP). This may be relapsing, chronically progressive, monophasic, or multifocal with persistent block [67, 115]. Although rare in childhood, it is seen in all ages, with peak incidence in the 5th and 6th decades. In most series males predominate. A history of antecedent infection or immunisation within a few weeks of the onset of symptoms or associated with relapses may or may not be present. ACDP may occur in the paraproteinaemias. Treatment with corticosteroids, azathioprine and plasmapheresis and of the underlying paraproteinaemia may be of benefit.

Diabetic Neuropathies

Diabetic neuropathies manifest as distal symmetrical PN (which is commonly mixed sensory-motor-autonomic PN, or may be predominantly sensory, motor or rarely autonomic); symmetrical proximal motor PN (diabetic amyotrophy); focal and multifocal PN (including asymmetrical motor neuropathy, cranial neuropathy, intercostal, other mononeuropathies and entrapment neuropathies). Distal symmetric polyneuropathy (DSPN) is the most common, and of the DSPN the frequencies of the various subtypes are as follows: sensorimotor autonomic neuropathy, 70%; predominantly sensory neuropathy 30% (large fibre loss 5%, mixed large and small fibre loss 15%, small fibre loss 10%); predominantly motor and autonomic PN each less than 1% [17].

The prevalence ratios of diabetic PN vary from 0% to 93%, depending on the selection of patients, the diagnostic criteria, and their sensitivity. The lowest ratios are obtained when diagnosis includes the presence of symptoms. In a study involving 4400 patients observed between 1947 and 1973 clinical evidence was present in 8% at time of diagnosis, increasing to 50% after 25 years duration: PN were rare in young diabetics [98]. Diabetic PN occur in every community: the prevalence, based on symptoms and signs, was 40% among 832 Nigerians [92], 21% among 137 Hopi and Navajo Indians [99], and 32% among 139 Tanzanians [77].

The risk factors for development of the common symmetrical PN include duration of diabetes, poor control of diabetic state, presence of microangiopathy, less obesity, higher mean blood pressure, lower haemoglobin concentration [95] and are unrelated to sex and type of diabetes [89]. Ischaemia and trauma are important in the pathogenesis of focal and multifocal PN. Hyperglycaemia, which reduces pain tolerance in both normal and diabetic subjects, is the major causal factor of acute painful diabetic PN [2, 81, 121]. Diabetic PN may however, predate the onset of glucose intolerance and symmetrical PN may rarely be precipitated by treatment of diabetes mellitus [34, 35, 92]. Genetic predisposition to PN in diabetics could be determined by: (a) slow acetylator phenotype, about which the findings are inconsistent [15, 73, 98]; and (b) chlorpropamide alcohol flushing which relatively protects against late complications including PN in diabetes [58].

The annual incidence rate of 2% is related to duration of diabetes. A survey of 995 patients with maturity-onset diabetes in Rochester, Minnesota, showed annual incidence rates as follows: distal symmetrical PN 7.8%; carpal tunnel syndrome 1.3%; other mononeuropathies 0.3% [97].

Axonopathy is the dominant lesion in distal symmetrical PN, with variable loss of large and small diameter fibres. Segmental demyelination secondary to both axonal degeneration and primary Schwann cell abnormalities also occurs.

Increased neural sorbitol associated with abnormal polyol pathway metabolism, altered myoinositol metabolism resulting in abnormal Na^+,K^+-ATPase activity and disordered axonal transport have been described in experimental and human diabetic PN [39, 72]. The relevance of these to the pathogenesis of diabetic PN receives support from the mild, though controversial, benefit shown in clinical trials of myoinositol supplement [120] and aldose reductase inhibitors [59].

Nutritional Neuropathies

When it causes neuropathy, a nutritional deficiency state is multifactorial, involving the lack of several vitamins and nutrients, with the possible exceptions of deficiency of thiamine and vitamin B_{12}. Even in addisonian pernicious anaemia, a factor such as cyanide has been incriminated as the cause of PN [129]. In nutritional neuropathies there is often involvement of the optic and auditory nerves, the spinal cord, and less frequently the basal ganglia and cerebral cortex. Axonopathy is the usual lesion.

Toxins from diet and other sources (e.g. drugs) may condition a nutritional deficiency state [3]. Isoniazid, hydralazine and oral contraceptives interfere with pyridoxine metabolism. Thalidomide inhibits riboflavin. Chloramphenicol and nitrous oxide cause vitamin B_{12} deficiency. Nitrofurantoin disrupts pyruvate oxidation by competing with cocarboxylase. Perhexiline interferes with lipid metabolism. The heavy metals which cause PN are general protoplasmic poisons and bind sulphydryl enzymes, causing impaired oxidative metabolism. Cyanide from cyanogenic glycosides present in many dietary items (especially cassava and millet) consumed in developing countries reversibly inhibits ferricytochrome oxidase, inactivates thiamine, pyridoxal phosphate-dependent enzyme systems, and oxidase activity of caeruloplasmin. Ethanol, though directly neurotoxic, causes deficiency of thiamine and possibly pyridoxine, folate and pantothenic acid.

Although exposure to nutritional deficiencies and malnutrition are common, especially in developing countries, not all subjects develop PN. Susceptible individuals may be identifiable, as shown in four subjects with Wernicke-Korsakoff syndrome who had a genetically determined abnormal form of transketolase [13]. Nutritional deficiencies are causal factors in 10%–40% of the peripheral neuropathies in Africa [7] and 2%–6% in India [124].

In some parts of the world epidemics of toxic-nutritional PN have occurred. Epidemiological investigations incriminated chronic cyanide intoxication (mainly from cassava, a root crop) as the major cause of a tropical nutritional PN (the prototype of the syndrome was first described among Jamaicans [114]), as seen in Nigeria [91] and in Mozambique [77]. Pyridoxine overdosage causes sensory PN [23, 103].

Toxic (Including Drug-Induced) Neuropathies

Large segments of the world population are exposed to toxic materials used in industry and agriculture or which are present in the environment (atmosphere, water) in some dietary items and in drugs used to treat diseases. In most cases exposure occurs at work or accidentally and several people are likely to be similarly affected. Exposure also occurs through the patients' life style and medication.

Concurrent involvement of parts of the central nervous system and other systems sometimes occur. In most toxic PN, axonopathy is common, but segmental demyelination occurs in a few conditions such as PN due to perhexiline and hexacarbon. Central-peripheral distal axonopathy occurs with certain toxins, such as TOCP [112]; clioquinol, causes a central distal axonopathy [102].

Toxic PN often occur in the industrialised world owing to exposure to acrylamide (used in mining and engineering works), carbon disulphide (in the viscose and rayon industry), hexacarbon solvents (used industrially and in domestic products such as glue), lead (in manufacture of batteries), organophosphates (used in insecticides, plasticisers and in lubricating oils), thallium (used as rodenticides), ethylene oxide (used to sterilise heat-sensitive materials) and arsenic (in insecticides and weed-killers). In some developing countries such as India, arsenic is an important component of opium, alcohol, and pills and powders administered by traditional medical practitioners [124].

Common drugs known to cause PN include amiodarone, dapsone, disulfiram, gold, isoniazid, metronidazole, ethambutol, phenytoin, perhexiline, vincristine, chloramphenicol, chloroquine and nitrofurantoin. Amiodarone causes corneal microdeposits in 90%, thyroid disorders and PN in 10% of patients [71]. Metronidazole causes potentially reversible sensory PN in about 50% of patients treated for 4 months or more [30] for encephalopathy and cerebellar ataxia. Perhexiline PN occurs in those with slow oxidation [106]. Dapsone produces a potentially reversible predominantly motor PN related to slow acetylation [44]. Platinum causes sensory PN and ototoxicity. Ethambutol predisposes to sensory PN and optic atrophy [118]. Vincristine causes a sensory PN characterised by a regressive axonopathy, early involvement of muscle spindles and absent tendon reflexes starting with the ankle jerk. Neuropathy due to chloramphenicol for the treatment of typhoid fever, which is highly prevalent in developing countries, is rare. Nitrofurantoin induces PN, especially in the elderly, in those with impaired renal function and as a result of prolonged therapy. Phenytoin has been associated with PN mainly in patients on long-term therapy [69] with the frequency of clinical PN varying from 0% to 33% and electrophysiological PN from 0% to 89%: some evidence suggests that phenytoin causes reversible slowing of nerve conduction and that PN is rare and may be related to duration of treatment, plasma levels of the drug, concomitant polytherapy with other anticonvulsants and folate deficiency [107]. A prevalence ratio of 16.7% for PN was found in 186 epileptic patients, but with no specific relationship to phenytoin usage [117]. Chloroquine PN is rare. A few toxins exert their neurotoxic effects in subjects with an independent metabolic abnormality, e.g. PN precipitated by barbiturates in acute intermittent porphyria.

Underlying disease may modify susceptibility to neurotoxins. Poor nutrition enhances neurotoxicity of cyanogenic glycosides, chemical solvents such as hexane, methyl-*n*-butylketone, organophosphates, nitrous oxide and isoniazid [3, 79]. Patients with lymphoma develop vincristine PN more often than those with other malignancies [126]. Patients with diabetes mellitus, alcoholism and cancer are susceptible since their peripheral nerves may already be affected. Strenuous exercise has been thought to predispose patients receiving sulphonamides to the development of PN [18].

Peripheral Neuropathies in Connective Tissue Disorders

Neuropathies, common in the connective tissue disorders, may be the initial manifestations, as mononeuritis simplex and multiplex, diffuse symmetrical PN (usually sensorimotor) or rarely demyelinating GBS type. Neuropathies are present in about 10% of patients with SLE [36]. The pathogenesis is mixed and apparently includes axonopathy, myelinopathy, vasculitis, mechanical effects of fibrinoid bodies compressing nerve fibres, deposition of immune complexes, humoral and cell-mediated immunity. Neuropathies are present in about 1%–10% of patients with rheumatoid arthritis [21], but are rare in scleroderma. In the vasculitides which represent a spectrum of disorders primarily characterised by inflammation and destruction of blood vessels and include classical polyarteritis nodosa, allergic granulomatosis (Churg-Strauss vasculitis), Wegener's granulomatosis and immune-complex-mediated destruction of vessel walls occur. Drugs and infectious agents, including hepatitis B may trigger off the autoimmune mechanism. About 50% of patients with polyarteritis nodosa develop PN, commonly as acute or subacute mononeuritis simplex or multiplex. In Reiter's disease and relapsing polychondritis, PN due to vasculitis may occur.

Neuropathies in Paraproteinaemias

Clinically obvious PN occur in 13% of patients with osteolytic myeloma (frequency of electrophysiological PN may be as high as 40%), 50% of osteosclerotic myeloma [64], 25% of macroglobulinaemia, 7% of cryoglobulinaemia, 10% of benign monoclonal gammopathy and 15% of patients with primary amyloidosis.

In the chronic demyelinating PN associated with the paraproteinaemias, a circulating antibody that binds to the myelin component may be demonstrable (hyperviscosity with ischaemia, toxins, metabolic disturbances are other postulated causes). There has been no consistent effect of plasmapheresis or immunosuppressive therapy [14]. Vasculitis occurs in cryoglobulinaemia. Both myelinopathy and axonopathy are present in primary amyloidosis and in monoclonal gammopathy of undetermined origin [62]: the latter often presents as cryptogenic PN and hence serum protein electrophoresis is necessary in the evaluation of idiopathic neuropathies [63]. Tumoricidal irradiation of solitary lesions of myeloma usually improves the PN although chemotherapy for multiple osteosclerotic lesions is less helpful [64].

Genetically Determined Neuropathies

Of the genetically determined syndromes associated with PN, in some, PN is the sole or predominant feature of the underlying gene mutation; in others PN is a significant component of pathological manifestations of multisystem disease.

The metabolic basis or enzymic defect in some is known: these include hereditary amyloidosis, the porphyrias, PN due to disorders of lipid metabolism (e.g. metachromatic leucodystrophy) and disorders associated with defective DNA repair such as ataxia telangiectasia.

For others the aetiology or metabolic basis is unknown: these include hereditary motor and sensory PN, hereditary sensory and autonomic PN, PN associated with hereditary ataxias, miscellaneous disorders such as giant axonal neuropathy, Chédiak-Higashi disease, chorea-acanthocytosis and hereditary susceptibility to pressure palsies.

Many of these conditions are extremely rare with less than 10–100 cases described or are confined to specific racial groups (e.g. abetalipoproteinaemia in Ashkenazi Jewish populations) or countries (e.g. variegate porphyria due to deficiency of protoporphyrin oxidase, a common condition among South African whites, but rare elsewhere apart from Finland and New England [82, 83].

On the other hand, some are not so uncommon, such as acute intermittent porphyria due to deficiency of porphobilinogen deaminase, described in virtually all races, with an incidence rate per 100000 per year of 7 in Sweden [127] and 6 in England [48]. It is the most common form of acute porphyria in North America. (Coproporphyria, due to deficiency of coproporphyrin oxidase, is the third form of porphyria which causes PN, but is extremely rare.)

The hereditary motor and sensory neuropathies (HMSN) are the most common disorders that give rise to the peroneal muscular atrophy syndrome or Charcot-Marie-Tooth disease, of which the prevalence ratio per 100000 is 41 in western Norway [108], 23.7 in Guam [19], 1.6 in Iceland [41] and 0.14 in Nigeria [1]. HMSN is subdivided into types I and II on the basis of motor nerve conduction velocity, usually below 30 m/s in type I and above 40 m/s in type II [16]. Type I is associated with demyelination and remyelination (and hence hypertrophied palpable nerves) and type II with axonal or neuronal atrophy. (HMSN type III or Dejerine-Sottas disease is a severe demyelinating PN which occurs in infancy.) Inheritance may be autosomal dominant or recessive in both types I and II and very doubtfully X-linked. Dominantly inherited HMSN type I is linked to the Duffy blood group locus whereas HMSN type II is not [12, 42]. Autosomal dominant HSMN type I occurs world-wide and is the commonest form of HMSN. Other rare forms of HMSN have been described in association with optic atrophy, deafness, pigmentary retinal degeneration and pyramidal features.

Infections, especially viral, may worsen or precipitate the onset of some hereditary PN such as Refsum's disease, PN of hereditary ataxias, and mononeuritis due to hereditary susceptibility to pressure palsies.

Neuropathies in Metabolic Diseases

Metabolic disorders commonly cause axonopathy, but myelinopathy may also occur. One of the best-studied metabolic PN is that due to renal failure and first reported in patients undergoing haemodialysis [5]. The PN, typically sensorimotor, is related to the duration and severity of renal failure, but not to the cause. Rapid improvement usually follows successful renal transplantation [84]. The pathogenesis is multifactorial, but no specific toxin has been implicated. Symptomatic compression mononeuritis such as carpal tunnel syndrome (CTS) is common in about 30% of chronic renal dialysis patients. Increasing time on dialysis was related to increased incidence of CTS; patients benefited from surgical release of thickened flexor retinaculum [45]. Hypothyroidism typically causes a sensory PN and was found in 6 (31%) of 19 patients in one series [132]. Predominantly motor PN may complicate hypoglycaemia associated with islet cell tumours [57].

Mild clinically important sensory or sensorimotor PN occur in about 50% of patients with acromegaly (also known to be associated with CTS) and in chronic liver disease, primary biliary cirrhosis, viral hepatitis, chronic cholestatic jaundice (which often causes vitamin E deficiency, a causal factor in predominantly sensory PN and cerebellar ataxia), gastrointestinal disorders associated with malabsorption, chronic obstructive pulmonary disease and acrodermatitis chronica atrophicans [49, 74].

Neuropathies in Malignancies

In carcinomas, predominantly sensory PN occur, but so also may mixed forms. In the lymphoproliferative disorders, including Burkitt's lymphoma, PN are typically sensorimotor, and may simulate GBS.

The frequency of PN in the malignancies ranges from 5% to 30%, although electrophysiological abnormalities are present in 30%–50% [75]. The pathogenesis of PN of malignancies is multifactorial and includes nutritional, metabolic, infective and autoimmune factors. The PN may antedate the malignancy.

Pressure Palsies and Entrapment Syndromes

Some nerves are anatomically vulnerable to external pressure and virgule or entrapment. Individual susceptibility also varies. Thus some patients with CTS have an anatomically small carpal space [27]. Some families have a genetically determined susceptibility to pressure palsies [33]. In some PN, e.g. due to diabetes, amyloidosis, hereditary and acquired demyelinating neuropathies, chronic renal failure, alcoholism, and malnutrition, the liability to local pressures is increased. Experimentally, diphtheritic PN predisposes to compression neuropathy [51]. Systemic disease such as hypothyroidism, acromegaly, or rheumatoid arthritis may predispose to entrapment syndromes in specific sites such as the carpal and tarsal tunnels.

Symptoms of local pressure are due to mechanical effects of the compression and, if severe enough, through ischaemia. Compression first causes conduction block, then demyelination, and next wallerian degeneration. The common entrapment compression syndromes have been described in all parts of the world. Compression of the median nerve at the wrist is the most common and usually affects healthy women. Obstetric neurapraxia, common in developing countries, is due to poor antenatal care, and follows prolonged labour [6].

Table 1. Peripheral neuropathy and parasitic infections

Parasitic infection	Geography	Type of neuropathy and pathogenesis	Frequency of neuropathy and comments
Trypanosomiasis			
American	Central and South America	Autonomic direct invasion of nerves. Myelinopathy	Always present in chronic phase of infection with neurotropic strain
African	West, Central and East Africa	Polyradiculopathy. Some autonomic involvement. Interstitial neuritis. Myelinopathy	Not always clinically obvious
Nosematosis			
(*Nosema connori*)	United States (DC)	Autonomic. Direct invasion of nerves	Very rare
Leishmaniasis	South and Central America, Africa, Asia, Europe (Mediterranean)	Polyneuropathy. ?Nutritional. Axonopathy	Common
Giardiasis	Tropical	Polyneuropathy (reversible). ?Nutritional. Axonopathy	Rare
Malaria	Tropical and subtropical (1 billion people at risk)	?Mononeuritis. ?Polyradiculopathy. ?Microvascular occlusion. ?Toxic	Rare. Occurrence disputable
Babesiosis	Tropical and subtropical.	Guillain-Barré syndrome	Rare
Toxoplasmosis	World-wide	Mononeuritis. Polyneuropathy. Interstitial	Congenital facial palsy common, otherwise neuropathy rare
Amoebiasis (especially *Naegleria fowleri*)	Tropical	Olfactory neuropathy	Rare
Schistosomiasis	Tropical and subtropical (400 million people afflicted)	Mononeuritis. Polyneuropathy. Compression and interstitial	Rare
Cysticercosis	Tropical	Mononeuritis. Compression	Rare
Angiostrongyliasis	South-East Asia and Oceania	Polyneuropathy. Axonopathy Direct Invasion	Common
Dracunculiasis	Africa and Asia	Mononeuritis. Compression	Rare
Toxocariasis	World-wide	Guillain-Barré syndrome	Rare
Trichinosis	World-wide	Mononeuritis. Compression	Rare
Ticks (Arachnida)	World-wide	Guillain-Barré syndrome. Botulinum-like intoxication. Spirochaetal and viral infection. Toxic	Rare

Neuropathies in Parasitic Diseases

The occurrence of neuropathies in parasitic diseases is shown in Table 1.

Isolated Cranial Neuropathies

Diabetes mellitus, infective and carcinomatous meningitides, vasculitides, paranasal sinus malignancies, aneurysms of the internal carotid and posterior communicating arteries, medial sphenoidal ridge meningiomas, pituitary tumours, ophthalmoplegic migraine and the painful ophthalmoplegic Tolosa-Hunt syndrome are common causes all over the world. Neurosarcoidosis is rare in India and black Africans. Burkitt's lymphoma is a common cause in areas of the tropics in which the disease is endemic. Haemoglobinopathies, especially (HbSS, HbSC) and migraine associated with sickle cell trait (HbAS) are also common causes in Africans.

Idiopathic acute facial palsy (Bell's palsy) is common all over the world, with an incidence rate per 100000 of 12–24 and doubtfully related to glucose intolerance. Trigeminal neuralgia on the other hand with an incidence rate of 2–4 per 100000 in whites [104], is virtually unknown in black Africans.

Miscellaneous: Neuropathies in AIDS

The acquired immune deficiency syndrome (AIDS) has over the past 5 years been reported in more than 12000 patients from all parts of the world. Some evidence suggests that the causative virus human T-cell lymphocytotropic virus (HTLV III) or lymphadenopathy associated virus (LAV) is native to Africa. Eight (16%) of 50 patients with neurological complications had painful sensorimotor symmetrical distal PN [110]. Recently, of 370 patients with AIDS, 178 had significant neurological complications: 37 (10%) had chronic inflammatory distal symmetrical PN; herpes zoster radiculitis was the presenting manifestation of AIDS in 6 young men [56]. The pathogenesis of PN could also involve nutritional deficiencies. GBS has been reported in AIDS [52]. Cranial neuropathies may be secondary to malignant and infective meningitides common in AIDS.

Conclusion

The methods for investigating the causes of PN have become increasingly helpful in elucidating aetiological factors. However, most of the information on PN is based on investigations in hospital populations. Further community-based and clinical epidemiological studies are needed to improve our knowledge of the prevalence, incidence, risk factors and natural history and our ability to manage effectively and prevent peripheral nerve disorders which as a group constitute one of the commonest afflictions of the nervous system.

References

1. Alyesimoju AB, Osuntokun BO, Bademosi O, Adeuja AOG (1984) The rarity of heredodegenerative disorders in Nigerian africans. Neurology 34:361–362
2. Archer A, Watkins PH, Thomas PK, Sharma AK, Payan AJ (1983) The natural history of acute painful neuropathy in diabetes mellitus. J Neurol Neurosurg Psychiatry 46:491–499
3. Argov Z, Mastalgia F (1979) Drug-induced peripheral neuropathies. Br Med J 1:663–666
4. Asbury AK (1981) Diagnostic considerations in the Guillain-Barre syndrome. Ann Neurol 9 [Suppl]: 1–5
5. Asbury AK, Victor M, Adams RD (1963) Uraemic polyneuropathy. Arch Neurol 8:413–428
6. Bademosi O, Osuntokun BO, van der Waal AL, Ojo OA (1980) Obstetric neuropraxia: a study of 34 patients at Ibadan. Int J Gynecol Obstet 17:611–614
7. Bademosi O, Osuntokun BO (1981) Diseases of peripheral nerves as seen in the Nigerian africans: a study of 358 cases. Afr J Med Sci Clin Med 10:33–38
8. Bak P (1985) Guillain-Barre syndrome in a Danish county. Neurology 35:207–211
9. Bassett ML, Danta G, Cook TA (1978) Giardiasis and peripheral neuropathy. Br Med J 2:19–20
10. Ben Hamida M, Bethi L, Ben Hamida C, Samoud S (1981 a) Les atrophies peronieres en Tunisie. J Neurol Sci 50:335–356
11. Ben Hamida M, Madani S, Zmerli et al. (1981 b) Les heredodegenerescences spino-cerebelleuses en Tunisie avec etude cystomanometrique des troubles sphincteriens. Rev Neurol (Paris) 136:495–508
12. Bird TD, Ott J, Giblett ER (1982) Evidence for linkage of Charcot-Marie-Tooth neuropathy to the Duffy locus on chromosome 1. Am J Hum Genet 34:388–394
13. Blass JP, Gibson JE (1977) Abnormality of a thiamine-requiring enzyme in four patients with Wernicke-Korsakoff syndrome. N Engl J Med 297:1367–1370
14. Bosch EP, Ansbacher LE, Goeken JA, Cancilla PA (1982) Peripheral neuropathy associated with monoclonal gammopathy. J Neuropathol Exp Neurol 41:446–459
15. Boulton AJM, Hardisty CA, Worth RC et al. (1982) Metabolic and genetic factors in diabetic neuropathy. Diabetologie 23:157–164
16. Brooks AP, Emery AE (1982) A family study of Charcot-Marie-Tooth disease. J Med Genet 19:88–93
17. Brown MH, Asbury AK (1984) Diabetic neuropathy. Ann Neurol 15:2–12
18. Brunn E, Hermann K (1942) Polyneuritis after treatment with sulphonamide preparations. Acta Med Scand 111:261–268
19. Chen K, Brody JA, Kurland LT (1968) Patterns of neurologic diseases on Guam. Arch Neurol 19:573–874
20. Chopra JS, Banerjee JM, Murphy JMK, Pal SR (1980) Paralytic rabies: a clinicopathological study. Brain 103:789–802
21. Conn DL, Dyck PJ (1975) Angiopathic neuropathy and connective tissue diseases. In: Dyck PJ, Thomas PK, Lambert EH (eds) Peripheral neuropathy. Saunders, Philadelphia, pp 1149–1165
22. Cruz M (1985) Personal communication of results of neuroepidemiological studies in South America
23. Dalton M (1985) Pyridoxine overdose in premenstrual syndrome. Lancet 1:1168–1169
24. Damluji S (1962) Mercurial poisoning from fungicide. Granosam. Med J Fac Med Baghdad 4:83–88
25. Dastur DK, Manghani DK, Osuntokun BO et al. (1982) Neuromuscular and related changes in malnutrition. J Neurol Sci 55:207–230
26. Dean G (1982) Porphyria variegata. Acta Derm Venereal [Suppl] (Stockholm) 100:81–85
27. Dekel S, Coates R (1979) Primary carpal stenosis as a cause of idiopathic carpal tunnel syndrome. Lancet 2:1024
28. Derlan LKA (1974) Outbreak of food poisoning due to alkylmercury fungicide on Southern Ghana State farm. Arch Environ Health 28:49–56

29. Dongre VY, Ganapati R, Chowala RG (1976) A study of mononeuritic lesions in a leprosy clinic. Lepr India 18:132–137
30. Duffy LF, Dalim F, Fisher SE et al. (1985) Peripheral neuropathy in Crohn's disease patient's treated with metronidazole. Gastroenterology 88:681–684
31. Dyck PJ (1982) Causes, classification and treatment of peripheral neuropathy. N Engl J Med 307:283–286
32. Dyck PJ, Oviate KF, Lambert EH (1981) Intensive evaluation of referred unclassified neuropathies yield improved diagnosis in neuropathies. Ann Neurol 10:222–228
33. Earl CJ, Fullerton PM, Wakefield GS, Schutta HS (1964) Hereditary neuropathy with liability to pressure palsies. Q J Med 33:481–498
34. Ellenberg M (1958 a) Diabetic neuropathy presenting as initial manifestation of diabetes. Ann Intern Med 49:620–625
35. Ellenberg M (1958 b) Diabetic neuropathy precipitating after institution of diabetic control. Am J Med Sci 236:466–470
36. Feinglass EJ, Arnett FC, Dorsch CA et al. (1976) Neuropsychiatric manifestations of systemic lupus erythematosus. Medicine (Baltimore) 55:323–329
37. Fite GL (1943) Leprosy from the histologic point of view. Arch Pathol 35:611–644
38. Gill GV, Bell DR (1982) Persisting nutritional neuropathy amongst former prisoners (in the Far East). J Neurol Neurosurg Psychiatry 45:861–865
39. Greene DA, DeJesus PV, Winegrad AI (1975) Effects of insulin and dietary myoinositol on impaired peripheral motor nerve conduction velocity in adult streptozotocin diabetes. J Clin Invest 55:1326–1336
40. Greenwood FJ, Newsom-Davis J, Hughes RAC et al. (1984) Controlled trial of plasma exchange in acute inflammatory polyradiculoneuropathy. Lancet 1:877–879
41. Gudmundsson KR (1969) Prevalence and occurrence of some rare neurological diseases in Iceland. Acta Neurol Scand 45:114–124
42. Guilof RJ, Thomas PK, Contreras M et al. (1982) Evidence of linkage of Type 1 hereditary motor and sensory neuropathy with the Duffy locus on chromosome 1. Ann Hum Genet 46:25–27
43. Guillain-Barre Syndrome Study Group (1985) Plasmapheresis and acute Guillain-Barre syndrome. Neurology 35:1096–1104
44. Gutmann L, Martin JD, Welton W (1976) Dapsone motor neuropathy – an axonal disease. Neurology 26:514–516
45. Halter SK, Delisa JA, Stolov WC, Scardafane DJ (1981) Carpal tunnel syndrome in chronic renal dialysis patients. Arch Phys Med Rehabil 62:197–201
46. Haq FU (1961) Agrosan poisoning in man. Br Med J 1:1579–1581
47. Harding AE, Thomas PK (1980) The clinical features of hereditary motor and sensory neuropathy types I and II. Brain 103:259–280
48. Hierons R (1957) Changes in the nervous system of acute porphyria. Brain 80:176–192
49. Hoff HC (1975) Peripheral neuropathy in acrodermatitis chronica atrophicans. J Neurol Neurosurg Psychiatry 38:452–458
50. Hogg JR, Kobrin DE, Schoenberg BS (1979) The Guillain-Barre Syndrome: epidemiology and clinical features. J Chron Dis 32:227–231
51. Hopkins AD, Morgan-Hughes JA (1969) The effect of local pressure in diphtheritic neuropathy. J Neurol Neurosurg Psychiatry 32:614–623
52. Horowitz SL, Benson DF, Gottlieb MS et al. (1982) Neurological complications of gay-related immunodeficiency disorder (Abstract). Ann Neurol 80:12
53. Hughes R, Newson-Davis J, Perkins G, Pierce J (1978) Controlled trial of prednisolone in acute polyneuropathy. Lancet 2:750–753
54. Impallomeni M, Kenny RA, Flynn MD et al. (1984) The elderly and their ankle jerks. Lancet 1:670–672
55. Jalili MA, Abassi AH (1961) Poisoning by ethyl mercury toluene sulphonalide. Br J Ind Med 18:303
56. JAMA (1985) Neurological complications appear often in AIDS. JAMA 253:3379–3383
57. Jaspan JB, Wollman RL, Bernstein L, Bernstein AH (1982) Hypoglycemic peripheral neuropathy in association with insulinoma. Medicine (Baltimore) 61:33–44

58. Jentorp P, Almer LO (1981) Chlorpropamide-alcohol flushing in relation to microangiopathy and peripheral neuropathy in non-insulin dependent diabetes. Acta Med Scand [Suppl] 656:33–36
59. Judzewitsch RG, Jaspan JB, Polonsky KS et al. (1983) Aldose reductase inhibition improves nerve conduction velocity in diabetic patients. N Engl J Med 308:119–125
60. Kaplan JE, Schoenberger LB, Hurwitz ES, Katona P (1983) Guillain-Barre syndrome in the United States 1978–1981: additional observations from the national surveillance system. Neurology 33:633–637
61. Kaur U, Chopra JS, Prabkar S, Radhakrishnan (1982) Clinical spectrum of peripheral neuropathies. Ind J Med Res 76:728–735
62. Kelly JR (1983) The diagnostic findings in peripheral neuropathy associated with monoclonal gammopathy. Muscle Nerve 6:504–509
63. Kelly JR, Kyle RA, O'Brien PC, Dyck PJ (1981) Prevalence of monoclonal protein in peripheral neuropathy. Neurology 31:1480–1483
64. Kelly JR, Kyle RA, Miles JM, Dyck PJ (1983) Osteosclerotic myeloma and peripheral neuropathy. Neurology 33:202–210
65. Kurland LT, Faro SN, Siedler H (1960) Minamata disease. World Neurol 1:370–378
66. Anonymous (1982) Chemotherapy of leprosy. Lancet 2:77–78
67. Lewis RA, Sumner AJ, Brown MJ, Asbury AK (1982) Multifocal demyelinating neuropathy with persistent conduction block. Neurology 32:958–964
68. Li SC, Schoenberg BS, Cheng XM et al. (1985) Epidemiology of neurologic disease in urban areas of the People's Republic of China (in press)
69. Lovelace RE, Horwitz SJ (1968) Peripheral neuropathy in long-term diphenylhydantoin therapy. Arch Neurol 18:69–76
70. Marra TA (1983) Recurrent lumbosacral and brachial plexopathy associated with Schistosomiasis. Arch Neurol 40:586–588
71. Martinez-Arizala A, Sobol SM, McCarty EM et al. (1983) Amiodarone neuropathy. Neurology 33:643–645
72. Mayhew JA, Gillon KRW, Hawthorne JN (1983) Free and lipid inositol, sorbitol and sugars in sciatic nerve obtained postmortem from diabetic patients and control subjects. Diabetologie 24:13–15
73. McLaren EH, Burden AC, Moorhead PJ (1977) Acetylator phenotype in diabetic neuropathy. Br Med J 2:291–294
74. McLeod JG, Pollard JD (1984) Neuropathies in systemic diseases: hidden and overt. In: Asbury AK, Gilliatt RW (eds) Peripheral nerve disorders. Butterworths, London, pp 92–126
75. McLeod JG, Tuck PR, Pollard JD et al. (1984) Chronic polyneuropathy of undetermined cause. J Neurol Neurosurg Psychiatry 47:530–535
76. Meyerhoff J (1983) Lyme disease. Am J Med 75:633–670
77. Mhando DA, Yudkins JS (1980) The pattern of diabetic complication in African patients in Dar Es Salaam. Trop Geogr Med 32:317–323
78. Ministry of Health, Mozambique (1984) Mantakassa: an epidemic of spastic paraplegia associated with chronic cyanide intoxication in a cassava staple area of Mozambique. Bull WHO 62:477–484
79. Money GL (1959) Isoniazid neuropathies in malnourished tuberculous patients. J Trop Med 62:198–204
80. Morgan JP, Penovich P (1978) Jamaica ginger paralysis. Arch Neurol 35:530–536
81. Morley GK, Mooradien AD, Levine AL, Morley JE (1984) Mechanism of pain in diabetic peripheral neuropathy. Effect of glucose on pain perception. Am J Med 77:79–82
82. Muhicaner JE, Pathak MA, Tishier PV, Fitzpatrick TB (1982) Variegate porphyria in New England. JAMA 247:3095–3102
83. Mustajoki P (1980) Variegate porphyria. Q J Med 49:191–203
84. Oh SJ, Clements RS Jr, Lee YW, Diethem AG (1978) Rapid improvement in nerve conduction velocity following renal transplantation. Ann Neurol 4:369–373
85. Oldfors A (1981) Nerve fibre degeneration of the central and peripheral nervous system of severe protein deprivation in the rat. Acta Neuropathol (Berl) 54:121–126

86. Oldfors A, Persson M (1982) Peripheral nerve fibre degeneration in protein deprived young rats: an ultrastructural study. Acta Neuropathol (Berl) 57:1–6
87. Ordonez JV, Carrillo JA, Miranda M (1966) Estudio epidemiologico de una enfermedad considerada como encefalitis en la region de Los Altos de Guatemala. Bol Of Sanit Panam 60:510–516
88. Osterman PO, Lundemo G, Pirskanen R et al. (1984) Beneficial effect of plasma exchange in acute inflammatory polyradiculoneuropathy. Lancet 2:1296–1298
89. Osuntokun BO (1970) The neurology of calcific non-alcoholic pancreatic diabetes mellitus. J Neurol Sci 11:17–43
90. Osuntokun BO (1980) Neuroepidemiology in Africa. In: Rose FC (ed) Clinical neuroepidemiology. Pitman Medical, London, pp 57–86
91. Osuntokun BO (1981) Cassava diet, chronic cyanide intoxication and neuropathy in the Nigerian Africans. World Rev Nutr Diet 36:141–173
92. Osuntokun BO, Akinkugbe FM, Francis TL et al. (1971) Diabetes mellitus in Nigerians: a study of 832 patients. West Afr Med J 20:295–312
93. Osuntokun BO, Schoenberg BS, Nottidge VA et al. (1982) Research protocol for measuring the prevalence of neurologic disorders in developing countries: results of a pilot study in Nigeria. Neuroepidemiology 1:143–153
94. Osuntokun BO, Adeuja AOG, Schoenberg BS et al. (1985) Prevalence of neurologic disorders in a Nigerian suburban community. In: Proceedings of the 13th world congress of Neurology. Abstract no 1913 (in press)
95. Paisey RB, Appendondo G, Villalobos A et al. (1984) Association of differing dietary metabolic and clinical risk factors with microvascular complications of diabetes: prevalence study of 503 Mexican type II diabetic subjects. Diabetes Care 7:428–433
96. Palmieri JC, LaChance MA, Connor DH (1983) Parasitic infections of the peripheral nervous system. In: Dyck PJ, Thomas PK, Lambert EH, Bunge R (eds) Peripheral neuropathy, 2nd edn, Saunders, Philadelphia, pp 1988–2008
97. Palumbo DJ, Elveback LR, Whisnant JP (1978) Neurologic complications of diabetes mellitus: transient ischemic attack, stroke and peripheral neuropathy. In: Schoenberg BS (ed) Neurologic epidemiology. Principles and clinical applications. Raven, New York, pp 593–600
98. Pirart J (1978) Diabetes mellitus and its degenerative complications: a prospective study of 4400 patients observed between 1947 and 1973. Diabetes Care 1:168–188, 252–263
99. Rate RG, Knowler WC, Morse HG et al. (1983) Diabetes mellitus in Hopi and Navajo Indians. Prevalence of microvascular complications. Diabetes 32:894–899
100. Ropper AH, Shahani BT (1984) Diagnosis and management of acute areflexic paralysis with emphasis on Guillain-Barre syndrome. In: Asbury AK, Gilliatt RW (eds) Peripheral nerve disorders. Butterworths, London, pp 21–45
101. Salako LA, Aderounmu AF (1978) Determination of the isoniazid acetylator phenotype in West African population. Tubercle 58:109–112
102. Schaumburg HH, Spencer PS (1980) Clioquinol. In: Spencer HS, Schaumberg HH (eds) Experimental and clinical neurotoxicity. Williams and Wilkins, Baltimore, pp 395–406
103. Schaumburg H, Kaplan J, Windebank A et al. (1983) Sensory neuropathy from pyridoxine abuse. N Engl J Med 309:445–448
104. Schoenberg BS (1983) Epidemiologic approaches to peripheral neuropathy. In: Dyck PJ, Thomas PK, Lambert EH (eds) Peripheral neuropathy, 2nd edn. Saunders, Philadelphia, pp 1191–1202
105. Senanayake N, Jeyaratnam J (1981) Toxic polyneuropathy due to gingili oil contaminated with tricresylphosphate affecting adolescent girls in Sri Lanka. Lancet 1:88–90
106. Shah R, Oates NS, Idle JR et al. (1982) Impaired oxidation of debrisoquine in patients with perhexiline neuropathy. Br Med J 284:295–299
107. Shorvon SD, Reynolds EH (1982) Anticonvulsant peripheral neuropathy: a clinical and electrophysiological study of patients on single drug treatment with phenytoin, carbamazepine or barbiturates. J Neurol Neurosurg Psychiatry 45:620–626
108. Skre H (1974) Clinical and genetic aspects of Charcot-Marie-Tooth disease. Clin Genet 6:98–118

109. Smith HV, Spalding JMK (1959) Outbreak of paralysis in Morocco due to ortho-cresyl-phosphate poisoning. Lancet 2:1019–1023
110. Snider WD, Simpson M, Nielsen S et al. (1983) Neurological complication of acquired immune deficiency syndrome: analysis of 50 patients. Ann Neurol 14:403–418
111. Softer D, Feldman S, Alter M (1978) Epidemiology of Guillain-Barre syndrome. Neurology 28:686–690
112. Spencer PS, Schaumburg H (1977) Ultrastructural studies of the dying back process. IV. Differential vulnerability of PNS and CNS fibres in experimental central-peripheral distal axonopathies. J Neuropathol Ex Neurol 36:300–320
113. Steere AC, Pachner AR, Malawista SE (1983) Neurologic abnormalities of Lyme disease: successful treatment with high dose intravenous penicillin. Ann Intern Med 99:676–762
114. Strachan H (1888) Annual of the Universal Medical Sciences, vol 1. Sajous, Philadelphia, pp 139
115. Sumner AJ (1984) Chronic demyelinating neuropathies. In: Asbury AK, Gilliatt RW (eds) Peripheral nerve disorders. Butterworths, London, pp 46–57
116. Susser M, Stein Z (1957) An outbreak of triortho-cresyl phosphate (JOCP) poisoning in Durban. Br J Ind Med 14:111–116
117. Swift TR, Gross JA, Ward LC, Grout BO (1981) Peripheral neuropathy in epileptic patients. Neurology 31:826–831
118. Takeuchi H, Takahashi M, Kang J et al. (1980) Ethambutol neuropathy: clinical and electromyographic studies. Folia Psychiatr Neurol Jpn 34:45–55
119. Tangchai P, Vejjajiva A (1971) Pathology of the peripheral nervous system in human rabies – a study of nine autopsy cases. Brain 94:299–306
120. Thomas DK, Elliasson SG (1983) Diabetic neuropathy In: Dyck PJ, Thomas PK, Lambert EH, Bunge R (eds) Peripheral neuropathy, 2nd edn. Saunders, Philadelphia, pp 1773–1810
121. Troni W, Carta O, Cantello R et al. (1984) Peripheral nerve function and metabolic control in diabetes mellitus. Ann Neurol 16:178–183
122. Van Voorhis WC, Kaplan A, Sarno EN et al. (1982) The cutaneous infiltrates of leprosy: cellular characteristics and the predominant T-cell phenotypes. N Engl J Med 307:1593–1597
123. Vora DD, Dastur DK, Braganca BM et al. (1962) Toxic polyneuritis in Bombay due to orthocresyl phosphate poisoning. J Neurol Neurosurg Psychiatry 25:234–239
124. Wadia NH (1984) Geographical patterns of neuropathy. India. In: Asbury AK, Gilliatt RW (eds) Peripheral nerve disorders. Butterworths, London, pp 287–302
125. Wadia NH, Swami RK (1971) A new form of heredofamilial spinocerebellar degeneration with slow eye movements (nine families). Brain 94:359–374
126. Watkins SM, Griffiths JP (1978) High incidence of vincristine-induced neuropathy in lymphomas. Br Med J 1:610–614
127. Wetterberg L (1967) A neuropsychiatric and genetical investigation of acute intermittent porphyria. Svenska Bokforlaget, Stockholm
128. WHO (1982) Chemotherapy of leprosy for control programmes. WHO Techn Rep Ser no 673
129. Wilson J, Langmans MJS (1966) Relationship of subacute combined degeneration of the cord to vitamin B_{12} deficiency. Nature 212:787–788
130. Winer JB, Hughes RAC, Greenwood RJ et al. (1985) Prognosis in Guillain-Barre syndrome. Lancet 1:1202–1203
131. Wulff CH, Hansen K, Strange P, Trojaborg W (1983) Multiple mononeuritis and radiculitis with erythema, pain, elevated CSF protein and pleocytosis (Bannwarth's syndrome). J Neurol Neurosurg Psychiatry 46:485–490
132. Yamamoto K, Saito K, Takai S, Yoshida S (1983) Unusual manifestations in primary hypothyroidism. Prog Clin Biol Res 116:169–187
133. Young RA, Mehra V, Sweester D et al. (1985) Leprosy outwitted. Nature 316:450–452

Epidemiology of Parkinson's Disease

R. J. MARTTILA and U. K. RINNE [1]

During the last three decades, there has been an increasingly productive interest in epidemiological research into Parkinson's disease (PD); as a result, a number of descriptive and analytical epidemiological studies have been recently completed. Although the epidemiological profile of PD is not yet fully elucidated, these studies have appreciably advanced our knowledge of the epidemiological indices and natural course of PD, and furnished some clues relating to the unknown cause of the disease.

Descriptive Epidemiology

Most of the studies have utilized the community survey approach, which is based on the ascertainment of all those affected in a defined area who have received medical attention. The result thus represents a minimum estimate of the frequency of the disease [19]. As an alternative approach, antiparkinsonian drug utilization has been tested as a measure of PD prevalence [32]. Obviously, this method can be successfully applied only in countries with a highly developed medical care system. A population-based survey is the preferable approach, and there are two recent examples of this type of study applied to investigating PD epidemiology [21, 40]. For practical reasons this method is feasible only when studying relatively small populations or samples of populations. In addition to differences in research design and inherent variability in the completeness of case detection, varying diagnostics may produce considerable variability in the morbidity figures. The original sample collected by community surveys often contains a large number of patients with an incorrect diagnosis of PD, as has been demonstrated in studies where a neurological examination of the cases has been carried out after the preliminary search [5, 8, 24, 33, 38]. The diagnosis of PD has also been subject to refinement during recent years, and many types of secondary parkinsonism or parkinsonism associated with neuronal system degenerations, as distinct from idiopathic PD, have been recognized, which the early studies were unable to take into account. For these reasons, the morbidity figures obtained in various studies are not strictly comparable, but have nevertheless established an overview of the epidemiological features of PD and identified some interesting trends.

[1] Department of Neurology, University of Turku, SF-20520 Turku, Finland.

Neurology
Ed. by K. Poeck, H. J. Freund, and H. Gänshirt

Prevalence

In the white race, the crude prevalence rates of PD vary from 66 to 187 per 100000 population (Table 1). Some studies also include cases with postencephalitic parkinsonism, but the variation does not essentially reduce if these are excluded. The studies come from geographically widely separated areas, but there appears to be no meaningful geographical pattern. Up to now, no clusters of PD have been detected, nor has it been possible to demonstrate any foci in the areas surveyed with an acceptable accuracy in case ascertainment [24, 38].

In the black race, considerably lower prevalence rates have been observed, even when the races live in the same geographical area [14, 37]. A rather low prevalence has also been found in the Sardinian population, which is ethnically mixed [38]. However, a recent study of a biracial community in the southern United States demonstrated rather similar prevalences in whites and blacks [39, 40]. The crude prevalence rates for the total population were 159 (whites) and 103 (blacks), but since the

Table 1. Epidemiology of Parkinson's disease

	Prevalence [a]	Incidence [a]
Whites		
United States		
Rochester 1955 [18] [b]	187 (167) [c]	23.8
Rochester 1965 [31]	157 (146)	19.3
Rochester 1967–1979 [36]		18.2
Baltimore 1967–1969 [14]	128 M, 121 F	
Mississippi 1978 [39]	159	
New Zealand, Wellington 1962 [33]	106 (97)	
Australia, Victoria 1962 [12]	85 (78)	7.0
England, Carlisle 1961 [3]	112	12.2
Scotland, Aberdeen 1984 [30]	164	
Iceland 1963 [8]	169 (163)	16.0
Finland, Turku 1971 [24]	120 (114)	14.8
Denmark, Aarhus 1972 [5]	84 (79)	8.7
Italy, Sardinia 1972 [38]	66 (63)	4.9
South Africa, Johannesburg 1970 [37]	159	
Blacks		
United States		
Baltimore 1967–1969 [14]	31 M, 4 F	
Mississippi 1978 [39]	103	
South Africa, Johannesburg 1970 [37]	4	
Asians		
Japan		
Kyoto 1978 [17]	46	
Kagoshima 1980 [17]	37	
Yonago 1980 [10]	81	10.2
China 1983 [21]	44	

[a] Per 100000 population.
[b] Reference.
[c] Postencephalitic cases excluded.

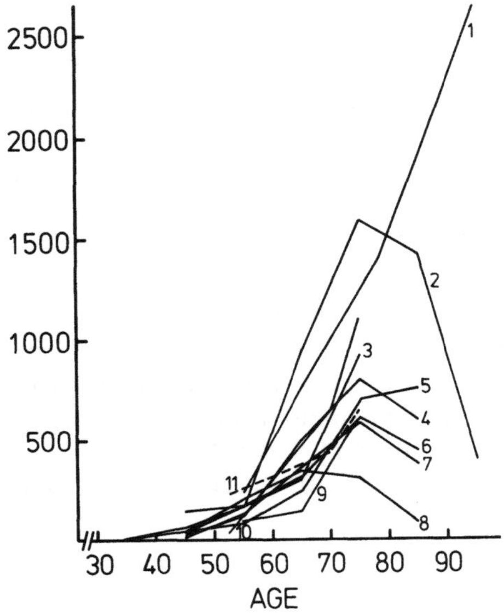

Fig. 1. Age-specific prevalence rates of Parkinson's disease per 100000 population. 1. Rochester, Minnesota [18]; 2. Iceland [8]; 3. Australia, Victoria [12]; 4. Finland, Turku [24]; 5. Japan, Yonago [10]; 6. England, Carlisle [3]; 7. Denmark, Aarhus [5]; 8. Italy, Sardinia [38]; 9. China [21]; 10. Copiah County, Mississippi, whites [40]; 11. Copiah County, Mississippi, blacks [40]

study was restricted to the population of 40 years or older, one should compare the prevalence rates for that part of the population alone, 352 for whites and 341 for blacks. Because this study utilized a population-based search it is probably not biased by medicosocial factors that may seriously affect studies based on the previous medical registration of the patients. The prevalence rates among the Japanese and Chinese are lower than most figures for the white race (Table 1), also suggesting that there may be racial differences in the occurrence of PD. Further studies are clearly needed to clarify epidemiological patterns of PD in different populations and races; aetiological clues may also emerge from such studies.

The age structure of PD patients appears to be broadly similar in all populations and races studied so far. The age-specific prevalence rates (Fig. 1) invariably show that the disease is rare before the age of 40–50 years, the prevalence then increasing with advancing age up to 70–80 years. After that age most studies indicate a declining tendency. In the majority of the remaining studies the evaluation of this point is not possible since the prevalence has been calculated for an open age group of over 70 years.

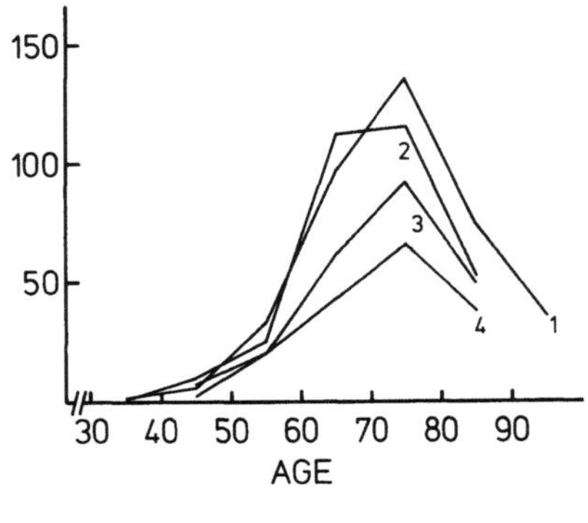

Fig. 2. Age-specific incidence rates of Parkinson's disease per 100000 population. 1. Iceland [8]; 2. Rochester, Minnesota [19]; 3. Finland, Turku [24]; 4. England, Carlisle [3]

Incidence

Incidence of PD has been studied less often than the prevalence, and in hardly any other race than the white. Similarly to the prevalence estimates, there is a large variation in the annual incidence rates, from 5 to 24 per 100000 population (Table 1). Age-specific incidence for onset, reported in four studies (Fig. 2), shows that the incidence is very low before the age of 40 years, followed by a sharp increase up to the age of 70–80 years, after which the incidence rapidly declines. A similar trend is also found in a study describing the age-specific incidence for diagnosis [36]. It has been speculated that PD might be somehow related to aging of the nervous system, but this incidence pattern is not consistent with an aging-associated pathogenesis.

Sex Distribution

In most clinical series, there has been a slight male predominance, suggesting a greater risk for men being affected, but several sources of bias may distort sex distribution in such series. Estimates from total prevalence rates are also susceptible to error because of the different age structures of male and female populations; this can be avoided by comparing age-adjusted or age-specific prevalence rates.

The best measure to evaluate the risk of PD in the sexes is incidence, and in particular, age-specific incidence. Prevalence studies suggest either a slight male predominance [14, 38], a slight female predominance [10] or show no difference [24, 40]. Two incidence studies with age- and sex-specific figures, however, do not indicate any significant difference between the sexes in the risk of being affected by PD [24, 36].

Temporal Pattern

Epidemiological studies of PD cover the last three decades. During that period of time, no evident temporal changes can be seen in the prevalence rates (Table 1). Similarly, incidence statistics from Rochester, Minnesota, have not indicated any substantial variation from 1935 to 1979 [31, 36]. A remarkable change in the epidemiological pattern, however, occurred during and shortly after the epidemic of lethargic encephalitis in the 1920s, when postencephalitic parkinsonism was about twice as prevalent as idiopathic PD [4]. Then, gradually, the proportion of postencephalitic parkinsonism decreased, and at present, only rare survivors with this condition can be encountered. However, it has been suggested that idiopathic PD could also be a result of subclinical lethargic encephalitis, and as the cohort exposed to the epidemic die, PD would disappear, or its prevalence would decline considerably during the present decade [34]. This assumption was based on the observation that the age at onset of patients with parkinsonism rose almost linearly with time during 1920–1995. Whether this increase was due to a cohort effect (the one-disease theory), or to a combined effect of two diseases, i.e. postencephalitic parkinsonism and idiopathic PD, has been debated for years. With the passage of time, the evidence appears to disprove the cohort theory; the number of cases with clinical signs of postencephalitic parkinsonism are disappearing, but there is no indication of decreasing incidence or prevalence of idiopathic PD.

Duration and Mortality

The duration of a disease with a stable prevalence and incidence can be estimated by dividing the prevalence rate by the annual incidence rate. In PD, such calculations produce figures from 8 to 10 years, which is close to several observations in clinical or pathological series prior to the levodopa era [11, 22, 35]. An excess mortality is also a necessary accompaniment of the natural course of PD. The relative 15 year survival rate of a cohort of PD patients was 67% [31], and Hoehn and Yahr [11] found in a large series of PD patients threefold increased mortality in comparison with the general population of the same age and sex. Although several studies have suggested that levodopa treatment reduces this excess mortality [23, 29, 41, 45], the impact of levodopa treatment has proved difficult to assess because of lack of comparability between the pre-levodopa figures and the recent series in terms of age structures and of disability of the patients. Nevertheless, after the introduction of levodopa treatment the average duration of PD increased from 9–10 years to 12–14 years; and at the same time, the average age at death had increased from 67–70 years [2, 11, 35] to 72–74 years [23, 29, 41, 45]. This may be interpreted to mean that levodopa treatment, in addition to improving the quality of life, concurrently ensures longer survival. As a result, the overall number of living patients with PD will probably increase in the near future [26].

Analytical Epidemiology

Analytical epidemiology, by identifying factors that are associated either with a low or high risk of a given disease, ultimately aims at the discovery of the cause of the disease. Principally, two types of approach are available: a prospective (cohort) study or a retrospective (case-control) study. Because of its relatively low incidence and long risk period for onset, PD is not easily amenable to a prospective study; all the studies reported so far have adopted the retrospective approach.

Genetics

The most intriguing problem in the aetiological exploration of PD is whether or not heredity has any significance. A number of studies have investigated familial occurrence of PD and produced highly conflicting results, permitting no definite conclusion. Recently, however, a low concordance for PD was found in monozygotic twins [43]. Being a powerful method to study the role of heredity, this twin study strongly suggests that heredity is not a decisive factor, but PD is probably an acquired disease caused by some environmental factor or factors.

Risk Factors and Associations

The lifetime risk of developing clinical PD can be estimated in a population when both age-specific incidence rates and life tables for that population are available. In different white populations, the risk has been found to be 1.4%–2.4% [8, 18, 24]. As yet, the search for risk factors and associations has not permitted identification of any group with a high probability of subsequent development of PD. PD does not correlate with sex, residence, social status or occupation [25, 38]. Nor has it been possible to detect any constant associations of PD with several other diseases [13, 16, 25]. Some studies tentatively suggest that PD patients may have experienced more head injuries than expected [7, 43], but the exposure to various environmental factors, except for smoking, appears to be no different from that of controls [13, 16, 43]. Several studies have confirmed that there is a lower number of smokers among PD patients than among the general population of comparable age and sex [1, 7, 15, 27, 43], and in particular, a significantly lower proportion of patients than their controls have ever smoked. It has been speculated that smoking protects against PD, but the finding that the amount of nicotine exposure of smokers who do subsequently develop PD is no different from controls [9] renders this explanation implausible. Furthermore, there are less smokers among women than men, yet the incidence of PD is similar in both sexes. Since smoking is usually started during adolescence or early adulthood, the low number of smokers is probably determined by some factor operating during that time. Clinical observations [42] and some case-control studies [44] suggest that there are distinct behavioural characteristics of parkinsonian patients that are evident even decades before the onset of the disease. Many patients have been introverted, inflexible, and susceptible to depression. Accordingly it has been suggested that these personality features could be responsible for abstaining from smoking, or that both abstaining and behavioural characteristics could be results of the same process, possibly of the subclinical PD.

Clues to Pathogenesis

These notions imply that there may be a subclinical period in PD, preceding the clinical onset by decades. In support of this, there are persons with Lewy bodies in the substantia nigra, but without clinical PD at death [22]. Neurochemical studies have shown that 70%–80% of the striatal dopamine is lost when motor symptoms appear, also suggesting a long subclinical period [2]. The length of the subclinical period is not known, but it has been estimated that the patients may be exposed to the cause of PD at least some 20–30 years prior to clinical symptoms [28]. As possible causes, two types of environmental factors, infections and toxic substances, have been most often suggested. Since there are examples of both causing parkinsonism in humans – postencephalitic parkinsonism [6] and MPTP-induced parkinsonism [20] – and both are compatible with the known epidemiological features of PD, they should be considered as serious candidates. Admittedly, there are no solid epidemiological clues in favour of either of them, nor are there any arguments that the future search for the cause should be restricted to these factors.

Acknowledgement. This study is supported by the Sigrid Jusélius Foundation, Finland.

References

1. Baumann RJ, Jameson HD, McKean HE, Haack DG, Weisberg LM (1980) Cigarette smoking and Parkinson's disease. 1. A comparison of cases with matched neighbors. Neurology 30:839–843
2. Bernheimer H, Birkmayer W, Hornykiewicz O, Jellinger K, Seitelberger F (1973) Brain dopamine and syndrome of Parkinson and Huntington. Clinical, morphological and neurochemical correlations. J Neurol Sci 20:415–455

3. Brewis M, Poskanzer DC, Rolland C, Miller H (1966) Neurological disease in an English city. Acta Neurol Scand [suppl 24]: 1–89
4. Dimsdale H (1946) Changes in the parkinsonian syndrome in the twentieth century. Q J Med 15: 155–170
5. Dupont E (1977) Epidemiology of parkinsonism: the Parkinson investigation, Århus, Denmark. In: Worm-Petersen J, Bøttcher J (eds) Symposium on Parkinsonism. Merck, Sharp and Dohme, Denmark, pp 65–75
6. Duvoisin RC, Yahr MD (1965) Encephalitis and parkinsonism. Arch Neurol 12:227–239
7. Godwin-Austen RB, Lee PN, Marmot MG, Stern GM (1982) Smoking and Parkinson's disease. J Neurol Neurosurg Psychiatry 45:577–581
8. Gudmundsson KRA (1967) A clinical survey of Parkinsonism in Iceland. Acta Neurol Scand 43 [suppl 33]: 9–61
9. Haack DG, Baumann RJ, McKean HE, Jameson HD, Turbek JA (1981) Nicotine exposure and Parkinson's disease. Am J Epidemiol 114: 191–200
10. Harada H, Nishikawa S, Takahashi K (1983) Epidemiology of Parkinson's disease in a Japanese city. Arch Neurol 40: 151–154
11. Hoehn MM, Yahr MD (1967) Parkinsonism: onset, progression, and mortality. Neurology 17:427–442
12. Jenkins AC (1966) Epidemiology of Parkinsonism in Victoria. Med J Aust 2:496–502
13. Kessler II (1972) Epidemiologic studies of Parkinson's disease. II. Hospital based survey. Am J Epidemiol 95:308–318
14. Kessler II (1972) Epidemiologic studies of Parkinson's disease. III. A community based survey. Am J Epidemiol 96:242–254
15. Kessler II, Diamond EL (1971) Epidemiologic studies of Parkinson's disease. I. Smoking and Parkinson's disease: a survey and explanatory hypothesis. Am J Epidemiol 94: 16–25
16. Kondo K (1984) Epidemiological clues for the etiology of Parkinson's disease. Adv Neurol 40:345–351
17. Kondo K, Shibasaki H (1981) Epidemiology of Parkinson's disease. Clues for etiology. 12th World congress of neurology, International Congress Series 548. Excerpta Medica, Amsterdam, p 233
18. Kurland LT (1958) Epidemiology: incidence geographic distribution and genetic considerations. In: Fields WJ (ed) Pathogenesis and treatment of Parkinsonism. Charles C. Thomas, Springfield, Ill, pp 5–49
19. Kurtzke JF, Kurland LT (1981) The epidemiology of neurologic disease. In: Baker AB, Baker LH (eds) Clinical neurology, vol 3, chap 48. Harper and Row, New York
20. Langston JW, Ballard P, Tetrud JW, Irwin I (1983) Chronic parkinsonism in humans due to a product of meperidine-analog synthesis. Science 219:979–980
21. Li S, Schoenberg BS, Wang C, Cheng X, Rui D, Bolis CL, Schoenberg DG (1985) A prevalence survey of Parkinson's disease and other movement disorders in the People's Republic of China. Arch Neurol 42:655–657
22. Lipkin LE (1959) Cytoplasmic inclusions in ganglion cells associated with parkinsonian states: a neurocellular change studied in 53 cases and 206 controls. Am J Pathol 35:1117–1133
23. Maier Hoehn MM (1985) Result of chronic levodopa therapy and its modification by bromocriptine in Parkinson's disease. Acat Neurol Scand 71:97–106
24. Marttila RJ, Rinne UK (1976) Epidemiology of Parkinson's disease in Finland. Acta Neurol Scand 53:81–102
25. Marttila RJ, Rinne UK (1976) Arteriosclerosis, heredity, and some previous infections in the etiology of Parkinson's disease. A case-control study. Clin Neurol Neurosurg 76:46–56
26. Marttila RJ, Rinne UK (1979) Changing epidemiology of Parkinson's disease: predicted effects of levodopa treatment. Acta Neurol Scand 59:80–87
27. Marttila RJ, Rinne UK (1980) Smoking and Parkinson's disease. Acta Neurol Scand 62:322–325
28. Marttila RJ, Rinne UK (1985) Clues from the epidemiology of Parkinson's disease. Adv Neurol (in press)
29. Marttila RJ, Rinne UK, Siirtola T, Sonninen V (1977) Mortality of patients with Parkinson's disease treated with levodopa. J Neurol 216: 147–153

30. Mutch W (1985) Parkinson's disease in Aberdeen; 1983–1984. In: Social, epidemiological and therapeutic aspects of Parkinson's disease. Abstracts. 5 Feb 1985, London
31. Nobrega FT, Glattre E, Kurland LT, O kazaki H (1969) Comments on the epidemiology of parkinsonism including prevalence and incidence statistics for Rochester, Minnesota, 1935–1966. In: Barbeau A, Brunetter JR (eds) Progress in neuro-genetics. Excerpta Medica, Amsterdam, pp 474–485
32. dePedro J, Rosenqvist U (1984) Tracers for paralysis agitans in epidemiological research. II. A model for indirect estimation of the prevalence of the disease. Neuroepid 3:97–107
33. Pollock M, Hornabrook RW (1966) The prevalence, natural history and dementia of Parkinson's disease. Brain 89:429–448
34. Poskanzer DC, Schwab RS (1963) Cohort analysis of Parkinson's disease. Evidence for a single etiology related to subclinical infection about 1920. J Chron Dis 16:961–973
35. Pritchard PB, Netsky MG (1973) Prevalence of neoplasms and causes of death in paralysis agitans. Neurology 23:215–222
36. Rajput AH, Offord KP, Beard CM, Kurland LT (1984) Epidemiology of parkinsonism: incidence, classification, and mortality. Ann Neurol 16:278–282
37. Reef HE (1977) Prevalence of Parkinson's disease in a multiracial community. In: den Hartog Jager WA, Bruyn GW, Heijstee APJ (eds) 11th World congress of neurology. Excerpta Medica, Amsterdam, p 125
38. Rosati G, Granieri E, Pinna L, Aiello L, Tola R, De Bastini P, Pirisi A, Devoto MC (1980) The risk of Parkinson disease in Mediterranean people. Neurology 30:250–255
39. Schoenberg BS, Anderson DW, Haerer AF (1982) Differences by race in the prevalence of Parkinson's disease. Abstracts of the 7th international symposium on Parkinson's disease, 27–30 June 1982, Frankfurt a. M., p 55
40. Schoenberg BS, Anderson DW, Haerer AF (1985) Prevalence of Parkinson's disease in the biracial population of Copiah County, Mississippi. Neurology 35:841–845
41. Sweet RD, McDowell RH (1975) Five years' treatment of Parkinson's disease with levodopa. Ann Intern Med 83:456–463
42. Todes CJ, Lees AJ (1985) The pre-morbid personality of patients with Parkinson's disease. J Neurol Neurosurg Psychiatry 48:97–100
43. Ward CD, Duvoisin RC, Ince SE, Nutt JD, Eldridge R, Calne DB (1983) Parkinson's disease in 65 pairs of twins and in a set of quadruplets. Neurology 33:815–824
44. Ward CD, Duvoisin RC, Ince SE, Nutt JD, Eldridge R, Calne DB, Dambrosia J (1984) Parkinson's disease in twins. Adv Neurol 40:341–344
45. Yahr MD (1976) Evaluation of long-term therapy in Parkinson's disease. Mortality and therapeutic efficacy. In: Birkmayer W, Hornykiewicz O (eds) Advances in Parkinsonism. Editiones Roche, Basle, pp 435–443

Epidemiology of Multiple Sclerosis

G. Pálffy[1]

The most important facts and views emerging from the observations described in surveys of the epidemiology of multiple sclerosis (MS) may be grouped as follows.
1. Geographic distribution and clustering
2. Migration and geographic isolation
3. Genetics, immunogenetics, and environmental factors
4. Comparative clinicopathology and special features
5. Source of data and diagnosis

Geographic Distribution and Clustering

The well-known thesis of the unequal geographic distribution of MS [20, 24], with a high prevalence in the temperate and cold zones, and medium frequency areas, e.g., in the Mediterranean basin, has to be reexamined and reevaluated. An epidemiologic study of MS performed over the past 5 years has confirmed an extremely high prevalence rate in northern Scotland [40], but thorough cooperative studies [13] have demonstrated that the prevalence of MS in southern Europe has previously been underestimated [15].

Kurtzke [24] has drawn attention to the relative paucity of good quality epidemiologic studies for eastern Europe. I quite agree with his criticism and have tried to collect as much reliable information from these countries as possible, beginning with my home town [37], county [36], and country. After examining all possible sources of medical information, including hospital files, data from all neurologists and general practitioners in the area, I found a prevalence of 56.9 per 100000 in the city of Pécs. The results in other areas of Hungary where studies based on similar methods have been done are as follows: in the county of Hajdu 30, Baranya 37, Vas 59, Fejér 61.85, and Makó district 93. The criteria for the diagnosis of MS were those suggested by Bauer [4]. In the other areas of Hungary data on the prevalence of MS are based on hospital files. In 1961 the prevalence of MS in Hungary was estimated at 20 per 100000 [28], at present it seems to be higher. The distribution of MS cases

[1] Department of Neurology and Psychiatry, University of Pécs Medical School Rét u. 2., Pécs 7623, Hungary

Neurology
Ed. by K. Poeck, H. J. Freund, and H. Gänshirt

in Hungary, with an area of nearly 100000 km^2, is uneven, more cases have been found in the industrial areas than in the agricultural ones [36]. Although the chief neurologists of each county and district in Hungary answered questionnaires willingly, only 18 Gypsy patients were found to suffer or to be suspected of suffering from MS. The Gypsy population in Hungary numbers about half a million at present.

As to the other countries of eastern Europe the prevalence of MS has been found to be 24.9 per 100000 for Istria, Yugoslavia [31], 26.6 for the northwestern areas of Transylvania [39], 43 for Halle, German Democratic Republic (Kissig, personal communication) 60.4 for Rostock, German Democratic Republic [33], 72.2 for western Poland and 38.6 for southeastern Poland [8]. The prevalence rate of 0.8–4.0 per 100000, a significant north-to-south gradient of MS prevalence in Japan [22], and a prevalence rate of approximately 1 per 100000 in Taiwan [44] has not changed in the past 20 years.

We are looking forward to obtaining the final result of an international cooperative study performed in Göttingen and the results of the fourth countrywide survey planned for 1986 to find out the change in MS frequency in Israel.

Clustering and epidemics lend further support to the view that MS is caused by an exogenous environmental factor. During the past 10 years several reports [12, 25] have been made on two epidemics, one of them was definite in the Faeroe Islands and the other was probable in Iceland. There have been reports on clusters from Finland [47]. In southern Hessen the distribution of cases points to the presence of some exogenous factors [27]; the highest prevalence rates were found in the southeastern montainous part of the region. The district has a lower annual mean temperature, more days of snow, and a higher annual precipitation compared with the other areas. The only area with a low frequency from where clusters have been reported is Africa, and the clusters are in places where whites live.

Migration and Geographic Isolation

The migration studies performed during the past 10 years in many countries: Finland [18], Federal Republic of Germany [48], Great Britain [10], Norway [26], and the United States [14] confirm the validity of observations made by Alter and coworkers [1, 2] in Israel, and Dean [9, 11] in South Africa two decades ago. Migrating adults carry the risk of their country of origin. Children and adolescents, however, are exposed to the risk of the country of adoption. Viischer, Bunner and Detels [45] have found multiple moves in MS patients. A case-control study of the number of changes of residence of MS patients in childhood shows that MS cases made significantly more moves than did controls. In the authors' opinion this difference may reflect a greater opportunity of exposure to a rare environmental agent or to agents closely related to MS. It is remarkable, however, that until 30 years ago the Gypsies in Hungary had been living in tents, continually wandering: nevertheless, until 1981 only one patient with MS had been detected in a Gypsy population of about 100000 in the south western part of Hungary [36].

Detels and co-workers [14] claimed that a careful clinical study of Asian MS patients born in the West was warranted. A study of three isolated communities deserves attention: the Parsi community in India, the Lapps in Norway, and the Gypsies in Hungary. The first is a small ethnic, Zoroastrian minority, which has remained substantially homogeneous since its migration from Persia around the seventh centruy A.D. The incidence of MS is higher in the Parsi community [46]. Not a single case of MS has been found among 26000 Lapps in Norway (S.I. Mellgren, personal communication). The Gypsy population in Hungary fulfills all the criteria of geographic isolation, viz., despite having been inhabitants of Hungary for centuries, for linguistic, social, and cultural reasons, and as a result of various prejudices, until 30 years ago the Gypsies of Hungary lived in clusters, apart from the adjacent population, dwelling in huts on the borders of villages or in tents in the forests, forming "Gypsy settlements," and marrying only within their communities. In the past 30 years the Gypsies in Hungary have been giving up their isolation. Most of them have abandoned their old way of life and many choose to be educated. They have moved into modern apartments and changed their dietary habits.

In 1973 Leibowitz, Kahana and Alter [29] suggested that the study of MS in countries undergoing rapid economic development might provide clues to the role of specific environmental factors. Nature is now offering us a unique opportunity to examine in isolation the environmental and genetic factors implicated in the pathogenesis of MS. The prevalence of MS in Gypsies is very low, it is worth studying thoroughly whether the rapid and very extensive changes of the last 30 years in housing, sanitary, and dietary circumstances have had any effect on the prevalence of MS. May I ask all experts in this field for help in the investigation of this problem.

Genetics, Immunogenetics, and Environmental Factors

The genetic and immunogenetic disposition to MS is supported by the difference in susceptibility to the disease observed in different races and families, by studies of twins, and by the demonstration of the fact that MS is frequently associated with certain histocompatibility antigens. In 1984 this topic was summarized excellently by McDonald [32]. The histocompatibility system of the members of an isolated community with a high frequency of MS was studied by Lowe and co-workers [30], and that of an isolated community with an extremely low frequency of MS by Gyódi and co-workers [16].

In 1962 Alter and co-workers reported [1] on their observation that consanguinity rates among the parents of patients were higher than in the general population. Intermarriage between close relatives is common even today in the Gypsies in Hungary, nevertheless the prevalence of MS is low.

Most of the reports on the epidemiology of MS supported the assumption that environmental factors, probably of a socioeconomic nature, play a role in the etiology of MS [3]. The role of precipitating factors, particularly that of some vaccinations [34, 38], should be reexamined by the same strict statistical method as was used by Kurland and co-workers in their work on swine flu vaccine [21].

Comparative Clinicopathology and Special Features

The comparative clinicopathology of MS in the eastern and western populations has been studied in several papers [23, 41, 44]; of outstanding quality is in the book *Multiple Sclerosis East and West,* edited by Yoshigoro Kuroiwa and Leonard T. Kurland. These studies are all in agreement with other reports from Asia [42, 43] where visual impairment at onset is more common, involvement of the optic nerve and spinal cord is predominant, and a higher occurrence of classical optic neuromyelitis is found. However, the pathogenesis of all kinds of leukoencephalitis is common [19].

Among the special features of MS, I wish to mention 62 patients with acute transverse myelitis treated in Israel from 1955 and studied by Berman, Feldman, Alter and co-workers [6]. The annual incidence was 1.24 per million. No significant difference between Euro-American born and Afro-Asian born populations has been found. In 37% of the patients a history of infection prior to acute transverse myelitis was reported. If other population-based studies were undertaken, a comparison with the results of the Israeli authors might throw light on the cause of this disorder.

Other special features, e.g., occurrence of MS in children [5, 7, 17] also deserve attention. The course of all patients with postvaccinal encephalomyelitis and other neurologic complications following the use of sera and vaccines should be followed for several years as some of them develop a disease which is indistinguishable from MS [38].

Source of Data and Diagnosis

The source of data should be reports from all general practitioners, all neurologists and ophthalmologists working in outpatient departments and hospitals of a certain area, and from all hospital files, and the autopsy material of all patients.

The diagnosis of MS is difficult to establish, and it is even more difficult to compare the results of different epidemiologic studies in which different diagnostic criteria have been used. A number of plans for diagnostic criteria have been put forward: none has met with universal acceptance. It would be worth defining the degree of confidence by comparing the correctness of the clinical diagnosis with the pathologic findings and then to make every effort to use those criteria whose confidence is the greatest. I have found the criteria proposed by Bauer [4] correct in every one of a series of 20 cases of MS autopsy material. The general use of these criteria would cause no problem to anyone.

Acknowledgments. I am indebted to J.A. Aarli, G. Ambrózy, M. Antony, H. Bauer, W. Cendrowski, G. Dean, S. Dobi, A. Fazekas, M. Gallai, G. Gátai, A. Guseo, Z. Haffner, L. Heiner, P. Johnson, E. Kahana, K. Karsay, E. Kluge, J. Kopa, H.J. Körting, G. Kovács, Y. Kuroiwa, L. Leel-Össy, A. Lipcsey, E. Mészáros, G. Németh, K. Onody, D. Péley, N. Pintér, J. Sepcic, Z. Somló, E. Szabó, J. Szántó, A. Szobor, G. Tass, Tsu-Pei Hung, and N.H. Wadia who made available data from studies performed in their epidemiologic areas. I am grateful to Mrs. A. Horváth for typing the manuscript.

References

1. Alter M, Halpern L, Kurland LT, Bornstein D, Leibowitz U, Silberstein J (1962) Multiple sclerosis in Israel. Prevalence among immigrants and native inhabitants. Arch Neurol 7:15–25
2. Alter M, Kahana E, Loewenson R (1978) Migration and risk of multiple sclerosis. Neurology 28:1089–1093
3. Antonowsky A, Leibowitz U, Medalie JM, Smith HA, Halpern L, Alter M (1967) Epidemiological study of multiple sclerosis in Israel, part 3. Multiple sclerosis and socioeconomic status. J Neurol Neurosurg Psychiatry 30:1–6
4. Bauer HJ (1980) IMAB-Enquête concerning the diagnostic criteria for MS. In: Bauer HJ, Poser S, Ritter G (eds) Progress in multiple sclerosis research. Springer, Berlin Heidelberg New York, pp 555–563
5. Bejar JM, Ziegler DK (1984) Onset of multiple sclerosis in a 24-month-old child. Arch Neurol 41:881–882
6. Berman M, Feldman S, Alter M et al. (1981) Acute transverse myelitis incidence and etiologic considerations. Neurology 31:966–971
7. Brandt S, Gyldensted C, Offner H, Melchior JL (1981) Multiple sclerosis in a two-year-old boy. Neuropediatrics 12:75–82
8. Cendrowski W, Wender M, Dominik W, Fleisierowicz, Owsianowski M, Popiel M (1969) Epidemiological study of multiple sclerosis in Western Poland. Eur Neurol 2:90–100
9. Dean G (1967) Annual incidence, prevalence and mortality of multiple sclerosis in white South-African born and in white immigrants to South Africa. Br Med J 2:724–730
10. Dean G (1982) Multiple sclerosis among Asian immigrants to England and multiple sclerosis in southern Europe-Sicily and Malta. In: Kuroiwa Y, Kurland LT (eds) Multiple sclerosis east and west. Kyushu University Press, Fukuoka, pp 195–200
11. Dean G (1984) Epidemiology of multiple sclerosis. Neuroepidemiology 3:58–73
12. Dean G, Goodall J, Downie A (1981) The prevalence of multiple sclerosis in the Outer Hebrides compared with North-east Scotland and the Orkney and Shetland islands. J Epidemiol Community Health 35:110–113
13. Dean G, Grimaldi G, Kelly R, Karhausen L (1979) Multiple sclerosis in Southern Europe I. Prevalence in Sicily in 1975. J Epidemiol Community Health 33:107–110
14. Detels R, Brody JA, Edgar AH (1972) Multiple sclerosis among American Japanese and Chinese migrants to California and Washington. J Chron Dis 25:3–10
15. Granieri E, Rosati G (1982) Italy: a medium- or high-risk area for multiple sclerosis, an epidemiologic study in Barbagia Sardinia southern Italy. Neurology 32:466–472
16. Gyódi E, Tauszik T, Petrányi Gy, Kotvász Á, Pálffy G, Takács I, Nemák P, Hollán SR (1981) The HLA antigen distribution in the gipsy population in Hungary. Tissue Antigens 18:1–12
17. Ishohara O, Yamaguchi Y, Matsuishi T et al. (1984) Multiple ring enhancement in a case of acute reversible demyelinating disease in childhood suggestive of acute multiple sclerosis. Brain Dev 6:401–406
18. Jokelainen M, Wikström J, Palo J (1984) Effect of birthplace on the development of amyotrophic lateral sclerosis and multiple sclerosis. A study among Finnish war evacuees. Acta Neurol Scand 60:283–288
19. Környey S (1952) Early stage of Schilder's disease and relation to other forms of leucoencephalitis. Arch Neurol Psychiatr 68:683–697
20. Kranz JS, Kurland LT (1982) General overview of the epidemiology of multiple sclerosis with emphasis on the geographic pattern and long-term trends. In: Kuroiwa Y, Kurland LT (eds) Multiple sclerosis east and west. Kyushu University Press, Fukuoka, pp 3–29
21. Kurland LT, Molgaard CA, Kurland EM, Wiederholt WC, Kirkpatrick JW (1984) Swine flu vaccine and multiple sclerosis. JAMA 25:2672–2675
22. Kuroiwa Y, Shibasaki H, Ikeda M (1983) Prevalence of multiple sclerosis and its north-to south gradient in Japan. Neuroepidemiology 2:62–69
23. Kuroiwa Y, Shibasaki H, Tabira T, Itoyama Y (1982) Clinical picture of multiple sclerosis in Asia. In: Kuroiwa Y, Kurland LT (eds) Multiple sclerosis east and west. Kyushu University Press, Fukuoka, pp 32–42

24. Kurtzke JF (1980) Multiple sclerosis, an overview. In: Rose FC (ed) Clinical neuroepidemiology. Pitman Medical, Bath, pp 170–195
25. Kurtzke JF, Hyllested K (1982) MS in the Faroes, an update. In: Kuroiwa Y, Kurland LT (eds) Multiple sclerosis east and west. Kyushu University Press, Fukuoka, pp 183–194
26. Larsen JP, Kvaale G, Riise T et al. (1984) An increase in the incidence of multiple sclerosis in western Norway. Acta Neurol Scand 70:96–103
27. Lauer K, Firnhaber W (1984) Epidemiological investigations into multiple sclerosis in southern Hesse. II. The distribution of cases in relation to exogenous factors. Acta Neurol Scand 70:266–273
28. Lehoczky T, Lehoczky-Halassy M (1961) Multiple sclerosis in Hungary. World Neurol 2:38–44
29. Leibowitz U, Kahana E, Alter M (1973) The changing frequency of multiple sclerosis in Israel. Arch Neurol 29:107–110
30. Lowe RF, Moore HH, Briggs BR (1980) The histocompatibility (HLA) antigen distribution in multiple sclerosis patients in Zimbabwe Centr. Afr. J Med 26:234–236
31. Materljan (1983) Epidemiology of multiple sclerosis in Istria (in Kroatian). Thesis, Medical faculty of the University Rijeka (summary in English)
32. McDonald MI (1984) Multiple sclerosis epidemiology and HLA associations. Ann NY Acad Sci 436:109–117
33. Meyer-Rienecker HJ, Buddenhagen F (1983) Grundlagen und Problematik der Epidemiologie der Multiplen Sklerose. Psychiatr Neurol Med Psychol 35:697–707
34. Pálffy G (1954) Neurologic complications following the use of sera and vaccines. Acta Med Acad Sci Hung 5:403–411
35. Pálffy G (1980) Some features of MS in Pécs, Hungary. In: Bauer HJ, Poser S, Ritter G (eds) Progress in multiple sclerosis research. Springer, Berlin Heidelberg New York, pp 549–550
36. Pállfy G (1982) MS in Hungary including the Gipsy population. In: Kuroiwa Y, Kurland LT (eds) Multiple sclerosis east and west. Kyushu University Press, Fukuoka, pp 149–157
37. Pálffy G (1982) The prevalence of multiple sclerosis in Pécs, Hungary.Ideggyógy Szle/ Hung Neurol Rev 12–17 (in Hungarian with summary in Russian and in German)
38. Pálffy G, Mérei FT (1961) The possible role of vaccines and sera in the pathogenesis of multiple sclerosis. World Neurol 2:167–171
39. Petrescu A (1977) Date actuale de epidemiologie a sclerosis multiple. Neurol Psychiat Neurochir 22:175–188
40. Shepherd DI, Downie AW (1980) A further prevalence study of multiple sclerosis in north-east Scotland. J Neurol Neurosurg Psychiatry 43:310–315
41. Shibasaki H, McDonald WI, Kuroiwa Y (1981) Racial modification of clinical picture of multiple sclerosis. J Neurol Sci 49:253–271
42. Singhal ES, Wadia NH (1975) Profile of multiple sclerosis in the Bombay region on the basis of critical clinical appraisal. J Neurol Sci 26:259–270
43. Trikannad VS, Wadia NH, Krishnaswany FR (1982) Multiple sclerosis and HLA B12 in Parsi and non-Parsi Indians. A clarification. Tissue Antigens 19:155–157
44. Tsu-Pei Hung (1982) Multiple sclerosis in Taiwan. A reappraisal. In: Kuroiwa Y, Kurland LT (eds) Multiple sclerosis east and west. Kyushu University Press, Fukuoka, pp 83–96
45. Viischer BR, Bunnel DH, Detels R (1981) Multiple sclerosis and multiple moves. An etiologic hypothesis. Am J Epidemiol 132:140–143
46. Wadia NH, Trikannad VS, Krishnaswamy PR (1981) HLA antigens in multiple sclerosis amongst Indians. J Neurol Neurosurg Psychiatry 44:849–851
47. Wikström J, Palo J (1976) Studies on the geographic clustering of multiple sclerosis and optic neuritis in Finland. J Neurol 213:79–85
48. Wikström J, Ritter G, Poser S, Firnhaber W, Bauer HJ (1977) Das Vorkommen von Multipler Sklerose in Südniedersachsen. Ergebnisse einer Feldstudie über 12 Jahre. Nervenarzt 48:494–499

Overview of Motor Neuron Disease

L. T. Kurland [1] and D. W. Mulder [2]

This overview is concerned with the epidemiology of motor neuron disease (MND) comprised of amyotrophic lateral sclerosis (ALS), progressive muscular atrophy (PMA), and progressive bulbar palsy (PBP). The mortality and morbidity distribution are described with emphasis on the geographic foci of the Western Pacific. The etiologic hypotheses are reviewed.

Over the years from 1949 through 1977, the annual crude death rate for MND per 100000 population in the United States has gradually increased from about 0.7 to 1.1 [1]. Although this upward trend may reflect a true increase, it is more probably related to aging of the population and to better diagnosis and reporting. The principal component of the MND group is ALS, which increased from 0.5 to 1.0 per 100000 population, while the rate for PMA and PBP decreased from about 0.2 to 0.1 in the same period. Thus it seems that the increasing proportion of deaths reported as ALS probably reflects a change in physicians' diagnosing patterns rather than a change in disease characteristics.

A detailed analysis of death rates in the United States by age, sex, and race was carried out for the period 1959 through 1961 [1]. Age-specific rates were highest at about the age of 70 years and decreased sharply beyond that age. The median age was approximately 62 years and the mean was 61 years. If the period of survival is 3 years, as is usually reported, the mean age at onset would have been about 58 years, although this is some 6 years older than that reported in some of the larger clinical series derived from referral practices [2]. The death rates by regions in the United States for the period 1959 through 1961 were nearly uniform; and when these were analyzed by states, there was remarkably little variation, with values in all but three of the states from 0.4 to 0.7 per 100000 population. More recent data with a breakdown by counties within the 50 states has been carried out by Bharucha [3]. This shows wider fluctuations in rates, as might be expected with the smaller county populations. However, there was no indication of foci of disease which are not explicable by chance or reporting variations.

A study of the Rochester, Minnesota, population covering 53 years indicated that the mean annual incidence for ALS averaged 1.8 per 100000, age-adjusted to

[1] Department of Medical Statistics and Epidemiology, Mayo Clinic and Mayo Foundation, Rochester, Minnesota, USA.
[2] Department of Neurology, Mayo Clinic and Mayo Foundation, Rochester, Minnesota, USA.

Neurology
Ed. by K. Poeck, H. J. Freund, and H. Gänshirt

the United States population of 1950. There was a small but not significant increase in the rates over this long period of time. The male to female ratio was about 1.6 to 1. A familial history is obtained in about 6% of the cases. The most notable aspect of the Rochester study, in contrast to every other study to date, is that incidence increased with increasing age [4, 5]. The median age at onset was 66 years; this is appreciably higher than the average of about 52 years from the clinical (referral) series at Mayo Clinic and other reported clinical series [2, 3, 6, 7]. These results contrast with the estimated median age of onset of the ALS cases on Guam (about 40 years) and that of the familial cases in the Mayo series (about 45 years) [6]. The median duration of the Rochester cases was about 2 years from onset to death, with longer durations occurring in the younger patients, i.e., those below the median age of 66 years at onset.

On the basis of epidemiologic and genetic features, three major types of ALS have been identified: 1) the classic and usually sporadic form; 2) the familial and presumably hereditary form; and 3) the Mariana Islands form, first described among the indigenous population (Chamorros) of Guam [8]. The specific features of these types have been described previously [9].

There is no general agreement on the cause or pathogenesis of ALS. The relatively stable death rates of the sporadic form suggest that a key etiologic factor is one that is uncommon, but evenly distributed throughout most of the world. The uniform male majority is a clue that remains unexplained. Confirmation of whether there is in fact a bias towards people of European origin, as against those of African or Asian ancestry, must await the results of additional population-based studies. The familial cases follow an autosomal dominant pattern which is probably due to some metabolic-biochemical disorder. A viral etiology for ALS seems unlikely on the basis of the persistently negative transmission experiments of Gibbs and Gajdusek [10] and also because no report has been substantiated of isolation or transmission of an infectious agent. The neurofibrillary tangles may be the basic and visible neuronal degenerative process and "common denominator" of ALS in the Mariana Islands and the Kii Peninsula foci [11, 12]. It is likely, but still unproven, that this is also the pathologic mechanism in the focus in West New Guinea [13]. The populations of these three foci differ so much that a simple Mendelian genetic mechanism seems unlikely. A more reasonable explanation is that exposure to some exogenous factor, most likely a toxin common to these areas, accounts for their status as endemic foci. It is also conceivable that the etiologic agents in these Western Pacific foci may be different but produce the same metabolic effect and end product in the victims of the disease. The hypothetical toxin, in smaller quantities, may also be consumed or absorbed by populations where ALS occurs sporadically and where only those excessively exposed or genetically predisposed are affected.

As increasing attention is focused on the high incidence in New Guinea, the rates in the Kii Peninsula and possibly on Guam appear to be decreasing. The films, photographs, and descriptions of the cases in West Irian remind us of the illness on Guam which we observed 30 years ago. The reduction in incidence and mortality rates on Guam has been noted for ALS but is less clear for parkinsonian dementia (PD), which has a later mean age of onset and may simply be lagging behind in the presumed gradual disappearance of the disease. The westernization of the cultures on Guam and the Kii Peninsula may be a factor coincident with or responsible for the decrease, although Gajdusek and associates and Yase continue to enunciate the hypothesis that low levels of calcium and magnesium in the soil and water are related to the etiology of the disease in those foci [14, 15].

We find it difficult to understand why calcium and magnesium intake would be low on an ocean island such as Guam, where, particularly in the earlier years, it is likely that the local population used sea salt which is relatively rich in calcium and magnesium on their food. Ground coral is used in betel chew and probably in food preparation as well. We have reviewed the paper by Yanigahara [16] and do not find convincing his suggestions that abnormalities in mineral metabolism are present.

The aluminum in the probes of affected neurons, as shown by Garruto [17], is indeed dramatic, but whether it is associated with cause or effect remains to be determined.

For the Mariana Islands form of ALS, a simple genetic explanation no longer seems applicable. The combination of the two prevalent neurologic diseases (which are now presumed to be clinical variants of a single disease entity), the described collagen changes in the skin, and the early description of multiple exostoses observed in a few families on Guam initially led us to search for some food or other vehicle with lathyrogenic properties. To date, no obvious source of lathyrogen has been found except for the small quantities of an aminopropionic acid in the nuts of *Cycas circinalis,* which has been a major food source of the Chamorros for more than a century and perhaps for several centuries [18]. We are not aware that the inhabitants of the Caroline Islands, to the south, had learned how to soak the cycad kernels adequately to remove most of the cycasin, a very potent toxin which the nut is known to contain. Caroline Islanders who had come to Saipan, the island north of Guam, in the early part of this century may have adopted and modified this process from the indigenous Chamorros. If the cycad toxin is an etiologic factor, it is of interest that ALS was found not only among the Chamorros of Saipan but also, to a lesser degree, among the Carolinian inhabitants of Saipan, although it has not been described as endemic in the Carolinians in their home islands. We have also seen among male Carolinians on Saipan, ages 40–65 years, several cases of a slowly progressive spastic paraparesis, often accompanied by muscle fasciculations and slight amyotrophy of the upper extremities. The cases differ from ALS in their very slow rate of progression; and cervical arthritis has not been ruled out as the cause. Unfortunately, the patients were not followed adequately to determine the exact nature of this small focus of cases on Saipan.

If cycad is the etiologic agent, must there be exposure in childhood or early adolescence? If cycad is a factor in the illness occurring among the Filipinos who settled in Guam as young adults, childhood exposure does not appear to be essential. The cycad nut contains large quantities of water-soluble cycasin, an exceedingly active hepatotoxic and carcinogenic agent, perhaps the most active such agent occurring in nature. In Guam, this was largely, if not entirely, removed by a ritual soaking in water changed daily for seven days. But there could conceivably be a small residue of the cycad toxin or of one of the fungi which grow on the surface of the nuts during the preparation of the flour into which they are made, which could perhaps interfere with the production of some liver enzyme essential for motor and other neurons. It is also possible that the practice of the herbalists in Guam, who for perhaps centuries before had used fresh cycad nut to poultice various skin lesions and tropical ulcers, could lead to the absorption of this agent, with ultimate damage to the hypothetical enzyme system [19, 20].

Although the aglycone of cycasin or methylazoxymethanol has produced cerebellar cell damage in newborn mice [21], there is only a suggestion that an analogue of ALS has been produced in primates. According to Dastur, a young rhesus monkey fed cycad-derived flour developed evidence of anterior horn cell degeneration. However, there was no cycasin detectable by the chemical method available at that time (1964), so that the possibility of another toxic agent had to be considered [22]. If cycad were causative of ALS and PD on Guam, the decreasing incidence of these disorders could be related to the westernization of Guam, with imports of wheat, corn, and other grain foods, as well as to other postwar changes [23]. There is at present no clear indication that cycad plays a similar role in the affected communities in the Kii Peninsula of Japan. Also, no azoxy compound or food which might have a nitrosamine-like or lathyrogenic-like effect has been described in the West Irian focus. Thus, we must conclude that there is a serious need to repeat and extend the primate feeding experiments initiated by Dastur to determine if indeed a constituent of cycad might be responsible for the ALS and PD on Guam.

It all seems unlikely, in view of the tremendous efforts that have been made to identify a slow virus or other infectious agent, that this would account for the extraordinary incidence of ALS in the three foci [10]. Thus, a combination of exposure to some agent and genetic variability in detoxifying the hypothetical agent may explain the population patterns and the form of ALS described here. Clarification of the etiology of ALS and PD in the Western Pacific foci or clarification of the biochemical defect of the familial cases can be expected to have widespread repercussions on the etiology not only of ALS but of parkinsonism and Alzheimer's disease as well.

References

1. Kurtzke JF, Kurland LT (1983) The epidemiology of neurologic disease. In: Baker AB (ed) Clinical neurology. Harper and Row, Philadelphia, chap 66
2. Mulder DW (1957) The clinical syndrome of amyotrophic lateral sclerosis. Proc Staff Meet Mayo Clin 32:427
3. Bharucha N (1985) Geographic distribution of motor neurone disease in the U.S. and correlation with possible aetiologic factors. Proceedings of the international symposium on motor neuron disease, Bangalore, India, 29–30 Oct 1984
4. Juergens SM, Kurland LT, Okazaki H, Mulder DW (1980) ALS in Rochester, Minnesota, 1925–1977. Neurology 30:463
5. Yoshida S, Mulder DW, Kurland LT, Chu C-P, Okazaki H (1986) Follow-up study on amyotrophic lateral sclerosis in Rochester, Minnesota, 1925 through 1984 (in press)
6. Mulder DW, Kurland LT, Offord KP, Beard CM (1985) Familial adult motor neuron disease (amyotrophic lateral sclerosis). Neurology (in press)
7. Mulder DW, Espinosa RE (1969) Amyotrophic lateral sclerosis: comparison of the clinical syndrome in Guam and the United States. In: Norris FH Jr, Kurland LT (eds) Motor neuron diseases: research on amyotrophic lateral sclerosis and related disorders. Grune and Stratton, New York, p 12
8. Kurland LT, Mulder DW (1954) Epidemiologic investigations of amyotrophic lateral sclerosis: preliminary report on geographic distribution, with special reference to the Mariana Islands, including clinical and pathologic observations. Neurology 4:355

9. Kurland LT, Choi NW, Sayre GP (1969) Implications of incidence and geographic patterns on the classification of amyotrophic lateral sclerosis. In: Norris FH Jr, Kurland LT (eds) Motor neuron diseases: research on amyotrophic lateral sclerosis and related disorders. Grune and Stratton, New York, pp 28–50
10. Gibbs CJ Jr, Gajdusek DC (1972) ALS, Parkinson's disease and the ALS parkinsonian dementia complex on Guam: a review and summary of attempts to demonstrate infectious etiology. J Clin Pathol [Suppl] 6: 132
11. Anderson FH, Richardson EP Jr, Okazaki H, Brody JA (1979) Neurofibrillary degeneration on Guam: frequency in Chamorros and non-Chamorros with no known neurological disease. Brain 102: 65
12. Shiraki H (1969) The neuropathology of amyotrophic lateral sclerosis (ALS) in the Kii Peninsula and other areas of Japan. In: Norris FH Jr, Kurland LT (eds) Motor neuron diseases: research on amyotrophic lateral sclerosis and related disorders. Grune and Stratton, New York, p 80
13. Gajdusek DC, Salazar AM (1982) Amyotrophic lateral sclerosis and parkinsonism syndromes in high incidence among the Auyu and Jakai people of West New Guinea. Neurology 32: 107
14. Gajdusek DC, Garruto RM, Salazar AM (1980) Ecology of high incidence foci of motor neuron disease in eastern Asia and the western Pacific and the frequent occurrence of other chronic degenerative neurological diseases in these foci. Tenth international congress on tropical medicine and malaria, Manila, 9–15 Nov 1980, p 382
15. Yase Y (1977) The basic process of amyotrophic lateral sclerosis as reflected in Kii Peninsula and Guam. Exc Med Int Congr Ser 434: 413
16. Yanigahara R (1982) Heavy metals and essential minerals in motor neuron disease. In: Rowland LP (ed) Human motor neuron diseases. Raven, New York, p 233
17. Garruto RM (1985) Deposition of calcium and aluminum in central nervous system neurons: a primary or secondary phenomenon? Proceedings of international symposium on motor neuron disease, Bangalore, India, 29–30 Oct 1984
18. Polsky FI, Nunn PB, Bell EA (1972) Distribution and toxicity of α-amino-β-methylaminopropionic acid. Fed Proc 31: 1473
19. Proceedings of the third conference on the toxicity of cycads, Chicago, Illinois, 17 April 1964. Fed Proc 23: 1337
20. Kurland LT (1972) An appraisal of the neurotoxicity of cycad and the etiology of amyotrophic lateral sclerosis on Guam. Fed Proc 31: 1540
21. Proceedings of the sixth international cycad conference, Chicago, Illinois, USA, 17 April 1971. Fed Proc 31: 1465
22. Dastur DK (1964) Cycad toxicity in monkeys: clinical, biological and biochemical aspects. Fed Proc 23: 1368–1369
23. Reed DM, Brody JA (1975) Amyotrophic lateral sclerosis and parkinsonism dementia on Guam, 1945–1972. I: descriptive epidemiology. Am J Epidemiol 101: 287

Discussion

Epidemiology of Peripheral Neuropathies

P. K. Thomas [1]

Osuntokun has provided a comprehensive survey of the occurrence and causation of peripheral nerve disorders, both in developed and developing countries. It is evident that neuropathies constitute a substantial medical and social problem. It is also clear that very few community-based surveys have been made. Osuntokun has emphasized one reason for this, namely the complexity of the manifestations that may occur, ranging from focal neuropathies to diffuse multifocal and generalized neuropathies.

One of the main problems in surveys of the prevalence of neuropathies relates to their definition. This has been particularly obvious in studies on diabetic neuropathy, for which estimates as to its prevalence have ranged from less than 5% to nearly 60% [9]. No doubt this partly reflects differences in the composition of various reported series in relation to factors such as the duration and severity of diabetes, the age of the subjects, etc., but to a major extent it must depend upon what the investigators choose to classify as neuropathy. Thus a proportion of diabetics will have abnormalities of nerve conduction in the absence of symptoms or signs of peripheral nerve disorder. Others will have clinical signs in the absence of symptoms. Dyck et al. [4] have recently addressed this problem in a prospective study in which correlations were sought between scored symptoms, scored neurological deficits, abnormalities of nerve conduction and changes on sural nerve biopsy. The morphological abnormalities were expressed as a single Index of Pathology (Ip) that combined the age-corrected loss of myelinated fibres with abnormalities in remaining fibres. The fifth percentile line of the Ip was found to provide a sensitive and reliable minimum neuropathological criterion for the diagnosis of neuropathy. The two clinical evaluations were found to discriminate between diabetic and nondiabetic subjects, as did abnormalities of nerve conduction. All these were associated statistically, although the correlation was not precise. It was therefore advised that adequate characterization of neuropathy should be based on the separate analysis of these three evaluations.

A detailed investigation of this type could pose considerable problems for field studies or under circumstances in which the expensive apparatus that is required or skilled and trained operators may not be available. Moreover, the examination

[1] Royal Free Hospital School of Medicine and Institute of Neurology, London, Great Britain.

Neurology
Ed. by K. Poeck, H. J. Freund, and H. Gänshirt

needs to be sufficiently comprehensive to allow for the substantial variations in clinical presentation that are encountered. What is undertaken is likely to have to be tailored to suit the type of neuropathy under investigation. Thus some neuropathies predominantly affect small fibres. An important aspect of the assessment would thus be the evaluation of autonomic function and pain and temperature sensibility. Impaired appreciation of pain is difficult to quantify, but satisfactory methods for the quantitation of thermal sensation are now available. In selective small fibre neuropathies, nerve conduction studies will tend to be an insensitive method of assessment as the standard current procedures reflect activity in fibres of larger calibre. In some conditions, sensory symptoms characteristic of peripheral neuropathy may be related to selective damage to the centrally directed axons of the dorsal root ganglion cells. Sensory conduction in peripheral nerves will be normal, but abnormalities in central conduction assessed from somatosensory evoked potentials will be informative. Such was the situation in subacute myelo-optic neuropathy related to clioquinol intoxication [8].

The level of functional deficit at which it is decided that a patient has a "neuropathy" must be somewhat arbitrary, as there will be a continuous gradation from normality to severe disease. Thus minor subclinical abnormalities of nerve conduction may be of importance in monitoring populations at risk from toxic exposure [3], whereas in the clinical situation, the development of symptoms or physical signs is the usual criterion. Gilliatt [5] argued that, for diabetic neuropathy, presentation of the patient with symptoms may be a suitable criterion for the acceptance of "neuropathy". This is perhaps not entirely satisfactory, as the degree of tolerance to symptoms varies considerably between subjects. Again the definition of neuropathy may have to take into consideration the nature of the abnormality that is present. Thus the common finding in patients with diabetes (and some other disorders) that there is an abnormal tolerance to ischaemic conduction failure (see [9]) probably depends upon metabolic changes rather than structural abnormalities and has a different significance. Again, the limits of a disorder which shows variable clinical features that may overlap with other syndromes may need to be defined quite precisely for epidemiological studies. This arose in relation to the Guillain-Barré syndrome [1].

A further difficulty in epidemiological studies relates to the selection of adequate control populations. Thus if the effect of a potential industrial hazard is being investigated, the proper control group must be other industrial workers and not a sedentary group. Common experience suggests that manual workers accumulate minor peripheral nerve injuries or develop subclinical entrapment neuropathies that are not encountered in office workers. A formal investigation of this clinical impression would be of value. It is also evident that control data should not be transferred too readily between different geographical areas. Osuntokun drew attention to his observation [6] that the ankle jerks may be absent in greater than 20% of healthy Africans aged 20–45 years in Nigeria and Tanzania, possibly related to subclinical nutritional deficiency.

An important aspect of the prevention of neuropathies to which Osuntokun drew attention is the identification of individuals at risk. This applies not only to populations as a whole, but to particular subpopulations who may display excessive susceptibility. He referred to genetic polymorphism for the detoxification of certain drugs. The demonstration that some individuals may be at particular risk for the development of the Wernicke-Korsakoff syndrome because of genetic polymorphism of transketolase activity [2] is of considerable interest. Alcoholic neuropathy is likely mainly to be the result of nutritional deficiency [11] and it would be of interest to know whether a similar individual susceptibility exists. Indication that genetic susceptibility to diabetic neuropathy exists is so far tenuous or poorly substantiated. Established diabetic sensory and autonomic neuropathy is often poorly responsive to currently available treatment, although a recent controlled study employing close glycaemic control with continuous subcutaneous insulin infusion has demonstrated modest improvement (F.J. Service et al., to be published). It is vital, therefore, that attention is given to defining the precise causative mechanisms and to try to identify which individuals are at particular risk.

Life does not stand still. Both small and large outbreaks of peripheral neuropathy related to the introduction of new drugs or industrial chemicals continue to occur and, in these, epidemiological studies are of paramount importance in establishing the nature of the responsible agent. The outbreak of the Guillain-Barré syndrome associated with vaccination against swine influenza in the USA in 1966 [7] is a conspicuous example. The toxic oil syndrome in Spain [10] is another. Continuous vigilance is necessary in order to contain such disasters.

References

1. Asbury AK, Arnason BG, Karp HR, McFarlin DE (1978) Criteria for diagnosis of Guillain-Barré syndrome. Ann Neurol 3:565
2. Blass JP, Gibson JE (1977) Abnormality of a thiamine-requiring enzyme in four patients with Wernicke-Korsakoff syndrome. N Engl J Med 297:1367
3. Buchthal F, Behse F (1979) Electrophysiology and nerve biopsy in men exposed to lead. Br J Ind Med 36:135
4. Dyck PJ, Karnes JL, Daube J, O'Brien P, Service FJ (1985) Clinical and neuropathological criteria for the diagnosis and staging of diabetic polyneuropathy. Brain 108: 861
5. Gilliatt RW (1965) Clinical aspects of diabetes. In: Cumings JN, Kremer M (eds) Biological aspects of neurological disorders, 2nd series. Blackwell Scientific, Oxford, p 117
6. Osuntokun BO (1980) Neuroepidemiology in Africa. In: Rose FC (ed) Clinical neuroepidemiology. Pitman Medical, London, p 57
7. Schonberger LB, Hurwitz ES, Katona P, Holman RC, Bregman DJ (1981) Guillain-Barré syndrome: its epidemiology and association with influenza vaccination. Ann Neurol [Suppl] 9:31
8. Thomas PK (1982) Selective vulnerability of the centrifugal and centripetal axons of primary sensory neurons. Muscle Nerve 5:S117
9. Thomas PK, Eliasson SG (1984) Diabetic neuropathy. In: Dyck PJ, Thomas PK, Lambert EH, Bunge R (eds) Peripheral neuropathy, 2nd edn. Philadelphia, Saunders, Philadelphia, p 1773
10. Toxic Epidemic Syndrome Study Group (1982) Toxic epidemic syndrome, Spain, 1981. Lancet 2:697
11. Victor M (1984) Polyneuropathy due to nutritional deficiency and alcoholism. In: Dyck PJ, Thomas PK, Lambert EH, Bunge R (eds) Peripheral neuropathy, 2nd edn. Saunders, Philadelphia, p 1899

Epidemiology of Parkinson's Disease – Relevance of the Risk Factors

K. KONDO[1]

In Parkinson's disease, indirect evidence suggests that (a) clinical manifestation is a threshold phenomenon conditioned by progressive neuronal loss no longer compensated for normal functioning; (b) neuronal loss is basically an aging process, (c) the process is influenced not only by inherited predisposition but by effects of life-long exposure to various environmental factors; and (d) whereas a single major factor may be decisive in a few individuals exposed, most cases are caused by the combined or cumulative effects of many relatively minor factors [1]. In what follows, the risk factors which adversely affect the process leading to Parkinson's disease are discussed, and our preliminary data for a better evaluation of such factors are presented.

Low Heritability in Parkinson's Disease

There are documented cases that Parkinson's disease runs in families, but the genetics of the disease is controversial. Irregular dominant inheritance has been rejected, but an alternative hypothesis of a multifactorial inheritance [4] was also unable to give a final answer. A study of twins may give a clue to the nature/nurture problem in a given disease. Ward et al. [6] reported that in 48 monozygotic pairs (MZ) with at least one co-twin affected with Parkinson's disease, only one was concordant, and three were accepted as concordant which included doubtfully affected co-twins. In 19 dizygotic pairs (DZ), only one co-twin had atypical features.

The prevalence rate of Parkinson's disease varies between 60 and 187 per 100000 in 16 reports for Caucasians. Taking 0.001 as the representative value, the observed frequency in DZ, 1/19, appeared grossly elevated. Frequency in MZ, 4/48, is still more than the value. Although these values are tentative because of small sample sizes, and because atypical cases were included, it is apparently premature to reject

[1] Department of Public Health, Hokkaido University School of Medicine, Kita-ku N15 W7, 060 Sapporo, Japan.

This study was supported by a grant from the Intractable Diseases Project, Japan Ministry of Health and Welfare.

Neurology
Ed. by K. Poeck, H. J. Freund, and H. Gänshirt

the role of genetic factors in Parkinson's disease. I fitted the twin data to a nomogram to estimate heritability based on Smith's theory [5]. The resulting value was 0.22, which is larger than the values for cancer all sites, and congenital heart diseases, but less than many other tested diseases showing unexplained familial aggregation. This result suggested that in Parkinson's disease nongenetic factors are more decisive although inherited factors play some role, and it is imperative to introduce surveys for a specific identification of the environmental risk factors.

There are several ways of "discovering" the risk factors to Parkinson's disease, including: (a) from its association with other diseases seen in clinical or pathological practice, (b) from its association with a patient history of particular lifestyle and environmental conditions (diet, residence, occupation, exposure to various agents, diseases, etc.) which are not necessarily etiological factors, but are often secondarily related with the factors, and (c) where the prevalence rate differs by area, time, or host attributes, from an association of the frequency with such group-specific factors. All these factors are usually "unilateral" when they are initially proposed, very often by alert clinicians.

Identification of the risk factors is probably one of the most important problems in the study of Parkinson's disease. A low heritability indicates that the factors are mostly environmental, and these are more easily manageable than the genetic factors. Identification of the high-risk individuals is then feasible which is realistic because Parkinson's disease is a common disease among the elderly, and it may be possible to develop a prophylaxis by controlling the risk factors in medical or even self-care.

Case-Control Studies

Case-control study is one of the standard methods to evaluate risk factors in a given disease. Available data including ours have been briefly reviewed [1]. Former studies mainly evaluated preceding diseases without rewarding results. Intertwin comparisons by Ward et al. [6] disclosed that affected monozygotic co-twins had less smoking history, rigid personality, and more head injuries. Our study included 271 questions covering a wide range of the factors emphasizing life-long behavioral histories [1]. Additional results will be quoted here which are based on the same data.

Sasaki (personal communication, 1984) applied a multivariate logistic model for both sexes to evaluate combined effects of three selected risk factors showing strongest associations identified in the case-control study. The relative risk increased dramatically in those who simultaneously have more risk factors than those without. In male individuals who have habitual constipation, Parkinson-prone personality, and no smoking history, the relative risk was 27.33, i.e., they are about 28 times more liable to get the disease than are those people who have none of the three factors. Females showed a similar fact. Details are presented elsewhere [3]. This result is what we expect from a multifactorial hypothesis, and if more suitable factors are selected which are more closely related with the pathomechanism of the disease, we would be able to identify a high-risk group more specifically.

Association with Other Diseases

Association of two diseases often indicates a common etiology or predisposition or that one prepares the other to occur. Many suggestions claimed that Parkinson's disease is associated with other disorders. Colorful interpretations have been made, while the facts themselves remained unestablished.

In comparing pathological findings in 236 proven Parkinson's disease autopsies with those in three control diseases (550 craniocervical injuries, 403 myocardial infarctions, and 440 autopsies with pulmonary tuberculosis), no evidence supported that the disease is associated with other disorders recognizable at the dissection [2].

Dose-Specific Incidence Rates Among Atomic Bomb Survivors

A study of dose-specific incidence rates among the atomic bomb survivors is under way by Dr. Wakabayashi of the Radiation Effects Research Foundation and myself. Studying the survivors in Hiroshima and Nagasaki provides an opportunity to evaluate whether the radiation influenced subsequent occurrence of neurodegenerative diseases like Parkinson's disease – possibly due to a premature aging of neurons associated with the radiation.

Cohorts, called the ME 200, established for the Adult Health Study were used for calculation of the dose-specific average annual incidence rate of Parkinson's disease per 100000 person-year (PY), 1958–1982. The ME 200 was established in 1958 involving 4998 residents in the two cities bombed within 1999 m of the hypocenters, along with age- and sex-matched subsamples from less-exposed residents and those who were not in the city (NIC). The cohorts involving a total of about 20000 residents have been subjected to a biennial medical examination. There were 22, 12, and 8 accepted cases among 269868, 143221, and 98131 PYs, who respectively received 0 (NIC), 1–99, and 100 or more rad estimated individually. The incidence rate was 8.15, 8.38, and 8.15, disclosing no significant differences ($P > 0.1$). Many survivors are not enough aged to develop the disease, and we will continue the study for at least 10 more years until the final conclusion is reached whether ionizing radiation is a risk factor to this disease.

Discussion

Prevention of Parkinson's disease is a further hope for beyond the levodopa treatment. Elimination of the causes and precipitating factors, either a single major cause such as viruses, toxins, etc. or a combination of numerous, less effective factors, is necessary for prevention. Identification of the manageable risk factors is extremely important for this purpose, not only for the elucidation of the pathomechanism.

Established risk factors to Parkinson's disease are: (a) elderly age, (b) less smoking, (c) particular personality, and (d) affliction of family members. Few small-scale studies refuted familial onset in which secondary cases have been directly reexamined, suggesting that reported secondary cases in other studies in fact have disorders other than Parkinson's disease. However, I accepted familial onset as established, because this bias implicates relatives of patients and controls equally, and there are many well-documented casuistic reports of the familial cases.

Tentative risk factors include: (e) head injury, (f) low blood pressure, (g) habitual constipation, (h) reduced physical activity. Surveys that support these claims are not quoted here, except that our study disclosed or reconfirmed the association of (f), (g), and (h) [1]. Among the stated factors, head injury is purely external, but all others are obscure in this respect. The strongest known risk factor is age, indicating that the underlying process to the disease is age-dependent, if it is not the aging process itself. Some authors postulate that association of the disease with a special premorbid personality suggests a common neurohumoral organization of the brain predisposing to the two conditions. It is possible that a similar mechanism is present behind other risk factors, especially (b), (f), (g), or (h). Further studies are urgently necessary to resolve these factors into more specific, hopefully manageable factors.

References

1. Kondo K (1984a) Epidemiological clues for the etiology of Parkinson's disease. In: Hassler RG and Christ JF (eds) Parkinson-specific Motor and Mental Disorders. Raven, New York, p 345
2. Kondo K (1984b) Motor neuron disease and Parkinson's disease are not associated with other disorders at autopsy. Neuroepidemiology 3:182–194
3. Kondo K (1985) Epidemiological evaluations of the risk factors to Parkinson's disease. In: Yahr MD (ed) Proceedings, the 13th International Symposium on Parkinson's Disease. Raven, New York (in press)
4. Kondo K, Kurland LT, Schull WJ (1973) Parkinson's disease, genetic analysis and evidence of a multifactorial etiology. Mayo Clinic Proc 48:465–475
5. Smith C (1970) Heritability of liability and concordance in monozygotic twins. Ann hum Genet 34:85–91
6. Ward CD, Duvoisin RC, Ince SE, Nutt JD, Eldridge R, Calne DB (1983) Parkinson's disease in 65 pairs of twins and in a set of quadruplets. Neurology 33:815–824

Discussion on Epidemiology of Motor Neurone Disease

M. GOURIE-DEVI[1]

Prevalence of Motor Neurone Disease

The prevalence of motor neurone disease varies from 1 to 7 per 100000 population in the developed countries, and a figure of 5 per 100000 population is an overall reasonable estimate [12]. The remarkable consistency of this figure was emphasised by Kurtzke [11], and he indicated the usefulness in determining the prevalence of other disorders from hospital-based statistics in countries where community data is not available. By taking the ratio of the cases of another disease to the cases of amyotrophic lateral sclerosis, an estimated prevalence for the disease under consideration can be determined [11].

The question arises whether there is predilection for people of European origin and those living in the developed countries compared to Asians in developing countries. Population-based studies are required to provide the answer. A house-to-house survey of a population of 57660 (semiurban 17734; rural 39926) of Gowribidanur town and 144 villages covering 622 km² in Karnataka State, South India, was done by non-professional grass root level workers using a simple questionaire (symptom check list) and final confirmation of the diagnosis by a neurologist [5]. The point prevalence of motor neurone disease was 4 per 100000 population, which is in conformity with the prevalence in the developed countries.

In the three endemic foci in the Western Pacific region, Guam, Kii peninsula of Japan and West New Guinea, the prevalence of ALS is 100 times or more than in the rest of the World. The declining trends in incidence and mortality in these "geographic isolates" has been attributed to westernization, change in food habits and occupation [1, 2].

Age at Onset

An interesting facet is the significant difference of age at onset in the West and in India. Many documented reports from the West show that the mean age at onset is

[1] Department of Neurology, National Institute of Mental Health and Neuro Sciences, Bangalore – 560029, India.

Neurology
Ed. by K. Poeck, H. J. Freund, and H. Gänshirt

Table 1. Neuroepidemiological study in Gowribidanur, State of Karnataka, India. Agewise distribution of population

Age group	Semiurban		Rural		Total	
	(*n*)	%[a]	(*n*)	%[a]	(*n*)	%[a]
0– 5	2396	13.5	6188	15.5	8584	14.9
6–10	2834	29.5	6408	31.5	9242	30.9
11–20	4344	54.0	8712	53.4	13056	53.6
21–30	3340	72.8	6776	70.3	10116	71.1
31–40	2318	85.9	5176	83.3	7494	84.1
41–50	1406	93.8	3849	92.9	5255	93.2
51–60	721	97.9	1866	97.6	2587	97.7
61 & above	375	100.0	951	100.0	1326	100.0
	17734		39926		57660	

[a] Cumulative percentage.

between 55 to 65 years [9, 10, 14]. In contrast our data of 124 cases of ALS in a 10-year period from 1973 to 1982 showed a mean age at onset of 46 years [6]. Thus the illness seems to make its appearance a decade earlier in India than in the West.

In this context it may be of interest to mention the age distribution of population in the neuroepidemiological study referred to earlier (Table 1): 30% were below the age of 10 years, 70% below 30 years, and 90% below 50 years. The earlier age at onset may either indicate that ALS truly starts at an younger age or since the life span is shorter than in the West, those with older age at onset are not being seen. It remains to be seen whether, with improvement of socioeconomic status and health care delivery system and consequent increase of survivorship, the trend would undergo alteration.

Atypical Forms of Motor Neurone Disease

Focal form with atrophy and weakness confined to one limb has been described from Japan [7] and subsequently from India [13, 15]. Since patients with atrophy of either one upper or one lower limb were seen, the condition was referred to as monomelic amyotrophy [3, 4]. Essentially this form is a benign condition with an initial slow progression for 2–4 years followed by a stationary phase, affecting young males predominantly. This type constituted 8.3% of a total of 323 cases of chronic anterior horn cell disease observed at the National Institute of Mental Health & Neuro Sciences, Bangalore, India, over a period of 10 years (1973–1982) (Table 2).

The second atypical form, the Madras pattern of motor neurone disease, formed 3.7%. Thus both atypical types together accounted for 12%. This entity was first described by Jagannathan and coworkers from Madras, India [8]. The clinical features of lower motor neurone signs in all four limbs, usually asymmetric in distribution, pyramidal tracts and cranial nerve involvement particularly sensory neural deafness, affecting young males and with a relatively benign course, distinguish it from the classical ALS.

Table 2. Classification of chronic anterior horn cell diseases – 1973 to 1982[a]

Type	*n*			Percentage
Amyotrophic lateral sclerosis (inclusive of progressive and pseudobulbar paralysis)	124			38.4
Progressive muscular atrophy (postpoliomyelitic progressive muscular atrophy – 2)	50			15.5
Spinal muscular atrophy	110			34.1
Atypical forms	39			12.0
a) Monomelic amyotrophy		27	8.3	
b) Madras pattern of motor neurone disease		12	3.7	
	323			

[a] National Institute of Mental Health & Neuro Sciences, Bangalore, India.

In conclusion, it may be emphasised that the global patterns of motor neurone disease are of considerable interest, requiring further in-depth study with special emphasis on search for the aetiological agent or agents.

References

1. Gajdusek DC (1984) Environmental factors provoking physiological changes which induce motor neurone disease and early neuronal aging in high-incidence foci in the western Pacific: calcium deficiency-induced secondary hyperparathyroidism and resultant CNS deposition of calcium and other metallic cations as the cause of ALS and PD in high incidence foci. In: Rose FC (ed) Research progress in motor neurone disease. Pittman Medical, London, p 44
2. Garruto RM, Yanagihara R, Gajdusek DC (1985) Disappearance of high-incidence amyotrophic lateral sclerosis and parkinsonism-dementia on Guam. Neurology (NY) 35:193–198
3. Gourie-Devi M, Suresh TG, Shankar SK (1984a) Monomelic amyotrophy. Arch Neurol 41:388–394
4. Gourie-Devi M, Suresh TG, Shankar SK (1984b) Monomelic amyotrophy – atypical and benign form of motor neurone disease in India. In: Chen KM, Yase Y (eds) Amyotrophic lateral sclerosis in Asia and Oceania. Shyan-Fu Chou, National Taiwan University, p 101
5. Gourie-Devi M, Rao VN, Prakashi R (1985a) Neuroepidemiological study in semiurban and rural areas in South India: Pattern of neurological disorders including motor neurone disease. In: Gourie-Devi M (ed) Motor neurone disease – global clinical patterns and international research. Oxford & IBH, New Delhi (in press)
6. Gourie-Devi M, Suresh TG, Shankar SK (1985b) Pattern of motor neurone disease in South India and monomelic amyotrophy (a benign, atypical form). In: Gourie-Devi M (ed) Motor neurone disease – global clinical patterns and international research. Oxford & IBH, New Delhi (in press)
7. Hirayama K, Toyokura Y, Tsubaki T (1959) Juvenile muscular atrophy of upper extremity: a new clinical entity. Psychiatr Neurol Jpn 61:2190–2197
8. Jagannathan K (1973) Juvenile motor neurone disease. In: Spillane JD (ed) Tropical neurology. Oxford University Press, London, p 127
9. Juergens MS, Kurland LT, Okazaki PHH, Mulder DW (1980) ALS in Rochester, Minnesota 1925–1977. Neurology (NY) 30:463–470
10. Kurland LT, Choi NW, Sayre GP (1969) Implications of incidence and geographic patterns on the classification of amyotrophic lateral sclerosis. In: Norris FH, Kurland LT (eds) Motor neurone disease. Grune and Stratton, New York, p 28

11. Kurtzke JF (1969) Comments on the epidemiology of amyotrophic lateral sclerosis (ALS). In: Norris FH, Kurland LT (eds) Motor neurone disease. Grune and Stratton, New York, p 85
12. Kurtzke JF (1982) Epidemiology of amyotrophic lateral sclerosis. In: Rowland LP (ed) Human motor neurone disease. Raven, New York, p 281
13. Prabhakar S, Chopra JS, Banerjee AK, Rana PVS (1981) Wasted leg syndrome: a clinical, electrophysiological and histopathological study. Clin Neurol Neurosurg 83:19–28
14. Rosati G, Pinna L, Granieri E, Aiello I, Tola R, Agnetti V, Pirisi A, De Bastiani P (1976) Studies on epidemiological, clinical and etiological aspects of ALS disease in Sardinia, Southern Italy. Acta Neurol Scand 55:231–244
15. Singh N, Sachdev KK, Susheela AK (1980) Juvenile muscular atrophy localised to arms. Arch Neurol 37:297–299

Clinical Trials

Clinical Trials Relating to Epilepsy

R.J. PORTER [1]

Introduction

As with all clinical trials, clinical trials in the epilepsies must, of necessity, be designed to deal with certain peculiarities of the disorder. The first important concept in the design of trials is the recognition that many different syndromes are included in the epilepsies and that meaningful data cannot be collected from an undifferentiated group of epileptic persons. Fortunately, very empirical information – the clinical seizure type – has rather good correlation with the various therapeutic measures and seizure classifications [2]. These data are useful as a first step in obtaining some form of homogeneity among the patients to be studied. This brief summary will concentrate on variables important in the clinical trials of new antiepileptic drugs; even though clinical trials of other therapeutic modalities (such as biofeedback or surgery) are quite important and remain in a relatively primitive state of development, most persons with epilepsy are treated with antiepileptic drugs, and most patients who remain uncontrolled on drugs are hopeful for the development of new, less toxic, and more effective medications. This communication will also be limited to a discussion of *controlled* clinical trials of antiepileptic drugs, in children and adults, exclusive of infantile spasms.

Patients

If the seizure classification is the first measure of suitability for clinical trials in epilepsy, one might logically ask how such a classification, properly applied, will assist in the selection of patients. Several major variables need to be considered in the planning stages of a clinical trial.

Preclinical Predictions

First, one must review the preclinical information on the compound and determine which human seizure type is most likely to respond to the medication. Unfortu-

[1] Chief, Medical Neurology Branch, Building 10, Room 5N-248, National Institutes of Health, Bethesda, Maryland 20205.

nately, only two preclinical tests have any clear-cut correlation with the activity of current antiepileptic medication against human seizures. The maximal electroshock test in rodents is useful in predicting activity against partial seizures and generalized tonic-clonic seizures; the subcutaneous pentelenetetrazol test is useful in predicting activity against absence seizures [6]. Many limitations of these procedures make them unattractive. They are old tests; their mechanism is obscure, and they do not provide a rational basis for drug development. Methods of evaluation with a more rational basis, however, suffer from inadequate validation – in most cases an enormous number of equally unsettling assumptions must be made. In spite of these difficulties, one must attempt to match the drug to a seizure type which seems most likely to respond.

Seizure Type

Second, one must choose a seizure type from the pool of epileptic patients. Obviously, a minimum number of patients with a shared seizure type must be available for a study to actually be performed. It is useless to speculate about the effect of a drug on a seizure type that is unavailable in sufficient quantities – either of seizures or patients – to test the drug. On those few occasions when a drug is especially effective against a rare seizure type, such as the amelioration by valproate of certain unusual myoclonias, the therapeutic effect may become immediately obvious, eliminating the necessity for a large patient sample. Such observations are unfortunately only likely to be made after the drug has been marketed for a different indication. Most commonly, however, vigorous bias control will be required to demonstrate unequivocal efficacy.

Given the limitations of finding sufficient patients of any reasonable homogeneity – using seizure type as the principle criterion – one naturally turns to what is available. Intensive monitoring may assist in the selection [5]. In children, studies are usually performed on absence seizures, if for no other reason than that the disorder is largely limited to children. Other studies have attempted to look at atonic seizures in children, though the best study (a negative study of cinromide) remains unpublished. Other controlled trials in children are quite sparse in number. In adults, the most frequent trials are carried out using patients with partial seizures, especially complex partial seizures. In Western countries partial seizures are the most common uncontrolled seizure type in adults. Generalized tonic-clonic seizures have also been studied, but have specific problems as noted below.

Patient Selection

After a seizure type has been chosen, based on both the preclinical expectations for the drug and the availability of patients with the chosen seizure type, one must further define the population to be studied. Of critical importance is the seizure frequency of the individual patients. This frequency must be high enough for a new compound to have an effect which can be measured with some degree of certainty. Factors that can compensate for a low seizure frequency in individual patients are (a) a larger number of patients and (b) a longer period of observation for each patient.

Different seizure types present different problems in evaluating seizure frequency and drug effect. The absence seizure has a very high frequency relative to other seizures and has a direct electroencephalographic (EEG) correlate. Anxiety about poor control and the possibility of harm to the patient during an absence seizure trial is low, though not nonexistent. As a result, trials can be shorter, can use objective EEG measurements as a criterion for drug effect, and can limit the overall exposure of each patient. Suitable patients are not exceedingly common, however, and the exact criteria for "typical" absence and "atypical" absence are controversial.

Studies of atonic seizures are difficult because of their inherent heterogeneity, as well as a lack of reliable EEG correlates and a need for continuous observation; self-reporting is rarely possible. No animal model has shown any promise in predicting effectiveness against atonic seizures.

The generalized tonic-clonic seizure has a major advantage: it is relatively easy to record. Also, a rather large segment of the population of patients with epilepsy has generalized tonic-clonic seizures. However, many such patients are not useful for clinical trials. Many patients, for example, have only a single generalized tonic-clonic attack and are never treated. Many others have attacks which are easily controlled on available medications. The therapeutic use of phenytoin and/or carbamazepine is highly effective in a very considerable number of patients with generalized tonic-clonic seizures [3, 4]. Others have uncontrolled attacks, but the attacks are sufficiently infrequent to require an investigation of enormous proportions – either in numbers of patients or duration of study. Anxiety about poor control is considerable, and maximal conventional therapy seems most appropriate at all times.

Finally, partial seizures in adults are available for study. The attacks are relatively easy to record, though some observation is necessary in most patients. Partial seizures are common and are often poorly controlled with available medications even when optimally prescribed. These seizures are often recurrent, and anxiety about uncontrolled seizures is less than for generalized tonic-clonic attacks, though greater than for absence seizures. Patients are, therefore, relatively easy to find and recruit. Disadvantages of clinical trials using partial seizures include within-group heterogeneity, especially if simple partial and complex partial seizures are studied together, and the need for a rather prolonged study. With patients who have three partial seizures per month, a study of 8 or 9 months' duration per patient must be expected in a study totaling about 50–60 patients.

Exclusion Criteria

Certain patients are ineligible for trials in epilepsy for reasons which go beyond their seizure disorder. Age and weight limits, for example, are typical for most clinical trials, and special permissions are usually needed to include children or adolescents.

The following patients were not considered suitable for participation in an actual trial of a new antiepileptic drug in partial seizures:

1. Patients with treatable causes of seizures, e.g., patients whose seizure etiology is metabolic, neoplastic, or infectious (a CT scan within the last 6 years is required to confirm absence of a treatable lesion, e.g., tumor, together with no new neurologic signs since the CT scan)

2. Patients who have received an investigational antiepileptic drug within 3 months prior to the beginning of baseline
3. Patients who are abusers of other drugs (e.g., narcotics), including alcohol
4. Patients who have progressive neurologic disorders
5. Patients who have a history of generalized tonic-clonic status epilepticus within 3 months prior to baseline, while receiving antiepileptic drug therapy
6. Patients who have other serious medical or psychiatric disorders (e.g., cardiac disease requiring drug therapy, a need for tranquilizers and psychotherapeutic agents, renal or hepatic disease)
7. Patients who have gastrointestinal abnormalities which are potentially capable of affecting drug pharmacokinetics
8. Patients receiving chronic therapy with nonantiepileptic drugs, including OTC ("over the counter") drugs (vitamins and mineral supplements are permitted)
9. Patients who have cancer with metastatic potential (does not include, e.g., skin cancer)
10. Patients with a history of poor compliance with past antiepileptic drug therapy, as judged by the principal investigator
11. Patients with abnormal laboratory values. (For entrance, a white count greater than $3000/mm^3$ with granulocytes greater than 50% will be considered normal. Patients should also be within their laboratory's upper limit for white count. Platelet counts are to be greater than $150000/mm^3$. Patients with elevated SGOT, SGPT, and alkaline phosphatase levels – up to two times the upper limit of normal – will be permitted to enter the study. However, if more than one baseline level doubles during the study, the patient must be removed. Patients may be retained in the study when *one* of these values is doubled, but if this value reaches three times baseline, the patient must be removed.)
12. Patients incapable of signing an informed consent
13. Patients unable to be hospitalized for a period of 2 weeks

Concomitant Medications

Ideally, a study of any disorder would permit a new therapeutic modality to be tested against either a placebo or against an active, already useful modality. Compromises are required in evaluating antiepileptic drugs because (a) uncontrolled seizures may be harmful, and (b) some effectiveness of currently available compounds exists for virtually all patients. The increasing sensitivity of institutional review boards to the ethics of "what is permissible" makes approval of epilepsy research protocols even more difficult [1]. In a definitive study of the effectiveness of valproate in absence seizures, for example, patients who were fully controlled on ethosuximide were not permitted to be crossed over to valproate (and vice versa). The initial plan for a simple crossover design was, of necessity, modified to a much more complicated response-conditional crossover study (Fig. 1). In this study of the relatively benign absence seizure, no patient went untreated at any time. Furthermore, the test medication – valproate – had demonstrated clear-cut efficacy in both pilot and foreign trials for absence seizures and was therefore a reasonable drug to apply as sole therapy in the study.

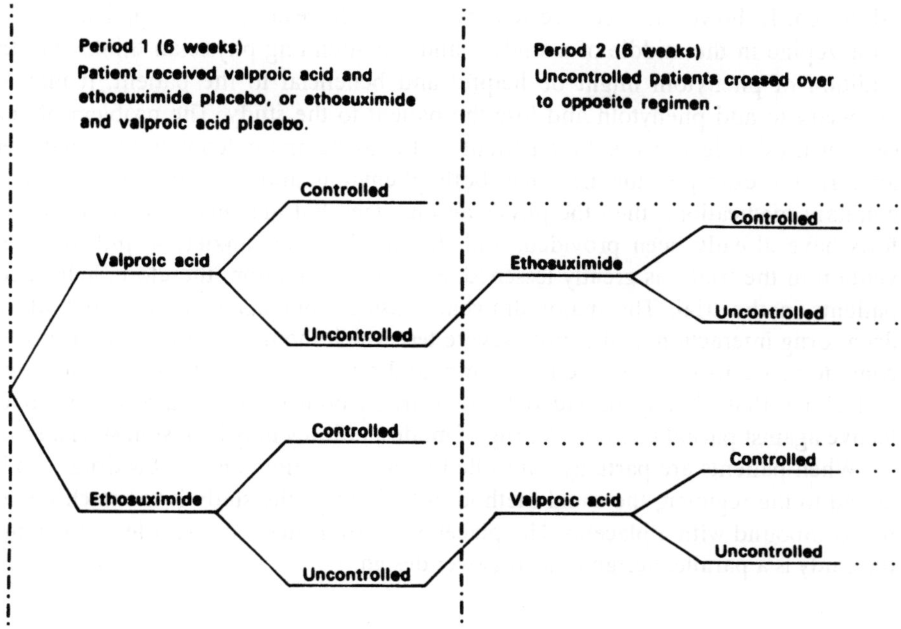

Fig. 1. This study design is an example of an incomplete (response-conditional) crossover in an investigation of valproic acid, which was being tested against the reference compound, ethosuximide. After period one, each patient who was controlled was dropped from further study. Only uncontrolled patients were crossed over to period two for the alternate medication. See text for discussion. (Based on study by Sato et al. [7])

Most such studies are not possible in epilepsy. The seizure type to be studied may be too severe to risk uncontrolled attacks, the drug's efficacy may not have been sufficiently proven, or both impediments may exist. For these reasons, in most early trials of a new antiepileptic drug, the new compound is "added on" to some other regimen. In pilot trials the add-on is often to existing medication; for controlled clinical trials one should attempt to obtain a homogeneity of concomitant medication in both the active group and the control group to eliminate puzzling variables such as drug–drug interactions.

The actual choice of concomitant medication can be very difficult if one is attempting to maintain homogeneity in the population under study. If, for example, one plans to conduct a study of a new drug in complex partial seizures, one must first decide which of the various possible concomitant therapies are most appropriate. If preclinical or pilot pharmacologic data indicate a prominent drug–drug interaction with certain marketed drugs, then these should be eliminated if possible. If the new compound has sedative side effects, then the concomitant use of primidone or phenobarbital may be relatively contraindicated. The usual concomitant drugs are carbamazepine or phenytoin or a combination of both. If the concomitant drugs are *too* effective (singly or in combination), the patients will have too few seizures on which to test the new compound. Patients having a tolerable but high seizure frequency (a state which is obviously difficult to define) on a single concomitant medication such as carbamazepine or phenytoin are ideal for the best, most uncomplicated design. If, however, excessive seizures occur – for example, in a patient on carbamazepine in the middle of a study – and the attending physician thinks that the addition of phenytoin might be helpful and beneficial to the patient, it may be necessary to add phenytoin and lose the patient to the study. The problem of "excess seizures" is less severe if the patient is already being treated with maximal therapy. If, for example, the trial has both phenytoin and carbamazepine as concomitant medications, then the physician may feel that maximal seizure control efforts have already been provided, and the threshold for anxiety – and for intervention in the trial – is greatly lessened. Such a combination, therefore, helps keep patients in the trial. The major drawback, aside from heightened probability of drug–drug interaction, is the more severe test which the new compound must overcome to prove its efficacy; the new compound must exert an efficacious effect over and above that already provided by two drugs, both of which are somewhat effective against partial seizures. A drug of modest efficacy may be lost in such a trial.

When patients are partially controlled by a medication, and a new drug is to be added to the regimen, the usual method of "blinding" the study is to match the active compound with a placebo. The placebo control is needed regardless of whether the study is a parallel design or a crossover design.

Seizure Frequency

As noted above, a minimal seizure frequency is necessary to obtain data. The fewer the seizures, the larger the trial must be, either in terms of number of patients or length of study. The ideal patient is one in whom the seizures are frequent but not severe, and whose seizures are likely to be drug-responsive; such patients, of course, are quite rare.

The effect on seizure frequency (or sometimes the percent reduction of seizure frequency) is usually the most meaningful outcome variable in trials of antiepileptic drugs. Improvement in the severity, i.e., a drug-induced decrement in seizure severity, is notoriously hard to quantify. Toxic effects of the new drug are also of great importance and must be recorded.

Dose of the Test Compound

Inadequate attention is often given to the problem of how much of the test drug to administer to patients in the clinical trial. It is naive to think that *any* dose will be effective; too often a dose is used which proves to be both ineffective and far below the maximal tolerated dose, i.e., that dose which reliably produces dose-related side effects. In order to give a new compound its best chance of success, especially in a trial in which concomitant medications are being used, the new drug (unless one is truly expecting miracles) should be administered near the maximal tolerated dose; otherwise, the efficacious effect may be lost and an expensive clinical trial will be wasted.

The argument that one should not approach the maximal tolerated dose in the study of a new antiepileptic drug because of unknown toxicity is faulty logic.

Although one must, especially at first, approach dose-related toxic effects slowly and carefully, there are several reasons why this maximally tolerated level should be achieved. First, the known dose-related side effects should have been recognized in pilot studies, allowing physicians to "know what to look for." Second, since every antiepileptic drug is "pushed to toxicity" in many patients by many physicians after marketing, these effects must be documented and catalogued before the drug becomes generally available. Finally, the required careful and close supervision of the patient during a clinical trial affords the logical opportunity to gather the much-needed information about dose-related side effects.

Having made strong arguments for using a high *dose* of the new drug – a premise which, it must be stressed, is quite independent of the *potency* of the drug – one must temper enthusiasm for obtaining the utmost efficacy from the drug with the unequivocal need to maintain the blind during the study. If a new compound has a distinctive dose-related side effect and if all patients experience this side effect while on the study drug, the blind will be broken in every patient. In general, distinctive dose-related side effects should not occur in more than about 20% of patients to preserve the blind.

Study Design

Assuming adequate bias control, that is, a randomized selection of patients and an unawareness on the part of both patient and evaluator of what the patient is taking at any particular moment in the trial, any number of actual trial designs are acceptable. Usually, however, antiepileptic drug trials are in one of two major categories: (a) parallel designs, in which a placebo group is compared to an active group or (b) crossover designs, in which each patient receives the active compound at some point in the trial and the placebo at a different point. Advantages and disadvantages of each are beyond the scope of this paper.

Summary

Controlled clinical trials of new antiepileptic drugs require an intimate knowledge of both preclinical testing and the heterogeneous disorder we call epilepsy. The preclinical data determine the nature of the seizure type to be tested although practical availability of patients is also of utmost consideration. Even though controlled trials in epilepsy are complicated by many variables unique to the disorder, bias control can indeed be accomplished to allow proper evaluation of new therapies.

References

1. Cereghino JJ, Penry JK (1982) Testing of antiepileptic drugs in humans: clinical considerations. In: Woodbury DM, Penry JK, Pippinger CE (ed) Antiepileptic drugs. Raven, New York
2. Dreifuss FE (1985) The medical management of partial and generalized tonic-clonic seizures. In: Porter RJ, Morselli PL (ed) The epilepsies. Butterworths, London

3. Mattson RH, Cramer JA, Collins JF, Smith DB, Delgado-Escueta AV, Browne TR, Williamson PD, Treiman DM, McNamara JO, McCutchen CB, Homan RW, Crill WE, Lubozynski MF, Rosenthal NP, Mayersdorf A (1985) Comparison of carbamazepine, phenobarbital, phenytoin, and primidone in partial and secondarily generalized tonic-clonic seizures. Engl J Med 313: 145–151
4. Porter RJ (1984) Epilepsy: 100 Elementary principles. Saunders, London
5. Porter RJ (1985) Intensive monitoring: epileptic and non-epileptic seizures. In: Porter RJ, Morselli PL (ed) The epilepsies. Butterworths, London
6. Porter RJ, Cereghino JJ, Gladding GD, Hessie BJ, Kupferberg HJ, Scoville B, White BG (1984) Antiepileptic drug development program. Cleve Clin Q Summer 1984: 293–305
7. Sato S, White BG, Penry JK, Dreifuss FE, Sachellares JC, Kupferberg HJ (1982) Valproic acid versus ethosuximide in the treatment of absence seizures. Neurology (Minn) 32: 157–163

Clinical Trials Relating to Head Injury

J. M. MINDERHOUD [1]

Introduction

The treatment of head-injured patients involves coping with a number of special difficulties, for example: the incompletely understood pathogenesis of cerebral edema, the fact that the brain is locked up in the bony skull (damaging itself if edema or intracranial hemorrhage cause shift and herniation), and the fact that treatment and management involves the most vital and complex part of the body.

In many instances treatment means prevention of the consequences of present lesions instead of treatment of these lesions themselves.

Certain aspects of head injuries, such as the severity, the kind of lesions, and the frequency and intensity of extracranial lesions can influence the results of clinical trials. Also important, however, is the nature of the patients themselves, including their social and economic background.

As the influence of age on the relation between the clinical state at admission or in the early days post trauma and outcome is well known, the importance of this factor on the results of trials has to be stressed. We found in our study on the epidemiological aspects of traffic accidents that the majority of these accidents were caused by males who were between 18 and 28 years old, riding under the influence of alcohol in the late evening or at night. In 1974 a majority of such injuries involved motorcycles. In the following years, when traffic laws forced motorcycle drivers to wear helmets, most head injuries occurred in car accidents, while recently an increasing majority of such injuries are the result of acts of violence in taverns.

It seems that in other countries as well this group constitutes a large part of the entire group of head-injured patients, influencing the outcomes and results of trials on treatment and management. An important age-dependent influence on the type and severity of injury is caused by brain swelling in children, which often (but not always) has a favorable outcome [6]. Another aspect which can influence the results of trials in head injuries is the type of brain lesion.

Gennarelli et al. published the results of a multicentered study on the influence of the type of intracranial lesions on outcome from severe head injuries [14]. They

[1] Academisch Ziekenhuis Groningen, Afdeling Neurologie, Oostersingel 59, 9713 EZ Groningen, The Netherlands.

Neurology
Ed. by K. Poeck, H. J. Freund, and H. Gänshirt

found that besides the seriousness of the injury as scored on the sum score of the Glasgow coma scale (GCS), the type of intracranial lesion also played an important role in determining the outcome of these severe head injuries. Their study proved that among patients with a total GCS < 9, mortality varied from 9% to 74%, depending on the principal lesion present. Lesions with a less favorable outcome were hematoma [48] and diffuse cerebral lesions with a coma longer than 24 h. So, in trials on the relation between cerebral lesions and outcome, eventually influenced by treatment, the location of the principal lesions, the severity of the lesions as scored with the sum score of the GCS, and the duration of abnormal scores, are all important factors.

In our study on the type of lesion, we raised objections to the use of the total GCS which withholds important information. Instead we used the separate scores of the eye-opening, and the motor and verbal functions to differentiate clinically between diffuse cerebral lesions and focal contusions (the so-called temporal contusions, [38]). Especially in moderately head-injured patients the relation between the GCS in the first days after trauma and outcome differed clearly in patients with a diffuse lesion and those with a focal or combined lesion.

While prevention of primary lesions to the brain seems to achieve some results, for example, in traffic accidents, the prevention of secondary lesions still needs improvement.

The influence of lesions caused by what Miller called "systemic insults to the brain" is very well known, and forms an important reason for prevention and treatment. Prevention should start at the spot of the accident, continue in regional hospitals, and be part of management in trauma centers.

In the past years management in trauma centers has changed from a rather conservative, cautious one to a more aggressive treatment [40]. For example, Hopkins et al. [24] published the results of an emergency resuscitation algorithm focussed on hypotension. Patients with trauma, hemorrhage, and sepsis whose care was in satisfactory compliance with the algorithm had shorter resuscitation times, lower times of low mean arterial pressure, and less shock-related complications. This algorithm, however, did not appear to be efficacious for patients whose trauma was primarily head injury. Since hypovolemia is usually not the major problem in these patients, a different algorithm is needed for them [24].

As many patients with severe head injuries are polytrauma cases, an algorithm focussed on the so-called secondary or systemic lesions to the brain seems to be worthwhile. Trials have been performed on the following general or special aspects of head-injured patients.

Infection

The risk of meningitis in head-injured patients is difficult to assess. It is, however, clearly related to open injuries, depressed fractures, and dural tears. A double-blind study was performed by Klastersky et al. in 1976 [32] on patients with a traumatic rhinorrhea or otorrhea. They found one case of meningitis in the placebo group (1/26) and none in the penicillin-treated group.

Similar results were obtained by MacGee et al. [33]. In retrospective studies by Braakman [4] and Jamieson and Yelland [26] on the infection rate in patients with depressed fractures, no relationship was found between the use of antibiotics and the infection rate, thus discouraging the use of antibiotics unless infection was suspected or debridement was delayed.

The results of a controlled study performed by Petersdorf et al. [42] even indicated that prophylactic antibiotic therapy is distinctly hazardous in unconscious patients.

Parenteral Feeding

Severe head injury is associated with a massive systemic metabolic insult and often a profound catabolism. It was found, for example, that decerebrate patients require as many calories as patients with major burn injuries and therefore it was suggested that early parenteral nutrition can aid in the recovery from cerebral edema. In a randomized controlled study Rapp et al. [43] found that in cases of early parenteral nutrition a more positive nitrogen balance was present together with a higher level of albumin and peripheral blood lymphocytes resulting in better resistance to infections, etc. and in general a favorable effect on the survival from severe head injury.

In 1985, however, Clifton et al. [9] reported that although it is possible to give feedings high in calories and proteins to these patients for prolonged periods, this did not result in a nitrogen equilibrium (although in some cases the use of steroids interfered with the trial).

One of the reasons for delaying nutritional support of severely head-injured patients is the presence of upper gastrointestinal complications. The brain-injured patient has increased gastric acid secretion and available evidence suggests that acid plays a key role in the genesis of stress-induced ulcera. Halloran et al. [21] in a double-blind study and more recently Holtermuller et al. [23] and Mouawad et al. [41] found that cimetidine reduced the number of complications. Cimetidine prophylaxis did not clearly reduce the incidence of gastric lesions, but did diminish gastric acidity, the severity of the gastric lesions, and the likelihood that they would complicate management of the patients.

Aggressive Treatment

Monitoring intracranial pressure (ICP) has been stressed as a very important part of management to reduce the mortality of severely head-injured patients and to improve their morbidity. In several reports, high ICP was found to correlate with high mortality [7, 36].

In 1977 Becker et al. [2], and in 1979 Marshall et al. [34, 35] published their results of aggressive treatment of severe head injuries in uncontrolled studies. After using dexamethasone, hyperventilation, mannitol, normothermia, and high-dose pentobarbital to control ICP, they compared their results with those of former studies [29] and concluded that their use of a more aggressive treatment early after injury was beneficial.

Saul and Ducker [44] compared the results of the management of severely head-injured patients in 1977–1978 with the results of the same management, now including the treatment of ICP, in 1979–1980. In the recent series, if ICP was normal (less than 15 mmHg) patients were treated with hyperventilation, steroids, and intensive care; if ICP was 16–24 mmHg, mannitol was administered and CSF was drained; if

ICP was 25 mmHg or greater the patients were randomized into a controlled barbiturate therapy study. This study reconfirmed that high mortality was related with high ICP, and that early aggressive treatment based on ICP monitoring significantly lessens the incidence of ICP of 25 mmHg or greater and reduces the overall mortality due to severe head injury without causing a disproportionate number of severely disabled or vegetative patients.

A number, but by no means all, of the aggressive managements-treatments have been subjected to controlled studies. Jane et al. [27] and Gelpke et al. [13] recently, compared the results of the more aggressive management regimes with the more conservative treatments.

Jane et al. compared the results from two relatively short consecutive periods in the same center and found a significantly lower mortality with the more conservative treatment. Gelpke et al. reached a similar conclusion when they compared the results from two centers, using the same scoring methods over the same period of time. These centers differed regarding their use of early hyperventilation (43% vs 14% of cases), ICP monitoring, etc., but not clearly in the attempts to avoid secondary and systemic insults to the brain in the early hours post trauma. As with other studies [27, 46], these results gave the impression that in order to improve the outcome of patients with severe head injuries, adequate measures taken within the first few hours after injury are more effective than whatever type of prolonged treatment given afterwards.

Seelig et al. [46] found that delays of more than 4 h in the treatment of acute subdural hematoma tripled the mortality rate.

Ventilation and Hyperventilation

Artificial ventilation with neuromuscular paralysis has become standard practice in many centers for patients thought to be in danger of intracranial hypertension. In these patients monitoring ICP may provide a good early warning of deterioration. In a noncontrolled prospective study in patients with isolated head injuries, Singbartl et al. [47] found that the posttraumatic course of the GCS values showed a temporary but statistically and clinically significant decrease in nonventilated patients, while deterioration was not encountered in ventilated patients.

Although a fall in mortality from 33% to 10% in patients treated with hyperventilation has been claimed by Gordon [17], and Rossanda et al. also reported beneficial effects of this treatment, reliable randomized controlled studies on the effects of hyperventilation are lacking, leaving the issue still under debate [22]. One of the difficulties in judging the effect of hyperventilation is that it is part of a total plan of aggressive treatment in which delay is reduced.

Another difficulty in judging the effect of artificial ventilation is the positive effect that can be expected in patients with a polytrauma in which pulmonary disturbances warrant ventilation. So ventilation or hyperventilation can also have an indirect influence on the ICP and thus on the outcome of the patients.

Steroids

One of the latest trials on the benefits of steroids in a normal dose was performed by Saul et al. [45] who treated patients either with 5 mg/kg/day methylprednisolone or with no steroids. The results did not differ significantly and although it appeared that probably some patients could benefit from this steroid treatment, they did not find the initial assessment of the patients to be useful in predicting the steroid effect.

In 1970 Gutterman and Shenkin [19] and in 1972 Alexander [1] denied a beneficial effect from conventional doses of dexamethasone phosphate. Gobiet et al. [16] could not detect a significant beneficial effect with conventional doses of dexamethasone (16 mg/day) either, but they did achieve a significant reduction in mortality and in the frequency of high ICP with high doses (48 mg initially and a total dose of 96 mg during the first day). Their control group, however, consisted of patients treated in previous years. Similar results were obtained in a double-blind study by Faupel et al. [12]. In a preliminary report James et al. [25] published the results of a small uncontrolled series of children with head injuries of varying severity and concluded that better quality of survival, shorter intensive care and hospital stay, and lower peak intracranial pressure were found in the high-dose dexamethasone group. In the same period, however, a number of rather open or controlled clinical trials failed to show that this therapy had a clearly beneficial effect on the clinical state and outcome of head-injured patients. In a prospective double-blind study, Cooper et al. [10], found no effect of dexamethasone, in either high or low dosages, on morbidity and mortality due to severe head injury. Similar results were obtained by Braakman et al. [5], Gudeman et al. [18], as well as others. The only clear effect of the treatment was the high incidence of gastric hemorrhage and hyperglycemia in these patients.

Barbiturates

The use of barbiturates to reduce increased ICP was based on the fact that they reduce cerebral metabolic rate and CBF by which intravascular pressure and the intracranial blood volume decrease, thereby reducing ICP. In the experimental setting, barbiturates reduce the lability and resting levels of ICP, decrease the formation of vasogenic edema, and prevent damage to endothelium. In 1979 Marshall, Smith, and Shapiro [34, 35] reported successful barbiturate therapy resulting in reduced ICP and satisfactory survival of the majority of patients so treated. The results of this therapy were first related to the effect on the ICP in patients in which artificial ventilation, surgical decompression, induced hypocapnia, CSF drainage, high-dose dexamethasone, and osmotherapy failed to control ICP. Although they found barbiturates successful in the majority of 25 patients in which other therapy failed to control ICP, this result could not be repeated by others [2].

In 1985 Ward et al. [49] from the same center (Richmond) published the results of a randomized, controlled trial of prophylactic pentobarbital therapy in a group of patients with very severe head injuries in which a high mortality could be expected. No clear differences were found between the treated group and the control group in the incidence of elevated ICP, the duration of the elevation, and the response of ICP elevation to treatment. The authors believed that barbiturates could even worsen the condition of the patient because arterial hypotension was frequently seen (54%) in the barbiturate-treated group. Recently Yano et al. found that barbiturate therapy had beneficial effect in patients with a GCS between 3 and 6 whose ICP was controlled below 20 mmHg. However, this trial was performed on treated patients and controls in different time periods.

Treatment and Prevention of Posttraumatic Sequelae

Sequelae of Severe Head Injuries

Although some claim that drugs and treatments can improve the outcome of patients with the sequelae of severe brain injuries, no randomized controlled studies have been performed to prove this statement. Based on the finding that in head-injured patients the metabolisms of dopamine and serotonin were decreased, severely injured patients were treated with neurotransmitters [51]. They claim, in an uncontrolled study, that by this treatment stimulation of the ARAS resulted in increased motor activity in nearly all patients and in improvement of consciousness in about half of them [3]. Similar results were achieved on an incidental basis with pyrithioxine by von Wild and Dolce [50] and Kitamura [31].

Posttraumatic Epilepsy

Opinions vary concerning the utility of anticonvulsant post trauma therapy after head injuries. As the incidence of early epilepsy (within the first week) was found to lay between 3.8% and 9% (4.1% was found recently [11]), preventive treatment could be worthwhile.

In patients with subdural or intracerebral hematomas, epidural hematomas, depressed skull fractures, cortical injuries, and posttraumatic amnesia lasting longer than 24 h, the incidence of early posttraumatic epilepsy is even higher, increasing the need for preventive therapy. Two-thirds of patients with a single posttraumatic seizure have additional seizures in the first week after injury. In a randomized, double-blind, placebo-controlled study in which (a) patients received phenytoin or placebo within 24 h after injury and (b) plasma concentration of at least 10 μg/ml was obtained in over 78% of treated patients, Young et al. [53] failed to find any difference between the two groups. The patients included in this study had either a penetrating missile wound or a blunt head injury with 10% or more probability of developing early posttraumatic epilepsy (as determined by Caveness et al. [8] and Jennett [28]).

Since the effectiveness of seizure prophylaxis was not established, the authors suggested that anticonvulsant drugs should be administered only after an early seizure had occurred. In contrast to reports by Wohns and Wyler [52] and others, they also failed to find any prophylactic influence on late posttraumatic seizures by phenytoin, but admitted that treatment with phenytoin because it induces higher plasma concentrations (12 μg/ml or more) could have a beneficial effect.

In 1983 Glotzner et al. [15] published their report on the prophylaxis of posttraumatic epilepsy with carbamezepine, which started immediately after injury and was continued for 1.5 to 2 years. Patients receiving carbamezapine showed a statistically significant lower probability of posttraumatic seizures than the placebo group with regard to early seizures within the first week, but not with regard to late posttraumatic seizures. Nevertheless, the authors emphasize that treatment should be continued for 1 year.

Postconcussional Syndromes

Long-lasting sequelae after minor head injuries have a multifactorial etiology; despite the organic basis, postconcussional symptoms become long-lasting complaints as a result of psychogenic, sociogenic, and iatrogenic factors [30]. Treatment of the syndrome with drugs such as Piracetam (a cyclic derivative of GABA [20]) and Pyritinol [31] was examined in double-blind studies. Minderhoud et al. [39] gave information, explanation, and encouragement to patients, in combination with the use of clear diagnostic criteria differentiating cerebral concussion from mild fronto-temporal contusions, on the one hand, and cervical whiplash and trauma capitis without cerebral involvement, on the other. In comparing the results of two consecutive series of patients, they were able to prove that a clear reduction of the number of patients with a postconcussional syndrome could thus be obtained.

References

1. Alexander R (1972) Medical management in closed head injuries. Clin Neurosurg 19:240–250
2. Becker DP, Miller JD, Ward JD et al. (1977) The outcome from severe head injury with early diagnosis and intensive management. J Neurosurg 47:491–502
3. Bioulac B, Richer E (1971) Tentative de traitement par la L-Dopa des troubles moteurs persistant au decours de comas prolonges. Bordeaux Med 4:1175–1178
4. Braakman R (1972) Depressed skull fracture: Data, treatment and follow-up in 225 consecutive cases. J Neurol Neurosurg Psychiatry 35:395–402
5. Braakman R, Schouten JA, Minderhoud JM (1983) Megadose steroids in severe head injury. Results of a prospective double-blind clinical trial. J Neurosurg 58:326–330
6. Bruce DA, Schut L, Bruno LA et al. (1978) Outcome following severe head injuries in children. J Neurosurg 48:679–688
7. Byrnes DP, Ducker TB (1980) Continuous measurement of intracranial pressure in 127 severe head injuries. In: Shulman et al. (eds) Intracranial pressure IV. Springer, Berlin Heidelberg New York, pp 73–78
8. Caveness WF, Meirowsky AM, Rish BL et al. (1979) The nature of posttraumatic epilepsy. J Neurosurg 50:545–553
9. Clifton GL, Robertson CS, Contant CF (1985) Enteral hyperalimentation in head injury. J Neurosurg 62:186–193
10. Cooper PR, Moody S, Clark K et al. (1979) Dexamethasone and severe head injury. A prospective double-blind study. J Neurosurg 51:307–316
11. Desai (1983) Epilepsia 24:289–296
12. Faupel G, Reulen HJ, Muller D et al. (1976) Double-blind study on the effects of dexamethasone on severe closed head injuries. In: Pappius HM, Feindel W (eds) Dynamics of brain edema. Springer, Berlin Heidelberg New York, pp 337–343
13. Gelpke GJ, Braakman R, Habbema DF et al. (1983) Comparison of outcome in two series of patients with severe head injuries. J Neurosurg 59:745–750
14. Gennarelli TA, Spielman GM, Langfitt TW et al. (1982) Influence of the type of intracranial lesion on outcome from severe head injury. J Neurosurg 56:26–32
15. Glotzner FL, Haubitz I, Miltner F et al. (1983) Epilepsy prophylaxis with carbamazepine in severe brain injuries. Neurochirurgia (Stuttg) 26:66–79
16. Gobiet W, Bock WJ, Liesegang J et al. (1976) Treatment of acute cerebral edema with high dose of dexamethasone. In: Beks JWF, Bosch DA, Brock M (eds) Intracranial pressure III. Springer, Berlin Heidelberg New York, pp 231–235
17. Gordon E (1971) Controlled respiration in the management of patients with traumatic brain injuries. Acta Anaesthesiol Scand 15:193–208

18. Gudeman SK, Miller JD, Becker DP (1979) Failure of high dose steroid therapy to influence ICP in patients with severe head injury. J Neurosurg 51:301–306
19. Gutterman P, Shenkin HA (1970) Prognostic features in recovery from traumatic decerebration. J Neurosurg 32:330–335
20. Hakkarainen H, Hakkamies L (1978) Piracetam in the treatment of the post-concussional syndrome. Eur Neurol 17:50–55
21. Halloran LG, Zfass AM, Gayle WE et al. (1980) Prevention of acute gastrointestinal complications after severe head injury. Am J Surg 139:44–48
22. Heffner JE, Sahn SA (1983) Controlled hyperventilation in patients with intracranial hypertension, review article. Arch Intern Med 143:765–768
23. Holtermuller K-H, Ebener B, Kuhl HJ et al. (1983) Stressulcerationen: Pathogenese und Prophylaxe. Z Gastroenterol [Suppl] 21:88–100
24. Hopkins JA, Shoemaker WC, Potter CC et al. (1983) Clinical trial of an emergency resuscitation algorithm. Crit Care Med 11:621–629
25. James HE, Madauss WC, Tibbs PhA et al. (1979) The effect of high dose dexamethasone in children with severe closed head injury. Acta Neurochir 45:225–236
26. Jamieson KG, Yelland JDN (1972) Depressed skull fractures in Australia. J Neurosurg 37:150–155
27. Jane JA, Rimel RW, Pobereskin LH et al. (1982) Outcome and pathology of head injury. In: Grossman RG, Gildenberg PL (eds): Head injury: Basic and clinical aspects. Raven, New York, pp 229–237
28. Jennett B (1974) Early traumatic epilepsy. Arch Neurol 30:394–398
29. Jennett B, Teasdale G, Galbraith S et al. (1977) Severe head injury in three countries. J Neurol Neurosurg Psychiatry 40:291–298
30. Kelly R (1975) The post-traumatic syndrome: An iatrogenic disease. Forensic Sci 6:17–24
31. Kitamura K (1981) Therapeutic effect of pyritinol on sequelae of head injuries. J Int Med Res 9:215–221
32. Klastersky J, Sadeghi M, Brihaye J (1976) Antimicrobial prophylaxis in patients with rhinorrheas or otorrheas: A double blind study. Surg Neurol 6:111–114
33. MacGee EE, Cauthen JC, Brackett CE (1970) Meningitis following acute traumatic cerebrospinal fluid fistula. J Neurosurg 33:312–316
34. Marshall LF, Smith RW, Shapiro HM (1979) The outcome with aggressive treatment in severe head injuries. Part I: Significance of intracranial pressure monitoring. J Neurosurg 50:20–25
35. Marshall LF, Smith RW, Shapiro HM (1979) The outcome with aggressive treatment in severe head injuries. Part II: Acute and chronic barbiturate administration in the management of head injury. J Neurosurg 50:26–30
36. Miller JD, Becker DP, Ward JD et al. (1977) Significance of intracranial hypertension in severe head injury. J Neurosurg 47:503–516
37. Miller JD, Sweet RC, Narayan R et al. (1978) Early insults to the injured brain. JAMA 240:439–442
38. Minderhoud JM (1979) Symptoms of temporal lobe contusions in the early period post-trauma. Acta Neurochir [Suppl] 28:63–65
39. Minderhoud JM, Boelens MEM, Huizenga J et al. (1980) Treatment of minor head injuries. Clin Neurol Neurosurg 82:127–140
40. Moss E, Gibson JS, McDowall DG et al. (1983) Intensive management of severe head injuries. Anaesthesia 38:214–225
41. Mouawad E, Deloof T, Genette F et al. (1983) Open trial of Cimetidine in the prevention of upper gastrointestinal hemorrhage in patients with severe head injuries. Acta Neurochir (Wien) 67:239–244
42. Petersdorf RG, Curtin JA, Hoeprich PD et al. (1957) A study of antibiotic prophylaxis in unconscious patients. N Engl J Med 257:1001–1009
43. Rapp RP, Young B, Twyman D et al. (1983) The favorable effect of early parenteral feeding on survival in head-injured patients. J Neurosurg 58:906–912
44. Saul TG, Ducker TB (1982) Effect of intracranial pressure monitoring and aggressive treatment on mortality in severe head injury. J Neurosurg 56:498–503

45. Saul TG, Ducker TB, Salcman M et al. (1981) Steroids in severe head injury. A prospective randomized clinical trial. J Neurosurg 54:596–600
46. Seelig JM, Becker DP, Miller JD et al. (1981) Traumatic acute subdural hematoma. Major mortality reduction in comatose patients treated within four hours. N Engl J Med 304:1511–1518
47. Singbartl G, Cunitz G, Hamrouni H (1983) Die qualitative Wirkung der Beatmungstherapie/kontrollierten Hyperventilation beim cerebralen Trauma. Anaesthesist 32:382–391
48. Stuart GG, Merry GS, Smith JA et al. (1983) Severe head injury managed without intracranial pressure monitoring. J Neurosurg 59:601–605
49. Ward JD, Becker DP, Miller JD et al. (1985) Failure of prophylactic barbiturate coma in the treatment of severe head injury. J Neurosurg 62:383–388
50. Wild Kv, Dolce G (1975) Pathophysiological aspects concerning the treatment of the apallic syndrome. J Neurol 213:143–148
51. Woerkom TCAM, Minderhoud JM, Gottschal T et al. (1982) Neurotransmitters in the treatment of patients with severe head injuries. Eur Neurol 21:227–234
52. Wohns RNW, Wyler AR (1979) Prophylactic phenytoin in severe head injuries. J Neurosurg 51:507–509
53. Young B, Rapp RP, Norton JA et al. (1983) Failure of prophylactically administrated phenytoin to prevent early posttraumatic seizures. J Neurosurg 58:231–241

Clinical Trials Relating to Peripheral Neuropathy

R. A. C. HUGHES [1]

Guillain-Barré Syndrome

Introduction

Controlled trials are particularly important in evaluating treatment in a condition such as Guillain-Barré syndrome (GBS), which has a high incidence of spontaneous recovery. Nevertheless analysis of 904 cases published in the last 15 years indicates the need for improved treatment since only two-thirds of patients had recovered by the end of a year, while 7% had died [15].

Corticoisteroids

In a small double-blind trial, nine patients were randomised to 100 units aqueous ACTH intramuscularly for 10 days and seven to placebo injections [24]. The mean time to recovery was shorter (4.4 months) in the treated than the placebo patients (9.0 months). Paradoxically the duration of hospitalisation was longer in the treated patients. The authors concluded from this double-blind study, their own experience with ACTH in other patients and a literature review that steroids are beneficial.

A larger randomised trial of prednisolone was conducted in London, England between 1974 and 1977 [16]. Forty-four patients were randomly allocated to receive either no steroids or prednisolone 60 mg daily for 1 week, then 40 mg daily for 4 days, then 30 mg daily for 3 days and then a regime reduced at discretion. The patients were scored at intervals by "blind" assessors according to a functional scale (Table 1). Four patients were withdrawn. According to most parameters, the outcome was not significantly different between the groups (Table 2). Where differences were discerned they favoured the control group. Those patients treated with prednisolone and entered into the trial in 7 or less days from the onset of symptoms had improved less at 3 months than the non-prednisolone group (Table 3). These results did not provide grounds for the use of steroids in GBS.

GBS has such a variable prognosis from complete recovery to persistent severe tetraparesis or death that it might be argued that this small trial (though the largest steroid trial available) happened to randomise more poor prognosis patients into the

[1] Department of Neurology, Guy's Hospital, London SE1 9RT, Great Britain.

Neurology
Ed. by K. Poeck, H. J. Freund, and H. Gänshirt

Table 1. Disability grade scale used in GBS prednisolone trial [16]

0	Healthy
1	Minor symptoms of neuropathy, but capable of manual work
2	Able to walk without support or a stick, but incapable of manual work
3	Able to walk with a stick, appliance, or support
4	Confined to bed or chairbound
5	Requiring assisted ventilation
6	Dead

Table 2. Randomised trial of prednisolone in GBS [16]

Findings	Prednisolone ($n=21$)	Control ($n=19$)
Median time to onset of improvement (days)	8	10
No. of patients with residual minor signs	17	13 [a]
No. of patients with residual inability to do manual work	7	2 [a]
No. of patients who relapsed within 1 year	3	0
No. of deaths	1	1 [a]

[a] Excluding one suicide during convalescence.

Table 3. Improvement in disability grade at 3 months in GBS prednisolone trial [16]

Delay from onset to entry		Prednisolone		Control	
days	No.	Degree of improvement	No.	Degree of improvement	Difference (P–C)
< 7	10	0.9	6	2.5	–1.6
8 – 14	11	1.0	14	2.0	–1.0
> 15	10	0.9	5	1.0	–3.0

prednisolone group. In this way it might have missed detecting a steroid-responsive subgroup within such a heterogeneous condition. Because of the uncertainties some authorities still favour the use of steroids in GBS and others have advocated high dose intravenous steroids on the basis of a successful outcome in individual cases.

It is worth emphasising that my own conclusion that the balance of evidence in GBS is against the use of steroids applies only to the acute form of the condition in which the peak deficit is reached within 4 weeks from onset of neuropathic symptoms.

Plasma Exchange

Following encouraging anecdotal reports and small series, plasma exchange (PE) has been the subject of five controlled trials in GBS. In the United Kingdom 14 patients were randomised to PE and 15 to no PE [13]. The patients were scored at intervals according to the functional scale used in the prednisolone trial (Table 1). At each follow-up assessment the PE group had improved slightly, but not significantly more than the control group. In this trial patients were randomly allocated, results were analysed by "intent to treat", which reduces potential bias, and two-tailed tests of significance were considered appropriate since PE might have made the patients worse rather than better. Major drawbacks of this trial were its small size and lack of "blind" observers.

The next trial to be published was from Sweden, where 38 patients were allocated alternately (a method which might not always be random) to PE or no PE. A slightly different disability scale was used dividing our category 2 into separate groups. Improvement began earlier and after both 1 and 2 months significantly more patients had improved one or more grades in the group receiving PE [21]. The mean fall in disability grades at 1 month was 2.1 ± 0.5 (SE) in the exchange and 0.6 ± 0.4 in the control group.

Two trials have only been published in abstract form. In one PE and prednisolone were compared. There were 12 patients in the PE steroid group and 13 controls and no significant difference in outcome was discovered [20]. The possibility that a deleterious effect of steroids counteracted the beneficial effect of PE has to be considered. A cooperative French group have reported preliminary results with 70 patients randomised to PE and 63 controls. The early phase of the disease appeared much more favourable in the PE group, but the definitive report must be awaited before the strength of the evidence can be judged [3].

The major evidence is from a North American multicentre study in which 245 patients were randomised to receive PE or not [14]. Patients were assessed daily by a trained, but not "blind", observer, usually a nurse, on the disability scale (Table 1). The characteristics of the PE and control groups at entry and the incidence of complications were similar. Four weeks after randomisation significantly more patients had improved one grade in the PE than in the control group (Table 4). Of the many other comparisons performed it was notable that of the ventilated patients the median time to come off the ventilator was only 24 days in the PE group compared with 48 days in the non-PE group ($P < 0.01$). For all the patients the median time to walk unaided was significantly shorter in the PE (53 days) than in the non-PE (85 days) group ($P < 0.001$). The difference between PE and control groups was more marked if randomisation occurred within 7 days of onset of the neuropathy (Table 5). Twelve patients were withdrawn because they did not complete the schedule for various reasons and data on these patients were incomplete. The results were

Table 4. Status of patients at 4 weeks after randomisation [14]

Group	Plasma exchange	Conventional	*P* value
All patients			
Improved at least 1 grade	64/108 (59%)	47/120 (39%)	<0.01
Mean grade change	1.1	0.4	<0.001
Respirator patient subgroup			
Improved at least 1 grade	26/52 (50%)	18/52 (35%)	=0.08
Mean grade change	0.8	0.1	<0.001

Table 5. Effect of length of illness before randomisation on time to improve one clinical grade: median times (days) (from [14])

Group	Plasma exchange	Conventional	*P* value
Randomised within 7 days of onset	23	68	<0.01
Randomised after 7 days	18	37	≅0.01

analysed separately with patients considered to have retained the grade when they were withdrawn. This analysis showed a difference which was still just significant with the one-tailed tests used.

Although each of these trials has its imperfections, particularly lack of any "blinding" technique, we do now have a substantial body of data suggesting that PE is effective. Although the pathogenesis of GBS is not known, the recent demonstration [19] of complement fixing antibodies to myelin in the serum during the earliest stages suggests a possible mechanism by which PE might work.

Immunosuppressive agents have been used in GBS in a few case reports, but have not been subjected to a controlled clinical trial.

Chronic Inflammatory Demyelinating Polyradiculoneuropathy

Introduction

Chronic inflammatory demyelinating polyradiculoneuropathy (CIDP) has been studied less than GBS to which it bears a pathological resemblance. It is defined by its progressive course usually reaching peak deficit over months or years, marked slowing of nerve conduction velocity indicating the presence of demyelination as the underlying pathology and elevated CSF protein [5]. The diagnosis depends on excluding other known causes of demyelinating neuropathy. CIDP is probably a heterogeneous group of conditions because it may run a varied clinical course, and be smoothly progressive, stepwise progressive, chronic relapsing or recurrent. All these patterns have usually been considered together in treatment trials.

Steroids

The usefulness of steroids in CIDP has been endorsed by many uncontrolled reports. Dalakas and Engel [4] reported that the majority of 25 patients improved on a regime of prednisone 100 mg daily for 1 month followed by gradual reduction to an alternate-day regime lasting more than 1 year. Although patients with CIDP have been considered to act as their own controls, spontaneous remissions do occur. The possible benefits of steroids have to be weighed against their serious side effects.

In the only controlled clinical trial of steroids in CIDP, 40 patients were assigned by restricted randomisation according to age, duration and sex into prednisone or no prednisone groups [6]. The prednisone group received 120 mg on alternate days for the first week and the dose was reduced by about 10 mg each week until the course finished after 12 weeks. Since 12 patients were withdrawn because of various departures from the protocol, only 14 patients were available for assessment in each group. Careful assessments were made on the basis of a neurological disability score (NDS) – a graded assessment of 35 aspects of the neurological examination on each side of the body (from 0 being normal to 4 representing no function), hand grip, computerised measurement of sensory threshold and nerve conduction velocity. Significantly greater but modest improvements in several parameters were noted in the treated compared with the untreated group. Neither the patients nor the investigators were reported to have been "blinded" in this study and it is difficult to blind observers in a trial of high dose steroids in which cushingoid side effects may become evident. Furthermore the patients withdrawn may have biased the result. Nevertheless the carefully measured effects support the general clinical experience that steroids are worth using when CIDP is severe enough to warrant running the risks of iatrogenic Cushing's syndrome.

Immunosuppressive Agents

Immunosuppressive agents have been tried in CIDP with conflicting reports of success. The only controlled trial assigned 30 patients by restricted randomisation to prednisone 120 mg every other day decreased over 9 months or to prednisone in the same dose plus azathioprine 2 mg/kg/day [8]. Two patients were withdrawn from the prednisone and one from the prednisone plus azathioprine group because of altered diagnoses. The same measures were assessed as in the prednisone trial described above. After 9 months both groups had improved by a median value of 100 points on the NDS and there was no significant difference between them in any parameter. The study therefore provided no evidence that azathioprine, at the rather small dose tested, was an effective adjunctive treatment to steroids. In their discussion the authors refer to their own experience, shared by the author, that azathioprine at higher doses may be beneficial.

Plasma Exchange

Plasma exchange has been reported helpful in some but not all patients with CIDP. Preliminary results from the only controlled trial support the idea that real is more effective than sham exchange. Fifteen patients received PE for 3 weeks and 14 sham PE; 5 of the 15 receiving PE showed greater improvement in their neurological disability score than the controls [7].

Diabetic Neuropathy

Hyperglycaemic Control

If the common sense and majority view, that diabetic neuropathy is more frequent and severe in poorly controlled diabetes, is correct [25], then it might be expected that improved hyperglycaemic control would result in improvement of neuropathy. This has not yet been convincingly shown. The best available study is a prospective randomised trial of rigorous vs conventional blood glucose control on 33 insulin-treated diabetic patients at the Mayo Clinic [23]. Even this study was confounded because eight of the patients in the conventional treatment group spontaneously achieved blood glucose levels which satisfied the criteria for the rigorous control group. Conversely five of the patients allocated to rigorous control never actually achieved rigorous control. Even if these patients were omitted from analysis, no statistically significant differences between the groups were discovered. It is too early to evaluate the effect of continuous insulin infusions on diabetic neuropathy.

Myo-Inositol

In streptozotocin diabetic rats, nerve *myo*-inositol concentrations fall and dietary inositol supplements prevent reduction of nerve conduction velocity. The fall in *myo*-inositol is thought to impair membrane bound Na-K ATPase, increase intra-axonal (Na) and reduce Na influx during voltage-dependent depolarisation. The few published trials provide little evidence that *myo*-inositol supplementation is an effective treatment for diabetic neuropathy. Treatment with 3 g daily for 6 months did not improve symptoms, motor nerve conduction velocity or vibration sense in a double-blind study of 55 patients, 30 treated with *myo*-inositol [11]. Treatment with 1 g daily for 2 weeks increased nerve action potential amplitude, but not conduction velocity in 7 patients [22]. A high *myo*-inositol diet was associated with significant but minor improvements in sensory and motor nerve conduction velocities in 10 patients with painful sensory neuropathy studied in a 16-week crossover trial [2]. Finally three of four patients randomised to *myo*-inositol by Greene et al. [12] exhibited clinical improvement after 6 months, compared with only one of five allocated to placebo. The main conclusion of this study was that clinical evaluation of small sensory nerve fibre function was more valuable than routine electrophysiological measurements in assessing the clinical course of diabetic neuropathy. Furthermore the time course of recovery of nerve function is so slow that 6 months is the minimum period in which it would be reasonable to expect improvement.

Aldose Reductase Inhibition

Since sorbitol concentration increases in the nerves of rats with alloxan-induced diabetes, it has been proposed that sorbitol accumulation in nerves may compromise nerve function. Sorbitol is generated from glucose by the action of aldose reductase present in nerves. Aldose reductase inhibitors also prevent the fall in nerve *myo*-inositol in experimental diabetes. Some small clinical trials suggest that aldose reductase inhibitors have a beneficial effect on human diabetic neuropathy. Thirty patients were treated with alrestatitin for 12 weeks in a double-blind trial [10]. Significant improvements occurred in sensory thresholds, particularly for vibration, together with a slight but significant increase in ulnar nerve-motor nerve conduction velocity. Three patients developed transiently elevated liver enzyme levels, one of whom had transient malaise and liver tenderness.

Another aldose reductase inhibitor (Sorbinil) has been reported to have minor beneficial effects in small studies of short duration. Sorbinil 250 mg daily for 9 weeks was compared with placebo in a randomised double-blind placebo-controlled crossover study of 39 patients [18]. None of the patients had clinical evidence of neuropathy, but there was a very small increase in motor and sensory conduction velocity during Sorbinil compared with placebo treatment. For instance, peroneal motor conduction velocity was 40.9 ± 0.76 m/s during Sorbinil treatment compared with 40.1 ± 0.73 m/s during placebo treatment ($P < 0.008$). Although statistically significant the biological meaning of this small change is difficult to interpret. In another double-blind placebo-controlled crossover study, 15 patients with chronic painful neuropathy were treated with Sorbinil 200 mg daily for 4 weeks [26]. The authors considered that the patients' report of improvement in pain was statistically greater during Sorbinil than placebo treatment, but most of the clinical and physiological variables showed no change. Sorbinil 250 mg daily for 3 weeks appeared more effective than placebo in relieving the pain of five of eight patients with severely painful neuropathy studied by Jaspan et al. [17]. Christensen et al. [1] randomised 37 patients with abnormal vibratory perception threshold to receive Sorbinil 200 mg or 50 mg daily for 4 weeks. No significant change in motor or sensory conduction velocity or vibratory perception threshold was detected. Fagius et al. [9] randomised 55 patients to Sorbinil 250 mg daily or placebo in a double-blind trial lasting 6 months. There were significant but small changes in three of nine electrophysiological tests, but no change in clinical symptoms, signs or sensory thresholds. Adverse skin reactions were encountered in 4/15 patients of Young et al. [26], 1/11 of Jaspan et al. [17] and 2/24 of Fagins et al. [9]. Clearer demonstration of efficacy and safety of aldose reductase inhibitors given for longer periods would have to be provided before they could be recommended for routine treatment of diabetic neuropathy.

Other Agents

Controlled trials of other agents have been reviewed by Thomas and Eliasson [25]. No benefit could be detected with vitamin supplementation. Amitriptyline and phenytoin have each been reported helpful for pain in one trial but not in others. Carbamazepine has also been reported useful.

References

1. Christensen J, Varnek L, Gregersen G (1985) The effect of an aldose reductase inhibitor (Sorbinil) on diabetic neuropathy and neural function of the retina: a double-blind study. Acta Neurol Scand 71:164–167
2. Clements RS, Vourganti B, Kuba T, Oh SJ, Darnell B (1979) Dietary *myo*-inositol intake and peripheral nerve function in diabetic neuropathy. Metabolism [suppl 1] 28:477–483
3. Cooperative French Group (1984) Cooperative randomised trial of plasma exchange in Guillain-Barré Syndrome. Preliminary results. Ann Med Interne (Paris) 135:8
4. Dalakas MC, Engel WK (1981) Chronic relapsing (dysimmune) polyneuropathy: pathogenesis and treatment. Ann Neurol [suppl] 9:134–145
5. Dyck PJ, Arnason BGW (1984) Chronic inflammatory polyradiculoneuropathy. In: Dyck PJ, Thomas PK, Lambert EH, Bunge R (eds) Peripheral neuropathy. Saunders, Philadelphia, pp 2101–2114
6. Dyck PJ, O'Brien PC, Oviatt KF et al. (1982) Prednisone improves chronic inflammatory demyelinating polyradiculoneuropathy more than no treatment. Ann Neurol 11:136–141
7. Dyck PJ, Pineda A, Daube J et al. (1984) Plasma exchange in chronic inflammatory demyelinating polyradiculoneuropathy, a controlled double blind trial. Ann Med Interne (Paris) 135:9

8. Dyck PJ, O'Brien PC, Swanson C, Low P, Daube J (1985) Combined azathioprine and prednisone in chronic inflammatory demyelineating polyneuropathy. Neurology (in press)
9. Fagius J, Brattberg A, Jameson S, Berne C (1985) Limited benefit of treatment of diabetic polyneuropathy with an aldose reductase inhibitor: a 24-week controlled trial. Diabetologia 28:323–329
10. Fagius J, Jameson S (1981) Effects of aldose reductase inhibitor treatment in diabetic polyneuropathy – a clinical and neurophysiological study. J Neurol Neurosurg Psychiatry 44:991–1001
11. Gregersen G, Borsting H, Theil P, Servo C (1978) *Myo*-inositol and function of peripheral nerve in human diabetics. A controlled clinical trial. Acta Neurol Scand 58:241–248
12. Greene DA, Brown MJ, Braunstein SN, Schwartz SS, Asbury AK, Winegrad I (1981) Comparison of clinical course and sequential electrophysiological tests in diabetes with symptomatic polyneuropathy and its implications for clinical trials. Diabetes 30:139–147
13. Greenwood RJ, Newsom Davis J, Hughes RAC et al. (1985) Controlled trial of plasma exchange in acute inflammatory polyradiculoneuropathy. Lancet 1:877–879
14. Guillain-Barré Syndrome Study Group (1985) Plasmapheresis and acute Guillain-Barré syndrome. Neurology 35:1096–1104
15. Hughes RAC, Winer JB (1984) Guillain-Barré Syndrome. In: Matthews WB, Glaser G (eds) Recent advances in clinical neurology, vol 4. Blackwells, Oxford, pp 19–49
16. Hughes RAC, Newsom Davis J, Perkin GD, Pierce JM (1978) Controlled trial of prednisolone in acute polyneuropathy. Lancet 2:750–753
17. Jaspan J, Maselli R, Herold K, Bartkus C (1983) Treatment of severely painful diabetic neuropathy with an aldose reductase inhibitor: relief of pain and improvement of somatic and autonomic nerve functions. Lancet 2:758–762
18. Judzewitsch RG, Jaspan JB, Polonsky KS, Weinberg CR et al. (1983) Aldose reductase inhibition improves nerve conduction velocity in diabetic patients. N Engl J Med 308:119–125
19. Koski CL, Humphrey R, Shin ML (1985) Antiperipheral myelin antibody in patients with demyelinating neuropathy: quantitative and kinetic determination of serum antibody by complement component 1 fixation. Proc Natl Acad Sci USA 82:905–909
20. Mendell JR, Kissel JT, Kennedy MS et al. (1983) Plasma exchange in acute inflammatory polyradiculoneuropathy: a controlled randomised trial. Ann Neurol 14:122
21. Osterman PO, Fagius J, Lundemo G et al. (1984) Beneficial effects of plasma exchange in acute inflammatory polyradiculoneuropathy. Lancet 2:1296–1298
22. Salway JC, Finneman JA, Barnett D et al. (1978) Effect of *myo*-inositol on peripheral nerve function in diabetes. Lancet 2:1282–1285
23. Service FJ, Daube JR, O'Brien PC et al. (1983) Effect of blood glucose control on peripheral nerve function in diabetic patients. Mayo Clin Proc 58:283–289
24. Swick RM, McQuillen MP (1976) The use of steroids in the treatment of idiopathic polyneuritis. Neurology 26:205–212
25. Thomas PK, Eliasson SG (1984) Diabetic neuropathy. In: Dyck PJ, Thomas PK, Lambert EH, Bunge R (eds) Peripheral neuropathy. Saunders, Philadelphia, pp 1773–1810
26. Young RJ, Ewing DJ, Clarke BF (1983) A controlled study of sorbinil, an aldose reductase inhibitor in chronic painful diabetic neuropathy. Diabetes 32:938–942

Discussion

The European Stroke Prevention Study

A. Lowenthal [1]

The European Stroke Prevention Study started in 1977 in Charing Cross Hospital, London, under the direction of Dr. Clifford Rose. Later on, other centers were included. In total this study now involves: three centers in Belgium, one in Denmark, one in Eire, one in Finland, six in The Netherlands, and four in the United Kingdom (Table 1). The activities of the different centers are correlated by a Coordinating Committee and by a Liaison Officer who visits these centers regularly. In general, meetings are held twice yearly, either by the Coordinating Committee or by the Steering Committee including all directors of the different centers.

All centers are working with the same design (Table 2). In summary this means that patients with ischemic lesions of the central nervous system, of duration 3 months or less, are included in the study and are to be followed for 2 years. Of these patients, 50% are administered 75 mg dipyridamole together with 325 mg aspirin three times a day. The other 50% are given a placebo. The study is carried out double-blind.

Examination and follow-up of the patients are regularly recorded in booklets. The data from these booklets are entered in a computer program and analyzed. The minimal clinical data base of this computer program consists of 12 elements. The compliance of the patients is followed by examining the presence of the drugs in the urine.

The study started in the different centers between 1977 and 1981, under the sponsorship of Boehringer Ingelheim. The last patients were recruited at the end of 1984 and the study will come to an end on 31 December 1985. Up to June 1985, data on 2533 patients had been entered in the computer program (Table 3).

Some remarks can already be made:

1. Concerning the randomization, one must take into account the fact that the number of dropouts is not to be underestimated. While the figure in Finland is only up to 12%, it increases up to 30% in other centers. We consider any patient who leaves the study for nonmedical reasons as a dropout.
2. The amount of end points is much lower than foreseen during the preparation of the study. Indeed, when one considers relapse of stroke or death, 13% was predicted, but only 8% or even 7% was observed in the study. As a consequence a

[1] Laboratory of Neurochemistry, University of Antwerp (UIA), Born-Bunge Foundation, Universiteitsplein 1, 2610 Wilrijk, Belgium.

Neurology
Ed. by K. Poeck, H. J. Freund, and H. Gänshirt

Table 1. Participating centers

Belgium	3	Start of trial	1977–1981
Denmark	1	End of recruitment	December 1984
Eire	1	End of trial	December 1985
Finland	1	Final results	1986
The Netherlands	6		
United Kingdom	4		
	16		

Table 2. Design

Aim	Prevention of death or stroke in patients with TIA, RIND, or recent stroke (less than 3 months)
Design	Randomized, stratified, double-blind, comparative treatment versus placebo
Medication	An association of dipyridamole (Persantin) 75 mg + acetylsalicylic acid 325 mg, t.i.d.
Duration of follow-up	2 years
Controls	At 1, 3, 6, 9, 12, 15, 18, 21 and 24 months

Table 3. Status June 1985

	Total (final) recruitments	Dropouts	(%)
Belgium	634	205	(32)
Denmark	7		
Eire	22	8	(36)
Finland	1319	166	(12)
The Netherlands	279	95	(34)
United Kingdom	272	91	(33)
Total	2533	565	(22)

larger number of patients had to be recruited during the study and the duration of the study had to be extended. The decline of the relapse of stroke is a general phenomenon in all western countries and thus not specific to our study.

3. As the study is carried out double-blind, it is impossible at the moment to comment on the effect of the prescribed medication.

Clinical Trials Relating to Epilepsy

J. M. MARTINEZ-LAGE[1]

Doctor Roger Porter, a major force behind the antiepileptic drug development program in the United States, is eminently qualified to deal with the subject of clinical trials of new antiepileptic drugs (AEDs). Our collective experience with the clinical evaluation of new AEDs has increased appreciably in the last 10 years. At least eight new chemical entities have reached the clinical phase of development. Problems in clinical development of AEDs are associated with patient selection, drug interactions, study design, and statistical analysis, as well as safety and efficacy evaluation.

I agree that one must attempt to match each drug to a seizure type which seems most likely to respond, according to the preclinical information on the compound. However, using seizure type as the only criterion to obtain homogeneity among the patients to be studied can bias the results. I think that it would be more useful to select a seizure type within a specific epileptic syndrome, as defined in the proposal for classification of epilepsies and epileptic syndromes (*Commission on Classification and Terminology of the ILAE,* 1985). By decreasing the heterogeneity, this dual criterion should decrease the number of patients required.

The more specific the epileptic syndrome, the more meaningful are the data collected. Take the case of absence seizures. They occur in patients suffering from childhood absence epilepsy, juvenile absence epilepsy, juvenile myoclonic epilepsy, and in other idiopathic and/or symptomatic generalized epilepsies and syndromes. How meaningful is it to try a new drug on the absence seizures of a pyknoleptic patient refractory to available AEDs as well as on those of a patient with Lennox-Gastaut syndrome?

Another important issue is the fact that the majority of clinical trials with new AEDs have been and are being carried out in drug-resistant patients. These are very severe cases with high seizure frequency, responding only partially to the conventional AEDs, despite plasma levels within the "therapeutic range." In fact, we are searching for a miraculous new drug which would even resolve intractable epilepsy.

Although naive epileptic patients cannot be located easily, the time has come to ask when new referral patients may be included in these clinical trials. Moral and

[1] Professor and Chairman, Department of Neurology, University Clinic and Medical School, University of Navarra, 31080 Pamplona, Spain.

Neurology
Ed. by K. Poeck, H. J. Freund, and H. Gänshirt

ethical considerations limiting testing of new drugs to subjects who are continuing to have seizures ought to be realistically and courageously revised.

Drug interactions are a complicating issue. Take the case of new drugs nafimidone and stiripentol. These are broad-spectrum inhibitors of drug metabolism. The levels of all AEDs with which they are coadministered increase appreciably. Any clinical trial with these drugs must allow for a strict control of levels of the associated AEDs. Otherwise results become difficult, if not impossible, to interpret.

I agree that any number of actual trial designs are acceptable. Nevertheless, it appears that studies of antiepileptic agents have not been innovative in their designs and analysis. More elegant and efficient designs with different end points and evaluation methods should be considered. The challenge is to identify and adopt those that offer real improvement in validity, efficiency, or operational ease.

The potential toxicity of new drugs deserves a few words. The unsatisfactory status or antiepileptic pharmacotherapy is more and more recognized. It is at the forefront of many doctors' minds. In parallel with the search for increased efficacy we should institute a search for less toxicity. However as Porter has pointed out, many compounds will be rejected as new drugs not because of inefficacy, but because of toxicity, especially neurotoxicity. Also, we must cautiously distinguish among these unfamiliar neurotoxic effects, determining which are important enough to halt further studies and which are unlikely to outweigh possible gains from the new drug. The risk-to-benefit ratio of a potential new drug is a function not only of its toxicity, but also of the severity of the disease to be treated by the new compound.

Some people with epilepsy may need to take antiepileptic medication for prolonged periods, in some cases for nearly a lifetime. Millions of patients worldwide are psychophysically and socially handicapped to an extraordinary degree. The ideal drug for them would be a completely active and nontoxic agent. Until that dream is realized, progress in the treatment of epilepsy will be made through new drugs which are either less toxic, but with the same efficacy as standard AEDs or more toxic but more efficacious than standard AEDs.

Controlled Clinical Trials of Head Injury

W. A. HAUSER [1]

Head injury is a major health problem internationally. Even though antecedent factors may vary between geographic areas, there are some epidemiologic characteristics which thus far are universal. Males are consistently more frequently affected than females, and the age group at highest risk is that between 15 and 35 years of age, a period of life in which those affected are entering their most productive years. For this group, permanent disability can mean many years of financial hardship and social burden.

Most clinical trials have been performed on patients with "severe" head injury. For this group, mortality is high even after hospitalization – depending upon the definition of "severe", upwards of 50% of patients may be expected to die. For this group, sufficient numbers of life or death events should be available to evaluate new therapies. In virtually all clinical trials in this field to date, major problems with study design exist, precluding interpretation of results, even with life or death as an outcome.

Sample Size

In few studies has the question of power and therefore sample size been addressed. If a new treatment or a modification of current therapy could be expected to have dramatic results, only a few cases in each treatment arm would be required to demonstrate effectiveness and to ensure that no evidence of benefit would be missed. None of the therapeutic approaches suggested to date appear to produce such results, however, be they to control intracranial pressure, infection, seizures, or the frequency of gastric bleeding. Sample size is dependent upon the number of possible outcome events expected in each treatment group: one must be certain that sufficient cases are enrolled to provide the appropriate outcome information. The greater the difference in expected outcome between treatment groups, the smaller the sample size needed to ensure an effect will be identified should one exist. Thus, if a treatment is expected to reduce mortality from 50% to 25%, an effect could be reliably shown with less than 100 patients. (Unfortunately, no therapy with such dramatic results is on the horizon.) A treatment reducing mortality or morbidity by

[1] Columbia University, 630 W 168th St, New York, NY 10032.

Neurology
Ed. by K. Poeck, H. J. Freund, and H. Gänshirt

10%–15% would still be of interest to neurosurgeons, but would require enrollment of 400 to 500 eligible and consenting patients. Since even major centers see no more than 100–200 severely head-injured patients a year, it is clear that cooperation between centers will be necessary, or an unduly long time will be required to complete a study.

While multicenter trials are complex to run, they do offer advantages in addition to more rapid patient recruitment. Patient populations differ, and methods of treatment not standardized by protocol will vary. A positive finding is therefore more likely to be universally applicable.

Follow Up

It is essential that the outcome be known for *all* patients entering a trial. Many of the studies of head injury with outcomes other than hospital death have suffered from lack of follow up and have lost further credibility through failure to take this lack into account during analysis.

Analysis Intervals

With regard to many of the studies, it appears that group differences have been repeatedly evaluated. While analytic methods exist to account for repeated evaluations, they are associated with considerable loss of sensitivity. Analysis intervals should be established at the design phase of a study and adhered to.

Controls

Many studies have attempted to use historical controls. The disadvantages are that patient populations may change over time, minor or major differences in treatment may take place, and worst of all, some crucial points of information may be missing. Such a procedure also precludes blinding. Collection of data on a smaller number of concurrent controls together with the use of historical controls has been advocated by some parties, but any differences in historical and concurrent controls may compromise interpretation.

Blinding

For some treatments in severe head injury, blinding of the physician is impossible – trials of barbiturate coma are one example. Nonetheless, trials resulting in outcomes other than death can still be assessed by a blinded evaluator, particularly when outcome measurements are subjective. If a clinician has the impression that one treatment is more beneficial than another, this bias can be reflected in many subtle ways.

End Point Definition

For some studies of severe head injuries, the end point can be defined as death. In many studies looking at other possible outcomes, however, end points have not been clearly defined. If end points are not well established at the onset of a study, and clearly defined so that they can be reproduced, the study will lack credibility.

Optimum Dose Levels

Any drug or treatment should be well understood before a trial is begun. Pharmacokinetics and toxicity must be understood so that the optimal dose can be prescribed. This may require pilot work, but it is essential in order to avoid later criticism that the dose, frequency, or mode of administration was inappropriate. Several otherwise well-designed studies in head trauma have been criticized because of this error.

Conclusions

Head injury is a major international problem, and the personal and social costs are great. Any improvement in outcome, whether in mortality rate, cognition, physical activity, social interaction, or employment, will have widespread benefits. It therefore behoves us to evaluate potential therapies appropriately, learning from the experiences of our associates studying cancer, cerebrovascular disease, and epilepsy.

Discussion of Clinical Trials Relating to Peripheral Neuropathies

A. K. Asbury [1]

Introduction

Two major types of peripheral neuropathy have been the subject of clinical trials. These are diabetic polyneuropathy and acquired demyelinating polyneuropathies, acute and chronic. The acute form is Guillain-Barré syndrome (GBS), and the chronic form is known as chronic inflammatory demyelinating polyradiculoneuropathy (CIDP). Hughes has, quite rightly, emphasized only the controlled studies of these polyneuropathies.

Guillain-Barré Syndrome

Of the several treatment modalities proposed for GBS, only plasma exchange has, so far, been shown to be of benefit [2]. One should be aware that, due to the design of the study, only severely weak patients unable to walk were selected for inclusion. Children, pregnant women, otherwise medically ill individuals, and patients previously treated by other means were excluded. Therefore, the conclusion of the study, that plasma exchange is beneficial, applies only to the types of patients studied. The value of plasma exchange in early, still mild GBS has not been studied. Nevertheless, the North American multicenter trial does show that plasma exchange was particularly effective for patients treated within 7 days of onset of GBS. Patients treated after 21 days did not differ significantly from patients receiving conventional treatment. Further, patients beginning plasma exchange prior to requiring ventilatory assistance improved significantly more rapidly than those respirator patients receiving conventional treatment, but those patients in whom plasma exchange was begun after they were on respirators did not differ from those treated conventionally. The lesson appears to be that plasma exchange should be started early in patients who are worsening rapidly and before they are respirator-dependent.

[1] Department of Neurology, Hospital of the University of Pennsylvania, 3400 Spruce Street, Philadelphia, PA 19104, USA.

Neurology
Ed. by K. Poeck, H. J. Freund, and H. Gänshirt

In the North American multicenter trial [2], differences between the plasmapheresis patients and the conventional therapy group persisted at 6 months, the cut-off date of this study. The failure rate at 6 months (failure to improve one grade or to regain the ability to walk unassisted) was significantly greater in the conventional therapy group than in the plasmapheresis group. But 6 months is not long enough to know whether the failures represented only slowness of recovery or fixed residual deficit. One would have needed examinations at 12 and possibly 18 months to determine the effect of plasmapheresis on eventual outcome. This and many other questions await further study.

Diabetic Polyneuropathy

Three major proposed treatment modes for diabetic neuropathy have been subjected to clinical trial, namely aldose reductase inhibitors, *myo*-inositol supplementation, and glycemic control itself. With respect to the first two, some controlled studies have yielded results which are encouraging, but as yet neither *myo*-inositol supplementation nor aldose reductase inhibitors can be recommended. Glycemic control, although exceptionally difficult to study in a controlled fashion [5, 7], may well bear a relation to diabetic neuropathy [3], and improved glycemic control has been shown recently to result in documentable improvement of some aspects of diabetic neuropathy [6].

The design of trials in diabetic neuropathy is of particular importance, aside from the usual considerations which are a requisite for any type of clinical trial. These are early biostatistical advice during the design phase and a randomized, controlled, and preferably double-blind design. Design aspects which are unique and necessary to trials of diabetic polyneuropathy are: (a) the duration of the trial should be no less than 6 or 8 months in order to allow regeneration and measurable recovery to occur, (b) the outcome measures should be clinical assessments, as quantitative as possible, of motor and sensory function and of pain, and should not rely heavily on electrophysiological measures, and (c) the patient groups to be studied should be relatively homogeneous, that is, severely enough affected to be able potentially to show measurable improvement, but not so severely affected as to be irreversible [1].

References

1. Asbury AK (1984) Strategies in the clinical investigation of peripheral neuropathies. In: Sobue I (ed) Peripheral neuropathy. Excerpta Medica, Amsterdam, pp 75–79 (International Congress Series 662)
2. GBS Study Group (1985) Plasmapheresis and acute Guillain-Barré syndrome. Neurology 35:1096–1104
3. Graf RJ, Halter JB, Pfeifer MA, Halar E, Brozovich F, Porte DF Jr (1981) Glycemic control and nerve conduction abnormalities in non-insulin dependent diabetic subjects. Ann Intern Med 94:307–311
4. Greene DA, Brown MJ, Braunstein SN, Schwartz SS, Asbury AK, Winegrad AI (1981) Comparison of clinical course and sequential electrophysiological tests in diabetes with symptomatic polyneuropathy and its implications for clinical trials. Diabetes 30:139–147

5. Service FJ, Dabue JR, O'Brien PC, Zimmerman BR, Swanson CJ, Brennan MD, Dyck PJ (1983) Effect of blood glucose control on peripheral nerve function in diabetic patients. Mayo Clin Proc 58:283–289
6. Service FJ, Rizza RA, Daube JR, O'Brien PC, Dyck PJ (1985) Near normal glycemia improved nerve conduction and vibratory sensation in diabetic neuropathy. Diabetologia (in press)
7. Windebank AJ (1983) Diabetic control and peripheral neuropathy – editorial. Mayo Clin Proc 58:344–346

Parkinson's Disease: Clinical Trials

J.K. TSUI, M. SCHULZER, and D.B. CALNE [1]

Introduction

Parkinson's disease has been one of the most meticulously measured of all neurological disorders. Clinical trials have repeatedly played a crucial role in improving treatment, and because drugs are frequently employed as tools for the analysis of biological mechanisms, clinical trials have also made important contributions to an understanding of Parkinson's disease. In this review of clinical trials in Parkinson's disease, we shall discuss the following: diagnostic criteria, design of studies, methods of evaluation and analysis of results.

Criteria for Diagnosis

Until recently, little attention has been focused on the diagnostic criteria for Parkinson's disease because most therapeutic clinical studies have involved patients with moderate or advanced disease, there being general agreement that mild disease does not normally justify treatment with the medications currently available. However, over the last few years speculations concerning aetiology have developed to such an extent that strategies for interfering with putative causal mechanisms are starting to be formulated, so that treatment of the underlying pathology now has to be considered, in addition to the conventional approaches to palliative therapy. If treatment is being studied to modify the progress of the disease, minimally affected patients are of major importance, so diagnostic criteria need to be defined. Schoenberg et al. [27], in their epidemiological study, defined Parkinson's disease as the presence of two or more of the following: resting tremor, bradykinesia, rigidity, parkinsonian gait or posture, retropulsion, mask-like facies, micrographia (after ruling out essential tremor, effects of drugs, and the "parkinsonian-plus" syndromes). They further defined possible Parkinson's disease as the presence of one of these definite signs with one or more equivocal signs, or two signs without adequate exclusion of

[1] Division of Neurology, Department of Medicine, University of British Columbia, Health Sciences Centre Hospital, 2211 Wesbrook Mall, Vancouver, British Columbia, V6T 1W5, Canada.

Neurology
Ed. by K. Poeck, H. J. Freund, and H. Gänshirt

other conditions. These criteria will probably undergo modification as the problem of early diagnosis becomes recognized more widely. For any clinical dilemma of this type, physicians with greater experience of Parkinson's disease may be able to make a firm diagnosis without meeting all of these stipulations, but experience is fallible so criteria must be set out, because there are no satisfactory laboratory tests for determining the diagnosis.

The problem of early diagnosis may be of less practical importance than expected, because the issue is mainly applicable to long-term prospective clinical trials, and here patients with probable or possible disease who subsequently evolve into another disorder can be omitted from analysis.

Design of Studies

Perhaps the first point to address in the design of clinical trials is the allocation of subjects. Patients should be assigned to treatment schedules at random, to avoid confounding factors such as intellectual ability or presence of concomitant disease. Where such bias is unavoidable, methods are available to minimize its impact [1, 6]. Sufficient replication of drug combinations (cells) should be undertaken to allow determination of treatment interactions; are multiple treatment effects additive, synergistic or inhibitory?

For Parkinson's disease, within-patient (longitudinal) comparisons are most commonly employed, where each patient receives drugs in random order, ideally under double-blind conditions. This requires sufficient "wash-out" periods to avoid carry-over effects from drug to drug. Special statistical analysis may be applied to check that no order effects are present (e.g. drug 1 before drug 2). Such analysis, "randomized blocks" in statistical jargon, provides precise comparative information on the drugs involved.

Between-patient (cross-sectional) comparisons (different patients allocated to different drugs) suffer from the obvious lack of homogeneity between the study groups; this weakens the drug effect determination, but studies can generally be improved by matching patients on relevant variables (such as age and sex), and using larger sample sizes to achieve the desired power (i.e. the ability to detect differences in treatment effects). Sample sizes can often be determined in advance for any appropriate design. To estimate adequate sample size one requires the desired significance level (P-value or type I error probability) and the magnitude of the effect which would be of sufficient biological interest to be detected with a high sensitivity. It is also essential to have some impression of data variability.

Occasionally experiments are performed on a sample of previously undetermined size – sequential analysis. For every comparative study, there is a null hypothesis (no difference) and an alternative hypothesis (some difference). In sequential analysis, a decision is made after each observation: reject the null hypothesis, reject the alternative hypothesis, or go on to the next observation. This method has the advantage that the sample size should turn out to be smaller than a predicted fixed sample size for the same significance level, sensitivity and data variability. Since there is, however, a small probability that this type of study could encompass excessively large samples, a modification may be introduced. This is known as Armitage's restricted procedure [2, 3], which terminates the experiment at an ultimate total sample end point if predetermined significance levels are not reached sequentially. Sequential methods are particularly useful when little is known about a drug, so that sample size cannot be fixed in advance. They are also preferable when ethical considerations demand that conclusions be drawn urgently. Most sequential methods have the disadvantages of requiring continuous monitoring for decisions, and of providing less precise conclusions on issues other than the simple question of choosing between the null and the alternative hypothesis.

In some situations, multicentre studies are designed. Their chief application is gathering information on rare conditions, where a single centre is not likely to provide a sufficiently large sample. The purpose is to pool the observations, which poses an obvious danger: intercentre variability. Different centres may deal with different populations, operate under different definitions of the disease, have different selection procedures, different techniques of evaluation, different follow-up policies and so on. Thus, centre-to-centre heterogeneity may become a serious confounding factor.

Another important choice in the design of drug studies is dosage. Should this be predetermined or titrated to an optimum level for each patient? If predetermined, should there be one dose, or a series of doses? The choice between a "fixed dose" and a "dose ranging" study will depend upon the extent of clinical experience with the drug, and the inter-individual variation in dosage expected to produce efficacy and toxicity. In Parkinson's disease, early drug studies tend to be dose ranging, whereas late studies can be based upon a body of knowledge that allows one or two fixed dose levels to be set, provided there is limited inter-individual variation. For example, drugs such as amantadine or deprenyl can be investigated in a fixed dose design, whereas dopamine agonists are more suitable for dose ranging studies, since it is known that the same oral intake can lead to a tenfold disparity in plasma concentrations among different subjects. Drugs that are subject to any major pharmacokinetic or pharmacodynamic variation between subjects will clearly require dose titration. Another specific problem for several antiparkinsonian agents is that increments in dosage may have to be undertaken slowly so that initial adverse symptoms have time to subside as a consequence of normal homeostatic adjustments.

Methods of Evaluation

Clinical Rating Scales. To be of value for the conduct of clinical trials, an ideal evaluation protocol should give measurements of parkinsonian features, functional disability, mental status and adverse reactions to treatment, averaged over the period between examinations. It should be possible to complete the evaluation within 15 minutes, without any expensive or elaborate equipment.

Many centres have developed their own rating scales based on various aspects of the disease: daily activities, symptoms, signs, mental status and the presence of dyskinesia. Most centres have adopted modifications of existing scales (Table 1), often combining them to take into account problems such as fluctuations of symptoms. A single total score from these scales frequently gives rise to misleading inter-

Table 1

	England and Schwab [10]	Hoehn and Yahr [16]	Webster [33]	Columbia University [8]	Mod. Columbia University [12]	University of British Columbia [23]	Bermuda
Clinical							
Tremor			+	+	+		+
Rigidity			+	+	+		+
Bradykinesia			+	+	+		+
Gait			+	+	+		+
Posture			+	+	+		+
Facies			+	+	+		+
Speech			+	+	+		+
RAM				+	+		+
Writing					+		+
Seborrhoea			+	+			
Sialorrhoea				+	+		+
Daily activities							
General	+	+	+		+		+
Dressing				+	+	+	
Feeding					+	+	+
Hygiene					+	+	+
Turning in bed					+		+
Rising from chair					+	+	+
Adverse reactions							
Dyskinesia					+	+	+
Fluctuation					+		+
Mental status						+	+ Hoehn and Yahr
Others							+ England and Schwab

pretation of clinical status because different aspects of the illness may give the same score, but may not carry the same weight. Larsen et al. [23] developed an assessment with reference to daily activities, dyskinesia, fluctuations in mobility, and mental status. They emphasized the argument for analysing separate scores for each deficit rather than a single total score.

A comprehensive rating scale for Parkinson's disease has recently been proposed that comprises scores for clinical features, disability and complications of therapy. The clinical features include mental status – intellectual impairment, thought disorder, depression and motivation. The Hoehn and Yahr staging [16] and the England and Schwab scale for activities of daily living [10] are included as indices of disability. Dyskinesia and clinical fluctuations are recorded separately. This "Bermuda" protocol is a useful broad-based evaluation which can be completed within 15 minutes.

Objective Assessment. Objective assessment of parkinsonian patients involves analysis of the pathophysiology of movement. Objective measurements are not suitable for the majority of clinical trials because they generally require elaborate, expensive equipment, and they tend to focus on limited aspects of the parkinsonian syndrome at a particular point in time. Their advantage is sensitivity, which exceeds by far anything that can be achieved clinically. They have a special place in the assessment of antiparkinsonian drugs – they are invaluable for early studies where a drug is undergoing initial dose ranging studies. Objective evaluation has been most extensively developed for measuring tremor, rigidity, speed and accuracy of movement, gait and balance.

Tremor can be measured by attaching accelerometers [22], ideally to record displacement in three planes. Electromyographic activity generating the tremulous movement can also be recorded. Whatever the detection system, analysis is facilitated by computerization. Telemetry is possible, but the results are difficult to interpret because of contamination by voluntary movement.

Measurement of rigidity involves quantifying the resistance to passive movement. The most widely used method is that developed by Webster and Mortimer [34], with a device that moves a joint through extension and flexion at fixed angular velocities. Through computer analysis, the results are expressed as the area of a hysteresis loop representing the work performed on the limb; this is more sensitive than measuring the torque alone; it is recorded with the patient relaxed, and repeated with activation by voluntary movement of the contralateral limb.

Speed of movement depends upon the reaction time (RT), and the velocity of displacement, which is calculated over a defined distance to give the movement time (MT). RT can be measured by the time taken to release a switch in response to visual or auditory stimuli. RT can be normal in parkinsonian patients, despite the presence of bradykinesia; it is a less sensitive index of parkinonism than MT [11, 32]. MT can be assessed by studying the time taken to move the hand between two targets a fixed distance apart [32]; this involves proximal motor activity and is an excellent measure of bradykinesia. Meaningful results can also be obtained with other rapid alternating movements (RAM), such as repetitive finger tapping or pronation–supination of the forearm. RAM and MT do not correlate well [29]; they probably reflect different aspects of bradykinesia.

Increased long latency reflexes have been reported in parkinsonian patients. The 50–120 ms electromyographic responses to stretch are increased in amplitude in the wrist extensors and flexors [28].

A range of techniques have been employed to measure gait. These include recording foot contact on a series of pressure-sensitive pads [21], and video or movie film analysis of limb swing [20]. Objective tests on other aspects of Parkinson's disease include measurement of saccades and smooth pursuit eye movements [30], analysis of handwriting [19] and balance [14, 17].

Biochemical Assessment. Biochemical indices of dopaminergic activity provide useful, though indirect measures of dopaminomimetic therapy. Suppression of plasma prolactin concentration is achieved by D2 activation of mammotropic cells in the anterior pituitary. Levodopa and D2 agonists produce a fall in plasma prolactin unless this is already too low to register a decrement. In parkinsonian patients, a useful measure can be achieved by studying prolactin concentrations in the plasma artificially elevated by thyrotropin-releasing hormone to a level against which the inhibitory action of dopaminomimetics can subsequently be recorded [9].

Another approach to study the action of dopaminomimetic agents is analysis of the major metabolite of dopamine, homovanillic acid (HVA), in the lumbar cerebrospinal fluid (CSF). D2 agonists reduce the HVA by stimulation of autoreceptors which decrease the release of endogenous dopamine [18]. Again, prior elevation of the level may facilitate detection of a dopaminomimetic effect, and such augmentation can be achieved with probenecid, which blocks the active transport system removing HVA from the CSF [21].

The newest biochemical technique having a potential role in the biochemical measurement of parkinsonism is positron emission tomography (PET). Methods are available for the semiquantitative analysis of fluorodopa and its metabolites in the striatum [24]. Attempts are also beginning to emerge for the study of ligands thought to bind to striatal dopamine receptors [31].

Analysis of Results

The most popular methods of data analysis are the classical, parametric techniques. There is a large body of flexible methodology available here for comparative studies, including the *t*-test and the analysis of variance, regression and covariance analysis, canonical and discriminant analysis, principal component analysis and other multivariate computations. The validity of these techniques rests on fundamental assumptions concerning the gaussian (normal) distribution of the data, constancy of the variance at different mean values, and independence (randomness) of the measurements. The methods are substantially weakened by departures from these assumptions; in particular, their validity becomes doubtful when outliers (unusually large or small observations) abound, or when variances differ widely, even without obvious outliers. Under these circumstances, a variety of approaches are available. One may begin by checking the outliers: are they correct? One can apply well-chosen transformations to the data (logarithmic, arc sine, square root) to stabilize the variances, reduce the perturbing effect of outliers and bring the data nearer to a gaussian distribution. More recent, "robust" statistical methods have been developed to handle the smoothing and analysis of "noisy" data with outliers; their main characteristic is the reduction of outlier effects on the calculated statistics. At present, many of these techniques are still somewhat controversial, primarily owing to their ad hoc quality [13, 15].

Another approach to difficult data is the application of a suitable nonparametric statistical technique. Common nonparametric methods are the sign test, the Wilcoxon (Mann-Whitney) test, the Kruskal-Wallis (nonparametric equivalent to analysis of variance) test, the Friedman test, the Spearman correlation coefficient, and nonparametric regression techniques. Nonparametric tests have proven particularly valuable for the analysis of clinical trials in Parkinson's disease because, as for most other neurological diseases, clinical scoring scales are not truly linear.

Binary data (yes–no observations) can be analysed using contingency tables (χ^2 tests). Recently developed multidimensional log-linear techniques and logistic regression methods are employed for more complex settings [7].

Correlated, non-independent observations (over time, for example) may be studied by techniques of "time-series analysis" [5]. Survival data and other measurements of time can be handled by a variety of methods often referred to as "survival analysis" [25].

In any of these comparisons, the alternative hypothesis (as opposed to the null hypothesis) may be formulated as a one-sided statement (new drug better than standard) or a two-sided claim (new drug different from standard, may be better or worse). A one-sided alternative hypothesis leads to a corresponding one-tailed test, which is more sensitive in identifying a difference suggested by the data in the direction of the alternative hypothesis, but is quite weak in detecting a departure in the opposite direction (new drug worse than standard).

The advantage of a two-tailed test is objectivity: a sufficiently large difference between the two drugs in either direction will be identified. Inevitably, a price must be paid for this objectivity: a two-tailed test is less sensitive in showing a one-way change with the new drug, since it looks both ways (is it better? is it worse?). In order to increase the sensitivity of the two-tailed test, the sample size must be enlarged.

Conclusions

While it is true that practical constraints may not allow all the goals expressed in this review to be attained, the formulation and execution of clinical trials can be a rigorous exercise of scientific and clinical technique. Because of the recent explosion of knowledge concerning the neuropharmacology of the basal ganglia, it is probable that over the last two decades more clinical trials have been conducted in Parkinson's disease than any other neurological disorder.

References

1. Anderson S et al. (1980) Statistical methods for comparative studies; techniques for bias reduction. Wiley, New York
2. Armitage P (1957) Restricted sequential procedures. Biometria 44:9–26
3. Armitage P (1960) Sequential medical trials. Blackwell, Oxford
4. Canter GJ, deLaTorre R, Mier M (1961) A method for evaluating disability in patients with Parkinson's disease. J Nerv Ment Dis 133:143–147
5. Chatfield C (1984) The analysis of time series: an introduction, 3rd edn. Chapman and Hall, London
6. Cochran WG (1983) Planning and analysis of observational studies. Wiley, New York
7. Cox DR (1970) An analysis of binary data. Methuen, London
8. Duvoisin RC (1970) The evaluation of extra-pyramidal disease. In: de Ajuriagerra J (ed) Monoamines: noyaux gris centraux et syndrome de Parkinson. Masson, Paris, pp 313–325
9. Eisler T, Thorner MO, MacLeod RM, Kaiser DL, Calne DB (1981) Prolactin secretion in Parkinson's disease. Neurology 31:1356–1359
10. England AC, Schwab RS (1956) Post-operative evaluation of selected patients with Parkinson's disease. J Am Geriatr Soc 4:1219–1232
11. Evarts EV, Teravainen H, Calne DB (1981) Reaction time in Parkinson's disease. Brain 106:167–186
12. Fahn S (in press) Methodology of drug trials in Parkinson's disease. In: Capilideo R (ed) Methodology of drug trials in neurologic disorders
13. Fienbery SE (1983) The analysis of cross-classified categorial data, 2nd edn. MIT Press, Cambridge, Mass
14. Folkerts JF, Njiokiktjien CJ (1971) The influence of L-dopa on the postural regulation of Parkinson patients. 1st Symposium international de posturographie, October 19–22, Madrid
15. Hoaglin DC, Mosteller F, Tukey JW (eds) (1983) Understanding robust and exploratory data analysis. Wiley, New York
16. Hoehn MM, Yahr MD (1967) Parkinsonism: onset, progression and mortality. Neurology 17:427–442
17. Jansen EC, Larsen RE, Olesen MB (1982) Quantitative Romberg's test. Acta Neurol Scand 66:93–99
18. Kartzinel R, Perlow MD, Carter AC, Chase TN, Calne DB, Shoulson I (1976) Metabolic studies with Bromocriptine in patients with idiopathic Parkinsonism and Huntington's Chorea. Trans Am Neurol Assoc 101:53–56
19. Knopp W (1968) Explorations in the assessment and meaning of the subclinical extrapyramidal effect of neuroleptic drugs. Pharmakopsychiatry 1:54–62
20. Knutsson E (1972) An analysis of Parkinsonian gait. Brain 95:475–486
21. Lakke JPWF, Van Praag HM et al. (1972) Predictive value of the probenecid test for the effect of L-dopa therapy in Parkinson's disease. Nature 236:208–209
22. Larsen TA, LeWitt PA, Calne DB (1983) Theoretical and practical issues in assessment of deficits and therapy in Parkinsonism. In: Calne DB, Horowski R, McDonald RJ, Wuttke W (eds) Lisuride and other dopamine agonists. Raven Press, New York, pp 363–373
23. Larsen TA, Calne S, Calne DB (1984) Assessment of Parkinson's disease. Clin Neuropharmacol 7 (2):165–169
24. Martin WRW, Stoessl AJ, Adam MJ, Ammann W, Bergstrom M, Harrop R, Laihinen A, Rogers JG, Ruth TJ, Sayre CI, Pate BD, Calne DB (1985) Positron emission tomography in Parkinson's disease. Glucose and DOPA metabolism. Adv Neurol (in press)
25. Miller RG Jr (1981) Survival analysis. Wiley, New York
26. Potvin AR, Tourtellotte WW (1975) The neurological examination: advancements in its quantitation. Arch Phys Med 56:425–437
27. Schoenberg BS, Anderson DW, Haerer AF (1985) Prevalence of Parkinson's disease in the biracial population of Copiah County, Mississippi. Neurology 35:841–845
28. Tatton WG, Eastman MJ, Bedingham W, Verrier MC, Bruce IC (1984) Defective utilization of sensory input as the basis for bradykinesia, rigidity and decreased movement repertoire on Parkinson's disease: a hypothesis. Can J Neurol Sci 11:136–143

29. Teravainen H, Calne DB (1980) Quantitative assessment of Parkinsonian deficits. In: Rinne UK, Klingler M, Stamm G (eds) Parkinson's disease: current progress, problems and management. Elsevier, North-Holland, pp 145–164
30. Teravainen H, Evarts EV, Calne DB (1980) Studies of Parkinsonian movement: 1. Programming and execution of eye movements. Acta Neurol Scand 62: 137–148
31. Wagner HN, Burns HD, Dannals RF, Wong DF, Langstrom B, Duelfer T, Frost JJ, Ravart HT, Links JM, Rosenbloom SB, Lukas SE, Kramer AV, Kuhar MJ (1983) Imaging dopamine receptors in the human brain by positron tomography. Science 221: 1264–1266
32. Ward CD, Sanes JN, Dambrosia JM, Calne DB (1983) Methods for evaluating treatment in Parkinson's disease. Adv Neurol 37: 1–7
33. Webster DD (1968) Critical analysis of the disability in Parkinson's disease. Mod Treat 5:257–282
34. Webster DD, Mortimer JA (1977) Failure of L-dopa to relieve activated rigidity in Parkinson's disease. In: Messiha et al. (eds) Parkinson's disease. Neurophysiological, clinical and related aspects. Plenum, New York, pp 297–313

Clinical Trials Relating to Multiple Sclerosis

J. F. KURTZKE[1]

The basic principles of treatment trials have been defined. Essentially, they consist of the concurrent observation of comparable groups of patients with the specified disease, treated in different ways, and assessed for a single primary end-point that defines "success." In multiple sclerosis (MS), the only way to assure comparability is to allocate each treatment by a strict randomization process. This ensures that every subject to be entered into the study has an equal chance of assignment to each therapy. If the alternative to a test agent is an equivalent placebo, and if the study is "double-blind," then, if the two groups differ significantly on the primary "success" criterion, we conclude *either* that they differ *because* of the treatment, *or* that a rare event has occurred by chance. The latter situation is defined by the probability level that is used to accept or reject the null hypothesis of no difference between the groups. If the study is *not* blinded as to both patient and doctor, then, should the groups differ significantly the only valid conclusion, other than a chance event, is that the results with a treatment regimen known to all to include treatment A differ from results with a treatment regimen known *not* to include treatment A. We can *not* assume that treatment A itself is the only reason for the differences.

Evaluating treatment in MS poses problems not met with in many other diseases. As with all, though, the goal of treatment must be defined. It is valid, for example, to assess means whereby patients with MS may better adapt to their environment, regardless of the disease. It is also valid to see whether specific disabilities, such as spasticity or incontinence, can be better managed. Each of these goals would require different methods of measurement. The aim of primary therapy, though, is to attack the disease itself. Now, we have no way of knowing in MS how much CNS tissue is involved with the disease process at any one time, but we can realistically assume that the greater in quality and quantity the neurologic dysfunction (as measured by the neurologic examination), the greater will be the amount of disease present. If neurologic dysfunction changes for better or worse, then we may conclude the disease has also changed in like manner.

We therefore require a system that will permit us to assess such neurologic impairment and the changes therein. There are a number of such schemes published. The problems they pose may perhaps be better illustrated with the specific treatment trials to be discussed. But the main problem may be illustrated by the dis-

[1] Neurology Service, Veterans Administration Medical Center, Washington, DC 20422, USA.

Neurology
Ed. by K. Poeck, H. J. Freund, and H. Gänshirt

DISCHARGE DSS	ADMISSION DSS 1	2	3	4	5	6	7	8	9	V	T
0		1	4	2		1					8
1	6	7	16	2	1	1		2			35
2	1	23	19	15	1	2		1			62
3		6	105	13	10	1	2				137
4		3	15	118	8	5		1			150
5			9	16	57	3		1			86
6				3	8	6	1		1		19
7					4	2	2	2			10
8			1	1	1	1	1	4			9
9				1							1
V		2	3	3	1					1	10
T	7	42	172	174	91	22	6	11	1	1	527

Fig. 1. Grid correlate of DSS at admission to and discharge from hospital for an early bout of MS: Army World War II series. Numbers along the main diagonal (0.0 . . . 9.9) indicate no change in DSS between admission and discharge: those above the diagonal improved and those below worsened, by the number of steps off diagonal for each locus [10]

ability status scale (DSS) [10]. DSS is a 0- to 10-step scale which was devised to incorporate all the deficits found in MS in the standard neurologic examination, this examination itself having been encoded into eight mutually exclusive functional systems. From the functional system scores and ambulation, a DSS step is assigned. Improvement or worsening would be *defined* as a gain or loss of one or more steps in the DSS between two points in time, for example, at entry into and completion of a drug trial (Fig. 1). Then, the numbers improved, unchanged, or worse on the DSS can be compared between the treatment regimens, and a decision made as to whether they differ significantly with the appropriate statistical test.

Of all the measurement schemes in use, this is the cleanest in providing mutually exclusive steps and in *not* repeatedly counting the same items. For example, there are systems that give separate points for each Babinski sign, for each spastic and/or weak limb; even for tendon reflexes. All these are really counting over and over evidence of involvement of the pyramidal tract.

The DSS also gives the best evidence that *all* the scales used in MS are at best rank-order scales – i.e., that a higher (or lower) number can only be considered "worse" than another number – for example, DSS 4 is worse than DSS 3. They are *not* true numerical scales which can be added and multiplied. DSS 5 does *not* equal DSS 3 + 2. DSS 6 is not twice as "bad" as DSS 3. Therefore, in *no* instance can one use parametric tests, such as comparisons of means, in *any* measurement scheme in MS. Perhaps all the schemes should have letters instead of numbers, so the DSS would be steps a to k. No one would infer that 2 "c"s equal 1 "f." Since this and all other schemes are nonparametric, then nonparametric statistics provide the only appropriate means of comparison.

However, if nonparametric rank-order tests are used, they must be made on the distributions themselves and *not* on the *differences* in the distributions, because by using score differences we are again falling into the trap of taking these scale scores as true numbers. While a change from DSS 5 to DSS 3 is greater than a change from 5 to 4, we have *no* assurance that 5 to 3 equals 6 to 4 or 3 to 1. That is, e minus c is more than e minus d, but its relation to f minus d or c minus a is absolutely unknown. Therefore *differences* in rank-order scores are not amenable even to rank-order tests. My own preference is to take DSS changes as better–same–worse – sometimes subdividing the first as "better 2+ steps" and "better 1 step," and then using a standard Chi-square analysis for differences between groups.

The simplest treatment goal in MS is to alter the acute bout itself. This was the aim of the randomized, double-blind, cooperative ACTH study of Rose et al. [15], where 80 units of ACTH or placebo were given daily for 1 week, tapering doses for the next week, and no drugs for the next 2 weeks (Fig. 2). Weekly assessments of neurologic status were made using several methods. Here we show the EOC (estimate of overall condition) and the DSS vs baseline; the weekly decision for EOC was whether patient and doctor thought the patient was better, the same, or worse. The DSS changes from baseline DSS scores are drawn on the right. Now both systems showed statistically significant differences between ACTH and placebo, but the differences seemed to narrow with time by EOC, while they remained constant by DSS changes. With the former, ACTH "hastens improvement"; with the latter,

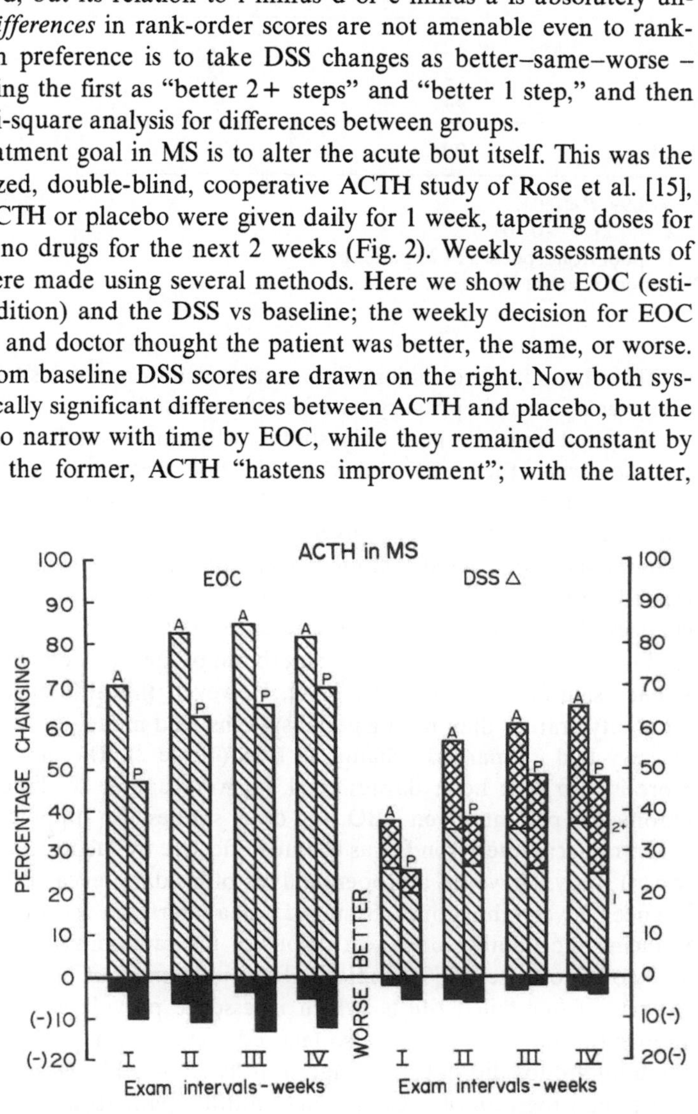

Fig. 2. Percentage frequency of patients improved and worsened vs baseline status after one (I) to four (IV) weeks of study. Therapy (ACTH, A or placebo, P) given one week (I) and tapered the next (II), with none thereafter (III, IV). Measurement systems are estimate of overall condition (EOC) on *left* and disability status scale (DSS) scores on *right*. Data of the nationwide Cooperative ACTH Study [15]; [11]

Table 1. Transfer factor (TF) in multiple sclerosis. DSS change in 2 years [2]

	Mean change[a] (±SD)	
	Placebo	TF[c]
	1.86±1.50	0.79±1.21
	Rank order[b]	
B	2	2
S	5	12
W	22	15
Total	29	29

[a] $t=2.99$, $P<0.01$.
[b] $X_2^2=4.21$, $P>0.10$.
[c] TF pool from spouses of 20 patients.
B, better; S, same; W, worse.

ACTH induces bout remission. The actual conclusion of this study, then, depends on what was a priori the primary criterion of success; for me, it was the DSS.

We shall consider here only studies wherein the authors concluded that their treatment was efficacious, and where the full papers have been published. First is transfer factor (Table 1). In Australia, Basten et al. [2] conducted an elegant double-blind study of transfer factor given for 2 years. By parametric *t*-tests of mean DSS changes, they considered that the placebo patients were significantly worse than the treated patients at the 1% level of probability. By the proper comparison of DSS changes, there was no significant difference between the groups.

Fisher et al. [4] asserted that hyperbaric oxygen was effective in MS, with a difference significant at the 0.1% level. However, the differences appeared to be in "mobility" rather than in functional systems, and in fact, only three "mild" patients at entry had a "marked" change in DSS (Table 2). The absurdity of a mean DSS score is also seen here. Barnes et al. [1] were unable to discern any difference in chronic MS patients given HBO, and other studies also support its lack of efficacy.

Intrathecal interferon B was claimed effective by Jacobs et al. [6] in a nonblinded (open) study. However, a proper analysis of his data revealed not even a hint of difference between the groups. Systemic alpha interferon was thought to be effective in reducing the number of exacerbations in the randomized, double-blind crossover study of Knobler et al. [9] (Table 3). Their judgement of "significance" was based on the use of one-tailed *t*-tests, which in essence provide a *P* value half that of the proper two-tailed test. They also ignored – even in that comparison – the fact that the total groups did not differ significantly ($P = 0.11$, one-tailed). Only when they chose the subgroup of exacerbating-remitting patients alone could they come to a one-tailed *P* of 0.04. However, as seen in the table, *all* of the apparent differences arose from one patient in the first year and one in the second.

Azathioprine was studied in an open study by Patzold et al. [14]. First it should be noted that the controls were clearly milder than the treated patients, and that this

Table 2. Hyperbaric oxygen (HBO) in MS [4]

Treated patients			Response[b]				
Entry DSS	n		None	Mild-S	Mild-L	Mkd-S	Mkd-L
6	11 (+2)[a]		4	5	2	–	–
5	1		–	–	–	1	–
4	0		–	–	–	–	–
3	5 (+1)		1	–	–	1	3
Mean	5.1	Σ	5	5	2	2	3
Entry DSS	n		Response by DSS change				
6	11 (+2)[a]		11	–	–	–	–
5	1		–	–	–	1	–
4	0		–	–	–	–	–
3	5 (+1)		1	–	–	1	3

[a] Drop-outs.
[b] Mild, FSΔ only; Mkd, 2+DSSΔ; S, short; L, long [4].

Table 3. Systemic alpha interferon (AIFN) in exacerbating-remitting MS; randomizing double-blind crossover [9]

Number of exacerbations in drug plus washout periods							
Drug first (1 year)				Placebo first (1 year)			
Patients (no.)	IFN	P1	Difference[a]	Patients (no.)	IFN	P1	Difference[a]
2[b]	2	NPP	–	1	0	0	0
3	0	4	4	5	1	2	1
4	1	2	1	6	0	0	0
8[b]	3	2	−1	7	0	0	0
10	0	0	0	9[b]	2	1	−1
11[b]	1	0	−1	12	0	0	0
14[b]	0	0	0	13[b]	0	0	0
16[b]	2	2	0	15	0	1	1
18[b]	2	2	0	17[b]	1	1	0
19	1	2	1	20	1	0	−1
22	0	1	1	21	0	0	0
23	1	0	−1	24	0	5	5
Σ	11+2	15	4	Σ	5	10	5
	Net differences 4/11				Net differences 5/12		

[a] Difference in bouts P1–IFN.
[b] ER + progressive.
NPP, no placebo period.
Not significant (P=0.22, paired t-test; 0.08 for 15 ER only); fatigue or malaise 23 IFN/2 P1; hair loss 18 IFN/0 P1.

Table 4. Azathioprine 2 mg/kg/day; open "randomized" [14]

	Results (completers)	
	AZ (*n*)	Control (*n*)
Relapse rates		
Intermittent	2.7 (22)	2.0 (31)
Intermittent-progressive	2.1 (32)	2.1 (20)
Change in severity score [a]		
Intermittent	2.8 (22)	3.8 (31)
Progressive	6.9 (6)	7.8 (4)
Intermittent-progressive [b]	5.8 (32)	17.5 (20)
(IP entry severity score)	(59.5)	(41.6)
(IP end severity score)	(65.3)	(59.1)

[a] Patzold 200-point scale.
[b] Only significant difference, AZ vs C.

difference was accentuated by the drop-outs. Their conclusion was that *only* the intermittent-progressive patients, and *not* the total group, differed significantly in mean score differences on a 200-point scale (Table 4). The big difference, though, was between their entry scores. In all other aspects the results were identical between the groups. The changes would seem even less impressive were one to recall that a 17.5 score difference is but 9% of the possible score of 200.

Thymectomy was added to azathioprine by Ferguson et al. [3], after they concluded that thymectomy alone was ineffective in MS. Benefit was claimed for remit-

Table 5. ACTH (A)-cyclophosphamide (C)-plasmaphereses (P) (randomized, not blind) [5]

	DSS			Amb. index		
	A	A+C [a]	A+C+P	A	A+C [a]	A+C+P
Results at 6 months						
B	1	5	3	1	7	5
S	11	15	10	7	11	7
W	8	0	5	12	2	6
Total	20	20	18	20	20	18
$X_4^2 = 10.90$, $P < 0.05$				$X_4^2 = 12.65$, $P < 0.02$		
Results at 12 months						
B	1	6	3	1	7	4
S	4	12	8	3	9	5
W	15	2	7	16	4	9
Total	20	20	18	20	20	18
$X_4^2 = 17.81$, $P < 0.01$				$X_4^2 = 14.67$, $P < 0.01$		

[a] "Best" R_X-authors.

ting patients, but again, the total groups did not differ significantly, and therefore subset analysis is not valid.

Azathioprine plus other agents was studied by Mertin et al. [13] in exacerbating-remitting MS. In my analysis of their results there were no significant differences between the patients and their controls, either as to DSS changes or relapses.

Tindall et al. [20] compared plasmapheresis plus azathioprine in chronic progressive MS with azathioprine alone. There was no suggestion that the groups differed – *even* by mean scores for a rating scheme that incorporated repeated counts of the same types of neurologic impairments.

In an open study, Hauser et al. [5] compared ACTH (A) with or without cyclophosphamide (C) and with or without plasmapheresis (P) in chronic progressive MS (Table 5). The groups differed significantly, and the A + C group appeared to have fared the best. Despite overall Chi-square values, the apparent benefit seemed to be lessening at 12 months, and this study was not blinded.

Contrary to this assertion, plasmapheresis plus cyclophosphamide in chronic progressive MS was claimed to be *more* efficacious than cyclophosphamide itself by Khatri et al. [7] (Table 6). In this well-done study, with sham plasmapheresis in the comparison group, the authors stated that changes in DSS were significant at $P < 0.007$ using the Wilcoxon rank-sum test. As seen, were the DSS changes themselves compared, there is no evidence of significant differences between the groups at either the 5- or the 11-month intervals. Weiner [21] had also pointed this out, but the authors insisted that the Chi-square analysis was incorrect in not taking into account the ordering of the changes [8].

My tests for several comparisons underlying their conclusions are presented in Table 7. I used the Mann-Whitney U test [18], since tables for exact P values were

Table 6. Randomized double-blind comparison of 20 TPV plasmaphereses vs sham phereses; all received cyclophosphamide (1.5 mg/kg/day), prednisone (1 mg/kg/a.d., taper), HISG (800 ml, total [7]

DSS change from entry	Results at 5 months[a]		Results at 11 months	
	Number of patients			
	PP[b]	Sham	PP[b]	Sham
B 3+	5	0	3	0
2	5	4	4	1
1	4	4	4	4
S 0	11	18	12	18
W 1	1	0	2	4
2+	0	3	1	2
Total	26[b]	29	26[b]	29

Each step[a]: $X_4^2=7.66$, $P=0.10$; $X_5^2=6.86$, $P=0.20$
B–S–W: $X_2^2=4.23$, $P=0.10$; $X_2^2=4.30$, $P=0.10$

[a] "W" combined for 5-month comparison.
[b] Excludes three drop-outs.

Table 7. PCP in chronic progressive MS; randomized, double-blind [7]

Significance of differences in rank order between regimens[a]

Comparison	z	p
DSS at 5 months	1.23	0.22
DSS at 11 months	0.72	0.47
DSS change 0–5 months	2.38	0.02
With drop-outs[b]	1.59	0.11
DSS change 0–11 months	2.17	0.03
With drop-outs[b]	1.45	0.15

[a] Mann-Whitney U-test, 2-tailed, corrected for tied ranks.
[b] Three MS PP drop-outs included as treatment failure with 1-step worsening on DSS assigned.

available to me; this should be equivalent to the Wilcoxon-White rank-sum test for unequal samples. It is not clear whether the authors used a one-tailed level of significance, but instead of $P < 0.007$, my assessment gave $P = 0.02$ at 5 months and 0.03 at 11 months. However, when three of the four treatment drop-outs were included in the comparisons (the fourth drop-out was a misdiagnosis), then no longer do the groups differ significantly even on this test – which has an innate fallacy.

We mentioned earlier that the DSS is a rank-order scale, but the DSS score *differences* can *not* be assumed to be ordered in similar fashion. If we compare on the Mann-Whitney test the *distributions* of DSS scores at 5 and 11 months – which *is* proper – then there is no hint of a difference between the groups. By the (incorrect) assessment of changes in DSS, as mentioned, there is no difference when drop-outs are included.

One last point needs to be raised in regard to the use of antimetabolites, such as azathioprine and cyclophosphamide. Lhermitte et al. [12] have been administering azathioprine for some time in rather low dosage (100 mg/day) to patients with MS. Among the 103 patients who had received only azathioprine and had been followed for at least 5 years, 10 carcinomas appeared – including five of the breast; for this last tumor this is a risk of 7%. The 10-year risk of breast cancer in US women of this age was less than 1.5% [17].

In conclusion, the only treatment which thus far has been shown to be effective in MS is the use of ACTH (or steroids) in the acute bout. This agent is not effective in chronic MS. No valid evidence of efficacy has been provided for transfer factor, hyperbaric oxygen, intrathecal or systemic interferon, azathioprine with or without other agents, cyclophosphamide with or without other agents, or thymectomy or plasmapheresis alone or in combination with the aforementioned drugs. It also appears that azathioprine may be carcinogenic in long-term usage.

References

1. Barnes MP, Bates D, Cartlidge NEF, French JM, Shaw DA (1985) Hyperbaric oxygen and multiple sclerosis: short-term results of a placebo-controlled, double-blind trial. Lancet 1:297–300
2. Basten A, McLeod JG, Pollard JD et al. (1980) Transfer factor in treatment of multiple sclerosis. Lancet 2:931–934
3. Ferguson TB, Clifford DB, Montgomery EB, Bruns KA, McGregor PJ, Trotter JL (1983) Thymectomy in multiple sclerosis. Two preliminary trials. J Thorac Cardiovasc Surg 85:88–93
4. Fischer BH, Marks M, Reich T (1983) Hyperbaric-oxygen treatment in multiple sclerosis. A randomized, placebo-controlled, double-blind study. N Engl J Med 308:181–186
5. Hauser SL, Dawson DM, Lehrich JR et al. (1983) Intensive immunosuppression in progressive multiple sclerosis. A randomized three-arm study of high-dose intravenous cyclophosphamide, plasma exchange, and ACTH. N Engl J Med 308:173–180
6. Jacobs L, O'Malley J, Freeman A, Murawski J, Ekes R (1982) Intrathecal interferon in multiple sclerosis. Arch Neurol 39:609–615
7. Khatri BO, McQuillen MP, Harrington GJ, Schmoll D, Hoffmann RG (1985a) Chronic progressive multiple sclerosis: Double-blind controlled study of plasmapheresis in patients taking immunosuppressive drugs. Neurology 35:312–319
8. Khatri BO, McQuillen MP, Harrington GJ, Schmoll D, Hoffman RG (1985b) Plasmapheresis in progressive MS. Neurology 35:614
9. Knobler RL, Panitch HS, Braheny SL et al. (1984) Systemic alpha-interferon therapy of multiple sclerosis. Neurology 34:1273–1279
10. Kurtzke JF (1983) Rating neurologic impairment in multiple sclerosis: An expanded disability status scale (EDSS). Neurology 33:1444–1452
11. Kurtzke JF (1984) Disability rating scales in multiple sclerosis. Ann NY Acad Sci 436:347–360
12. Lhermitte F, Marteau R, Roullet E, De Saxcé H, Loridan M (1984) Traitement prolongé de la sclérose en plaques par l'Azathioprine à doses moyennes. Bilan de quinze années d'expérience. Rev Neurol 140:553–558
13. Mertin J, Rudge P, Kremer M et al. (1982) Double-blind controlled trial of immunosuppression in the treatment of multiple sclerosis: final report. Lancet 2:351–354
14. Patzold U, Hecker H, Pocklington P (1982) Azathioprine in treatment of multiple sclerosis. Final results of a 4½-year controlled study of its effectiveness covering 115 patients. J Neurol Sci 54:377–394
15. Rose AS, Kuzma JW, Kurtzke JF, Namerow NS, Sibley WA, Tourtellotte WW (1970) Cooperative study in the evaluation of therapy in multiple sclerosis: ACTH vs placebo. Final report. Neurology 20 (part 2): 1–59
16. Rose J, Klein H, Greenstein J, McFarlin D, Gerber L, McFarland H (1983) Lymphocytapheresis in chronic progressive multiple sclerosis: Results of a preliminary trial. Ann Neurol 14:593–594
17. Seidman H, Sylberberg E, Bodden A (1978) Probabilities of eventually developing and dying of cancer. Cancer 28:34–44
18. Siegel S (1956) Nonparametric statistics for the behavioral sciences. McGraw-Hill, New York
19. Sipe JS, Knobler RL, Braheny SL, Rice GPA, Panitch HS, Oldstone MBA (1984) A neurologic rating scale (NRS) for use in multiple sclerosis. Neurology 34:1368–1372
20. Tindall RSA, Walker JE, Ehle AL, Near L, Rollins J, Becker D (1982) Plasmapheresis in multiple sclerosis: prospective trial of pheresis and immunosuppression versus immunosuppression alone. Neurology 32:739–743
21. Weiner HL (1985) An assessment of plasma exchange in progressive multiple sclerosis. Neurology 35:320–322

The Clinical Relevance of Neuroepidemiology

B. S. SCHOENBERG[1]

Despite the fact that neuroepidemiology is a relatively new field, contributions to clinical neurology have already been many. Neuroepidemiologic research requires neither expensive nor sophisticated equipment, and the skills to implement investigations successfully are present worldwide, as evidenced by the reports in this volume. The developments in the epidemiologic study of neurologic disease have contributed significantly to the evolution of neurology as a scientific discipline. At first, we were capable only of making a correct diagnosis and offering a prognosis. Studies of large populations forced us to establish a common nomenclature, diagnostic criteria, and systems of classification to be certain that we were all describing the same clinical entity. As neuroepidemiologists carefully studied the entire spectrum of disease in the community, it became possible to provide the clinician with more accurate information on natural history and the identification of factors important in prognosis.

Unlike the laboratory investigator, who is able to manipulate experimental conditions precisely, the epidemiologist studies disease occurrence in people who during the course of their lives are exposed to a multitude of circumstances and factors, some of which play a role in disease etiology. However, it is possible to apply carefully designed analytic research strategies to these "experiments of nature" in order to yield important clues concerning causation. In this way, analytic epidemiologic techniques make it possible to recognize characteristics associated with a high risk of developing neurologic disease.

As clinical neurology evolved, investigators introduced new therapies for a number of disorders of the nervous system, such as epilepsy and Parkinson's disease. But we required methods to evaluate both the safety and effectiveness of new therapeutic modalities. Certain neurologic diseases, such as multiple sclerosis, are characterized by a fluctuating course involving exacerbations and remissions. Hence, it becomes difficult to evaluate the results of therapy. Does improvement represent the natural history of the disease, the result of treatment, or some combination of the two? By using the techniques of controlled clinical trials (i.e., experimental epidemiology) it is possible to make rational decisions about the usefulness and safety of

[1] Neuroepidemiology Branch, NINCDS, National Institutes of Health, Room 804, Federal Building, 7550 Wisconsin Avenue, Bethesda, MD 20892, USA.

Neurology
Ed. by K. Poeck, H. J. Freund, and H. Gänshirt

new drugs and procedures. It is just as important to be able to document the *lack of effectiveness* of a new drug as it is to demonstrate a positive result.

Perhaps the most exciting era in the modern evolution of clinical neurology is the current opportunity to practice *preventive neurology*. By identifying the risk factors for neurologic disease (derived from analytic epidemiologic studies) and by reducing or eliminating these factors, it has become possible to reduce the incidence of new cases of neurologic disease. For example, by detecting and treating hypertension, it is now possible to lower the risk of stroke. The value and possible harmful effects of prevention programs can also be formally tested utilizing the techniques of experimental epidemiology.

With descriptive epidemiologic studies, the magnitude and distribution of neurologic disease can be documented, and misconceptions concerning disease frequency can be corrected. For example, it has long been a clinical dictum that Parkinson's disease is rare among blacks in the United States. A careful door-to-door survey demonstrated that this is not the case. Blacks with Parkinson's disease are simply not going to clinicians with neurologic expertise, so that the disease is not being correctly diagnosed.

Analytic epidemiologic studies enable us to identify characteristics of the individual or the environment which are associated with a high risk of disease. It is important to emphasize, however, that association should *not* be equated with cause. A particular characteristic being investigated may only be indirectly related to a biologically significant factor. There are a number of features of epidemiologic associations which suggest causal inferences. For example, one must consider whether the disease appears to follow exposure to a given agent after an appropriate period of time consistent with current knowledge concerning the latency of the agent's known effects. One must consider also the strength of the association and whether exposure to the given agent appears to lead to a specific neurologic disease. If the link between a given factor and a specific disease is consistent with available knowledge of pathogenesis, the possible causal role of the factor is more likely. Finally, one must look at the results of multiple studies to verify the consistency of a reported association between a particular agent and a specific disease. Analytic epidemiologic investigations can also be helpful in other ways. By following cases over time in a prospective study, we can identify factors which best predict disease outcome.

Hypotheses related to strategies for treatment or prevention can be tested under controlled conditions, employing the principles of experimental epidemiology. Both positive and negative results serve as a useful guide to the clinician in deciding whether to utilize a new drug or procedure.

Studies of the international distribution of cerebrovascular disease have demonstrated very high rates in both Japan and China. Investigations of Japanese migrants appear to indicate the importance of environmental factors in influencing the risk of completed stroke.

Both case-control and prospective studies consistently demonstrate the significance of hypertension, heart disease, and diabetes mellitus in increasing the risk of stroke. Despite the large number of studies in this area, there are many strokes which we cannot explain on the basis of known risk factors, suggesting that the search must continue if we hope to maintain the current trend in the reduction of incidence rates in many parts of the world.

Epilepsy appears to be a major public health problem in several areas of Latin America and Africa, with prevalence figures there considerably higher than those reported from North America and Western Europe. Case-control studies are critical in these high-prevalence regions in order to design rational programs of prevention. Many of the cases in developing countries go without treatment, and special efforts are under way to test safe, effective, and inexpensive methods of providing anti-epileptic therapy to affected individuals.

Studies of head injury continue to demonstrate its importance as a major cause of both morbidity and mortality, wherever it has been studied. More recently, through the efforts of the World Health Organization, it has been possible to begin to obtain data from both urban and rural communities in developing countries. Based on the public health importance of head injury, we must concentrate on efforts to prevent this condition.

Peripheral neuropathies which have been more easily studied epidemiologically include those occurring in clusters (e.g., neuropathy secondary to organic mercury intoxication), those with an acute onset and clear-cut symptoms (e.g., Bell's palsy and trigeminal neuralgia), and those resulting in potentially life-threatening situations (e.g., the Guillain-Barré syndrome). Among the most fruitful contributions of epidemiology has been the investigation of clusters of peripheral neuropathy due to environmental agents. The identification of toxins within the food supply or within industrial settings represents the success of such studies.

Recent epidemiologic studies of Parkinson's disease are changing long-held concepts related to the occurrence of this disorder. Although heredity was thought to play a major etiologic role, a careful study of monozygotic twins revealed very low concordance. Clinicians in the United States have felt that Parkinson's disease is relatively uncommon among blacks, but a recent community survey revealed that this is not the case. Analytic studies have been fairly consistent in reporting an inverse association between cigarette smoking and the risk of Parkinson's disease. This relationship is probably unrelated to pathogenesis, however. Smoking patterns have been changing over the last 40 years, while the incidence rate of Parkinson's disease has apparently remained stable over this same period.

When the discipline first began, neuroepidemiology was almost synonymous with investigations of multiple sclerosis. Studies have yielded a number of intriguing clues (e.g., the distinct distribution of the disease geographically, the changing risk depending on age of migration and place of migration, the cluster of cases in time and place in the Faroe Islands, etc.). To date, however, there is no single factor which can account for all these observations. Some have suggested that perhaps it is a combination of factors acting in a particular sequence which leads to the clinical disease.

In contrast to multiple sclerosis, the geographic distribution of motor neuron disease has been fairly uniform. The only well-documented exceptions occur in geographic isolates in the western Pacific. Studies of these isolates have led to testable hypotheses concerning the possible role of certain cations (e.g., calcium and aluminum) in the etiology of the disease.

As new therapeutic possibilities are introduced in neurology, the role of controlled clinical trials has grown considerably. It is no longer adequate to test a new drug in three or four patients and make pronouncements concerning its usefulness or lack of effect. In the area of cerebrovascular disease there are a number of currently used therapies for which efficacy has not been scientifically established (e.g., anticoagulants or carotid endarterectomy). Recent advances demonstrate the feasibility of large-scale clinical trials documenting (a) the effectiveness of aspirin in secondary stroke prevention, and (b) the lack of any benefit relating to stroke reduction from anastomosis of the superficial temporal artery to the middle cerebral artery.

The large number of drugs being screened for epilepsy requires efficient and effective techniques for clinical testing. Preclinical data must be utilized in the design of the trial. It is also important that one deals with homogeneous seizure types in any given evaluation. In carrying out controlled clinical trials for antiepileptic medication, the design must guard against possible observer bias and a potential placebo effect.

The many advances in modern neurosurgical techniques and the opportunities for sophisticated monitoring of the patient with a head injury offer opportunities to test the value of possible therapies for this major cause of morbidity and mortality.

As potential therapies become available for peripheral neuropathies, the methods of controlled clinical trials are being specially adapted to measure safety and efficacy. This is particularly difficult with a disease such as the Guillain-Barré syndrome, which is usually characterized by a spontaneous remission of some degree. The recent trial relating to the value of plasmapheresis in this condition is an excellent example of how such investigations can be implemented.

An important problem in carrying out controlled clinical trials of neurologic diseases is a decision concerning what measurements will be used to determine whether a form of treatment is effective. Whatever one chooses to measure, one must be certain that the measurement is relevant to the clinical course of the disease. One must also take into account the accuracy and reproducibility of the outcome measurement. Studies of new therapies for Parkinson's disease have provided a number of innovative techniques for objectively evaluating the patient's current clinical status.

The problems in attempting to judge the value of potential therapies for multiple sclerosis have already been mentioned. Objective, reproducible measurements of clinical course have been especially difficult with this disorder. To date, controlled clinical trials relating to multiple sclerosis have been generally helpful in demonstrating the *lack* of effectiveness of several suggested therapies.

In conclusion, one must be aware that studies of people cannot achieve the rigid controls available to the laboratory investigator. Because of this, every effort should be made to avoid the many potential biases which can lead to faulty conclusions. Such studies (especially controlled clinical trials) are often difficult to carry out, particularly if they involve multiple centers. In fact, the various stages in the "natural history" of a controlled clinical trial have been facetiously described as follows: (a) enthusiasm, (b) disillusionment, (c) panic, (d) search for the guilty, (e) punishment of the innocent, and (f) praise and honors to the nonparticipants. Despite these difficulties, such investigations have been successfully implemented as demonstrated by the reports in this volume.

Discussion

Clinical Trials in Parkinson's Disease

M. D. YAHR [1]

I shall limit my remarks to some of the pitfalls and difficulties encountered in undertaking a clinical trial in Parkinson's disease and offer some suggestions as to how they can be minimized. Time is insufficient to address the equally important issues of experimental design, applicable statistical methods, and interpretation of results.

Essential prerequisities for implementing a controlled clinical trial are a well-defined patient population in whom the diagnosis is firmly established; the natural evolution of the disease process known; and precise, objective quantitative methods of measuring the effectiveness of available therapeutic agents in impeding its progressive course or controlling its symptoms. Investigators assessing the effectiveness of therapeutic agents in Parkinson's disease are confronted by a number of problems in attempting to comply with these requirements.

Though Parkinson's disease is a distinctive pathological entity, firmly establishing its clinical diagnosis may be difficult. Autopsy reports suggest that misdiagnosis may be as high as 10%–15% [3]. There are a number of disorders of the nervous system which can produce a similar set of symptoms and early phases of these disease processes as well as Parkinson's disease itself may lack distinguishing hallmarks. Differentiating these so-called secondary forms of parkinsonism as well as conditions akin to Parkinson's disease, whose therapeutic responses differ markedly, presents a special challenge to the clinician. Though in a few instances diagnostic tests have been developed to identify some of these disorders and in others diagnosis can be established on a clinical basis after extended serial observation over time, there are some whose true nature is only recognized at necropsy. The use of PET scanning as indicated by Dr. Calne may well become a useful tool for resolving the issue of diagnosis, but this still requires validation. More often than not reports of clinical trials fail to indicate the steps taken to assure that secondary forms of parkinsonism have been eliminated from the study group involved in the clinical trial. With no intent of downgrading the clinical accumen of those responsible for clinical trials, it should be stated: recognition of the Parkinson syndrome presents little difficulty, establishing the diagnosis of Parkinson's disease does and warrants careful consideration.

[1] Professor and Chairman, Department of Neurology, Mount Sinai School of Medicine, 1 Gustave Levy Place, New York, NY 10029, USA.

Neurology
Ed. by K. Poeck, H. J. Freund, and H. Gänshirt

Presuming an established diagnosis of Parkinson's disease, the next consideration in assessing effectiveness of therapy is its variable nature as regards type, severity, and rate of progression of symptoms. Admixtures of the classical signs are such that in some tremor predominates, while in others rigidity or akinesia is the overriding symptom. Rate of progression for the disease as a whole, as well as for individual phenomena, may occur independent of each other in any patient; and when minimal symptoms are present, difficulties arise in assessing therapeutic effect. The implications of these for evaluating therapy are obvious. Patients with slowly advancing disease may well respond differently than those in whom the disorder is rapidly fulminant, and those in whom tremor predominates may have differing responses than those who are rigid or akinetic. It is essential that these numerous variables be adequately represented in the population chosen for study. I believe this would be a more frequent occurrence if an agreed classification which included the major subgroups were established.

In an effort to deal with these numerous and variable factors we have resorted to the following procedures. Subjects selected for clinical trial are limited to those who have been under observation for a sufficient period of time to allow the major manifestations of their disease to become fully apparent and evaluable. In this regard we maintain a patient registry where patients are enrolled, subject to periodic and uniform evaluations, and available for therapeutic trials as they fulfill certain criteria. Patients are classified as primary Parkinson's disease or secondary parkinsonism. Those in the former category are further subdivided into definite, possible, or probable. Only those who fall into the definite category are used for clinical trials. Detailed cataloging of symptoms as to time of occurrence, degree of severity, and rate of progression is performed. Further, scores on a rating scale designed to assess the overall degree of severity of the Parkinson state, with indices indicative of the extent and type of bodily involvement as well as the resultant disability (Table 1) are kept current for each patient [2]. For most studies those whose severity of disease falls into Stages 2, 3, and 4 are particularly suitable. Their symptoms are manifest to a degree that valid assessment is possible. This scheme can also be utilized to track the progression of the disease and is useful as an overall measure of effectiveness of therapy. Reversing severity by one stage has proven to be a reliable indication of therapeutic effectiveness of a particular treatment program.

Table 1. Parkinson's disease – stages of severity

Stage	
I	Unilateral involvement only, with minimal or no functional impairment
II	Bilateral or midline involvement, without disturbance of balance; minimal or no functional impairment
III	Bilateral and midline involvement with impaired righting reflexes and postural stability; functional impairment mild to moderate – capable of leading independent life with work potential
IV	All of above – severe disabling disease – able to walk and stand with assistance; markedly incapacitated
V	Fully developed disease with complete incapacity; confinement to bed or wheelchair – assistance needed in all activities of daily living

Table 2. Rated Parkinson exam

Ht .... Wt .... Temp .... Resp ....
BP (supine) .... (seated) .... (ortho) ....
PR (supine) .... (seated) .... (ortho) ....

1.	Facial expression		
2.	Seborrhea		
3.	Salivation		
4.	Speech		
5.	Rigidity	RUE	
6.		LUE	
7.		Face (lips, tongue, etc.)	
8.		RLE	
9.		LLE	
10.	Tremor	RUE	
11.		LUE	
12.		Neck	
13.		RLE	
14.		LLE	
15.	Finger tapping, right		
16.	Finger tapping, left		
17.	Succession movements, RUE		
18.	Succession movements, LUE		
19.	Foot tapping, right		
20.	Foot tapping, left		
21.	Arising from chair		
22.	Standing posture		
23.	Stability		
24.	Gait		
25.	Bradykinesia		
		Total	

More frequently used for this purpose, however, are rating scales of the major symptoms of Parkinson's disease. All of these share in common an attempt to quantitate the degree of severity of each symptom by assigned numerical value. Though differences exist among investigators as to which of the pleomorphic manifestations of Parkinson's disease are most important in contributing to disability, and the best manner of their assessment, overall there is general agreement in the design of these rating scales. Our own is indicated in Table 2. We have chosen 25 items which lend themselves to this type of quantitation using a scale of 1 to 4 which indicates increasing severity. In our hands the scale is reproducible, rapidly performed, and when expressed as a percentage change has good interinvestigator reliability [1]. A 25% improvement in the rated exam has significance as to a beneficial therapeutic effect. Validating single observer reliability as to ratings is essential and must be carried out prior to undertaking any study. This scale suffers from shortcomings characteristic of all such rating scales in that it is subjective on the examiner's part and highly dependent on patient cooperation, motivation, and environmental factors. Yet it has served our purpose well and to date we have not found that any of the numerous mechanical devices which purport to measure these symptoms in a more objective, quantitative fashion generate more reliable data. However, here again, what is needed is standardization of rating scales which will be uniformly applied by investigators.

Lastly, a comment about the effectiveness of pharmacologic agents presently in use is appropriate. Validation of therapeutic efficacy of these drugs is based on their ability to provide symptomatic relief – since none alter the underlying disease process. Their mechanism of action is primarily the reestablishment of homeostasis between the neurotransmitters dopamine and acetylcholine. This is most effectively accomplished by agents that enchance striatal dopamine activity such as levodopa or dopamine-receptor agonists. Curiously, these agents have their optimal effects during the first few years of their administration [4]. Subsequently, not only does therapeutic efficacy decline, but a host of untoward reactions become apparent. To assess these variables and determine the full usefulness of a drug in Parkinson's disease requires an extended period of observation. If such was done, one would avoid the not infrequent occurrence of initial enthusiastic reports which then must be tempered or withdrawn at a later date.

In summary, I have outlined some of the difficulties which confront investigators in carrying out clinical trials in Parkinson's disease, including those relative to diagnosis, patterns of evolution of the disorder, and methods of assessing alteration in the state of Parkinson symptoms and overall severity of Parkinson's disease.

References

1. Duvoisin RC (1971) The evaluation of extrapyramidal disease. In: de Ajuriaguerra J, Gauther G (eds) Monoamine noyaux gris centraux et syndrome de Parkinson. Masson, Paris, pp 313–325
2. Hoehn MM, Yahr MD (1967) Parkinsonism: onset, progression, and mortality. Neurology 17, 5:427–442
3. Jellinger K (1985) An overview of morphological changes in Parkinson's disease. In: Yahr MD, Bergmann K (eds) VIII Proceedings of the VIII international symposium on Parkinson's disease. New York, p 2
4. Yahr MD (1984) Limitations of long term use of antiparkinson drugs. Can Sci Neurol 11 1:191–194

Discussion on Kurtzke's: Clinical Trials in Multiple Sclerosis

S. Poser [1]

As a clinician involved with the actual work within these trials I would prefer not to argue with John Kurtzke about statistics, but let me make a few remarks from a practical point of view.

It is our hope that we can obtain a parameter of how much CNS tissue is involved with the disease multiple sclerosis through magnetic resonance imaging (MRI). At present this procedure cannot assess the state of the blood-brain barrier and the age of different lesions, but perhaps this can be achieved in the future.

For the time being we have no better parameter than the neurologic examination, and everyone involved in clinical trials is familiar with the difficulties encountered in appropriate recording of symptoms and signs and the problems of scoring them.

Any system based on a summation of signs and symptoms has the disadvantage of repeatedly counting the same items and of adding "apples and pears." The disability status scale (DSS) is an attempt to overcome this problem while paying the price of being rather insensitive to change. Sipe et al. [6] correlated their score with the DSS for individuals. A number of patients with changing signs and symptoms did not show a corresponding change in the DSS.

In a double-blind study of cyclosporin A vs azathioprine [1] we are now employing a whole battery of tests including the functional groups and the DSS of Kurtzke. It has been our experience that the DSS – even in its expanded form – is quite difficult to apply in some patients. For instance, you obtain a score of 6 in the visual system for patients with bilateral vision of less than 0.1. If they have only slight or moderate disturbances of gait, you just cannot score them satisfactorily with the DSS, which is based on ambulation exclusively in the higher degrees of disability. We feel that some kind of scoring of the original signs and symptoms is necessary in addition to Kurtzke's bifid system.

In the reanalysis of studies, John Kurtzke said he selected those wherein the authors concluded that their treatment was efficacious. At least two of the authors and their co-workers [3, 7] did not claim a significant advantage of the treatment tested over placebo or another treatment method. Others were very cautious in the interpretation of their results. For instance, Ferguson et al. [2], who tested thymecto-

[1] Department of Neurology, University of Göttingen, FRG.

Neurology
Ed. by K. Poeck, H. J. Freund, and H. Gänshirt

my with or without azathioprine, concluded: "Because of the small numbers, lack of randomization and single-blind nature of our study these data can only be considered to be suggestive, but this is the nature of a preliminary trial."

But even if we accept all of John Kurtzke's criticism there still remains the possibility of viewing the literature "the other way round": How many studies using the DSS did not give a significant result because the DSS was not sensitive enough to change?

But let us consider the case that such analyses would not deliver a different result. The conclusion that the only treatment which thus far has been shown to be effective in MS is the use of ACTH in the acute bout might also be criticized. The original conclusions drawn by Rose et al. [4] are that "ACTH hastened the evidences of improvement of symptoms and signs but it cannot be stated from the data of this study that the ultimate extent of improvement was greater than that attained by placebo." Criticism came from different sides [5] about the low dose of ACTH, the short period of follow-up, and the inclusion of patients already improving spontaneously.

Let me mention one last point. I know of no study which used mortality as the parameter of therapeutic efficacy. It is evident that this is a life-long job, but when you consider that had a study comparable to the ACTH project, which started in 1965, been continued up to now, mortality may have been the best parameter.

For everyone who is currently involved in a therapeutic trial and feels somewhat discouraged by John Kurtzke's contribution, a little comfort might be given by the following: In a double-blind study Zeeberg et al. [8] were not able to find a difference between patients on azathioprine and placebo, but both groups did better than untreated patients. This effect permits a number of interpretations. The important message, however, is clear: keep up the work!

References

1. Dommasch D, Kappos L, Patzold U, Poser S, Haas I, Krauseneck P, Malin I (1984) The cyclosporin A/azathioprine study: A double-blind controlled trial comparing therapeutic effects of immunosuppression in MS. Max Planck Society Clinical Research Unit for Multiple Sclerosis, Annual Report 2:9–12
2. Ferguson TB, Clifford DB, Montgomery EB, Bruns KA, McGregor PJ, Trotter JL (1983) Thymectomy in multiple sclerosis. J Thorac Cardiovasc Surg 85:88–93
3. Mertin J, Rudge P, Kremer M, Healey MJR, Knight SC, Compston A, Batchelor JR, Thompson EJ, Halliday AM, Denman M, Medawar PB (1982) Double-blind controlled trial of immunosuppression in the treatment of multiple sclerosis: final report. Lancet 2:351–354
4. Rose AS, Kuzma JW, Kurtzke JF, Namerow NS, Sibley WA, Tourtellotte WW (1970) Cooperative study in the evaluation of therapy in multiple sclerosis. ACTH vs placebo. Neurology 20(2):1–59
5. Schumacher GA (1974) Critique of experimental trials of therapy in multiple sclerosis. Neurology 24:1010–1014
6. Sipe JC, Knobler RL, Braheny SL, Rice GPA, Panitch HS, Oldstone MBA (1984) A neurologic rating scale (NRS) for use in multiple sclerosis. Neurology 34:1368–1372
7. Tindall SA, Walker JE, Ehle AL, Near L, Rollins J, Becker D (1982) Plasmapheresis in multiple sclerosis: prospective trial of pheresis and immunosuppression vs immunosuppression alone. Neurology 32:739–743
8. Zeeberg I, Heltberg A, Kristensen JK, Raun NE, Fog T (1982) A long-term double-blind, controlled trial – of azathioprine vs placebo – in treatment of progressive multiple sclerosis. In: Hommes O, Mertin J, Tourtellotte WW (eds) Immunosuppression in multiple sclerosis. Proceedings of the Nijmegen Workshop June 10–12, 1982 (to be published)

4 Neuroimaging

Neuroimaging: Preface

F. GERSTENBRAND [1]

The World Federation of Neurology (WFN), which follows all new developments in neurologic science and its applications, realized the significance of modern brain imaging technologies and the need to stimulate neurologic interdisciplinary influence on these new approaches. In anticipation of further developments, the WFN responded to the proposals of a group of experts in 1981 by organizing a new research group on neuroimaging within the research committee of the WFN.

In our century new imaging technologies represent the most dramatic progress in neurological diagnostic procedures. After the revolutionary detection of X-ray in 1895, it took more than five decades to develop a second way of imaging, i.e., nuclear medicine. Ten years later the ultrasound technique was put into diagnostic use. Some 15 years ago computer tomography (CT) was invented, and 5 years later the principle of magnetic resonance (MR) was described (Fig. 1).

The term "neuroimaging" designates the capacity to visualize the morphological and functional features of a pathological condition within the CNS. Enclosed and hidden within the osseous structure of the skull and vertebral column, the CNS is withdrawn from direct examination.

For a long time the neurologic examination indicated the topographical feature of a lesion, and classical radiology brought a certain degree of visualization of lesions within the CNS, but the image showed mostly a silhouette of lesion or a compressive distortion of certain structures. Angiography came closest to producing a direct, positive image; however, the increased accuracy achieved was accompanied by increase in the agressiveness of the procedures.

The capability of CT to demonstrate the geography and character of both normal and abnormal intracranial structure, without the necessity of intrathecal or intra-arterial contrast studies, has altered the approach of the neurodiagnosis to clinical CNS problems dramatically. MRI has made further major contributions in both basic neuroscience and clinical use.

MRI has appeared far more sensitive in detection of a lesion than CT, but at present the histologic specifity and tissue characterization of MRI appears to be less than that of CT. However, CT and MRI now represent the standard imaging method for in vivo neuropathology or "living neuropathology." The introduction of

[1] Department of Neurology, University Hospital, Medical School, Innsbruck, Austria.

Neurology
Ed. by K. Poeck, H. J. Freund, and H. Gänshirt

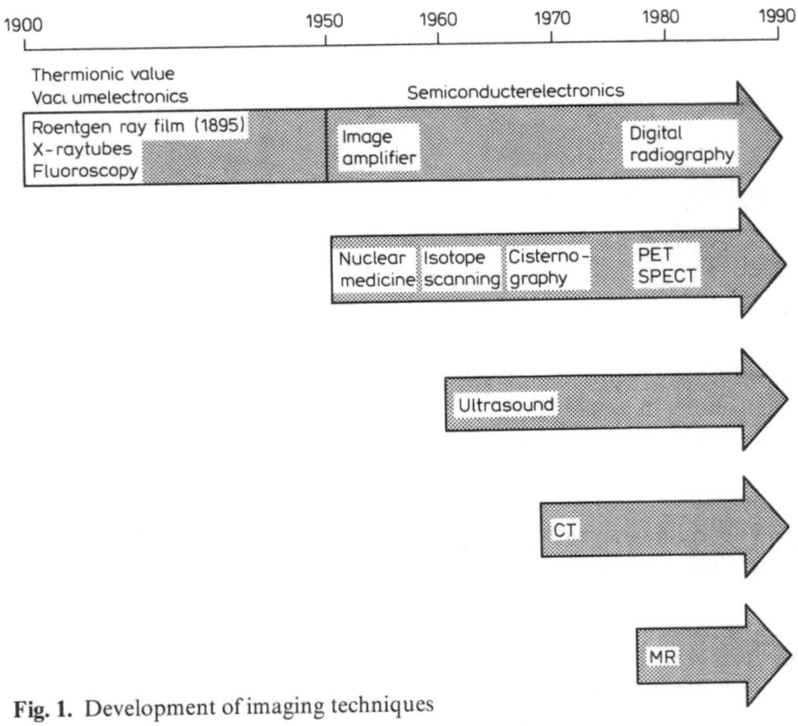

Fig. 1. Development of imaging techniques

MRI in neurologic practice has added an important and valuable diagnostic role to our armamentorium [1].

During the last two decades, clinical brain research has taken a step forward because of the development of methods for measuring regional brain functions. The practical applications of positron emission tomography (PET) in the diagnosis of brain disease are limited to tumors, certain types of epilepsy as well as cerebrovascular disease (CVD). The hopes that PET might enable us to unravel some of the secrets of the brain has attracted to it researchers in areas of physics, electronics, radiochemistry, biochemistry, physiology, and the clinical neurosciences.

In this enthusiasm, very few have called attention to the very serious threat posed by the uncontrolled utilization of this procedures to the education and training aspects of neurology, as well as to the health and welfare of patients. How frequently does the practitioner get a sense of false security about his headache or seizure patient when told that the MR scan is normal? How many patients are told that the MR scan will save them the expense of a neurologic consultation, when in fact they pay more? Is the MR and PET scan indeed better in the detection of early lesions than the CT scan? Are they reducing the cost of health care, or adding to it?

The worldwide increasing number of neurologists includes the risk of overuse of the new technologies. While in 1963 only 1822 neurologists were registered in the USA, this number has increased to 5142 in 1980 [2]. The increased and generous use of the new imaging technologies does not lead congently to the benefit of the patients. Many additional examinations seem to add little information that cannot be obtained from a careful neurologic history and examination. Many neurologists expect their patients' problems to be solved by MR scanning and every patient demands it.

There is a serious need to find a middle course between blind acceptance of the new technologies as routine investigations, valuable procedures for an individuals' problem, and experimental studies research. In the years since the introduction of MRI, a multitude of studies have described the appearance of the MR image in a specific clinical condition. Few studies have attempted to analyze the overall clinical value of this new neurodiagnostic technique; in particular no study is available analyzing the influences and implications of MRI on therapy of neurologic disorders, which seems to be of great importance. Journalists have pointed to MR scanning as the latest example of technology run amok, driving up the cost of medical care [3]. The economic concern and controversy associated with the rise of new imaging technologies will be discussed in some of the following chapters.

All these considerations and others must cross the mind of the clinical neurologist who is concerned about mechanodiagnosis replacing his skill and experience in the diagnosis and management of neurologic disease, and the neurologic teacher who sees students opt for the MR scan instead of the more traditional approach. I believe that the following papers render an important service to neurologists and their patients by soliciting contributions from various groups and scientists able and willing to shed some light on these new important problems.

References

1. Gerstenbrand F, Grćević N, Aichner F (1985) Neuroimaging. Fischer, Stuttgart
2. Menken M, Sheps CG (1985) Consequence of an oversupply of specialists. The case of neurology. JAMA 253: 1926–1928
3. Anonymous (1984) Voll marschieren. Spiegel 32: 132–134

Impact of Computerized Tomography in Neurology

W. R. Kinkel [1]

In considering the impact of computerized axial tomography (CAT or CT) in neurology, it became evident to me that a scientific approach in the usual fashion of statistics and references from the literature would not due this topic justice, nor is it necessary. There is a period before CAT (BC) and a period after CAT (AC) (Fig. 1). This capsulizes the talk completely. It reminds me of the very early period in CT when the question would come up, How do you know what we see is actually true? How many postmortem correlations do you have? It is interesting how few postmortem correlations actually appeared in the literature after the very initial publications [1]. What we saw was quickly accepted as "in vivo brain cutting." What I will present here is a philosophical and personal review of the past decade of CT.

For some 20 years I have given the final lecture to the freshman medical students in neuroanatomy at the State University of New York at Buffalo. This lecture has gradually turned into a review of the historical perspective of neuroscientists in their attempt to clinically view what was inside the skull. After Bill Oldendorf wrote his excellent monograph labeled a "Quest for an image of the brain" [2], I borrowed his title for my yearly talks to the freshman medical students. The lecture has gradually changed. CT was added to it in 1973 and more recently all the other new modalities such as positron emission tomography (PET) and nuclear magnetic resonance (NMR) have been included. The progress over the past decade with the advent of the CT is amazingly rapid considering the slow progress from the first pneumoencephalograms and angiograms.

The clinical diagnostic standards against which CT was compared in the formative years are outlined in Table 1, showing the number of special neurodiagnostic tests done during 1973 (the last year before the CT scanner was in use) and 1976 (a year in which CT was in full operation after 2 years' experience). It should be noted that these figures represent a prospective study. They reflect what actually happened at a neurologic diagnostic center without influence of subspecialities. Ultrasound midline was abandoned completely. Pneumoencephalography almost disappeared (actually completely disappearing the following year). The isotope brain scan then in vogue quickly felt the impact of CT. For those actively involved with CT a comparative analysis between these two noninvasive neurodiagnostic techniques was

[1] Dent Neurologic Institute, 3 Gates Circle, Buffalo, NY, USA.

Neurology
Ed. by K. Poeck, H. J. Freund, and H. Gänshirt

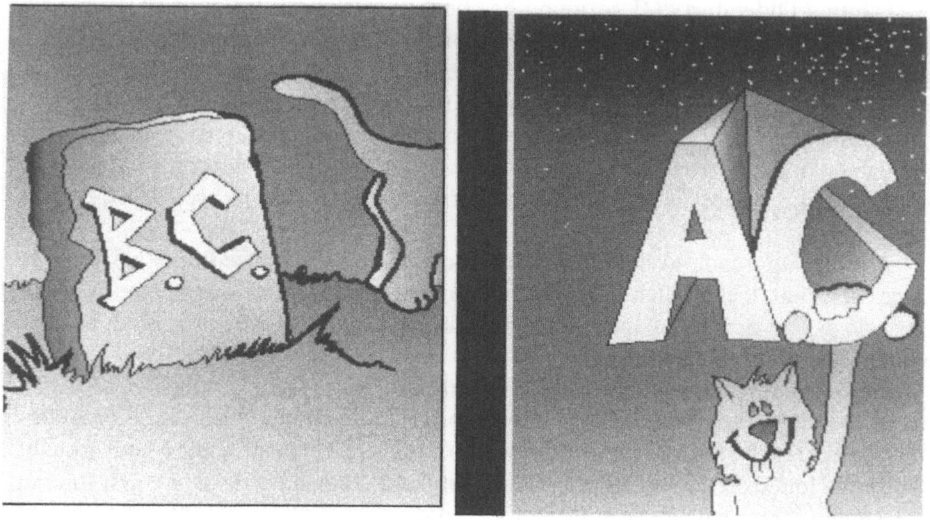

Fig. 1

Table 1. Effect of CT on various procedures at the Dent Neurological Institute, Buffalo, NY

Procedures	1973 (pre-CT)	1976 (post-CT)	Decrease
Echoencephalograms	189	0	
Pneumoencephalograms	39	5	87%
Isotope brain scans	579	157 (16)[a]	73%
Lumbar punctures	425	167	60%
EEGs	1047	731	30%
Angiograms	111	87	22%
Hospitals admissions	355	393	
Patients seen in ER	222	291	
Office consultations	668	1087	
In-patient consultations	812	1208	

The numbers below the line indicate that, despite the reduction of tests, the total patient workload increased by 31% between 1973 and 1976.
[a] Sixteen tests were required by neurosurgeons and neurologists.

not even a worthwhile undertaking. In medicine it is rewarding on occasion to have results so obvious that one does not have to get into statistical analysis to know the answer. Actually only 16 of the 157 isotope brain scans ordered post-CT were ordered by neurologists or neurosurgeons, representing a 97% reduction in isotope brain scanning after CT was available.

In this study the overwhelming reduction in the then standard clinical neurodiagnostic techniques is accentuated by the overall 31% increase in hospital admissions and emergency room, office, and hospital consultations.

How much impact CT has on diagnostic tests ordered in the neurologic work-up of patients will vary from institution to institution and over time as further experience is gained in CT.

Quoting Oldendorf "CT scanning has become such a crucial part of diagnostic neurology and neurosurgery that it is possible to compare it to shadow radiography for the orthopedic surgeon, who uses it to evaluate fractures, arthritic changes, tumors, demineralization, etc. It is generally understood that it would be virtually impossible to practice orthopedic surgery without shadow radiography of bones, and a similar pivotal role now exists for CT scanning in the clinical neurospecialties. Accordingly, it is impossible to practice modern neurology without access to CT scanning" [2].

Another approach to this presentation today is a personalized one. No proof is necessary that the impact has been monumental. Each and every one of us in neurology has personal experiences that although anecdotal cannot be denied as cumulative proof of the impact.

My first experience with CT came by chance. I was taking a refresher course in neuroradiology in New York City in May of 1972. I had never heard of computerized tomography. As a surprise addition to the refresher course they had brought Godfrey Houndsfield over from London, England, and showed for the first time in the United States, images seen using CT. It did not take much of a genius to realize that this was revolutionary and essential for the practice of neurology. In August of 1972, I was in England, looking at the equipment and from then on I was trying to raise money to get a CT scanner at our institute. This we accomplised by December of 1973; this is my AC, after CAT.

The new neurology that ensued cannot be overstated. Again to personalize this presentation I would like to just briefly tell about some of my early experiences which still seem amazing to me. As I show this series of cartoons of some of my recollections, perhaps you will be reminded of similar experiences.

A month before installation of our CT scanner in 1973, I was visiting the Massachusetts General Hospital to see their CT which was already in use. I recall vividly looking at an image of a patient with an intraparenchymal hemorrhage extending into the ventricles. I said, "the patient must be dead" (Fig. 2). In response I was told that he was very much alive and in the other room being scanned. I went in to see and talk to the patient, and it dawned on me that until then I had only seen hemorrhages in the ventricles at postmortems. The assumption that the above patient was dead was based on a false premise.

At the first presentation on CT at our hospital, one of the physicians present came up afterwards and asked me whether I thought CT might be helpful in a patient with proptosis without a known etiology. I said I would certainly like to find out, and saw the first cavernous hemangioma of the orbit (Fig. 3). This was the beginning of what turned out to be a rather extensive study of the orbit at our institute [3].

Our interest then and now has also been with stroke [4, 5]. How interesting it was to find out that many of our previous concepts concerning the clinical approach to stroke were erroneous. Probably none are more striking than our ignorance prior to CT with respect to hemorrhagic and nonhemorrhagic strokes (Fig. 4). It didn't take us long to be a little more circumspect in our differential diagnosis prior to having the CT done. Some clinical observations resulting from CT studies in stroke deserve mention. In our series of 111 patients with cerebrovascular disease, 21 had intracerebral hemorrhage. Only 48% of the patients with hemorrhage had hypertension at

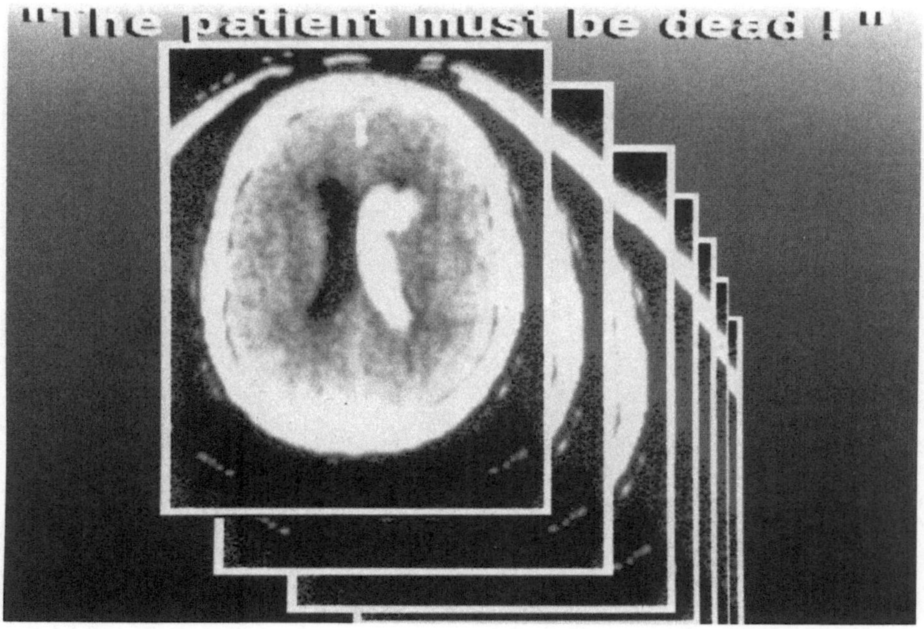
"The patient must be dead ! "

Fig. 2

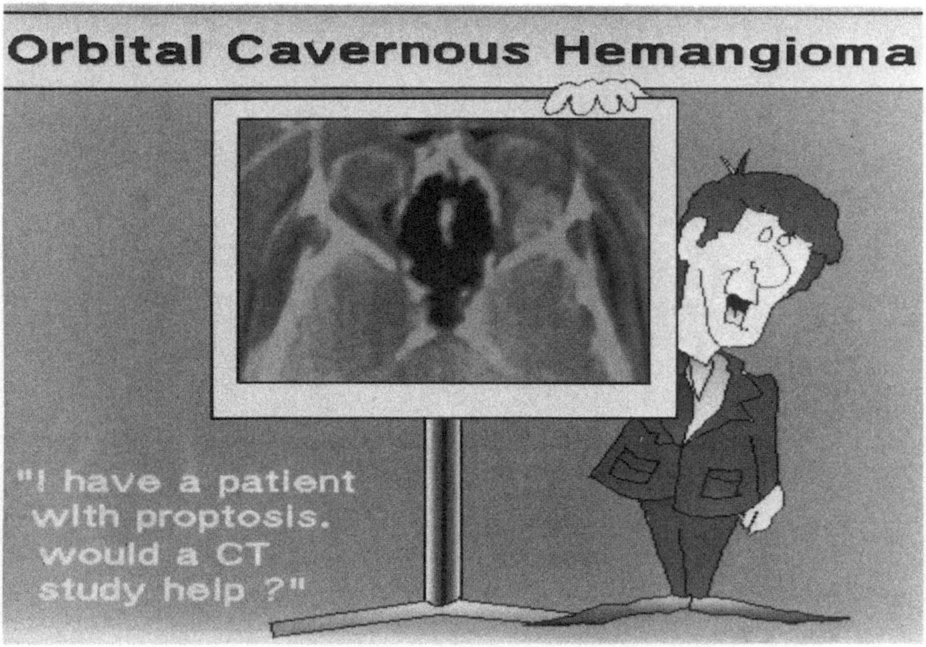
Orbital Cavernous Hemangioma
"I have a patient with proptosis. would a CT study help ?"

Fig. 3

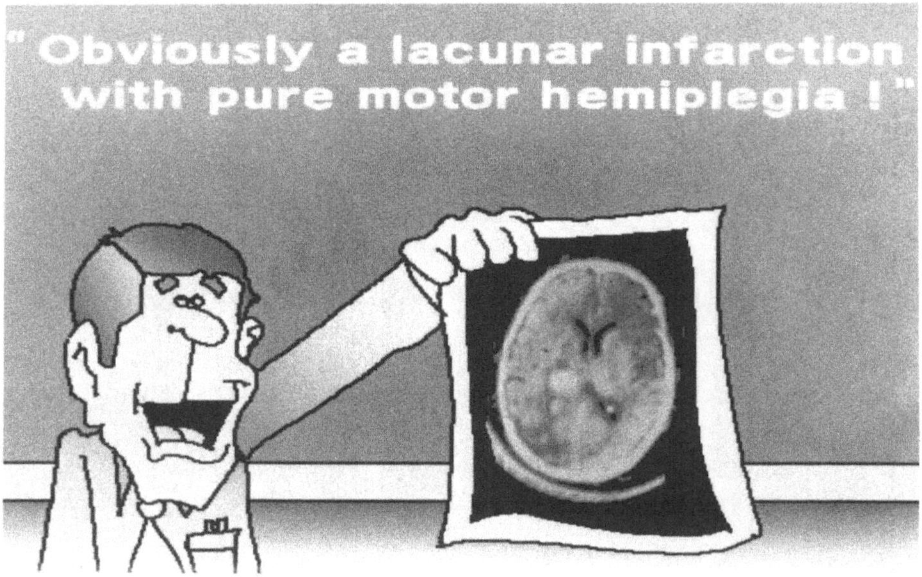
" Obviously a lacunar infarction
with pure motor hemiplegia ! "

Fig. 4

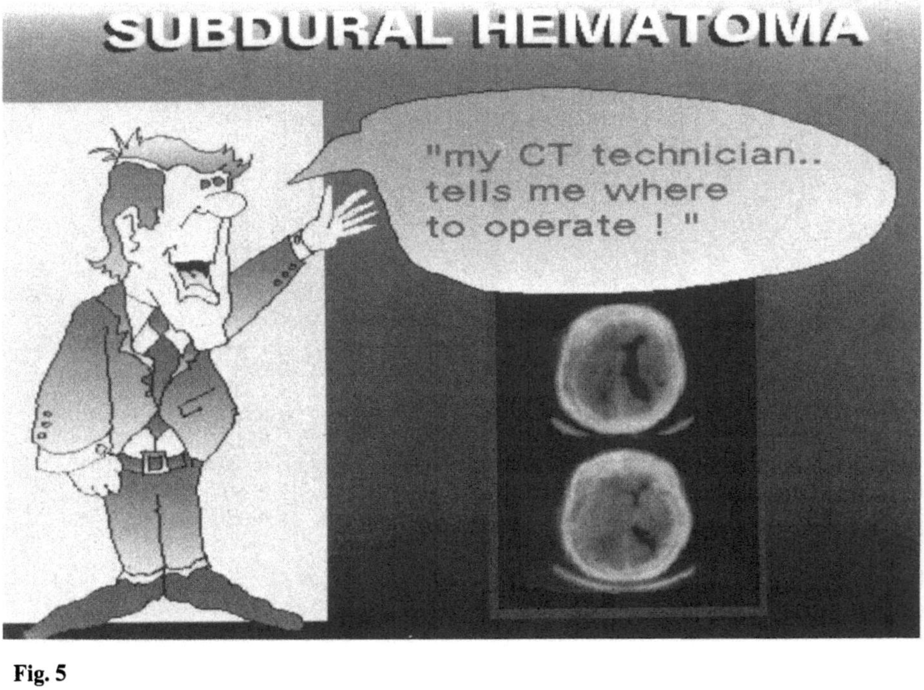
SUBDURAL HEMATOMA
"my CT technician..
tells me where
to operate ! "

Fig. 5

the time of admission, a finding that differs widely from previous statistics indicating almost all patients have hypertension. Only 28% of the patients died, a mortality far below the quoted 75%–95%. Moreover, the fact that only 40% of patients with intraventricular extensions of the hemorrhage died is contrary to the belief that such hemorrhage is almost always fatal. These surprising observations may relate to the fact that infarction was the clinical diagnosis by neurologists in 43% of the patients whose subsequent CT scan showed hemorrhage. In many of these patients, the hemorrhages shown by CT were not suspected clinically [4].

Another incident that comes to mind is a dinner party where a very well-known neurosurgeon knowing of my interest in CT chidingly and irritatingly voiced his opinion on CT interpretation (Fig. 5). The neurosurgeon really does not need the neurologist in many cases the way that he may have needed him in the past, since quite frequently the diagnosis by CT is obvious. This is unfortunately true of many other physicians who also by-pass neurologists.

Then again many neurologists believe that the time-honored and very skillful clinical history and exam is better than it really is at times. A comment that I have heard quite frequently by very capable neurologists is that if they had taken the history and done the exam, they would have found something (Fig. 6). How much have we missed over the years and just didn't know it?

In resident training the CT is all important. There is no use trying to hide CT from the residents (Fig. 7). We encourage and at times insist that the neurology residents do their neurologic evaluation and formulate their opinion prior to seeing the

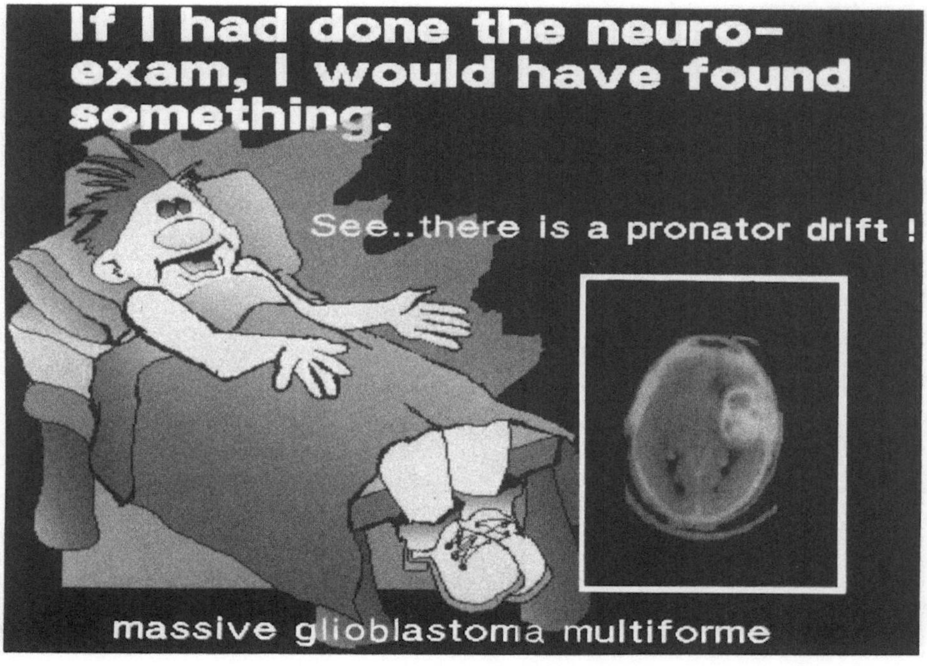

Fig. 6

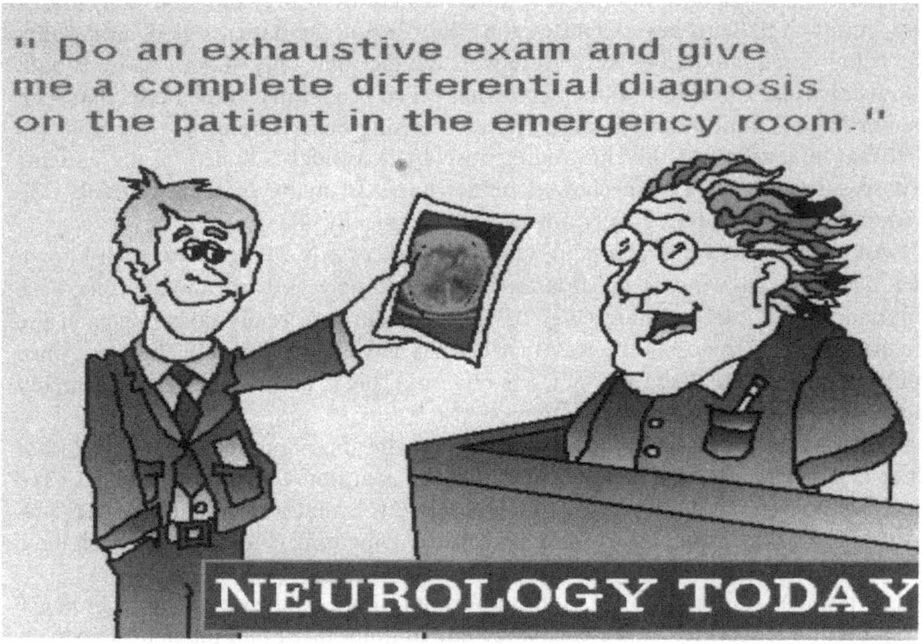
" Do an exhaustive exam and give
me a complete differential diagnosis
on the patient in the emergency room."
NEUROLOGY TODAY

Fig. 7

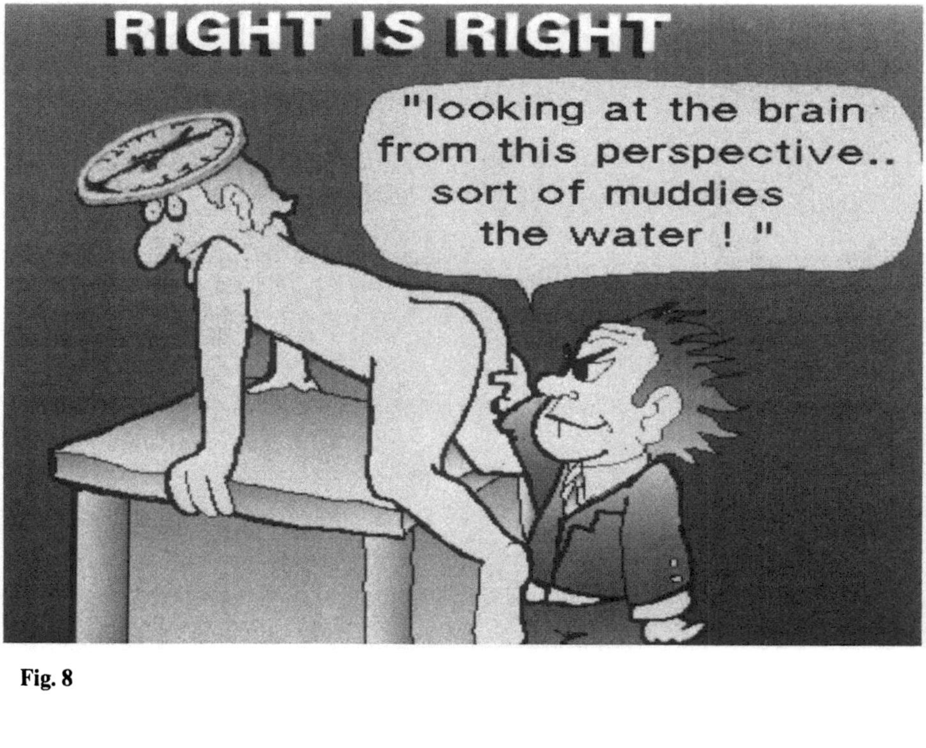
RIGHT IS RIGHT
"looking at the brain
from this perspective..
sort of muddies
the water ! "

Fig. 8

CT. The CT is located in the department of neurology with all the other neurodiagnosis equipment. The CT reading room is the center of activity for the entire Neurologic Institute.

The impact of CT has many other ramifications. One that is particularly irksome to me, and has been for a decade, is the question of how to view the brain [6]. In one of the very early meetings on CT, the radiologists unilaterally decided that the brain should be viewed as a proctologist would view it (Fig. 8). I am amazed how many neurologists tolerate this ridiculous approach. In the United States it has raised a very serious question to neurosurgeons. With multiple hospitals being serviced and viewing CT in two perspectives, there unfortunately are a significant number of operations recorded that have been done on the wrong side of the brain.

One really has to mention also yet another ramification, namely the political bureaucratic problems that have occurred not only in the United States but all over the world concerning this diagnostic tool unjustly labeled as super expensive. There can be no question that CT has saved more money than it has cost and more importantly has helped more people than could have been helped without it. In the United States CT and a national health-planning system were developed at the same time. Out of some of the chaos that ensued there is one incident I would like to share with you. In the State of New York there were no rules or regulations for the first CT scanner to be installed in the state and in typical bureaucratic fashion, the government insisted that we lead-line the CT room in spite of all scientific facts to the contrary. This led to the president of our medical staff referring to the new installation at the Dent Institute as Kinkel's CAT house, the only lead-lined CAT house in the world (Fig. 9).

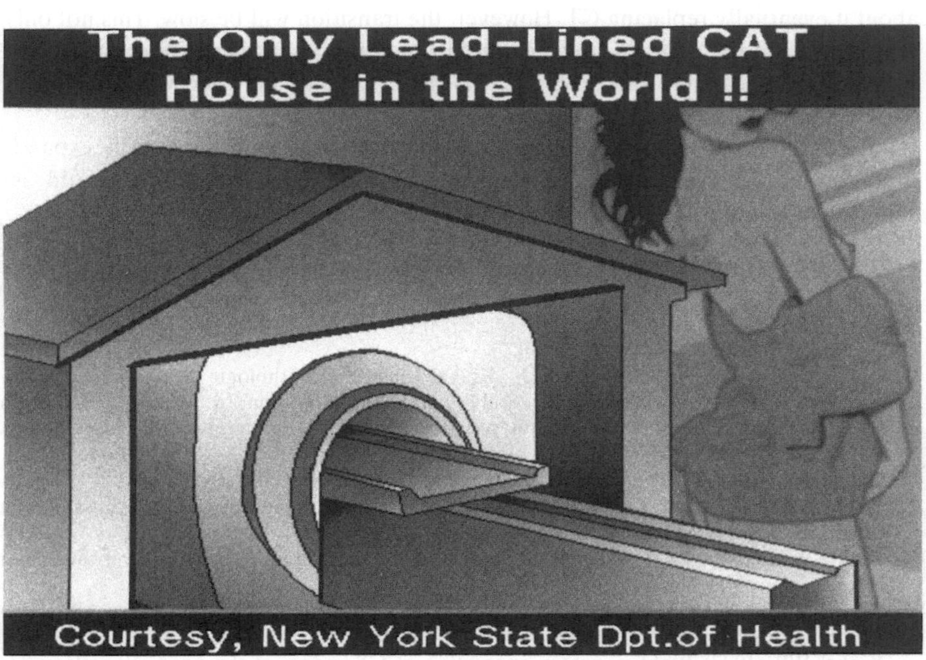
The Only Lead-Lined CAT
House in the World !!
Courtesy, New York State Dpt.of Health

Fig. 9

The State of New York is keeping up its reputation however now that we enter the new era of NMR. Contrary to what is known about NMR and to be sure that NMR is of some clinical value for the State of New York (forgetting about the other states in the Union and the rest of the world), and also to protect the health costs in the state, they have allowed only the very expensive big super-conducting magnets to be used on a trial basis.

In conclusion, the impact of CT has been monumental and in its brief decade has changed the approach of the neurosciences in the study of the brain. We as neurologists cannot afford to be left behind, but we have been. In this sense there has been a negative impact on neurology. Although numerous battles have and still are taking place to keep the study of the central nervous system in the hands of those physicians who have specifically trained themselves in the neurosciences, for reasons often out of our control all over the world neurology as a specialty of medicine has too often been the loser. We must insist that CT be emphasized in our neurology residency training programs and that neurologists be actively involved in this subspecialty of neurology. The examinations given neurology residents should include CT in as much detail as the other neurology subspecialties covered. It is imperative that a fully trained neurologist be able to interpret CT scans equal to any other clinical subspecialty of the neurosciences, and much better than physicians that have not been specifically trained in the clinical neuroscience subspecialties.

In our "quest for an image of the brain" we are again standing where we were a decade ago with the introduction of the revolutionary CT scanner. The introduction of NMR however has not been quite as dramatic as CT, because CT already exists. This time we are not, for example, comparing CT with isotope brain scanning. However, after over 2½ years' experience with NMR, there is no question in our minds about it eventually replacing CT. However, the transition will be slow. This not only relates to economic factors and health care controls, but also to the established worldwide CT scanners and experience. NMR is in its infancy and will take longer to develop.

To survive as a subspecialty, neurology must catch up with the rapidly expanding scientific achievements in neuroimaging. Furthermore, neurology should assume a leadership role.

References

1. Kinkel WR, Jacobs L, Heffner RR Jr, Kinkel PR (1981) Pathologic correlations of computerized tomographic images in cerebral ischemia and infarction. In: Moossy J, Reinmuth OM (eds) Proceedings of the twelfth research conference on cerebral vascular disease. Raven, New York, pp 157–180
2. Oldendorf WH (1980) The quest for an image of the brain. Raven, New York
3. Jacobs L, Weisberg LA, Kinkel WR (1980) Computerized tomography of the orbit and sella turcica. Raven, New York
4. Kinkel WR, Jacobs L (1976) Computerized axial transverse tomography in cerebrovascular disease. Neurology 26:924–930
5. Kinkel WR (1983) Computerized tomography in clinical neurology. In: Baker AB, Baker LH (eds) Clinical neurology. Harper and Row, Philadelphia, pp 1–115
6. Kinkel WR (1977) Right is right – orientation of CT images of the head. Neurology 27/No 1:98

Transition from Computer Tomography to Nuclear Magnetic Resonance Scanning

W. OLDENDORF

Since it became commercially available in 1973, X-ray computer (axial) tomography (CT) scanning has revolutionized the practice of neurology and neurosurgery because it has allowed direct visualization of brain tissue structures without the introduction of any significantly toxic contrast media. A CT scan is actually a map of specific gravity, the local tissue density. Bone appears white because it is significantly more dense than brain tissue. Brain tissue in turn is slightly more dense than the cerebrospinal fluid which fills the ventricles and the subarachnoid space. Within the hemispheres, white matter appears darker since it is slightly less dense than the surrounding gray matter.

There is just enough difference in specific gravity of the various brain tissues that some structural correlations can be made, and different pathological lesions may be less dense or more dense than healthy brain. By noting the shape, size, and location of the lesion, and whether it is less or more dense than the healthy brain, much clinically valuable information can be inferred.

Remarkable as the X-ray CT scanner is, it represents a map of local tissue density, and only that. It is limited technically because X-rays, which serve as a probe of the tissues, can have only very simple interactions with tissues. We might imagine three X-rays entering the head, on a path which would take them to an X-ray detector if nothing within the tissues interfered with them. The first X-ray persists in its path to the detector. The second X-ray is deflected by an elastic collision with one of the electrons of a tissue atom; this is Compton scatter. The X-ray in this case is deflected through enough of an angle that it misses the detector; the detector is then able to tell the computer to which it is attached that the X-ray beam has lost an X-ray. The third X-ray is in a full collision with an electron in a brain atom; its energy is completely lost to this electron, and the X-ray disappears. This is called photoelectric capture. This X-ray also fails to arrive at the detector.

Whether it is a Compton or a photoelectric interaction, neither of the latter two X-rays arrive at the detector. In CT scanning (and traditional radiography), X-rays of a relatively high energy are used; high energy is required to ensure that some of the X-rays will completely traverse the body. According to the laws of physics, for

[1] The Centre of the Health Science, Los Angeles, CA 90024, USA.

Neurology
Ed. by K. Poeck, H. J. Freund, and H. Gänshirt

an X-ray of this high energy to be photoelectrically captured requires an atom of high atomic number. Body tissues are made up largely of light elements: carbon, hydrogen, oxygen, phosphorus, and calcium. The interaction of X-rays with these elements is largely by Compton scatter. Since the Compton interaction is directly proportional to the mass through which the X-ray passes, the final computer map in an uncontrasted scan is very closely a map of specific gravity of the tissues.

When heavy atoms such as iodine are introduced into the brain after intravenous injection of a contrast medium, a significant amount of photoelectric capture of these energetic X-rays occurs; this capture is in addition to the Compton interaction due to the ordinary atoms making up the tissues. In the uncontrasted scan, almost all of the deletion of X-rays from the beam is by Compton interaction; and in the contrasted scan, there is an additional photoelectric interaction due to the iodine in the tissues. In the contrasted scan, the CT image consists of a map of specific gravity on which is superimposed an image of the distribution of the iodine.

The interaction of X-rays with tissues is therefore correspondingly simple, being either by capture or by deflection, and the possible diagnostic strategies for learning about brain by X-rays are quite simple. As we proceed, and see the complex interactions of magnetic fields with tissues, we will be able to make the comparison that X-ray CT is to the simple game of checkers as nuclear magnetic resonance (NMR) is to chess. This comparison suggests the much more complex strategies possible with NMR.

NMR involves the interaction of a magnet and a magnetic field. The most familiar magnet is a compass needle, the most familiar magnetic field is the earth's field, and the most familiar interaction of the two is the alignment of a compass needle directed toward the north and south magnetic poles. The earth's field comes out of a relatively small region at the magnetic poles, spreads out through space and over the surface of the earth, and converges on the other magnetic pole. For this reason, the strength of the magnetic field on the surface of the earth is not constant, being maximal at the poles and lowest at the equator. The common unit of magnetic field strength is the gauss; at the equator the field strength is about 0.3 gauss, progressively increasing as one travels toward, for instance, the north pole, where it is about 0.7 gauss. This gradual transition from one field strength to another is an example of a magnetic field gradient, or simply a magnetic gradient. Field gradients are the key to NMR imaging since they allow localization of the "compass needles" in the body by relating resonant frequency to position in space.

If a compass needle were taken to the equator, allowed to align itself north and south, and then pulled off center and released, the earth's magnetic field would pull it back toward north. It would then overshoot and oscillate back and forth at some particular frequency that depends upon its size and other physical characteristics.

Suppose a magnet of a particular size oscillates at the equator at one cycle per second or one hertz. This same magnet carried north to higher latitudes would be found to oscillate at a progressively higher frequency. The frequency of this oscillation is directly proportional to the field strength in which the compass finds itself. If it oscillated at one hertz at the equator, it would oscillate at about 2.3 hertz at the magnetic pole, where the field is about 2.3 times stronger than at the equator. At points in between the pole and equator, the compass would oscillate at intermediate frequencies, depending on the steepness of the earth's magnetic gradient. The compass needle could, theoretically, be used as a navigational aid. Its frequency of oscillation, or resonant frequency, would indicate the parallel of latitude on which it was located.

Since any one of these compasses is itself a magnet, a voltage would be induced in a coil of wire (antenna) placed near it, as the needle swung back and forth. If one were to remove this antenna to some great distance, such as in a stationary orbit, no single compass needle could be expected to induce a measurable voltage in it. However, if many compasses were set in motion simultaneously, and remained synchronized in their swings, it should be possible, with enough compasses, to detect their combined signals, even at a great distance.

In this model, all of the basic components of NMR scanning are represented: compass needles which align themselves with a strong orienting magnetic field, a means of generating this field with its gradients (together with a mechanism for kicking these compases off alignment simultaneously), and a method for detecting their subsequent oscillations.

In the body, the "compass needle" of greatest interest is the nucleus of the hydrogen atom. The hydrogen nucleus consists of one proton; often in discussing NMR, "proton" is used interchangeably with "hydrogen nucleus." The hydrogen atom is the commonest atom in the body. In brain it makes up, by number, roughly two-thirds of all of the brain atoms. Because they are so numerous, the hydrogens in brain water are of greatest interest; it is these hydrogens that are imaged in NMR.

A magnetic field is always the result of moving electrical charges. Within the hydrogen nucleus, there is a positive charge at some position. The hydrogen nucleus is spinning about an axis. The positive charge, being somewhere off this axis, is carried in an approximately circular path. As a result, it generates a magnetic field, identical in principle to a loop of wire carrying negative charges (electrons) in a circular path.

The following is a listing of the major components of an NMR scanner. The first requirement is for a very strong and very uniform main orienting magnetic field. This is several thousand times stronger than the earth's magnetic field, and in some machines may be as much as 15000 gauss. Usually, though, it is of the order of 1500 to 5000 gauss. To this main, uniform field, secondary, nonuniform fields are added. These secondary fields are much weaker than the main field, and serve to partially cancel or add to it, thus creating gradients in different directions. In this way a gradient, typically 1% of the main field, can be created between one edge of a body section and the other. With a main field of perhaps 1000 gauss, for instance, the addition of secondary fields would produce a gradient with 1000 gauss on one edge, and increasing to 1010 gauss on the other.

An excitation coil is also required to kick the hydrogen nuclei out of alignment with the main field. This excitation coil is on only about 1% of the time, in a series of pulses. These pulses are quite intense, but the total amount of power put into the body by the excitation coils is actually quite small, because they are on for such a short period of time. A receiving coil is also necessary, to pick up the signal put out after the excitation coil is turned off. A short-wave receiver is needed to amplify these very feeble signals, and finally a computer with software and display are necessary to reconstruct the image of the inside of the body from these signals.

The physical appearance of an NMR scanner is somewhat like that of a CT scanner, the major obvious difference being the shape of the gantry. The gantry of an

NMR scanner is a relatively long cylindrical tube, perhaps three times as long as the thickness of an X-ray CT gantry. The patient is relatively inaccessible while in the scanner. Associated with the scanner are a computer, a control console, and a complex of power supplies and amplifiers providing current to the various coils in the gantry. In the NMR gantry, there is no X-ray tube.

The magnetic gradients are turned on and off in a complex cycle which is synchronized with the excitation pulses. This allows the localization of hydrogen within the body. Excitation coils, which transmit radio frequency energy into the tissues, are wrapped around the part to be examined. Because the transmission occurs only for brief periods, in pulses, these same coils can serve as receiver coils to pick up the signal that comes back out of the body after the excitation pulse throws the hydrogens out of alignment with the main field.

There is entirely different shielding required for an NMR gantry than for an X-ray CT gantry. Since there are no X-rays or other ionizing radiations emitted by the NMR gantry, no dense lead shielding is required. However, shielding from radio frequency short-wave signals is necessary, both to prevent the NMR gantry coils from interfering with other electronic devices in the building and to keep extraneous radio frequency signals from being mixed with the feeble imaging signals coming out of the body.

Using multiple applied pulses it is possible to emphasize the two factors determining the observed rate of decay of the emitted radio frequency signal. These factors, T_1 and T_2, provide information about tissue characteristics.

Current Status of NMR Imaging

In mid-1985 there are approximately 200 NMR scanners in operation, about 60% of them in the USA. There are approximately 7000 CT scanners, but there is some evidence that the USA market for these is weakening, largely due to restriction in hospital reimbursements. Many state-of-the-art CT scanners are being offered at substantially lower prices than 2 years ago. Some of this trend in CT sales is the result of concern on the part of potential customers over the immediate future of NMR and the possible unpredictable obsolescence of CT scanners before they are paid for.

Purchasers of new, state-of-the-art NMR scanners feel intimidated by the complexity of the theory and practice of scanning. An NMR scanner costs roughly twice as much (installed) as a CT scanner. The throughput of patients is about half that of a CT scanner. Its upkeep is two to three times as expensive, and interpretation of its image is perhaps 5–10 times more complex. Much of this complexity of interpretation can be simplified if the NMR scanner is treated like a fifth-generation CT scanner, and it is used simply as an indicator of morphology with the additional ability to make high resolution sections directly in coronal and sagittal planes.

The unfortunate reversal of left and right head images is being perpetuated in NMR scanning as it was short-sightedly introduced into CT.

Future Directions of Clinical Applications of NMR

Most of the research efforts in clinical applications have been directed toward elaborating on weighted T_1 and T_2 images for tissue characterization. There are several other areas which are likely to be fruitful.

The rapid movement of blood, particularly arterial and cardiac, makes it visible as a low signal region and thus offers great potential for arteriography. With further progress in respiratory and heart motion gating, visualization of the blood in the major coronary arteries could become routine. In the head, thick sections (4–5 cm) which would allow continuity in following the undulating course of an arterial tree, and pulse sequencing to emphasize blood movement, could probably replace much invasive arteriography.

Bone marrow has never been globally accessible to any means of assessment, even postmortem. Its ready accessibility in NMR imaging should spawn a new field of interest to hematologists. Are some myelogenous leukemias regional early in their course?

Cortical bone is usually considered as producing no signal because of its reputed low hydrogen content. This is true if the matrix display is windowed for soft tissue detail. Cortical bone has, however, 12%–13% water content (in the human adult) with up to 25% in childhood. This is in addition to the hydrogen content of collagen and other organics in bone. This should offer many possibilities of characterizing cortical bone and its many disease states.

Chemical shift hydrogen spectra (proton spectra) should be of enormous benefit in characterizing tissues. The lactate buildup in brain and heart ischemia is immediate. By suppressing water hydrogens, other chemically shifted peaks become recognizable. The three methyl hydrogens of lactate accumulate to 20–30 mM in dangerously ischemic tissues; the high efficiency with which hydrogen nuclei resonate will probably cause lactate mapping to become of value. It appears that the imaging of ordinary sodium will offer an early indicator of ischemia.

Specialized surface coils will be developed to provide high resolution images and measurements in small anatomical regions. They could include orbit, sella turcica, posterior fossa, and spine.

Patient movement is probably the limiting factor in spatial resolution with modern NMR scanners. In a sick hospitalized population, limited attention span, respiratory difficulties, pain, etc., would cause 25%–50% of patients to be unscannable. One must be cautious in assessing commercial images which usually are made on healthy or chronically ill patients who can lie still for the prolonged scan periods currently required. Some method which will monitor patient movement and, through the computer, correct for it, probably will be forthcoming.

Prices of scanners will come down, probably through refinement of systems based on resistive and permanent magnets. It is quite possible that, a decade hence, the commonest NMR scanner in clinical use will have a main field strength in the range of only 200–500 gauss (0.02–0.05 T).

There is a turf battle now being waged in the USA between nuclear medicine, radiology, and other disciplines in which NMR is of great interest (such as those concerned with the nervous system). The attempt to introduce the term magnetic resonance imaging (MRI) emphasizes the imaging aspect and minimizes the nuclear medicine aspect. For greatest simplicity, the term "magnetic tomography" (MT) should probably be used since neither "nuclear" nor "resonance" is relevant to everyday usage. To abolish this purposeless battle we must recognize that all of the clinicians involved are physicians first and disciples of a specialty second. There is an urgent need for some ethical statesmanship by the involved factions.

This is a field with such enormous complexity that it is unsure where it will go, technically or politically. The diagnostic potential and complexity of NMR are so great that it is uncertain at present if it appropriately falls within any current specialty. It is not inherently a radiological device because there is no ionizing radiation. It may be in order to form an entirely new specialty which, like nuclear medicine, would be fully interdisciplinary.

Correlative Neuropathology in Neuroimaging

N. GRČEVIĆ[1]

The ultimate goal of clinical examination is identification of the pathological background of a particular clinical picture or syndrome. In this process the *inspection*, i.e., the visualization of the morphological features of the pathological lesions is a very desirable and extremely informative category. Pathological anatomy has traditionally been the main descriptor of morphological phenomena of the disease processes and creator of criteria for classification and nomenclature of diseases. Since clinical "inspection" is based on morphology, it is logical that it should follow the principles and approaches of pathological anatomy to the diagnostic conclusions. This applies to superficial processes accessible to direct inspection as well as deep lesions accessible to endoscopic procedures. Thus, the correlation with pathology is practically integrated in every clinical examination in which the pathological process is exposed to visualization. Medicine has always tried to invent the methods of visualization of the processes hidden in the depths of the body, in the regions which are not accessible to the direct or indirect visual inspection.

A great revolution in this respect was the introduction of radiology. As soon as the first X-ray recording of an otherwise hidden process became available, a correlative pathological approach to its identification received immediate attention. As better image and more details were demonstrated, more pathological correlations became possible and were practically employed.

Unable to enter the skull or vertebral canal unaggressively, i.e., unable to apply any method of inspection of the pathological process within the CNS, neurology has traditionally strived to develop indirect methods of identification of such a process. In spite of an impressive progress in clinical neurophysiology and neurobiochemistry, the lack of practically any reliable visual information about the pathological process in the CNS kept neurological examination defective in a very important aspect: the identification of the pathological background of the clinical syndrome. The X-ray, by the native recording gave little morphological information, but the application of air and the contrast media brought forth a certain degree of visualization. Another step forward was gamma scintigraphy, but the morphological information was still limited in scope and details. An entirely new horizon opened with the introduction of computerized axial tomography (CT), which provided the

[1] Department of Neuropathology, Clinical Medical Center, 41000 Zagreb, Yugoslavia.

Neurology
Ed. by K. Poeck, H. J. Freund, and H. Gänshirt

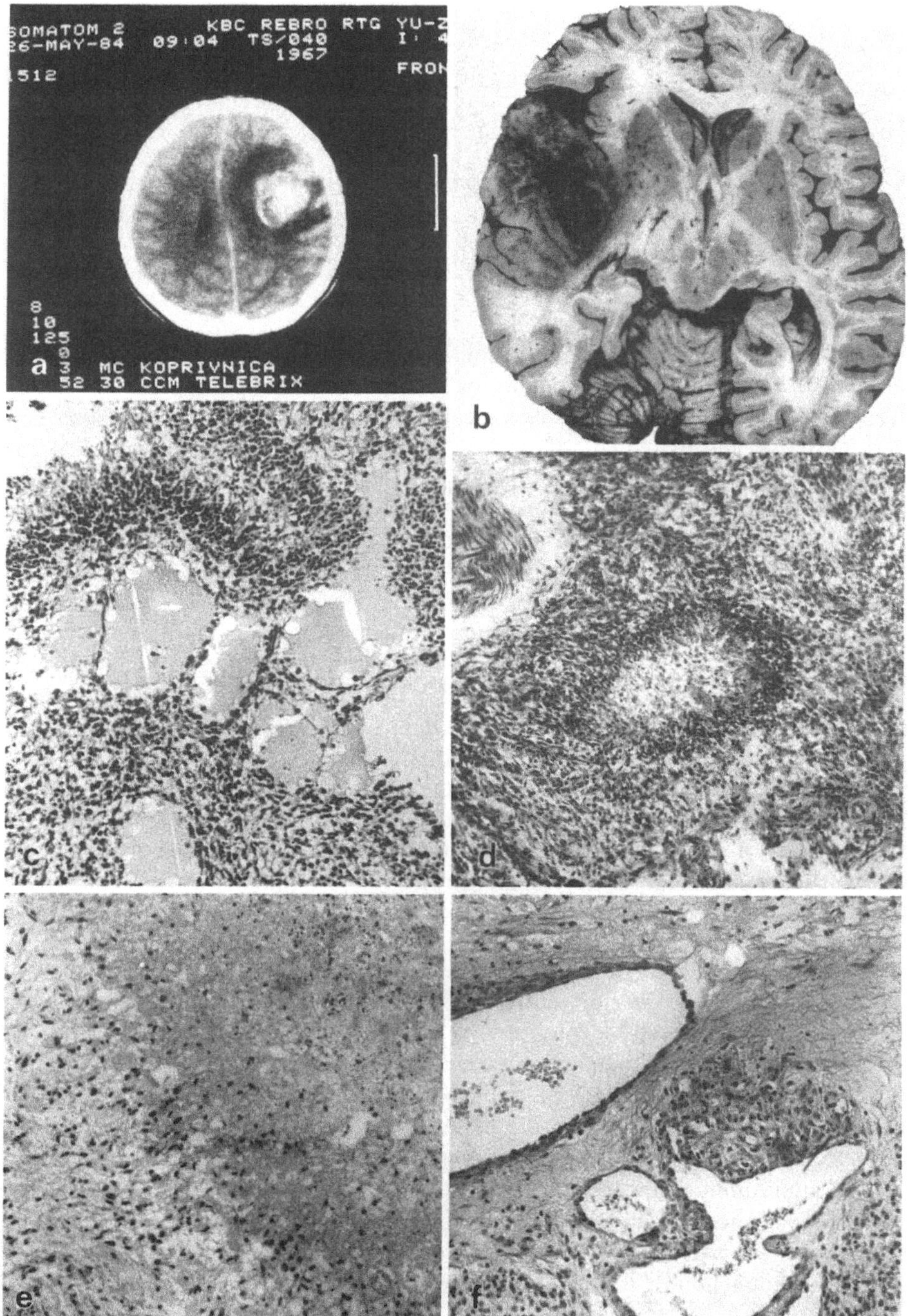

Fig. 1 a–f. Glioblastoma. Variegated structure with microcysts (**c**), necrosis (**d, e**), edema (**e**), and pathologic vascularization (**f**)

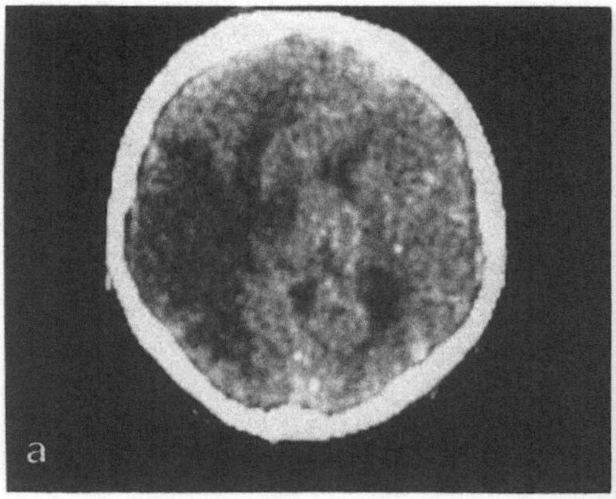

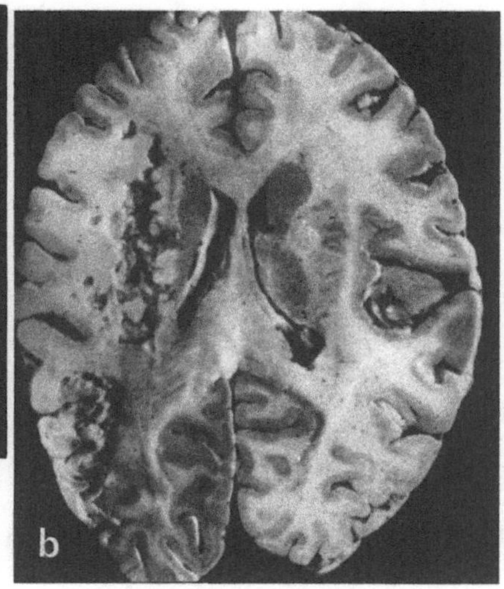

Fig. 2a, b. Large ischemic infarction in the acute stage (**a**), and subacute stage 12 days afterwards (**b**)

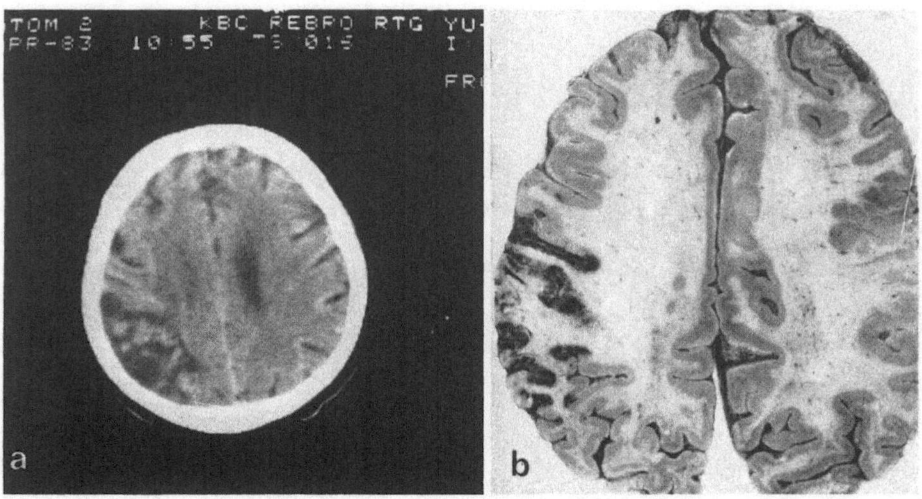

Fig. 3a, b. Acute ischemic infarction with hemorrhagic border zones

first actual "image" of a pathological condition inside the brain and spinal cord. The morphological information became so accurate that a neuropathological correlation followed as a logical consequence. Technical advances of the new generations of the CT, and especially the introduction of magnetic resonance imaging (MRI), are bringing improvements in the clarity and quality of the image to levels beyond anticipation just a few years ago. The modern "neuroimage" may give morphological information of high reliability and of great help in forming anatomopathological conclusions.

This applies primarily to *topography* of the pathological process. Sometimes it is possible to obtain more complete topical information by studying a CT or MR

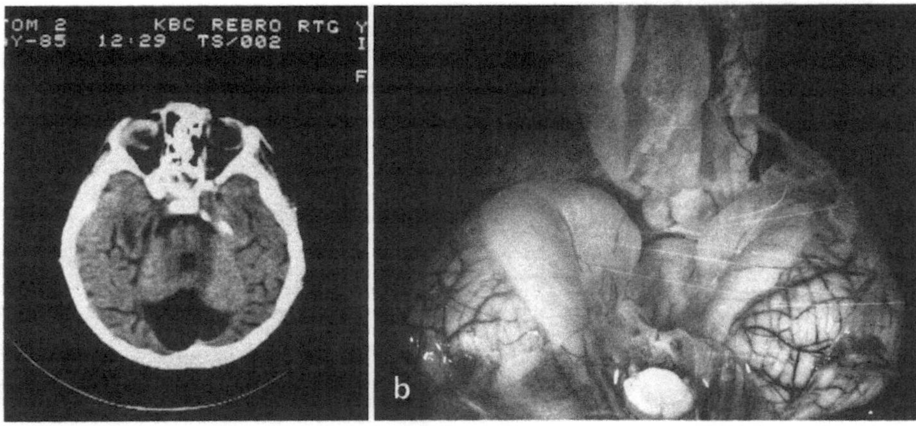

Fig. 4 a, b. Dandy-Walker syndrome; aplasia of the vermis

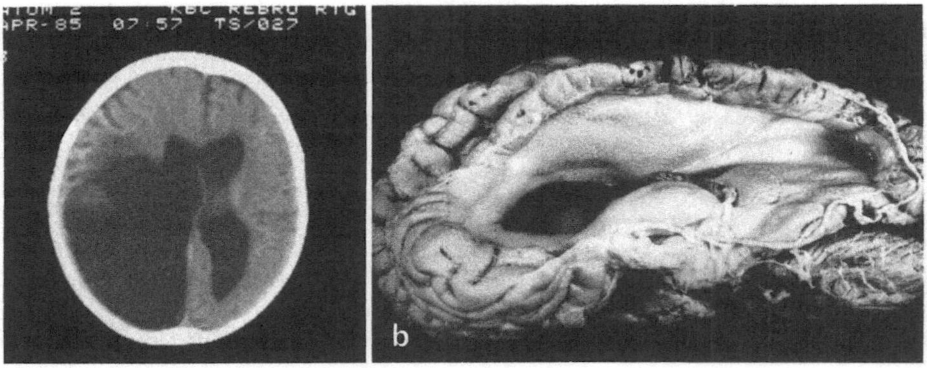

Fig. 5 a, b. Large porencephalic cyst

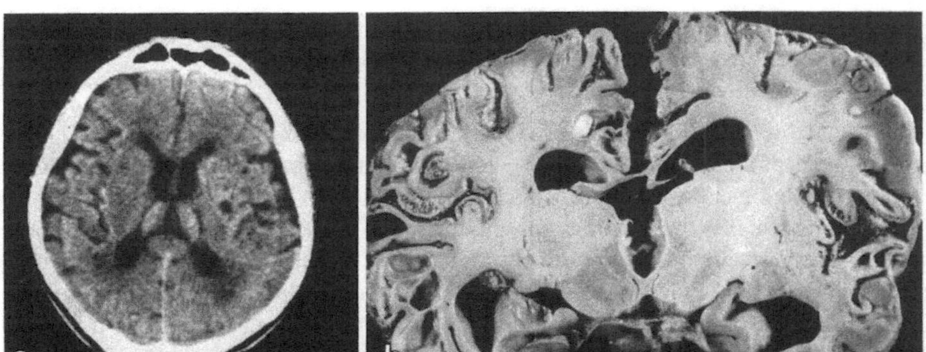

Fig. 6 a, b. Ulegyria; postnecrotic scarring process

Fig. 7a–d. Hemorrhagic infarction of the periventricular zone due to thrombosis of vena magna Galeni

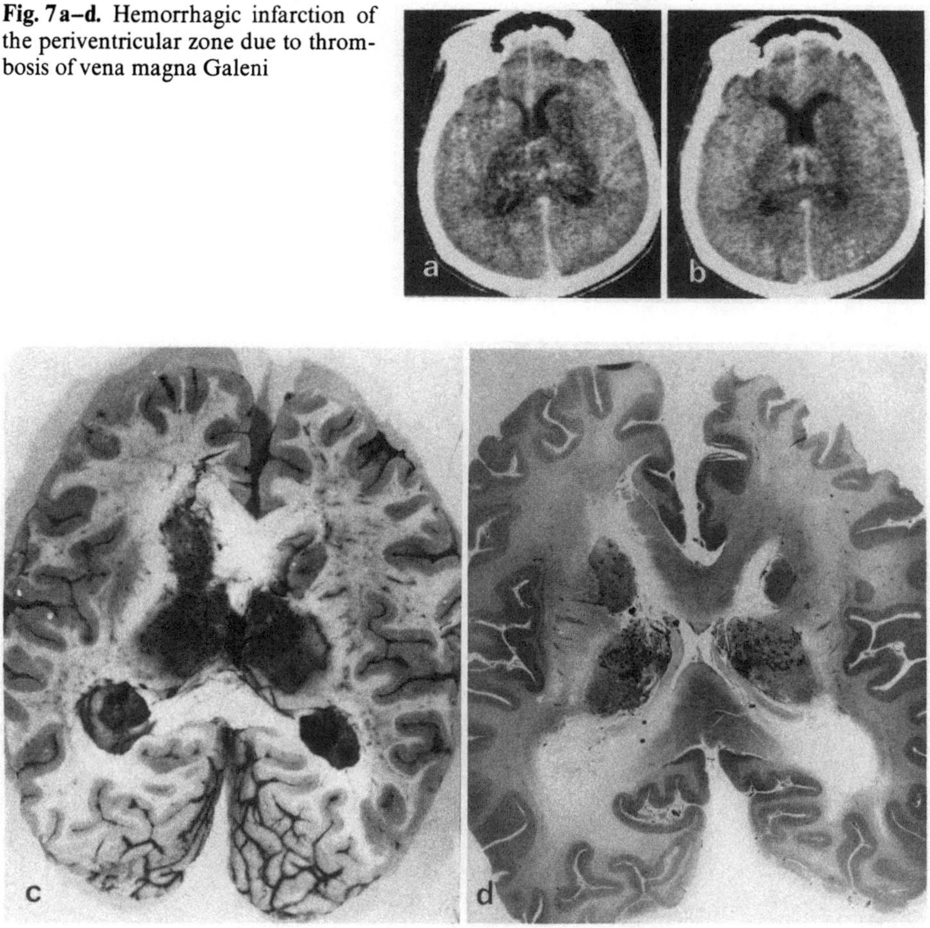

image than by naked-eye examination of sections of the formalin-fixed brain, because the CT and MRI offer various possibilities of reproduction and threedimensional reconstruction of the image, and because some lesions and tissue alterations are better visible in an adequate neuroimage than in a gross pathological specimen (e.g., edema, early necrosis, demyelination, etc.). This fact led us to introduce the term "living pathology" meaning that the intravital information on morphological features of a pathological process can be, and should be, used also as a complementary neuropathological method. Correlation between the postmortem findings and the CT or MR image may bring important data on dynamics of development and spread of a pathological process (Figs. 1–6). It can also make sampling of the tissue for histological examination easier and more accurate. In addition to the capacity of definition of localization, size and form of a single lesion, neuroimaging offers superb possibilities of visualizing and reconstruction of a "pattern" of distribution of multiple lesions. Recognition of a number of coexisting lesions as a "pattern of predilection" typical for a certain disease rather than just an accidental dissemination of a process may be a decisive diagnostic point. There is no doubt that

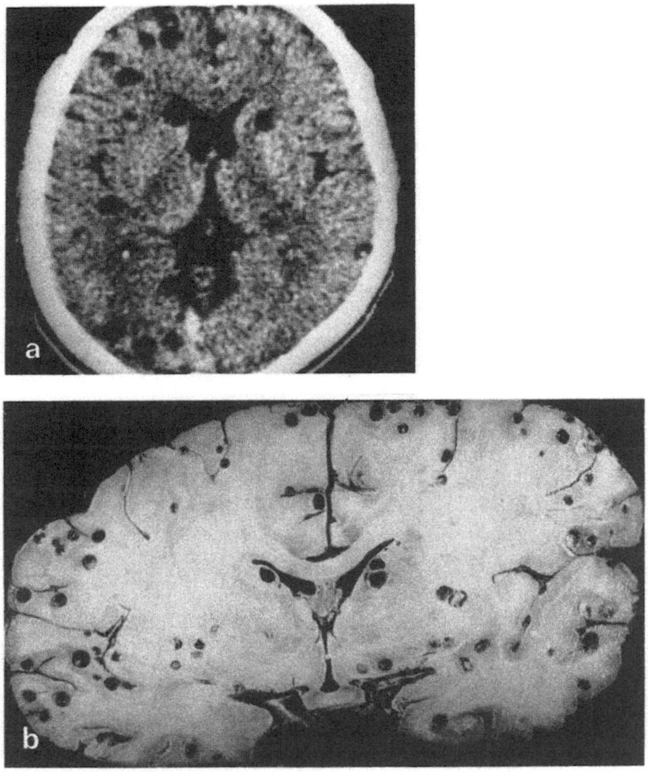

Fig. 8 a, b. Typical pattern of dissemination of cysticercosis

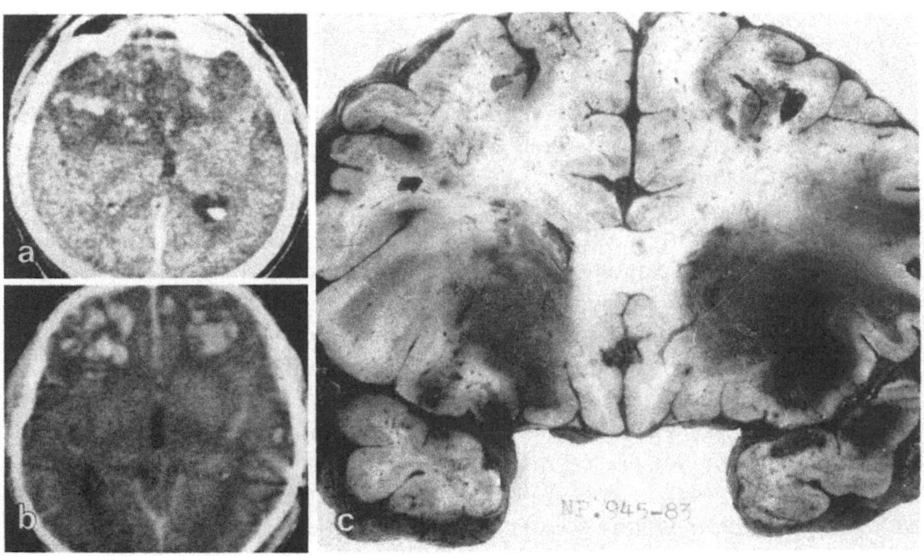

Fig. 9 a–c. The pattern of traumatic "contre-coup" lesions; hemorrhagic necrosis and edema

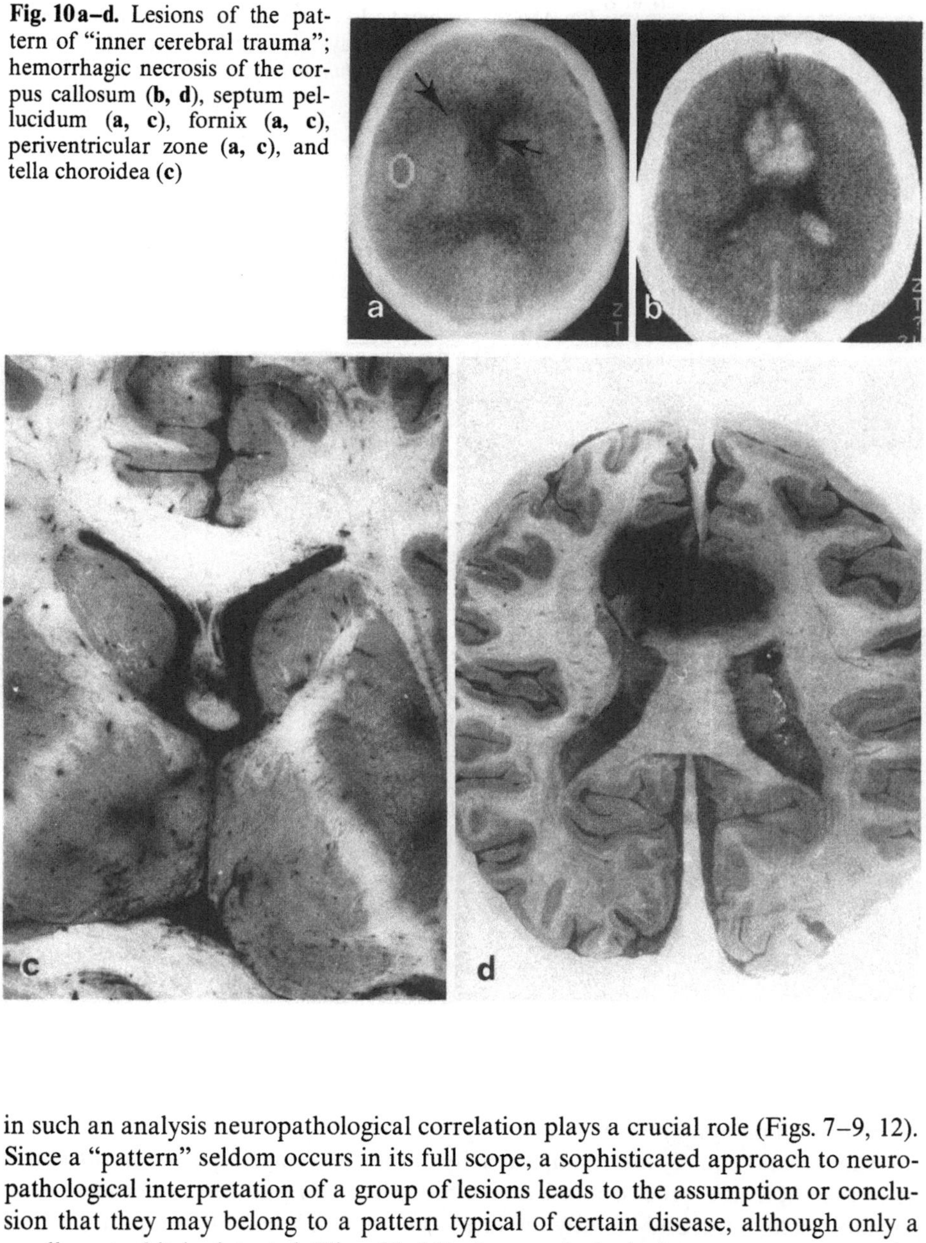

Fig. 10a–d. Lesions of the pattern of "inner cerebral trauma"; hemorrhagic necrosis of the corpus callosum (**b, d**), septum pellucidum (**a, c**), fornix (**a, c**), periventricular zone (**a, c**), and tella choroidea (**c**)

in such an analysis neuropathological correlation plays a crucial role (Figs. 7–9, 12). Since a "pattern" seldom occurs in its full scope, a sophisticated approach to neuropathological interpretation of a group of lesions leads to the assumption or conclusion that they may belong to a pattern typical of certain disease, although only a small part of it is detected (Figs. 10, 11). As a pathological process progresses, its pattern undergoes changes. The same is true with each individual lesion, which also displays changes related to its age, the process of healing, or the process of complication. A reliable interpretation of such variations is incomplete without application of correlative neuropathological doctrine (Figs. 2, 11, 12). The neuroimage as a complementary gross neuropathological method is of great help in surgical pathology. An intraoperative neuropathological diagnosis of a tumor with variegated structure, based on just a small piece of tissue, is more reliable if the pathologist is

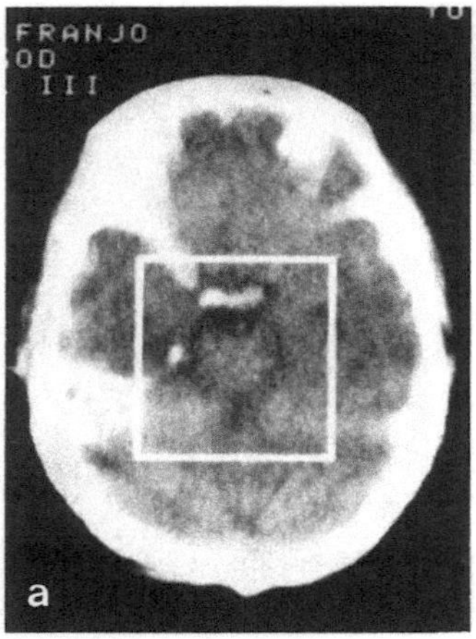

Fig. 11a–c. Traumatic lacerations in the midbrain. Recent stage (**a, b** – *arrows*); 7 days afterwards, necrosis (**c** – *thick arrow*), hemorrhage (**c** – *thin arrow*)

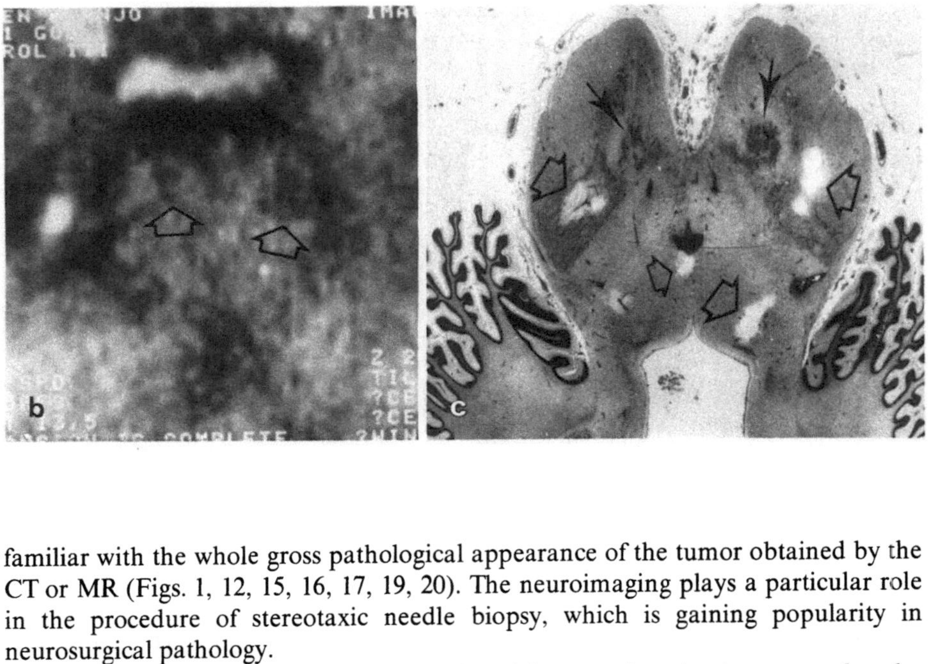

familiar with the whole gross pathological appearance of the tumor obtained by the CT or MR (Figs. 1, 12, 15, 16, 17, 19, 20). The neuroimaging plays a particular role in the procedure of stereotaxic needle biopsy, which is gaining popularity in neurosurgical pathology.

Another and equally interesting capacity of the neuroimaging is *structural* analysis of a pathological process in a living subject. Both CT and MRI offer increasing possibilities to detect and identify the fine structure of a lesion, its composition, and character. Here a neuropathological correlation is especially valuable. One may say that the more neuropathology is used in the analysis of this aspect of an image, the more details and fine structural characteristics of the disease process will be detected.

If we take only the *density,* as a basis of analysis of a CT image, the neuropathological correlation offers valuable information. The following features of the structure of a pathological process may be correlatively identified in a CT scan: The *general composition* of the lesion, meaning either an even or variegated texture (Figs. 1,

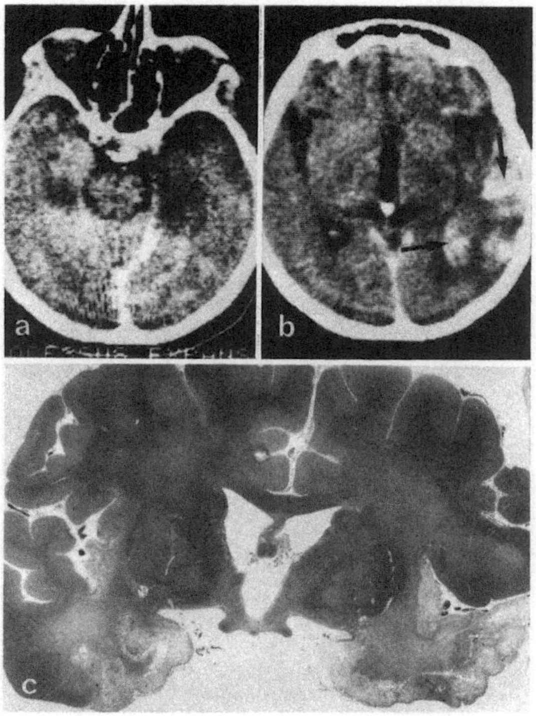

Fig. 12 a–c. Typical pattern of predilection of herpes simplex encephalitis. Recent stage, hemorrhagic necrosis (**a**, **b** – *arrow*) and edema (**a**, **b**). Subacute stage (3 weeks survival), necrosis, gliosis, granulation (**c**)

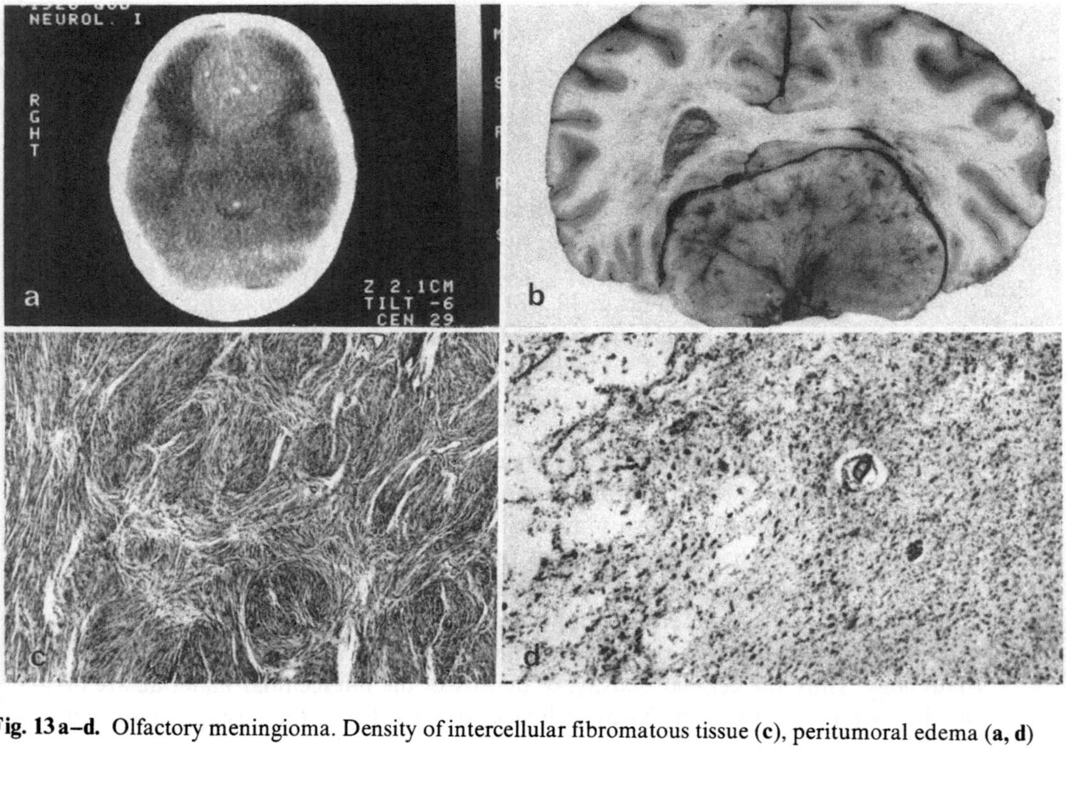

Fig. 13 a–d. Olfactory meningioma. Density of intercellular fibromatous tissue (**c**), peritumoral edema (**a**, **d**)

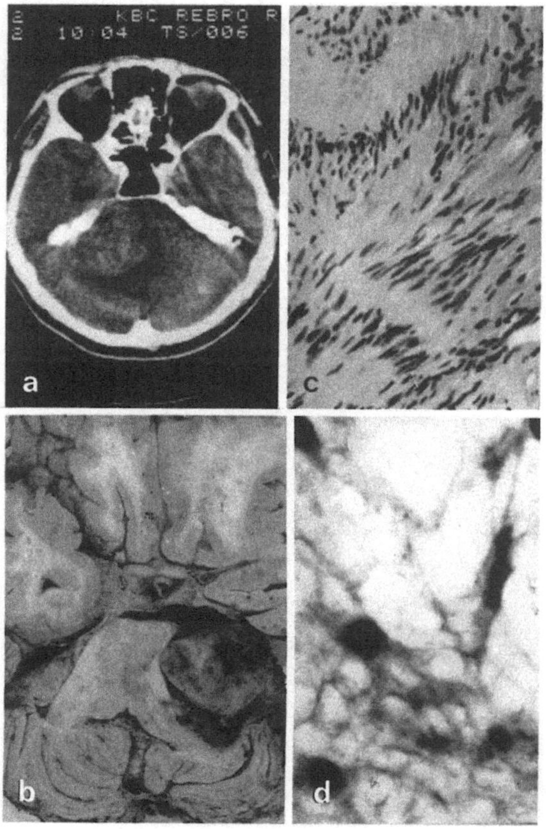

Fig. 14a–d. Variegated structure of a pontocerebellar neurinoma. Dense fascicular type A tissue (**c**), and reticular hydropic type B (**d**)

7, 11, 12, 13, 15, 19). In each of these two basic categories a number of *microfeatures* may be identified. These include the density of the cellular population (Fig. 16); the density of the intercellular material (Figs. 13, 16); the integrity of the tissue specified as (a) colliquative necrosis (Figs. 2, 12, 18), (b) coagulative necrosis (Fig. 1), (c) hydropic alteration (Figs. 14, 15), (d) edema (Figs. 1, 2, 3, 9, 10, 11, 12, 13), (e) cystic disintegration (Figs. 2, 6, 12, 17, 18, 20), (f) scar formation (Fig. 6), (g) calcification (Figs. 17, 19, 20), or (h) hemorrhage (Figs. 3, 7, 9, 10, 12). If the contrast media are applied, a number of other features may be identified, such as (j) type of vascularization or (k) condition of microcirculation, etc.

The *MRI image* is based on different principles of recording and the approach to the analysis of the image is also somewhat different. The anatomical details of the CNS are in the MRI better demonstrated and more sharply outlined. This makes the *topographic* analysis of the image more precise – if the lesion itself is well presented. The latter is not always the case, and there are many examples of better effects in structural presentation of a process with the CT than the MRI, especially in tumoral pathology. Thus, the cellular density, or density of the intercellular material, are often better reflected using the X-ray technique of the CT scan than using the magnet-

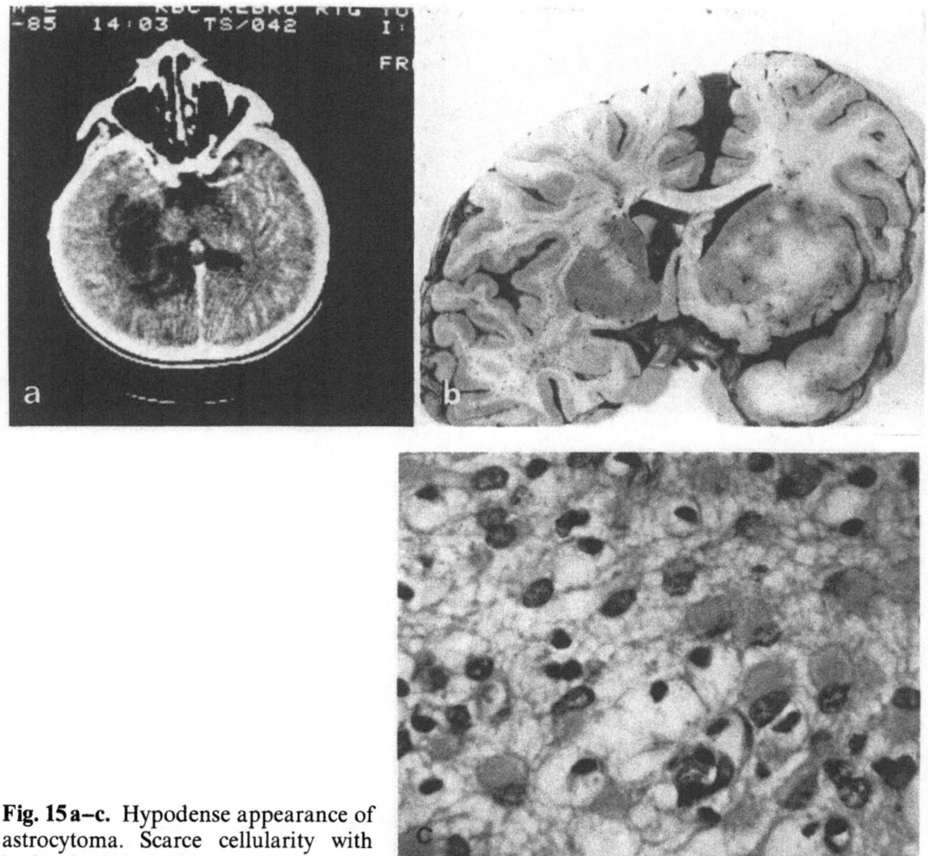

Fig. 15 a–c. Hypodense appearance of astrocytoma. Scarce cellularity with hydropic changes (**c**)

ic response of the hydrogen compound in the first generation of the MRI. However, recent stages of hypoxic, toxic, and inflammatory processes featuring significant changes in water content display MR images which often clearly surpass the capacity of the CT scan. Neuropathological correlations in such cases can naturally go further than with the CT scan and even better confirm the contribution of "living pathology" to the diagnosis. A significant advantage of the MRI vs CT is also the possibility of making cuts at very small distance, thus providing substantially more information available to digital reconstructions at various planes of sections (sagittal, coronal, horizontal). A threedimensional experience of a disseminated process of good MRI sensitivity gives almost optimal possibilities for understanding a "pattern of distribution" of lesions (e.g., multiple sclerosis). The other important advantage of the MRI procedure lies in the possibility of repetition of recording at short time intervals and in practically unlimited ways because it is not aggressive to the cerebral tissue. This can give invaluable information on the dynamics of the pathological process, the course of development, the secondary complications as well as the follow-up of therapeutic procedures. In all this, the neuropathological correlation is indispensable and, especially at this stage of development of the MRI,

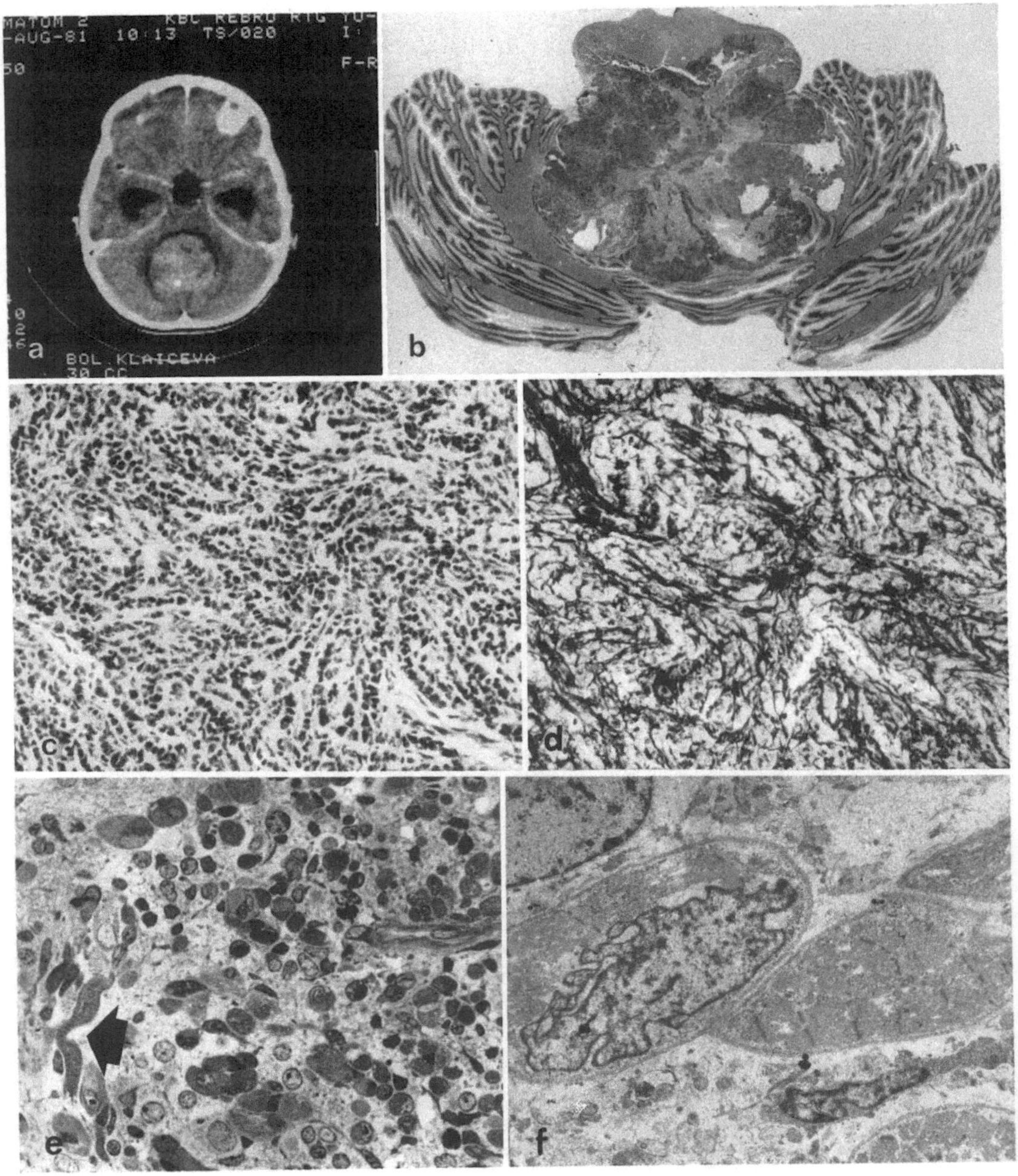

Fig. 16 a–f. Cellular (**c**) and interstitial (**d**) density of tissue of the cerebellar medullomyoblastoma; myoblastic elements (**e, f**)

Fig. 17a, b. Cystic and calcified tissue of craniopharyngioma

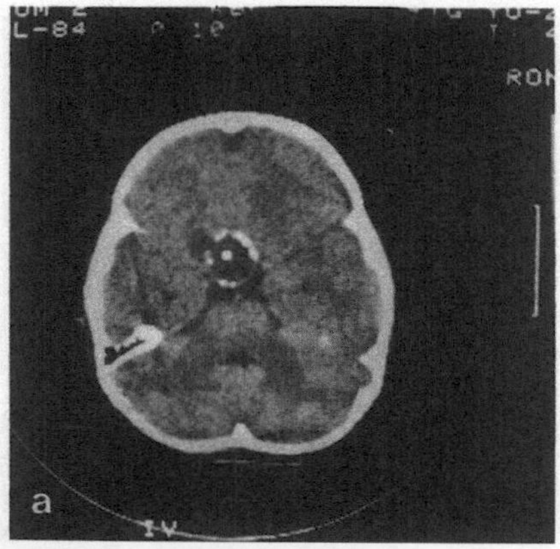

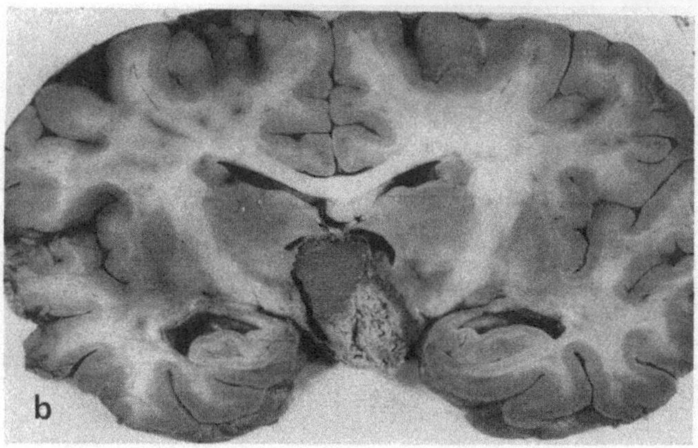

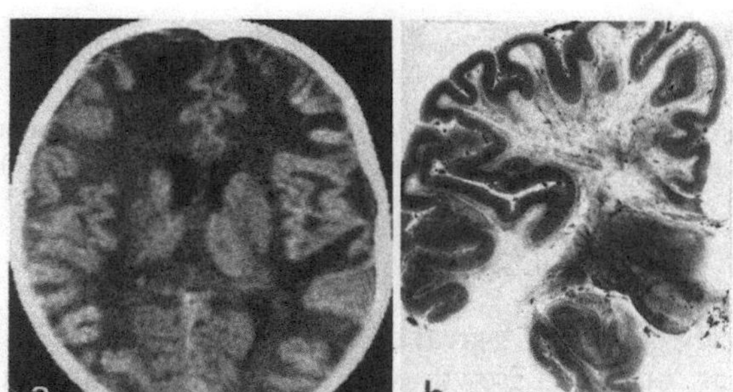

Fig. 18a, b. Sudanophilic leukodystrophy. Hypodense (**a**) appearance of the white matter due to extensive demyelination and cystic destruction (**b**)

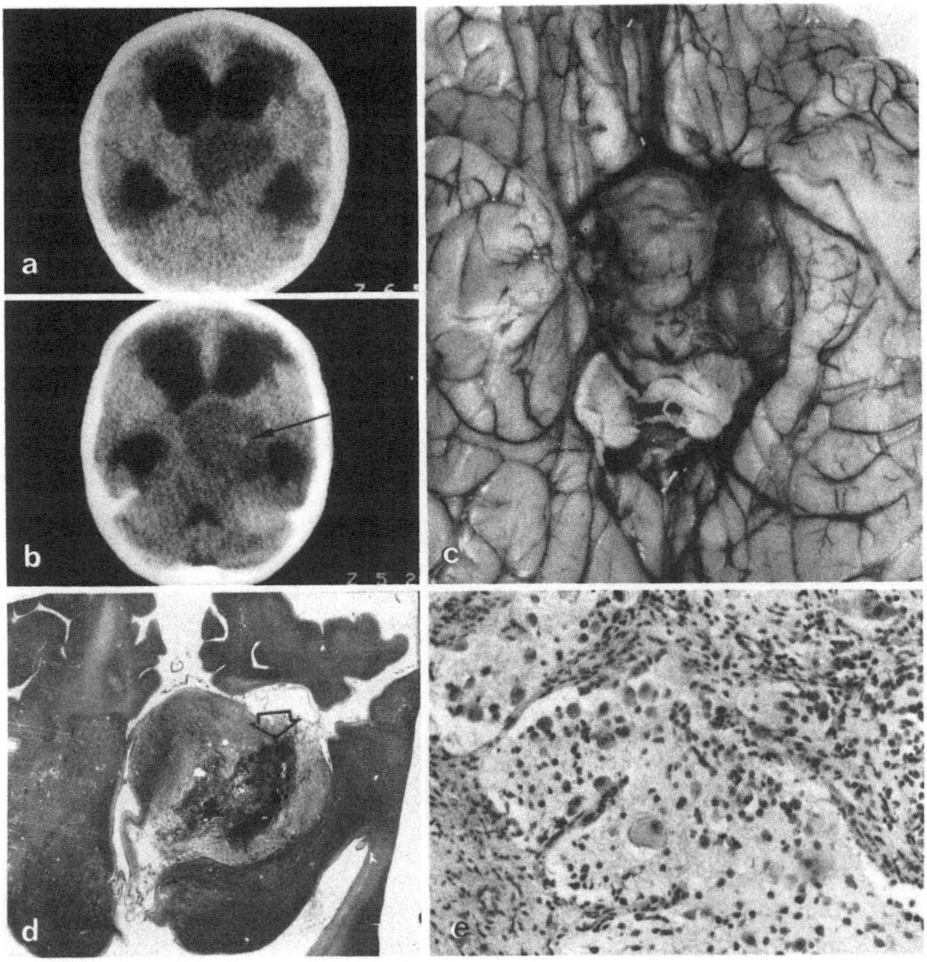

Fig. 19 a–e. Mostly hypodense appearance of ganglioneuroblastoma of the floor of the third ventricle. Loose tumoral (**e**) and dense-calcified (**d**, *arrow*) areas; hydrocephalus

very desirable. A great deal of neuropathological correlation of the MRI is still missing, but rapid growth of this field is under way. It is the correlation with neuropathology which has to provide data and evidence regarding the advantages of one or another system of imaging. The judgements will always remain subject to new technological developments, which will presumably bring better images providing more information applicable in the process of neuropathological correlation and identification of the character and kind of the disease.

Neuroimaging is an interdisciplinary method or field, which is still growing and taking shape. Technical systems develop rapidly and new discoveries in such a dynamic field are difficult to anticipate. But one essential principle remains and with

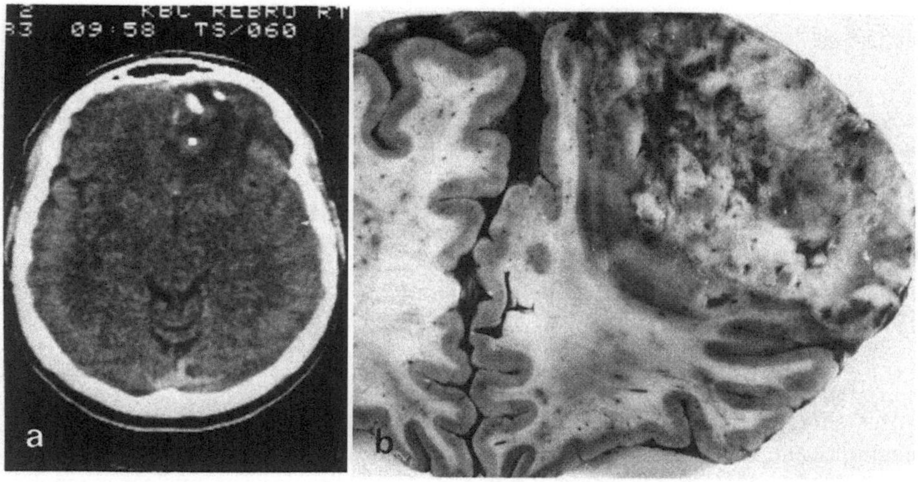

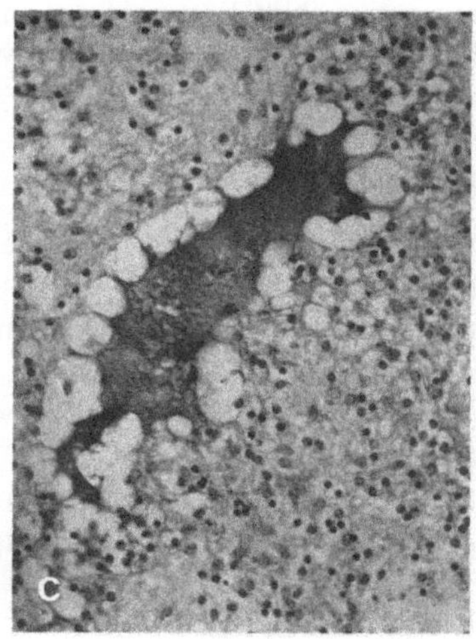

Fig. 20 a–c. Frontal oligodendroglioma with pronounced calcifications (**a**) and hypodense hydropic and cystic tumoral tissue (**a, c**)

every new technique gains in significance – the principle of pathological analysis of a disease in a living subject. In order to apply the doctrine of "living pathology" to the process of interpretation of a neuroimage, and to be able to use the neuroimage as a complementary neuropathological method, we have to keep the interrelation between the imaging and pathology permanently active.

Nuclear Magnetic Resonance Imaging of the Central Nervous System

R. E. STEINER [1]

In this short chapter, recent clinical developments in magnetic resonance (MR) imaging of the brain will be discussed. The technical developments have been reported previously [1] and there are a number of recent reviews on nuclear magnetic resonance (NMR) imaging of the brain [2, 3]. A new development which has not been covered previously deals with paramagnetic contrast agents which are of potential importance in MRI of the central nervous system.

Paramagnetic Contrast Agents

Soft tissue contrast on MR images is largely due to the difference in tissue relaxation times T_1 and T_2. Paramagnetic contrast agents have the ability of changing these relaxation times. Most paramagnetic contrast agents are metallic and therefore toxic, in a chelated form however, toxicity is markedly reduced. Gadolinium DTPA (Schering) is the first compound used in clinical practice. It is administered intravenously and retained in the vascular compartment and eventually excreted by the kidney [7]. It is capable of crossing the abnormal blood-brain barrier and to date appears to be safe in its clinical application [8].

Demyelinating Disease

It has been shown that MRI is most effective in demonstrating demyelinating disorders and its first application was in the diagnosis of disseminated sclerosis [10]. The sensitivity of MRI to demonstrate demyelinating plaques in MS is high, but its specificity is relatively low since identical features may be seen in systemic lupus erythematosus [11], sarcoidosis, infective conditions and periventricular oedema. The principal advantage of MRI however is the ability to demonstrate small lesions in clinically silent areas in patients whose symptoms or signs are minimal (Fig. 1). The MRI appearances of a wide range of other demyelinating diseases have been described. Some diseases have fairly characteristic appearances, as for instance the leukodystrophies displaying symmetrical confluence patterns [12].

[1] NMR Unit, Royal Postgraduate Medical School, DuCane Road, London W12 OHS, Great Britain.

Neurology
Ed. by K. Poeck, H. J. Freund, and H. Gänshirt

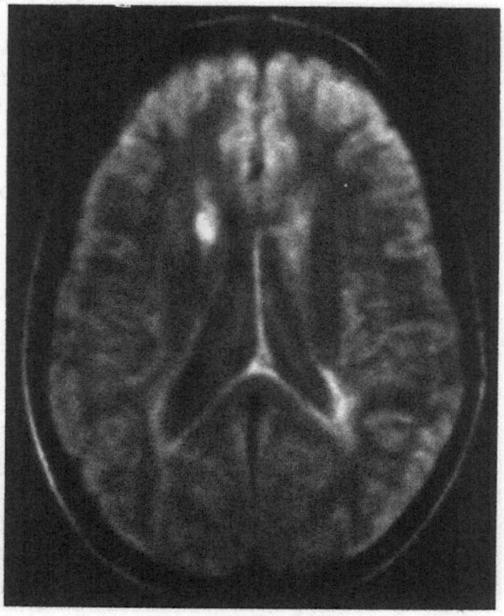

Fig. 1. SE 544/22 scan. Early disseminated sclerosis. Two small demyelinating plaques can be seen periventricularly

Cerebral Vascular Disease

From a clinical point of view some difficulties have been reported in recognising haemorrhage in the acute or subacute phase, particularly since the time course of intracranial haemorrhage relates to considerable variations in T_1 and T_2 values. Sipponen et al. [13, 14] have shown prolonged T_1 and T_2 in the early phase after a haemorrhage with a subsequent decrease within days or weeks and followed later by an increase in T_1. In the later phase of the haemorrhage, characteristic features can be observed to enable one to distinguish haemorrhage from other space-occupying lesions [15].

Cerebral infarction in the brain stem is more readily recognised with MRI than with computer tomography (CT) and periventricular lesions can be frequently observed in the elderly [16]. The lesions may well represent subclinical infarction. Subarachnoid haemorrhage and subdural haematoma are clearly diagnosed on MRI by the characteristically long T_2 and relatively short T_1 (Fig. 2a, b, c).

Infectious Disorders of the Central Nervous System

MRI is sensitive to abnormalities caused by infections, either focal or generalised. The temporal lobe effects in herpes simplex encephalitis are well recognised. On the other hand, generalised infections are often less specific and of a periventricular distribution, an abnormal appearance. Abscesses are well displayed, but have no specific signs to separate them from other mass lesions; associated calcification is not clearly visible.

Benign Brain Tumours

Meningiomas have a wide variety of presentation in MRI imaging. Unfortunately some meningiomas do not have an increased T_2, the commonly used screening se-

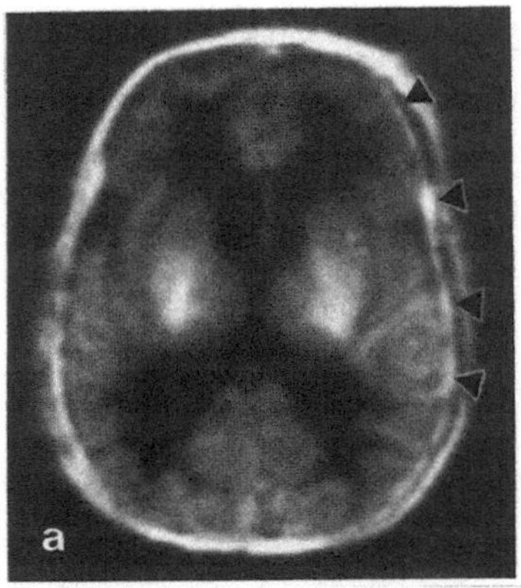

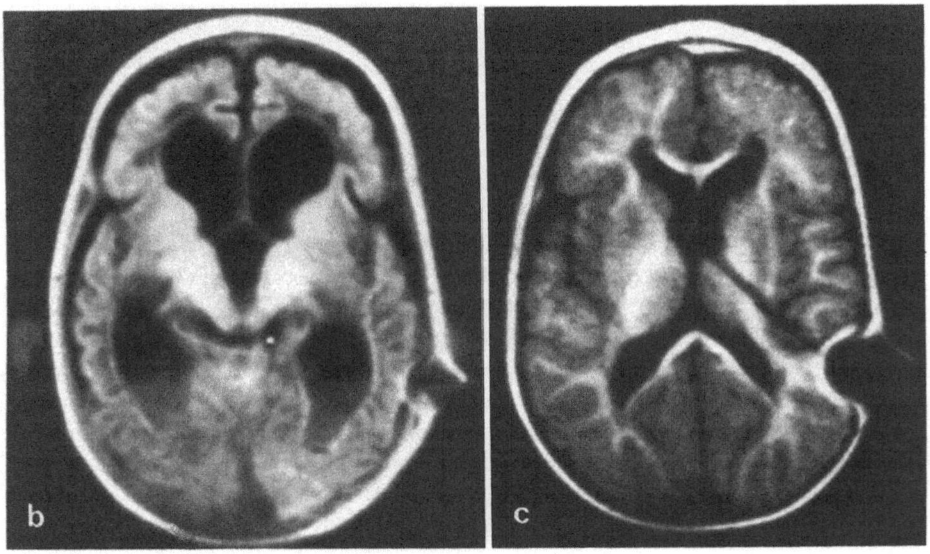

Fig. 2. **a** SE 1800/600 scan. One-week-old baby with a small subarachnoid haemorrhage, thin white line *"arrowed"*. Myelination in the internal capsule only, some ventricular dilatation. **b** At 3 months. The hydrocephalus was shunted. Some delay in myelination in the occipital region. **c** Hydrocephalus now disappeared, shunt track clearly visible, myelination has now progressed normally

quence, so that they may be missed on this particular investigation. The inversion recovery sequence, however, is much more sensitive than the spin echo sequence in detecting meningiomas and is also sensitive to contrast enhancement so that its use together with contrast enhancement results in a better diagnostic yield than that obtained using CT [17] (Fig. 3a, b).

Acoustic Neuromas

The internal auditory canal is easily seen so that soft tissues may be detected within the canal or cerebellopontine angle. Acoustic neuromas show a variable appearance with a minority not demonstrating an increase in T_2. A comparison with CT studies suggests that MRI is more sensitive in the diagnosis of both large and small acoustic neuromas [18]. Acoustic neuromas enhance with contrast media, thus further improving the diagnostic yield (Fig. 4a, b).

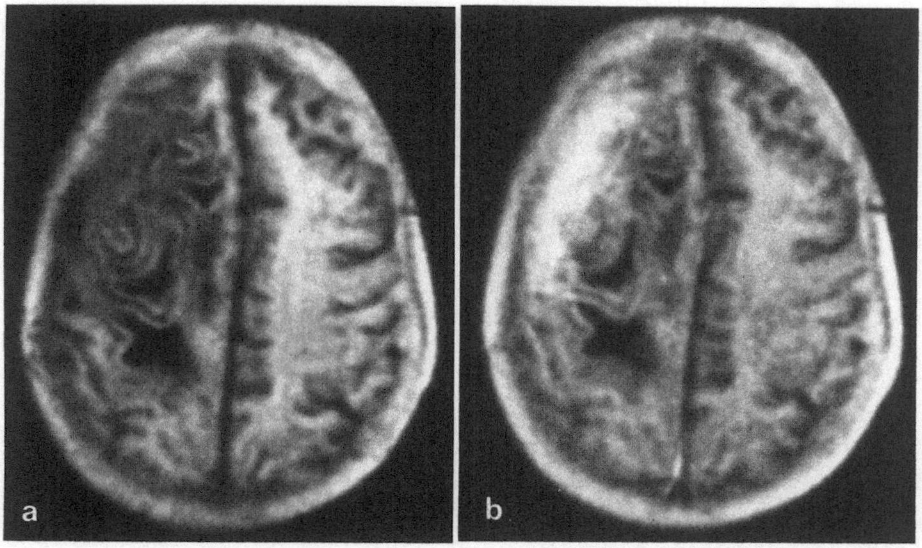

Fig. 3. **a** IR 1400/400 scan. Left frontoparietal meningioma. Large area of reduced signal in the frontoparietal lobe. Slight midline shift. Impossible to differentiate tumour from oedema. **b** Following administration of paramagnetic contrast medium (Gadolinium DTPA), relaxation time of the tumour greatly reduced, highlighted in *white,* surrounding oedema is *dark grey*

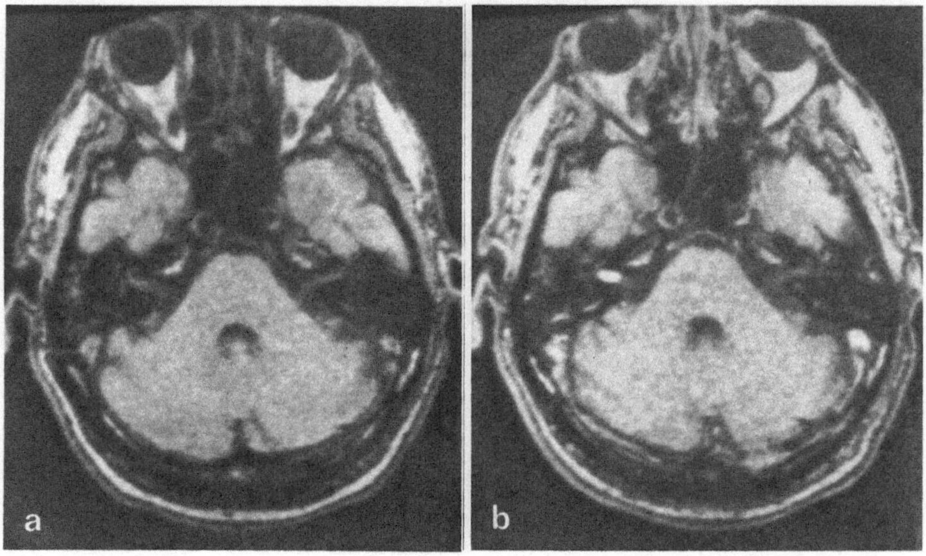

Fig. 4. **a** SE 544/22 scan. Intracanalicular acoustic neuroma of the left 8th nerve. In comparison with the rightside there is slight expansion of the nerve. **b** After administration of paramagnetic contrast medium. Tumour now highlighted

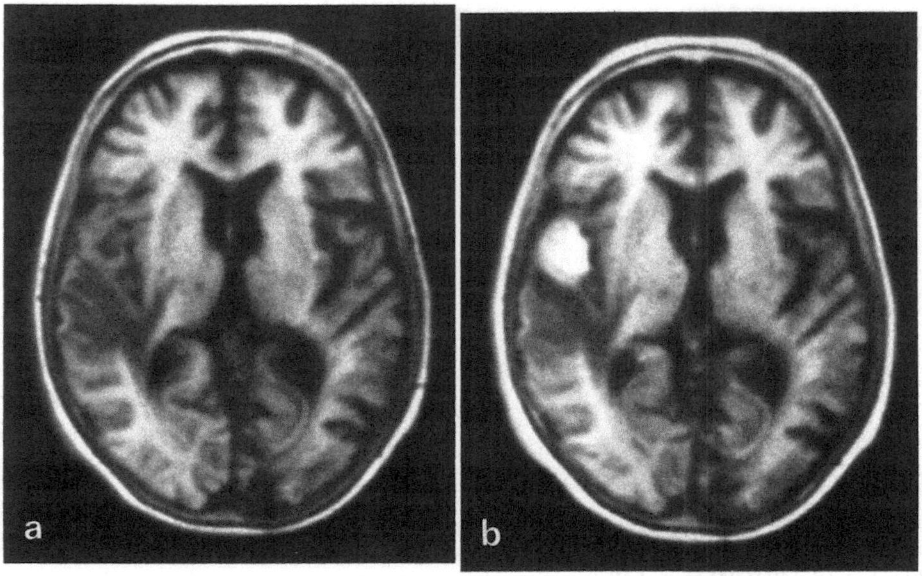

Fig. 5. a IR 1400/400 scan. Left temporal lobe metastasis, primary in the breast. Tumour indistinguishable from oedema. **b** After administration of paramagnetic contrast medium. Metastases highlighted in *white,* surrounding oedema in *dark grey*

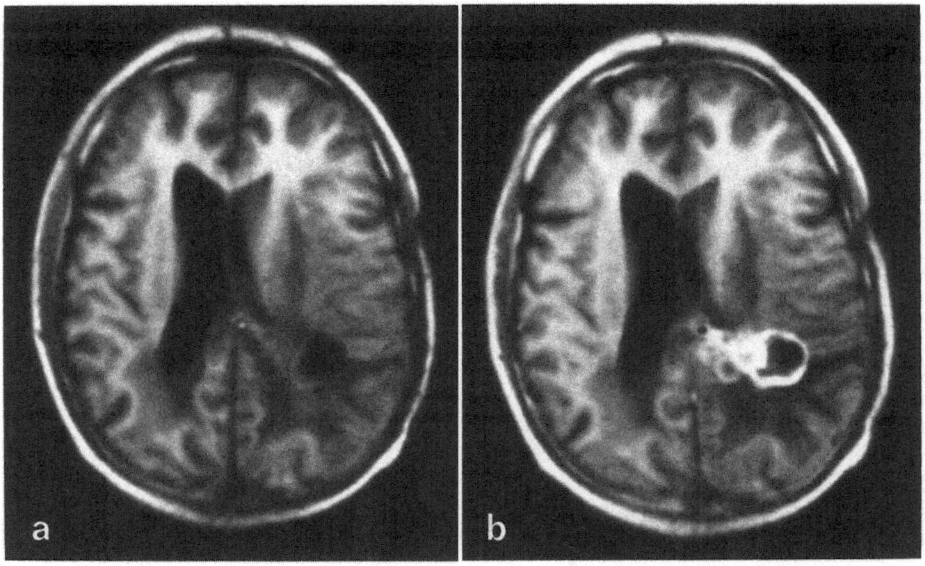

Fig. 6. a IR 1400/400 scan. Ependymoma right parietooccipital region with low signal in *black.* Surrounding oedema *dark grey.* **b** Following paramagnetic contrast medium ring enhancement of the mass lesion, central area necrotic, in addition tumour spread towards the ventricle. Surrounding oedema *dark grey*

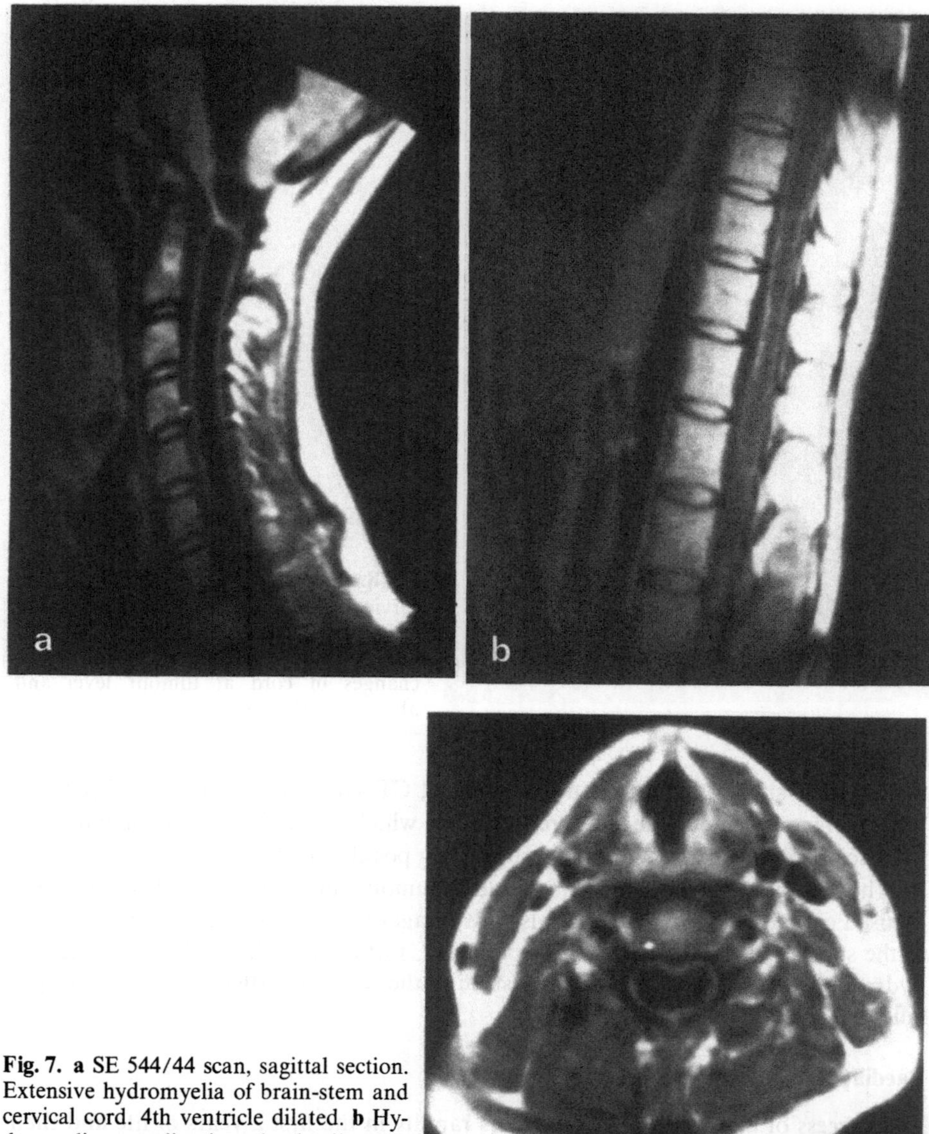

Fig. 7. a SE 544/44 scan, sagittal section. Extensive hydromyelia of brain-stem and cervical cord. 4th ventricle dilated. **b** Hydromyelia extending into the dorsilumbar region. **c** Transverse section cervical region, demonstrating extent of the hydromyelia

Malignant Tumours

The majority of malignant tumours on MRI have an increased T_1 and T_2. There are however some exceptions [19], including malignant melanoma, tumours containing lipid [20] and some other types. Prior to the use of paramagnetic contrast media the separation of tumour from cerebral oedema was a disadvantage for MRI compared with CT, but with its use better results are now being obtained (Fig. 5a, b). Graif et

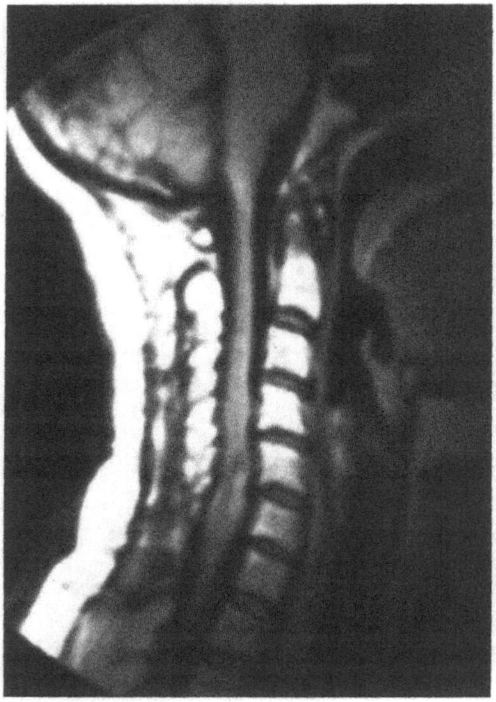

Fig. 8. SE 544/44 scan, sagittal section, cervical region, demonstrating expanded lesion of the cervical cord at C6/7 level due to intra-axial glioma. Note cystic changes in cord at tumour level and above in *dark grey*

al. [21] have shown that on contrast-enhanced CT scans from a number of patients with malignant tumours, the apparent oedema which was visible on the unenhanced MRI scan enhanced after contrast – suggesting possible tumour infiltration (Fig. 6 a, b). The advantage of MRI in demonstrating tumours in the posterior fossa was recognised early on [22, 23]. MRI has also advantages for patients presenting symptoms in the supratentorial region. In these patients CT often only shows the mass effect of hydrocephalus without clearly demonstrating the tumours. MRI is much more specific in displaying tumour size and site.

Paediatrics

The process of myelination which occurs rapidly in the first 2 years of life and then continues into the second decade is readily demonstrated using MRI (Fig. 2 a, b, c). Delay in myelination or deficity has been reported by Johnson et al. [12]. A general range of pathologies has been shown in infants and children, including vascular and ischaemic disorders, anoxic changes, haemorrhage and infarction, periventricular leukomalacia, hydrocephalus and periventricular oedema. Tumours are well demonstrated and the essential features are not too different from those noted in adults.

Spinal Cord

With the development of localised radio-frequency receiving surface coils, image quality of the cervical cord has improved considerably, and to some extent also of the thoracic and lumbar regions. The demonstration of the cranio-cervical junction is yet another advantage of MRI, avoiding bone artefacts seen on CT. A large variety of disease processes have been reported, for instance, syringomyelia (Fig. 7a, b, c) and intra- and extra-axial tumours (Fig. 8) [24].

MRI does not require an intrathecal contrast injection, but the use of gadolinium DTPA has shown some useful enhancement of tumours and vascular abnormalities. Large disc protrusions are well demonstrated using MRI [25], but there is still some difficulty in clearly defining small disc lesions.

References

1. Gore JC (1983) Physical principles of nuclear magnetic resonance imaging. Recent Adv Radiol Med Imaging 1:1–13
2. Brant-Zawadzki M, Davis PL, Crooks LE, Mills CM, Norman D, Newton TH, Sheldon P, Kaufman L (1983) NMR demonstration of cerebral abnormalities: comparison with CT. AJR 140(5):847–854
3. Zimmerman RA, Bilaniuk LT, Goldberg HI, Grossman RI, Levine RS, Lynch R, Edelstein W, Bottomley P, Redington R (1983) Cerebral NMR imaging: early results with a 0.12 T resistive system. AJR 141:1187
4. Bydder GM, Pennock JM, Steiner RE, Orr JS, Bailes DR, Young IR (1984) The NMR diagnosis of cerebral tumors. Mag Res Med 1:5–29
5. Bydder GM (1984) NMR imaging of the brain. Br Med Bull 40(2):170–174
7. Schorner W, Felix R, Lawiado M, Lange L, Weinmann H-J, Claussen C, Fiegler W, Speck U, Kazner E (1984) Testing the nuclear magnetic resonance tomography contrast medium gadolinium-DTPA in tumours: Tolerance, alteration of contrast and first clinical results. RÖFO 140:493–500
8. Carr DH, Brown J, Bydder GM, Weinmann H-J, Speck U, Thomas DJ, Young IR (1984) Intravenous chelated gadolinium as a contrast agent in NMR imaging of cerebral tumours. Lancet i:484–486
9. Carr DH, Brown J, Bydder GM, Steiner RE, Weinmann H-J, Speck U, Hall AS, Young IR (1984) Gadolinium-DTPA as a contrast agent in MRI: Initial clinical experience in 20 patients. AJR 143:215–224
10. Young IR, Randell CP, Kaplan PW, James A, Bydder GM, Steiner RE (1983) NMR imaging in white matter disease of the brain using spin-echo sequences. J Comput Assist Tomogr 7(2):290–294
11. Vermess M, Bernstein RM, Bydder GM, Steiner RE, Young IR, Hughes GRV (1983) NMR imaging of the brain in systemic lupus erythematosus. J Comput Assist Tomogr 7(3):461–467
12. Johnson MA, Pennock JM, Bydder GM, Steiner RE, Thomas DJ, Hayward R, Bryant DRT, Payne JA, Levene MI, Whitelaw A, Dubowitz LMS, Dubowitz V (1983) Clinical NMR imaging of the brain in children: normal and neurologic disease. AJNR 4:1013–1026 and AJR 141:1005–1018
13. Sipponen JT, Sepponen RE, Sivula A (1983) Nuclear magnetic resonance (NMR) imaging of intracerebral hemorrhage in the acute and resolving phases. J Comput Assist Tomogr 7:954–959
14. Sipponen JT, Sepponen RE, Sivula A (1984) Chronic subdural hematoma: demonstration by magnetic resonance. Radiology 150:79–85
15. Bailes DR, Young IR, Thomas DJ, Straughan K, Bydder GM, Steiner RE (1982) NMR imaging of the brain using spin-echo sequences. Clin Radiol 33:395–414
16. Bradley WG, Waluch V, Yadley RA, Wycoff RR (1984) Comparison of CT and MR in 400 patients with suspected disease of the brain and cervical spinal cord. Radiology 152:695–702
17. Bydder GM, Kingsley DPE, Brown J, Niendorf HP, Young IR (1985) MRI of meningiomas including studies with and without Gadolinium-DTPA. J Comput Assist Tomogr 9(4):690–697

18. Curati WL, Graif M, Kingsley DPE, Niendorf HP, Young IR (1986) Magnetic resonance imaging: contrast enhancement of acoustic neuromas with intravenous gadolinium-DTPA. Radiology 158:447–451
19. McKay IM, Bydder GM, Young IR (1985) MRI of central nervous system tumours which do not display evidence of an increase in T_1 or T_2. J Comput Assist Tomogr 9 (6):1055–1061
20. Davidson HD, Ouchi T, Steiner RE (1985) NMR imaging of congenital intracranial germinal layer neoplasms. Neuroradiology 27:301–303
21. Graif M, Bydder GM, Steiner RE, Niendorf HP, Thomas DGT, Young IR (1985) Contrast enhanced MRI of malignant brain tumors. AJNR and AJR 6:855–862
22. MacGinnis BD, Brady TJ, New PFJ, Buonanno FS, Pykett IL, DeLaPaz RL, Kistler JP, Tavernas JM (1983) Nuclear magnetic resonance (NMR) imaging of tumors in the posterior fossa. J Comput Assist Tomogr 7:575
23. Randell CP, Collins AG, Young IR, Hayward R, Thomas DJ, McDonnell MJ, Orr JS, Bydder GM, Steiner RE (1983) NMR imaging of posterior fossa tumors. AJR 141:489–496
24. Norman D, Mills CM, Brant-Zawadski M, Yeates A, Crooks LE, Kaufman L (1983) Magnetic resonance imaging of spinal cord and canal: potentials and limitations. AJR 141:1147–1152
25. Modic MT, Pavlicek W, Weinstein MA, Boumphrey F, Ngo F, Hardy P (1984) Magnetic resonance imaging of intravertebral disc disease: Clinical and pulse sequences consolidation. Radiology 152:103–111

Positron Emission Tomography and Nuclear Magnetic Resonance Imaging: New Perspectives in Neuroimaging

G. Di Chiro[1]

The rise of nuclear magnetic resonance imaging (NMR or MRI) to a preeminent position among the neuroimaging methods has brought about lively debate among the cognoscenti on the advantages, if any, of this diagnostic modality. For reasons which are rather complex, and not always solely "science motivated," MRI is being frequently pitted against positron emission tomography (PET). This is indeed an unlikely and, superficially, an unevenly matched confrontation. MRI has already recruited legions of practitioners with experts, or soi-disant experts, multiplying by the day. In contrast, the number of investigators who actually deal with PET represents an exiguous maniple. The MRI systems in operation worldwide are already many more than the pitifully few PET units which are mostly "research" dedicated. Also, relatively few neurologists and neurosurgeons, and even fewer neuroradiologists, could point to clinical applications of PET useful in the everyday practice of medicine. Thus the contraposition MRI–PET must find its justification in different aspects than the relative diagnostic merits.

A possible explanation of this puzzling trend toward MRI–PET comparison may reside in the grossly exaggerated, almost hyperbolic, claims and expectations in the NMR technology. The precedent of the MRI success in, at least partially, dethroning computer tomography (CT) as the "optimal" imaging technique, may easily lead to other anticipations. NMR can and will be used for assessment of flow and metabolism, profess some self-appointed advocates. Of course, study of flow and metabolism is just the area in which PET can offer, and indeed has already offered, distinct advantages. If these advantages have not been fully exploited in the clinical area, this is not for the PET technique having been found wanting, but is related to some idiosyncratic features of the PET community. At any rate, PET represents the only methodology which so far has shown credible possibilities in the combined exploration of form (images) and function (metabolic data). This exploration is also possible, according to some investigators, by means of NMR, with the added benefit of the exquisite display of anatomical detail which PET, with its inherently poor spatial resolution, can not possibly match.

[1] Neuroimaging Section, National Institutes of Health, Bethesda, MD, USA.

Neurology
Ed. by K. Poeck, H. J. Freund, and H. Gänshirt

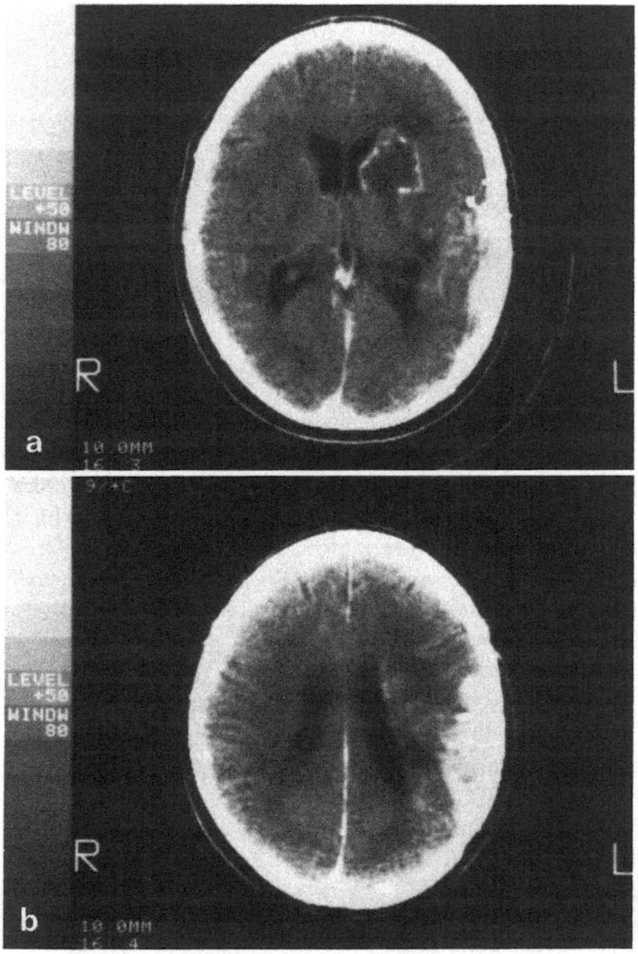

Fig. 1 a, b

Fig. 1 a–g. Patient with high grade astrocytoma on the surface of left cerebral hemisphere; necrosis in the left basal ganglia area has occurred following selective intraarterial BCNU infusion. In post-contrast CT scans, note rim enhancement of deep necrotic area (**a**) as well as blush of superficial tumor (**b**). T2-weighted MRI images (**c** and **d**) of corresponding levels do not permit discrimination between necrotic area and tumor. PET scans with FDG (**e, f** and **g**) show hypometabolism of entire left cerebral hemisphere except for markedly hypermetabolic tumor (**e** and **f**). Note profound hypometabolism of left basal ganglia region, whereas right basal ganglia display normal glucose utilization (**e** and **f**). Lower scan (**g**) reveals crossed-cerebellar diaschisis as well as contrast between two anterior temporal lobes, with the left being hypometabolic and the right normometabolic. (Surgeon Dr. E. H. Oldfield)

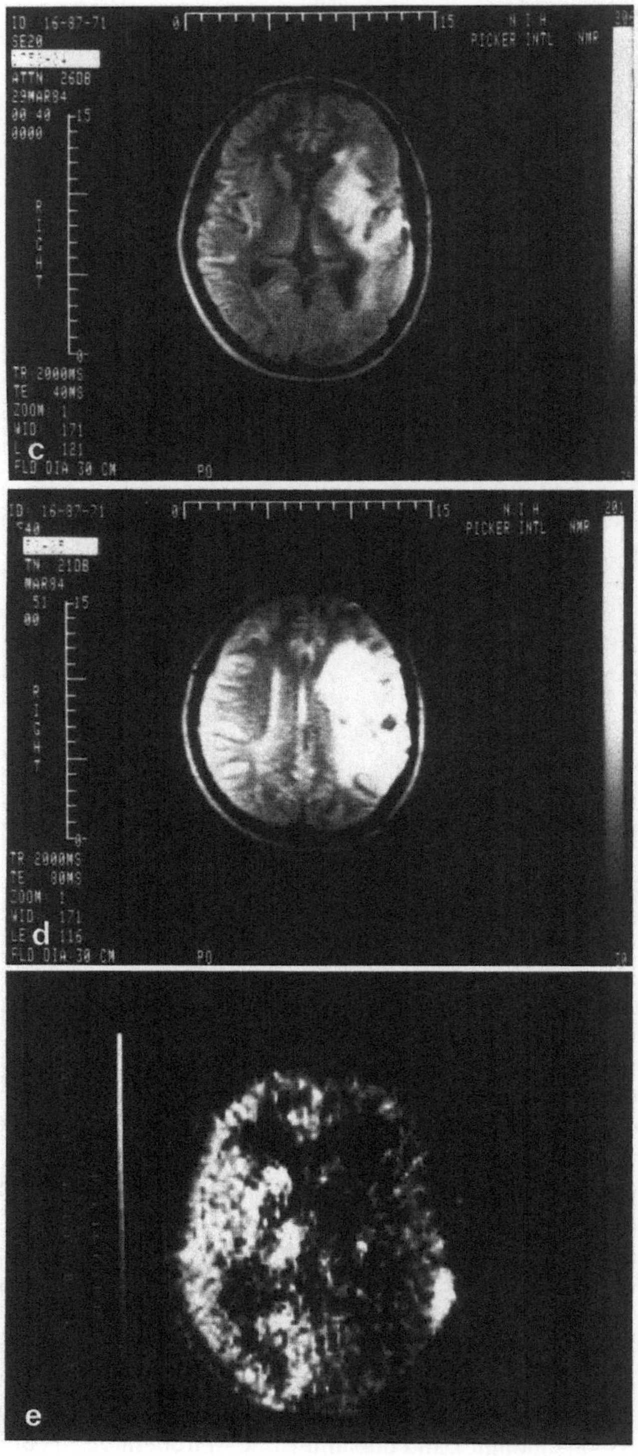

Fig. 1 c–e

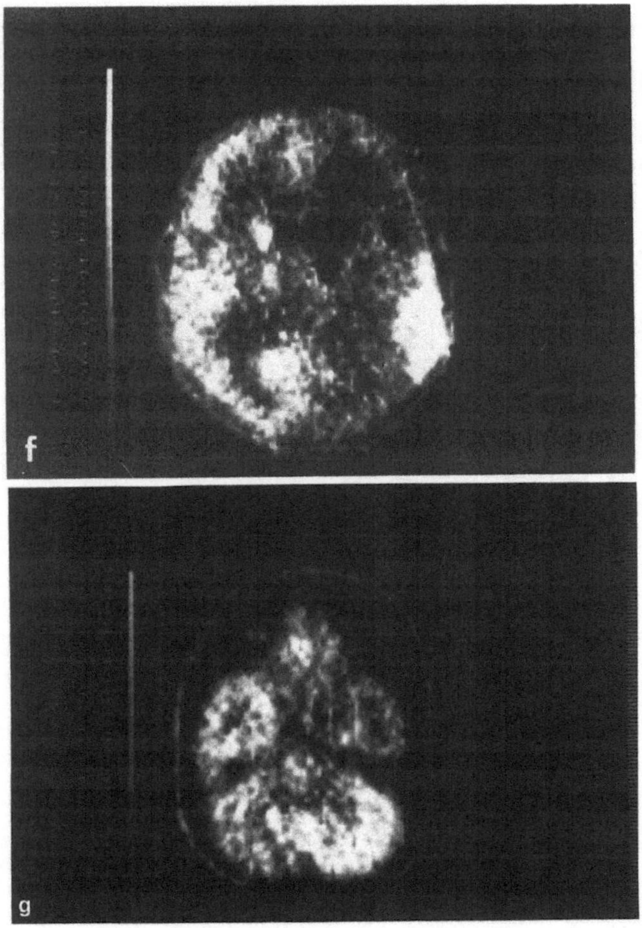

Fig. 1f, g

Positron Emission Tomography

Cerebral PET allows imaging of brain structures and measurement of local tissue concentration of injected radioactive tracers. This quantitation capability, together with appropriate kinetic models, permits measurement of cerebral physiological processes and their derangements. Positron emission tomography may be looked at as a form of in vivo noninvasive autoradiography, and, in fact, some of the PET methods, e.g. the ^{18}F-2-deoxyglucose technique (FDG) for estimating the cerebral metabolic rate for glucose, are directly derived from autoradiographic studies.

Applications of PET include the evaluation of *cerebral blood flow* ($H_2{}^{15}O$, $C^{15}O_2$, ^{77}Kr), *cerebral blood volume* (^{11}CO), oxygen transport and metabolism ($^{15}O_2$), glucose utilization (FDG, ^{11}C-deoxyglucose, ^{11}C-glucose), amino acid transport and metabolism (^{13}N or ^{11}C tagged amino acids), protein synthesis (^{11}C-leucine, ^{11}C-methionine), and dopamine (^{11}C-spiroperidol, ^{11}C or ^{18}F-L-dopa) and opiate receptors (^{18}F-acetylcyclofoxy, ^{11}C-carfentanil). As a research tool to investigate the workings of the brain, PET is promising. For example, it has been possible to delineate neural pathways (e.g., visual) through an analysis of local energy metabolism modifications after sensory stimulation or motor activation. One should note, however, that such findings have been primarily confirmatory and have not in substantial ways modified our knowledge or conceptions of neural function. In the clinical area, PET evaluation of oxygen metabolism has proven useful in the evaluation of cerebrovascular diseases, and PET assessment of glucose utilization has been helpful in the diagnosis of complex partial epilepsy, in grading primary cerebral tumors, and in distinguishing Alzheimer's disease from other forms of dementia. The differentiation between tumor recurrence and postradiation or postchemotherapy cerebral necrosis is currently possible only using the PET-FDG technique (Fig. 1). Preliminary observations indicate that neuroreceptor studies may well assist us in the management of patients with extrapyramidal disorders, such as Parkinson's disease.

Nuclear Magnetic Resonance

In proton magnetic resonance imaging (MRI), which is currently the one used most widely, the detected signals will differ depending upon the physicochemical properties of the tissue and the manipulation of the applied radio frequency (RF) pulses. These signals, with proper spatial encoding, can be processed by techniques for reconstruction from projections to yield tomographic images with high contrast and spatial resolution and oriented in the axial, coronal, or sagittal planes.

Many factors affect the NMR image: excited proton density and its rate of change (flow or diffusion), the longitudinal (spin-lattice) relaxation time T1, the

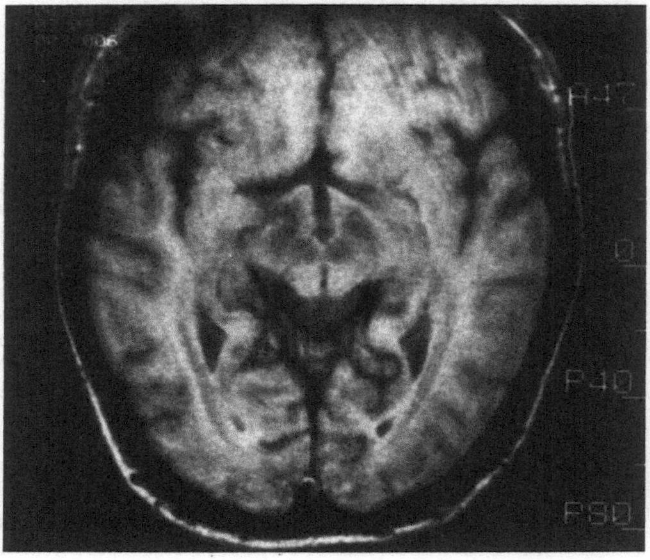

Fig. 2. MRI demonstration of substantia nigra and red nucleus

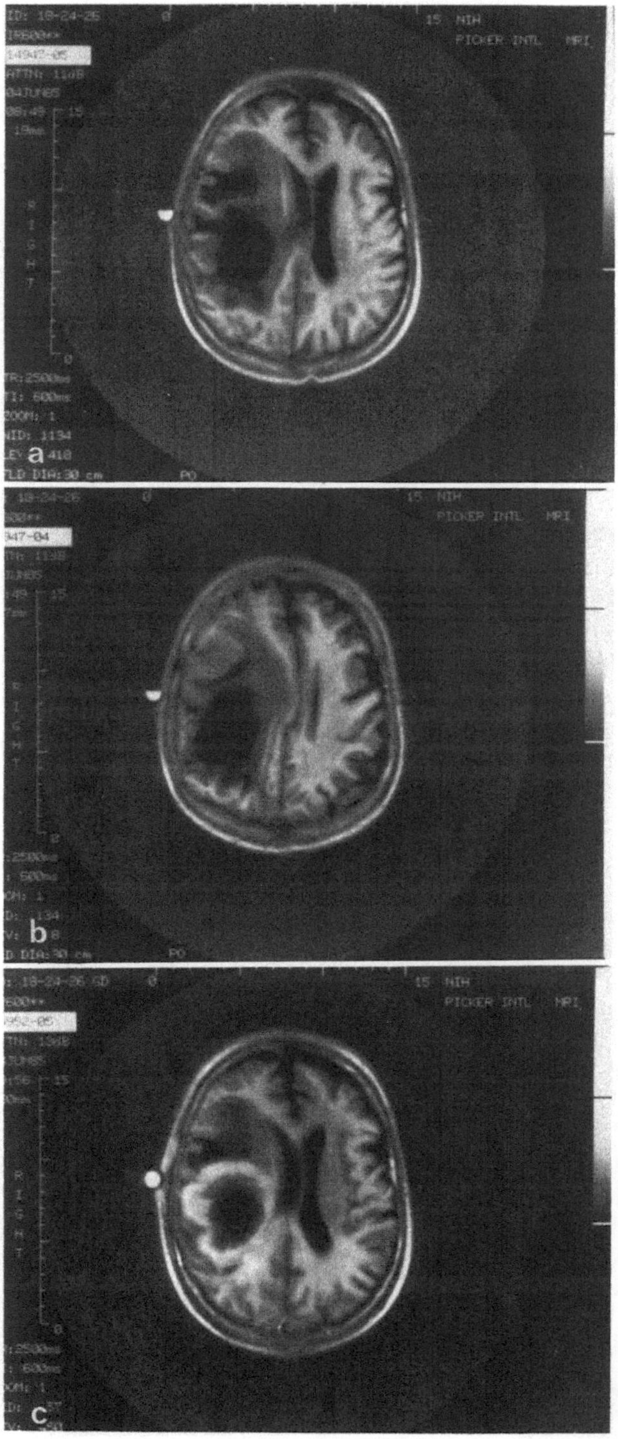

Fig. 3 a–i. Gd-DTPA MRI study in a case of high-grade astrocytoma. Pregadolinium (**a** and **b**) and postgadolinium (**c** and **d**) inversion recovery axial scans; postgadolinium spin-echo axial (**e**) and coronal (**f**) scans; pre- (**g**) and postgadolinium (**h**) spin-echo axial scans. Postgadolinium scans allow better differentiation of viable tumor, necrotic center, and surrounding edema. PET scan with FDG (**i**)

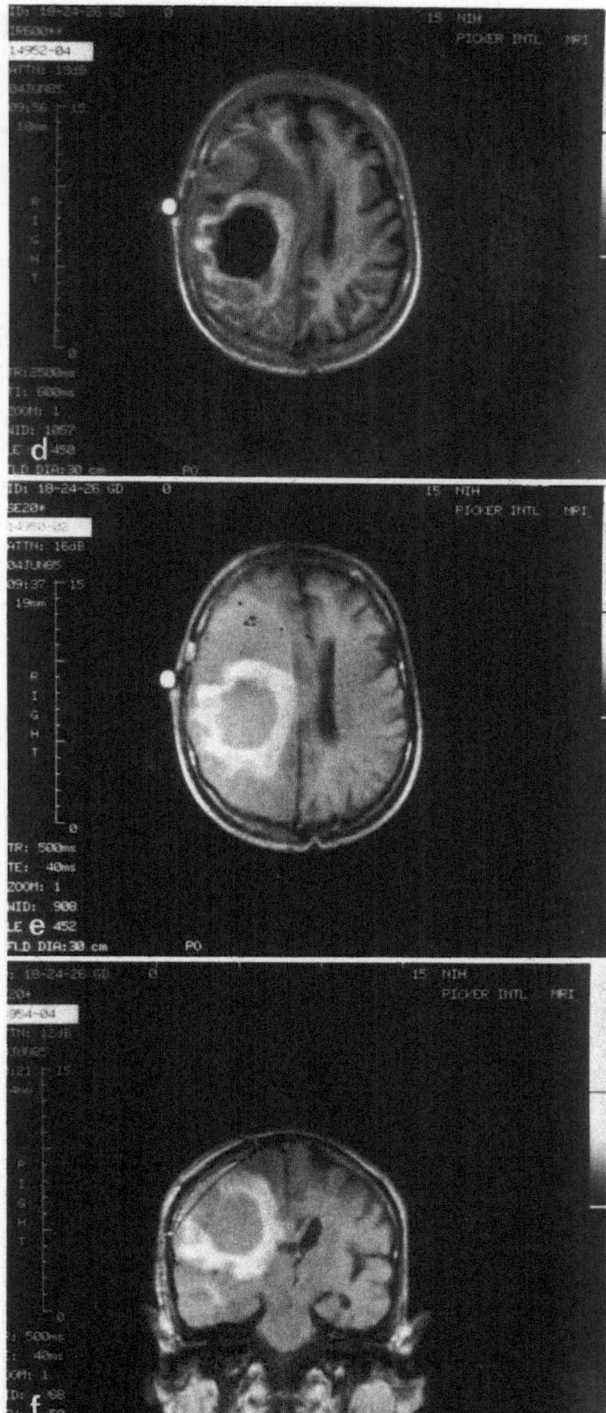
ID: 18-24-26 GD
15 NIH
PICKER INTL MRI
14952-04
d
ID: 18-24-26 GD
15 NIH
PICKER INTL MRI
ATTN: 16dB
04JUN85
09:37
19mm
R
I
G
H
T
TR: 500ms
TE: 40ms
ZOOM: 1
WID: 908
LE 452
e
FLD DIA:30 cm
PO
15 NIH
PICKER INTL MRI
f

Fig. 3d–f

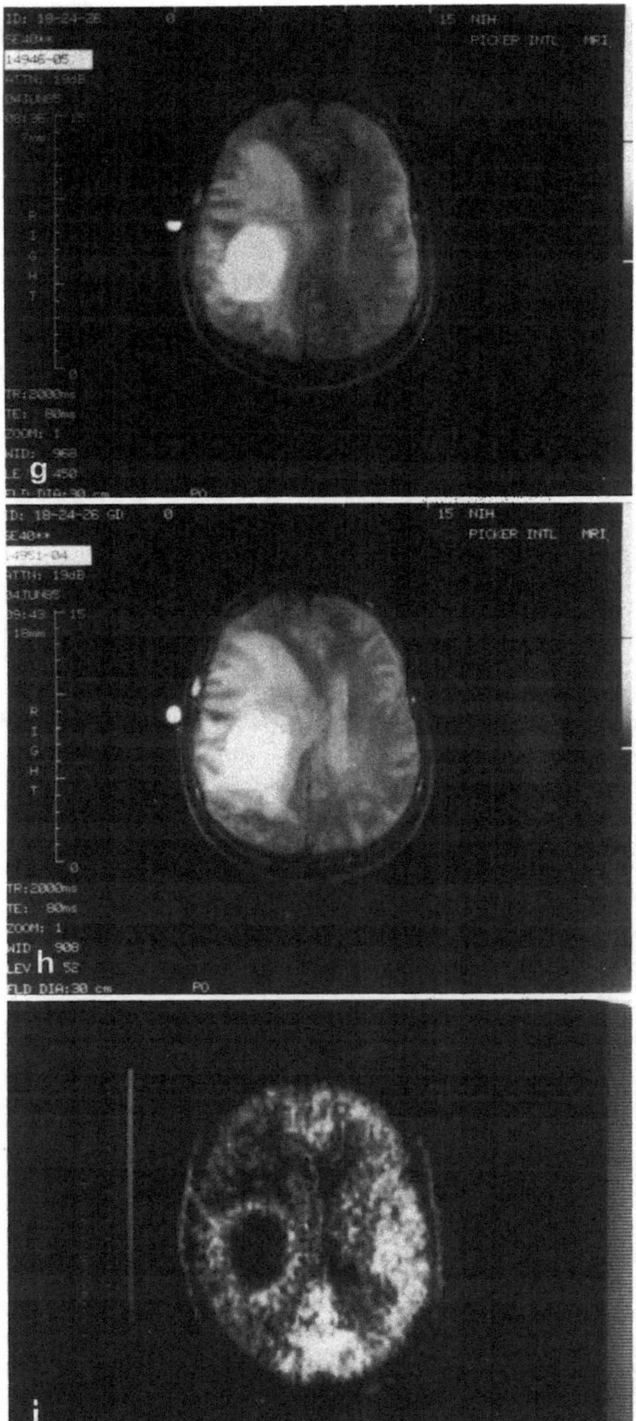

Fig. 3g–i

transverse (spin-spin) relaxation time T2, and flow. Differences in tissue relaxation times are the main determinants of image contrast. Therefore, a priori knowledge of the relaxation behavior of different tissues is important in the selection of the proper RF pulse sequence for obtaining optimal images. The two most commonly used imaging techniques utilize the spin-echo and inversion recovery. The RF pulses which tilt the nuclear spins 90° or 180° may be injected at various times, with various sequences, and with various frequencies. The terms TE-echo time, TR-repetition time, and TI-inversion time are used to indicate some of these parameters. Finally the signal-to-noise ratio is favorably affected by higher field strength and by the usage of the surface coils.

The resolution of the proton NMR images of the brain allow us, with the newer scanners, to recognize such fine normal structures as the substantia nigra and the red nucleus (Fig. 2). In selected cases we may also distinguish the various thalamic nuclei separated by myelin strips and, in axial images of the spinal cord, the H-shaped central distribution of the gray matter.

Pathological lesions of the CNS are often characterized by long T1 and T2. Particularly advantageous is the long T2, which in T2-weighted spin-echo techniques elicits a strong signal from the abnormality. In fact, one of the commonly adopted strategies to visualize pathology of the CNS is the usage of a spin-echo technique with late echoes: due to the long T2 of the lesion its signal tends to persist, while the signal from surrounding tissues vanishes.

The sensitivity of MRI in the detection of CNS lesions is superior to that of CT. This is exemplified by the MRI's capability to identify multiple sclerosis plaques, a capability unmatched by the best CT studies, including those with double dosage of intravenous contrast medium. The ease with which we may obtain NMR sagittal images is of great help in examinations of the spinal cord. Tumors, syrinxes, compression (discal, traumatic), and atrophy, as well as congenital abnormalities (such as the tethered cord), are easily recognized. In the posterior fossa, due to the absence of bone-derived beam-hardening artifacts, the MRI are often more informative than CT. For tumors in the supratentorial region, CT and MRI are about equivalent, although the similarity of the NMR signal originating from the neoplasm and the surrounding edema makes it difficult to assess the tumoral extent. This shortcoming will be alleviated when the usage of magnetic contrast agents, such as gadolinium-DTPA, become widespread (Fig. 3).

The diagnostic weakness of MRI is undoubtedly its poor specificity. Tumors, infarctions, hematomas, demyelinating foci, and edematous areas all give similar signals and, further, calcific deposits cannot be identified as in CT. Also, functional measurement such as O_2 metabolism or glucose utilization, and assessment of neurotransmitter concentrations are beyond the capabilities of MRI. One should note however that MRI is in a state of transition with advances being made at a bewildering pace. New developments are taking place in subtechnologies such as surface coils, magnetic field strength, imaging pulse sequences, contrast media, chemical shift imaging, multinuclear imaging (^{23}Na, ^{19}F), spectroscopy (^{31}P), and flow studies. Finally, it should be emphasized that no biological hazards are known to exist at the magnetic field strengths and RF pulse sequences currently employed in MRI; this is certainly an advantage as compared with the risks of ionizing radiation associated with CT and PET.

Positron Emission Tomography with Oxygen-15 Radiopharmaceuticals

M. E. RAICHLE [1]

Introduction

The initial development of tracer strategy for the measurement of brain oxygen utilization and blood flow with positron emission tomography (PET) was designed to accommodate the slow data gathering capabilities of the early PET tomographs (e.g., PETT III, ECAT II). Thus, data from equilibrium images of inhaled gases such as oxygen-15-labeled carbon dioxide and molecular oxygen, obtained at relatively low counting rates, were used for the computation of these important measurements [17]. Although important new data have been acquired using these techniques in humans, significant performance shortcomings detract from their usefulness [5]. The recent development of tomographic systems capable of acquiring a large number of events over relatively short periods of time [18] permits the development of tracer techniques for the measurement of oxygen consumption and blood flow that can be executed over relatively short periods of time [6, 12, 14]. These techniques, if properly implemented, come closer to the ideal of capturing a physiologic steady state and appear to perform well under a variety of conditions likely to be encountered in studies of human subjects, permitting not only rapid measurements because of their ease of preparation and analysis (Table 1) but also multiple sequential studies in the same subject because of rapid radioactive decay (i.e., 2 min; Table 1) and low radiation dose (Table 2). Presented below are descriptions of three methods which employ data collection times of less than 1 min following the administration of radiotracers either by intravenous bolus injection ($H_2{}^{15}O$) or single breath inhalation ($O^{15}O$, $C^{15}O$).

Measurement of Cerebral Blood Flow

In 1951, Kety [9] presented a theory of inert gas exchange in the lungs and tissues and its possible application to the measurement of tissue blood flow [8]. A short time

This research was supported by NIH Grants NS06833, NS03991, HL13851, and NS14834 and the McDonnell Center for Studies of Higher Brain Functions.

[1] Division of Radiation Sciences, Washington University School of Medicine, 510 South Kingshighway, St. Louis, MO 63110, USA.

Neurology
Ed. by K. Poeck, H. J. Freund, and H. Gänshirt

Table 1. Time (approximate) required for a complete study (i.e., a single measurement) in human subjects utilizing ^{15}O-radiotracers

Measurement	Tracer	Cyclotron bombardment (min)	Chemistry preparation (min)	Data collection	Clearance of residual tracer[a]	Total (min)
Blood flow	$H_2{}^{15}O$ (i.v. bolus)	4	2	40 s	10 min	17
	$CO^{15}O$ (bolus inhalation)	4	0	40 s	10 min	15
	(continuous inhalation)	11	0	15 min	10 min	36
Blood volume	[^{15}O]carbon monoxide	6	2	5 min	10 min	23
Metabolism	[^{15}O]oxygen[b] (single breath)	6 ($O^{15}O$)	2	40 s	10 min	
		6 ($C^{15}O$)	2	5 min	10 min	
		4 ($H_2{}^{15}O$)	2	40 s	10 min	
		16	6	6 min	22 min	60
	[^{15}O]oxygen (continuous inhalation)	11 ($O^{15}O$)	0	15 min	10 min	
		11 ($CO^{15}O$)	0	15 min	10 min	
		6 ($C^{15}O$)	2	15 min	10 min	
		28	2	45 min	30 min	105

[a] Calculation based on five half-lives of physical decay beginning at the termination of data collection.
[b] The two $C^{15}O$ oxygen methods for measuring oxygen utilization require the separate administration of three separate tracers and provide measurements of blood flow, blood volume, oxygen extraction, and oxygen utilization.

Table 2. Radiation doses to critical organs for oxygen-15 radiopharmaceuticals

Labeled compound (route of administration)	Critical organ	Administered activity (mCi)	Total dose (rads)	Permissible dose[a] (rads)
[^{15}O]Water (intravenous)	High flow organs[b]	70	0.5	5
[^{15}O]Oxygen (single breath)	Trachea	50	1.0	5
[^{15}O]Carbon monoxide (single breath)	Trachea	50	0.6	5

[a] Code of Federal Regulation, Title 21, page 161, April 1, 1981.
[b] Heart, lungs, brain, kidney, gastrointestinal tract.

later, he and his colleagues described, in detail, [10, 11] a tissue autoradiographic technique for the measurement of local brain blood flow in laboratory animals based on this theory of inert gas exchange and a simple, one-compartment model which assumes that tracer equilibrates instantaneously throughout all areas of the tissue (i.e., vasculature, extra- and intracellular spaces). The technique has been widely applied and revised on several occasions [15, 16] as newer radiotracers were substituted for the one initially employed – volatile, and difficult-to-handle trifluoroiodomethane. Because PET provides a quantitative measure of local tissue radioactivity and, hence, an in vivo autoradiograph, it was reasonable to suppose that local cerebral blood flow can be measured in human subjects using the principles of the Kety autoradiographic technique in conjunction with PET and a freely diffusible, inert radiopharmaceutical labeled with a positron emitter [13]. Such an approach has been developed, implemented, and validated in human subjects using $H_2{}^{15}O$ as the diffusible tracer [6, 14]. For the measurement of regional CBF with PET an emission scan (scan length, 40 s) is performed following an intravenous, bolus injection of 12 ml saline containing 50–100 mCi $H_2{}^{15}O$ (half-life, 124 s). Arterial blood samples are drawn about every 5 s during the scan.

There is one very important constraint that must be placed on the use of this technique as well as on the classic tissue autoradiographic technique [10]. The duration of the study must not exceed 1 min as originally prescribed by Kety and others. Any collections in excess of this time period show an underestimation of CBF that increased with time [14]. This phenomenon is also shown in the data of Eklof et al. [1]. In the latter study, the classic autoradiographic technique was used, but direct tissue sampling was substituted for the actual tissue autoradiography. Examining several tracers with differing permeabilities, the investigators observed a decline in the measured blood flow as the tissue data collection was delayed from 30 s to 60 s or 120 s. This phenomenon is quite clearly not related to any aspect of the PET adaptation of the original Kety autoradiographic technique because it occurs in applications of the original technique [1] as well as in our work [14]. It is definitely not due to the permeability of a particular tracer and it is not due to tissue inhomogeneity as Eklof et al. [1] discusses in detail.

The most likely explanation for this phenomenon is the inadequacy of a simple, one-compartment model as a description of the complex events occurring to an inert, diffusible tracer such as $H_2{}^{15}O$ as it passes through brain tissue. Such a model assumes, quite unrealistically, that tracer concentrations are, everywhere, the same when, in fact, that is unlikely to be the case. Variable gradients of tracer activity in tissue are undoubtedly produced by vascular endothelial and cell membrane permeability limitations to the inert, diffusible tracer as well as the size of the spaces (i.e., extra- and intracellular) into which the tracer distributes. The higher the blood flow in relation to these variables the greater the departure of the tracer behavior from the predictions of a single, well-mixed compartment. The consequences of this problem seem intuitively obvious; that is, there is less tracer in the tissue with time after injection than would be expected on the basis of predictions from the one-compartment model. Estimates of blood flow using this one-compartment model would be expected, therefore, to progressively underestimate blood as data sampling times lengthened. In effect, the Kety tissue autoradiographic method [10, 11] and its PET adaptation [6, 14] perform satisfactorily only when tissue sampling times are sufficiently short to preclude significant tracer egress from the tissue (i.e., less than 1 min after tracer administration). Under such circumstances, an inert, diffusible tracer is treated like, and functions as, a microsphere. Thus, its distribution within the microenvironment of the brain capillary becomes unimportant.

There are several important consequences of this problem. Investigators employing the Kety autoradiographic technique [10, 11] or its PET adaptation [6, 14] must employ data collection times of less than 1 min for accurate results. In order to ensure PET images of high statistical quality with such a short data collection time it is, therefore, necessary to inject rather substantial quantities of $H_2{}^{15}O$ (i.e., 50–100 mCi). It is very important to employ an imaging device capable of handling the resulting very high counting rate. Investigators already aware of this problem of high counting rates when employing the PET adaptation of the Kety autoradiographic technique have suggested alternative tracer strategies employing lower dose, bolus injections of $H_2{}^{15}O$ followed by several sequential PET scans from which estimates of blood flow and distribution volume are estimated [7, 8]. Although superficially appealing, this approach is flawed in exactly the same manner as the Kety autoradiographic technique and its PET adaptation, namely, reliance on the assumptions of a single compartment model. Until a more satisfactory model can be developed (e.g., a distributed model) that presents a more realistic description of the tracer behavior in tissue and can, also, realistically be implemented with PET, the PET adaptation of the original Kety autoradiographic strategy is the technique of choice for measurement of local CBF with PET.

It is important to emphasize the advantage of $H_2{}^{15}O$ over alternative inert tracers, labeled with longer lived radionuclides, that might be selected because of their greater blood-brain barrier permeability (e.g., ^{11}C-butanol). Because the data collection time for this technique must be short (i.e., less than 1 min; see above) approximately equivalent millicurie doses of radiopharmaceutical must be used regardless of the radionuclide. This results in an appreciably higher dose to the subject when long lived, positron-emitting radionuclides are used and more prolonged residual background activity must be tolerated. The consequence of these effects is to reduce greatly the number and frequency of measurements that can be made safely in a single subject. Using $H_2{}^{15}O$, for example, we routinely make as many as eight sequential measurements of CBF in a single setting with the measurements spaced about 12–15 min apart [2, 3]. Such a protocol, used in our case for functional mapping of the brain would be difficult, if not impossible, with tracers labeled with ^{11}C, ^{13}N, ^{15}O, or ^{18}F. The relatively low radiation dose of $H_2{}^{15}O$ has also permitted satisfactory studies of very young infants to be safely performed [19, 20] well within the guidelines for such studies prescribed by the Food and Drug Administration (i.e., 10% of the doses shown in Table 2).

Measurement of Cerebral Oxygen Utilization and Blood Volume

The introduction of molecular oxygen-15 into the vascular compartment of the body results in the distribution of the labeled oxygen to the tissue where it is converted to $H_2{}^{15}O$ metabolism. This labeled water then redistributes to all tissues by the same vascular compartment. Unmetabolized labeled molecular oxygen is ultimately removed by respiration. We have incorporated these properties of the oxygen-15 tracer into a two-compartment model that corresponds to the different molecular forms, $O^{15}O$ and $H_2{}^{15}O$, found in the brain [12]. The first compartment containing $O^{15}O$ physically corresponds to the intravascular space. The molecular oxygen enters via the arterial input and leaves by the venous drainage. It is assumed that the diffusion of $O^{15}O$ into the tissue space can be expressed by a fractional extraction, E, specific for a given region, times the arterial input. Once it is extracted from the vascular space, the $O^{15}O$ is assumed to be immediately metabolized to $H_2{}^{15}O$ and enters the second compartment. Thus the extravascular tissue oxygen content is assumed to be zero.

The second compartment for $H_2{}^{15}O$ physically corresponds to the free water distribution space in the brain including all vascular spaces. The entrance of tracer occurs from the arterial input carrying $H_2{}^{15}O$ redistributing from all tissues, and from $H_2{}^{15}O$ of metabolism created locally. The latter amount is, of course, equal to the product of the local extraction fraction and the $O^{15}O$ arterial input curve as described above. The exist of $H_2{}^{15}O$ occurs by a venous drainage at a concentration equal to the product of the tissue concentration and the blood/brain partition coefficient for water. Except for additional input from extracted $O^{15}O$, this half of the model is identical to the classic one-compartment Kety model designed to measure blood flow (see above). Implementation of our mathematical model to calculate the local extraction of oxygen and, ultimately, the $CMRO_2$ requires the successful execution of several steps.

1. The adequate inhalation of $O^{15}O$ as a single breath and subsequent PET scan of sufficient length to assure statistical accuracy (scan time, 40 s)
2. Description of the $O^{15}O$ and $H_2{}^{15}O$ arterial blood activity curve
3. Determination of blood flow and blood volume in all regions of interest
4. Measurement of the arterial total oxygen content at the time of the scan

Using these data, the $CMRO_2$ is computed as the product of the local extraction of oxygen, the local cerebral blood flow, and the arterial oxygen content [12].

Table 3. Comparison of labeled oxygen and substrate analogs (e.g., ^{18}F-2-deoxy-D-glucose) for measurement of metabolism with positron emission tomography

Compound	Advantage	Disadvantage
Labeled oxygen	1. Tracer and tracee are identical 2. No unknown model parameters 3. Rapid radioactive decay and lower dose; easily repeatable	1. Blood volume and blood flow must be measured 2. In-house cyclotron required 3. Subject must be able to take a single breath of labeled gas on command
Labeled deoxyglucose	1. Efficiently trapped in tissue 2. Blood volume and blood flow need not be measured 3. In-house cyclotron not required	1. Tracer and tracee are not identical 2. Long measurement time (> 30 min) 3. Relatively larger radiation dose [a] and slow decay; not easily repeatable 4. Model parameters must be assumed

[a] The absorbed dose of radiation (whole body as well as critical organ) is directly related to the half-life of the radionuclide used. ^{18}F has a half-life of 110 min compared with 2 min for ^{15}O.

It should be noted that measurement of local cerebral blood volume, which is a necessary component of the measurement of $CMRO_2$ using our approach, is accomplished by the separate inhalation of a single breath of air labeled with trace quantities of $C^{15}O$ [4]. Allowing approximately 2 min for tracer equilibrium to be achieved, images of local cerebral blood volume are then obtained over a period of 5 min.

Several points should be made about this approach to the measurement of $CMRO_2$. First, this model is relatively simple and lacks limiting assumptions. The local cerebral blood flow which determines the entrance and exit behavior of the only metabolite $H_2{}^{15}O$, is measured explicitly. Since no average value is assumed for local flow, the model is equally useful in varying areas of high, normal, and low blood flow. The local cerebral blood volume which is necessary for determining the amount of $O^{15}O$ tracer in the vascular compartment is also measured explicitly resulting in similar versatility. Recirculating water of metabolism contributing to the overall arterial blood activity curve, is measured explicitly. Thus, few assumptions are made regarding the subject's general metabolic rate or physiology as it pertains to these variables (Table 3).

References

1. Eklof B, Lassen NA, Nilsson L, et al. (1974) Regional cerebral blood flow in the rat measured by the tissue sampling technique; a critical evaluation using four indicators C^{14}-antipyrine, C^{14}-ethanol, H^3-water, and $xenon^{133}$. Acta Physiol Scand 91:1–10
2. Fox PT, Raichle ME (1984) Stimulus rate dependence of regional cerebral blood flow in human striate cortex demonstrated by positron emission tomography. J Neurophysiol 51:1109–1120
3. Fox PT, Raichle ME (1985) Stimulus rate determines regional brain blood flow in striate cortex. Ann Neurol 17:303–305
4. Grubb RL Jr, Raichle ME, Higgins CS, et al. (1978) Measurement of regional cerebral blood volume by emission tomography. Ann Neurol 4:322–328
5. Herscovitch P, Raichle ME (1983) Effect of tissue heterogeneity on the measurement of cerebral blood flow with the equilibrium $C_{15}O_2$ inhalation technique. J Cereb Blood Flow Metab 4:407–415
6. Herscovitch P, Markham J, Raichle ME (1983) Blood flow measured with intravenous $H_2{}^{15}O$. I. Theory and error analysis. J Nucl Med 24:782–789
7. Huang S-C, Carson RE, Phelps ME (1982) Measurement of local blood flow and distribution volume with short-lived isotopes: a general input technique. J Cereb Blood Flow Metab 2:99–108
8. Huang S-C, Carson RE, Hoffman EJ, Carson J, MacDonald N, Barrio JR, Phelps ME (1983) Quantitative measurement of local cerebral blood flow in humans by positron computed tomography and ^{15}O-water. J Cereb Blood Flow Metab 3:141–153
9. Kety SS (1951) The theory and application of the exchange of inert gas at the lungs and tissues. Pharmacol Rev 3:1–41
10. Kety SS (1960) Measurement of local blood flow by the exchange of an inert, diffusible substance. Methods Med Res 8:228–236
11. Landau WM, Freygang WH Jr, Rowland LP, et al. (1955) The local circulation of the living brain; values in the unanesthetized and anesthetized cat. Trans Am Neurol Assoc 80:125–129
12. Mintun MA, Raichle ME, Martin WRW, Herscovitch P (1983) Brain oxygen utilization measured with O-15 radiotracers and positron emission tomography. J Nucl Med 25:177–187

13. Raichle ME (1979) In vivo autoradiography with positron emission tomography. Brain Res Rev 1:47–68
14. Raichle ME, Martin WRW, Herscovitch P, Mintun MA, Markham J (1983) Brain blood flow measured with intravenous $H_2{}^{15}O$. II. Implementation and validation. J Nucl Med 24:790–798
15. Reivich M, Jehle J, Sokoloff L, et al. (1969) Measurement of regional cerebral blood flow with antipyrine-^{14}C in awake cats. J Appl Physiol 27:296–300
16. Sakurada O, Kennedy C, Jehle J, et al. (1978) Measurement of local cerebral blood flow with iodo[^{14}C]antipyrine. Am J Physiol 234:H59–H66
17. Subramanyam R, Alpert NM, Hoop B Jr, Brownell GL, Taveras JM (1978) A model for regional cerebral oxygen distribution during continuous inhalation of $^{15}O_2$, $C^{15}O$, and $C^{15}O_2$. J Nucl Med 19:48–53
18. Ter-Pogossian MM, Ficke DC, Hood JT Sr, et al. (1982) A positron emission tomograph utilizing cesium fluoride scintillation detectors. J Comput Assist Tomogr 6:125–133
19. Volpe JJ, Herscovitch P, Perlman JM, Raichle ME (1983) Positron emission tomography in the newborn: extensive impairment of regional cerebral blood flow with intraventricular hemorrhage and hemorrhagic intracerebral involvement. J Pediatr 72:589–601
20. Volpe JJ, Herscovitch P, Perlman JM, Kreusser KL, Raichle ME (1985) Positron emission tomography in the asphyxiated newborn: parasaggital impairment of blood flow. Ann Neurol 17:287–296

PET Studies of Local Brain Metabolism During Sensory and Motor Tasks: Strategies, Results and Applications in Neurologic and Psychiatric Diseases

J. C. Mazziotta [1]

Positron emission tomography (PET) provides a means of studying local sensory, motor, memory, and cognitive functions in normal subjects in vivo. Such tasks have been used to define the functional neuroanatomy of the human brain. Once consistent and interpretable data from normal individuals have been obtained, these can be applied in abnormal populations to test the functional reserve and recovery capacity of patients with various types of neurological and psychiatric disorders. In our laboratory we have begun to put together relevant data on normal populations in various stimulated and resting states [5–15]. These investigations reflect four specific aims:

1. To accumulate data in populations of normal subjects using the most accurate measurement specifications possible (e.g., the highest spatial resolution available)
2. To explore normal cerebral responses to sensory, motor, memory, and cognitive tasks
3. To design, develop, and validate the stimulation tasks and the resultant normal data base to use as probes in studying patients with minimal abnormalities seen on "resting" PET studies
4. To use these probes as a means of studying the functional recovery or maintenance of cerebral processes following brain injury. Hence, these investigations are a necessary prelude to the full exploitation of PET metholodology in patients, while simultaneously providing previously unavailable information about normal cerebral function.

We have explored the use of PET for measuring changes in local cerebral metabolic rate for glucose utilization (LCMRGlc) in normal individuals and in select patient groups who have lesions disrupting systems that we have studied in normal subjects. Most of our results have been reported at length elsewhere [5–15] and will be described only briefly here in order to detail current results, strategies, and applications in patient populations.

[1] Department of Neurology, Department of Radiological Sciences, UCLA School of Medicine, Laboratory of Nuclear Medicine, Los Angeles, CA 90024, USA.

Neurology
Ed. by K. Poeck, H. J. Freund, and H. Gänshirt

The following is a summary of neurobehavioral PET results using measurements of cerebral glucose metabolism:

1. Progressive increase in local cerebral metabolic rate for glucose with increases in stimulus complexity (visual system [14, 17])
2. Topographic cortical responses to selective sensory receptor stimulation (visual system [10])
3. Excellent clinical/PET correlations of sensory pathway lesions (visual system [16])
4. Hemisphere lateralization effects that vary with stimulus content (visual system [9] and auditory system [6])
5. Lateralization effects in response to subject strategy on a behavioral task (auditory system [6])
6. Subcortical (caudate, thalamus) responses to sensory and motor stimuli (auditory system [8], motor system [5])
7. Changes in magnitude and symmetry (anterior–posterior and left–right) of local cerebral metabolic rate for glucose with changes in baseline ambient test states [7]

Stimulation Studies in Normal Subjects

Visual Stimuli

Our initial studies of the visual system were designed to demonstrate the effect of the stimulus complexity on the metabolic responses of the visual cortex [14]. These studies were performed in normal individuals and were expanded to include a group of patients with homonymous hemianopia. The patients had structural lesions that involved the optic radiation, but that spared the occipital cortex itself [17]. In addition, high resolution metabolic investigations were used to examine the topographic distribution of selective central visual stimulation vs full-field stimulation [10].

The effect of stimulus complexity was examined by comparing studies in normal subjects who had their eyes closed with stimulation experiments in which the same subjects were exposed to either white light, alternating black and white checkerboard patterns, or a complex moving color scene [16, 17]. Stimuli were presented binocularly in all cases. Five subjects had a third study done, in which monocular checkerboard stimuli were presented and were compared with the binocular condition [14, 17]. The results demonstrated that the LCMRGlc increased from the eyes-closed to the stimulated state in all cases. There was a graded increase in metabolic response, with the white light producing the most minimal response, the complex scene producing the maximal response, and the checkerboard stimulus producing an intermediate response. Binocular stimulation produced a greater increment in LCMRGlc than monocular stimulation when both were compared with the eyes-closed control state [14, 17]. The rate of increase for the secondary visual areas (Brodmann areas 18 and 19) was greater than for the primary visual cortex (area 17). In addition, LCMRGlc responses (closed and stimulated, monocular and binocular) were symmetrical, confirming a 50% functional input from each eye to both visual cortices [14, 17].

All hemianopic patients exhibited reduced LCMRGlc in the visual cortex contralateral to the visual field defect. The average LCMRGlc of the involved primary

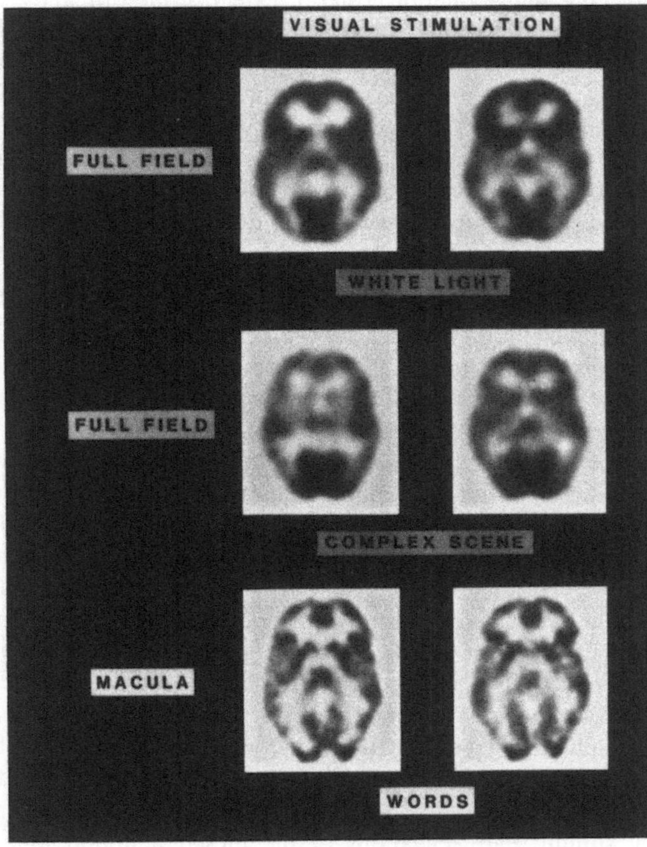

Fig. 1. Three separate fluorine-18 labeled fluorodeoxyglucose PET studies demonstrating the human cortical topographic response to selective visual stimuli. The *top* and *middle* sets of images were obtained in normal subjects receiving full-field visual stimuli consisting of either simple white light or a complex moving color outdoor scene. The images, which were obtained with the ECAT II PET device, demonstrate that the full anterior-posterior extent of the medial occipital cortex responds to both types of full-field stimuli. The *bottom* set of images is from a subject seeing symbols presented to the central 2 degrees of vision. The resultant images demonstrate relative activation of only the occipital poles, consistent with the expected topographic distribution for central retinal projections. The improved spatial resolution of the *bottom* set of images results from the fact that the images were obtained with the NeuroECAT PET device. (From [10], with permission)

and secondary visual cortical areas, respectively, was 32±7% and 44±6% lower than that of the normal, contralateral side [17]. The metabolic response of the visual cortex was normal on the unaffected side. The metabolic values of the involved visual cortex in these patients were lower than those found in unstimulated normal subjects with their eyes closed and patched. High-resolution studies of the topographic response of the visual system to selective central retinal stimulation revealed the expected distribution for the metabolic response mapped onto the visual cortex. For individuals receiving full-field checkerboard, white light, or complex scene stimulation, the entire anterior-posterior extent of the primary visual cortex responded. With selective stimuli (central 2 degrees of vision) the cortical metabolic response was limited to the occipital poles (Fig. 1) [10].

Thus, for the human visual system, PET stimulation studies have demonstrated (a) an increasing LCMRGlc that varies with the complexity of the stimulus, (b) equal cortical functional inputs from each eye to each visual cortex, (c) excellent clinical/PET correlations of visual pathway lesions, and (d) the expected topographic cortical distribution for central and peripheral retinal stimulation [9, 10, 14, 17].

Auditory Stimuli

The human auditory system has been examined with PET and these studies indicated a correlation between the distribution of glucose utilization and the content of the stimulus and, in some cases, the strategy used by the subject to solve the task [6]. While complex patterns of responses to auditory stimuli were observed, verbal stimuli caused asymmetric increases in glucose utilization that were greater in the left hemisphere in right-handed individuals. Nonverbal stimuli, such as chords, activated primarily right hemisphere areas particularly in the inferior frontal, parietal, and superior temporal regions. In subjects who listened to sequences of notes and were asked to determine whether notes in one sequence differed from those in another, the pattern of glucose utilization correlated with the strategy used by the subject. Individuals who used specific visual imagery and analytic strategies ("visualizing" frequency histograms or musical scales in their minds) had predominantly left hemisphere asymmetries and increases in glucose utilization in the posterior temporal region. Subjects who did not use this strategy to solve the task, but rather used mental "resinging" of the notes had activations in the inferior parietal regions of the right hemisphere. In addition, subjects who were asked to recall specific aspects of auditory stimuli, had activations of the mesial temporal lobe (hippocampus, parahippocampus) that were never seen in situations where auditory perception without memory tasks was required (Fig. 2) [6].

Motor Stimuli

A battery of relatively simple motor tasks has been developed and evaluated using PET and fluorodeoxyglucose (FDG) to study the effects of activation in the motor system on normal volunteers [5, 12]. The same task was used to evaluate patients with Huntington's disease and metabolic abnormalities of the striatum [12] (see below).

Two motor tasks (sequential finger movements and signature writing) were studied in normal volunteers ($n = 11$). All subjects were strongly right-handed and served as their own control by also having a baseline (no movement) PET-FDG study. All subjects were blindfolded for both control and stimulation studies (ears unoccluded, equipment noise only, dim lighting). Results were compared by obtaining the percent increase of the maximal responses in each state.

In normal subjects both tasks resulted in significant increases in glucose metabolism in the primary sensorimotor cortex contralateral to the moving hand at an axial level that coincided with the cingulate cortex medially. While no other significant regional metabolic rate changes were found with the finger sequence task, bi-

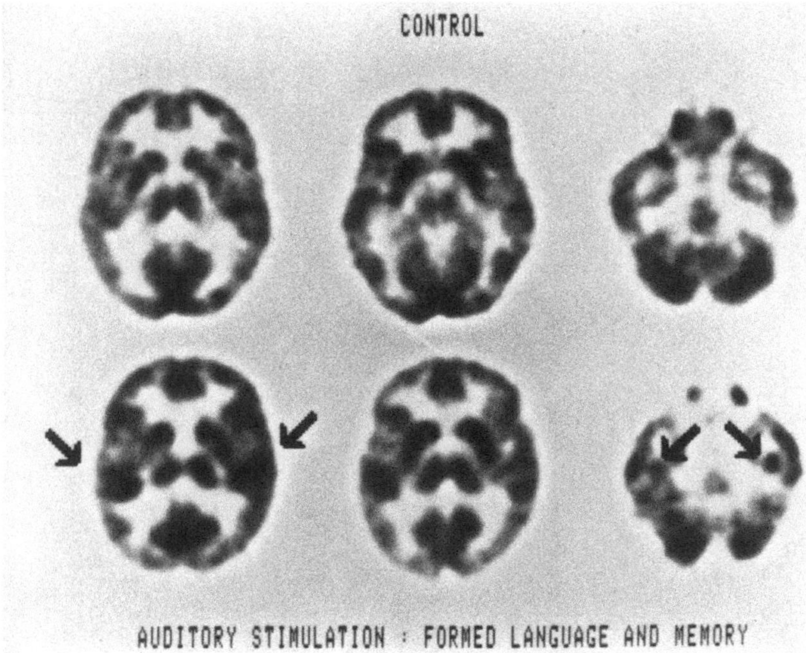

Fig. 2. Two sets of images from two normal subjects studied with FDG to determine glucose metabolism in a control (*top row*) and auditory-stimulated state (*bottom row*). The *top row* of images was obtained from a subject with no auditory stimulation. The *bottom row* was obtained from a second subject listening to a factual story monaurally. Note the activation of the primary auditory cortex situated bilaterally in the posterior transverse, temporal cortical zone. The left-right asymmetries closely parallel known anatomical asymmetries for these areas in the human brain (i.e., the region on the left is larger, wedge-shaped, and more posterior than its counterpart on the right). Note also in the lowest image (*rightmost*) the activation of the hippocampus during the verbal task. The subject was instructed to remember specific phrases of the auditory stimulus material (a Sherlock Holmes story) and told that he would be paid in proportion to his performance on an examination following the stimulation task. (From [6], with permission)

lateral striatal increases in metabolic rate were found with the writing paradigm. In addition, a few subjects had increases in metabolic rate for glucose in the contralateral thalamus (2/11 subjects) and ipsilateral cerebellar cortex (3/11), but these were not significant when the entire group of subjects was considered. The magnitudes of the increases were as follows: contralateral sensorimotor cortex 18.6 + 6.9%, contralateral striatum 19.0 + 10.2%, ipsilateral striatum 18.3 + 8.4%.

In a poststudy interview of the subjects, all normal controls indicated they performed the task in a largely subconscious and automatic way. Since the writing task is very overlearned and a semiautomatic motor activity and the finger sequence task is relatively novel, it was hypothesized that the basal ganglia involvement in the writing task may be a product of the motor learning process. Studies are presently under way to see if this programming capacity of the basal ganglia can be induced

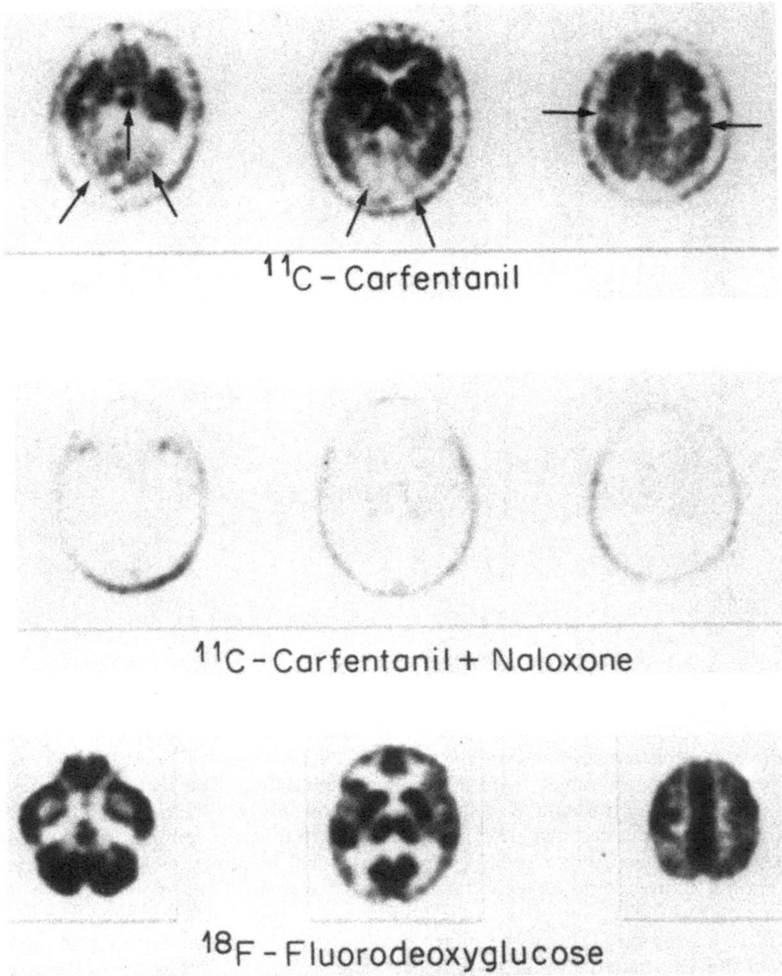

Fig. 3. In vivo pharmacology with PET. Opiate receptors in human brain. The PET images in the *top row* were obtained 30–60 min after intravenous administration of 25 mCi [^{11}C]-carfentanil (80 ng/kg) a mu opiate antagonist. The three images are 7.2 cm, 4 cm, and 0.8 cm above the canthomeatal line. Images in the *middle row* were acquired 30–60 min after intravenous administration of (1 mg/kg) naloxone (+isomer), an opiate antagonist, and the same dose of [^{11}C]-carfentanil used in the first study. In the *top row,* a preferential accumulation of activity is seen in the areas rich in opiate receptors such as the thalamus, basal ganglia, and frontal cortex (*center* and *right-hand* images) and pituitary gland (*left-hand* image, inner *arrow*). Low activity is seen where opiate receptors exist in low concentration, such as the occipital cortex (*center* image, *arrows*), the postcentral gyrus (*right-hand* image, *arrows*) and the cerebellum (*left-hand* images, *arrows*). Images in the *middle row* demonstrate the low level of nonreceptor binding when labeled carfentanil binding is blocked with naloxone. Approximately 90% of specific opiate receptor binding in the thalamus and basal ganglia is blocked. Outer ring in images is from ^{11}C activity in the scalp. *Bottom row* of images are of glucose utilization obtained using FDG for approximately the same levels as the opiate receptor distribution study. (From [15], with permission; carfentanil study courtesy of J. Frost, Johns Hopkins University, with permission)

by serially studying with PET normal volunteers who learn how to write their signature with the nondominant hand.

Pharmacologic Stimuli

While the use of PET to investigate in vivo pharmacology is not completely developed in terms of validated tracer kinetic methods, some exciting new approaches have been examined. Two different strategies can be used. In the first, pharmacologic doses of drugs can be administered to normal subjects and patients with cerebral disorders and the effect on processes such as blood flow and metabolism can be examined to determine the anatomic sites where drug-induced alterations in these processes occur. Alternately, the drug itself can be labeled with a positron emitting isotope and its pharmacokinetic behavior examined directly in vivo (Fig. 3). Either way, biochemical assays can be performed to determine the pharmacologic effects of specific agents on behavior, symptoms, and structure–function relationships in the human brain, and to identify neurotransmitter systems involved in specific diseases.

The emphasis on the development of appropriate PET compounds has led to the capacity, in the dopaminergic system, to examine both the presynaptic and postsynaptic components of the neurotransmitter-receptor system. In such studies, ^{18}F-L-dopa was used to examine the presynaptic distribution of stored neurotransmitter via this positron-labeled precursor compound. The postsynaptic receptor distribution has been examined using the positron-labeled ligand ^{11}C-methylspiperone [18]. Additional studies have been performed using ^{11}C-carfentanil to determine the distribution of opiate receptors [2]. Using this compound, the specific distribution of the appropriate subclass of opiate receptors (mu) was identified in PET images obtained 30–60 min following the intravenous administration of the compound. It was also demonstrated that binding of the labeled compound could be blocked by the antagonist compound naloxone (Fig. 3). Studies have been performed or are under way to examine not only opiate and dopaminergic systems but also cholinergic, benzodiazepine, and adrenergic neurotransmitter-receptor complexes.

Applications in Patients

Since all diseases of the brain result from or produce biochemical alterations, functional images that depict such processes have demonstrated earlier, larger, and more distributed lesions than those found in anatomically oriented techniques and even in detailed postmortem evaluations. Examples of mismatches between structural and functional lesions have been demonstrated in patients with seizure disorders, cerebral infarction, dementing processes, and neuropsychiatric diseases [15, 16]. Since the brain consists of large numbers of interconnected substructures, damage to one substructure or its interconnecting fiber bundles will also result in functional effects at multiple sights throughout any given network (Fig. 4). PET has revealed this distributed organization, leading to a more comprehensive view of human functional brain systems in health and disease. Traditional clinical-pathologic correlations that have been the mainstay of symptom-lesion localization in the brain may

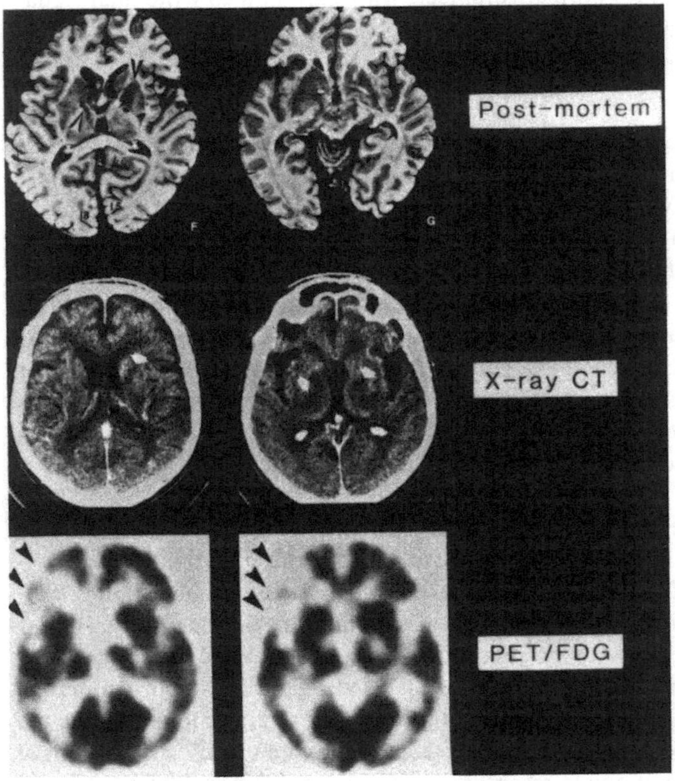

Fig. 4. Structural vs functional anatomy. Image obtained with three different methods from a patient with multiple infarct dementia. Patient had X-ray computed tomography (*center row*) and PET studies of glucose utilization with FDG (*bottom row*) on the same day. Seven days later the patient died of nonneurological causes and gross and microscopic evaluation of the brain (*top row*) was performed. Both forms of structural imaging (X-ray CT and postmortem) and the metabolic study with PET demonstrated multiple small infarctions of deep structures of the brain (striatum, thalamus, and internal capsule). Neither structural imaging technique demonstrated abnormalities of the cortex. PET, however, demonstrated widespread abnormalities of frontal cortex particularly on the *left*. These distant effects probably represent disruption of afferent and efferent fiber systems between the frontal cortical areas and subcortical zones, most likely resulting from small subcortical infarcts seen structurally and metabolically. (From [15], with permission)

soon give way to "clinical-physiologic correlations" that can be performed in vivo with PET.

Through a comprehensive investigation of stimulation tasks such as those previously described in normal populations, sets of paradigms have been and will continue to be developed which predictively activate cortical and subcortical brain regions. These paradigms can then be used in patient populations to unmask more subtle alterations in physiologic variables that might go undetected in simple resting PET studies. The use of such provocative behavioral, and potentially pharmacologic stimuli, can enhance the diagnostic specificty and anatomic localization of functional lesions thus far disclosed by PET in patients with various forms of neuropathology.

Lastly, stimulation paradigms can be used to study the recovery of the brain function following injury. Such studies should not only provide insight into the fundamental processes of cerebral reorganization after injury, but can also potentially provide guidelines for the pathophysiologically oriented rehabilitation of such brain-injured individuals.

Huntington's Disease

Glucose utilization has been determined in patients with Huntington's disease (HD) and indicates a marked hypometabolism of the striatum in all symptomatic patients [3]. In patients with early manifestations of the disease, structural imaging techniques such as X-ray CT were normal, but investigations of glucose metabolism still revealed profound reductions in glucose utilization in the caudate and putamen [3]. In a group of 15 asymptomatic individuals who were at-risk for HD, approximately half demonstrated mild to moderate reductions in glucose utilization in the caudate nucleus [3]. Three of the four individuals with the most abnormal metabolism in the caudate have subsequently developed symptoms [4]. Thus, it appears that PET can identify functional lesions of Huntington's disease that precede gross structural changes in the brain (as determined by X-ray CT) and perhaps can identify abnormalities in patients even before the symptoms of the disease are manifest. Correlation of these presymptomatic changes identified with PET and the presence of the abnormal gene determined from genetic linkage studies is presently under way in a number of laboratories. The study of at-risk individuals is not purely of academic interest since experimental treatments for such disorders would be most useful when applied in symptomatic or early stage subjects. PET may be useful in identifying those subjects and providing an objective means of monitoring whether therapeutic interventions are beneficial or harmful.

As was described above, normal subjects performing signature writing demonstrated bilateral metabolic increases of approximately 20% in the contralateral sensorimotor cortex and bilateral activations of the same magnitude in the striata [5, 12]. Since HD subjects have marked hypometabolism of the striatum in the resting state and can perform the writing task reasonably efficiently, we evaluated three HD patients at rest and during the writing task with FDG and PET [12]. The HD patients had marked reductions in striatal glucose utilization in the baseline, resting study despite minimal or no atrophy of these structures on X-ray CT imaging. The HD patients differed from normal in their metabolic responses to the writing tasks. While their contralateral sensorimotor cortex had increases in glucose metabolism that occurred at the same site but at a larger magnitude when compared with controls, no response was found in their striata; a pattern which mimics that seen in normal subjects when they performed a novel finger sequence task. The magnitudes of the responses were: contralateral sensorimotor cortex $31.9 \pm 2.7\%$, contralateral striatum $2.1 \pm 3.7\%$, ipsilateral striatum $0.2 \pm 9.8\%$ relative to the resting state in the same subject. In the poststudy interview, the HD subjects indicated that they had to concentrate specifically on the task and at the same time suppress involuntary movements. The behavioral characterization and pattern of responses seen in the

HD patients suggests the loss of automatic motor programming ability secondary to the disease process. The continued ability to perform the motor task in the face of this disease may result from the use of motor networks normally reserved for more novel motor activities. The fact that the cortical responses were of greater magnitude in the HD group (31.9±2.7% vs controls 18.6±3.9%) may be indicative of the neuronal effort required by these patients to perform the task faithfully and to suppress other unwanted motor activity [12].

Similar tasks could be developed and used in patients with strokes and motor weakness or language disorders assuming that baseline study in normal populations provided the range and magnitude of the normal responses to these tasks. Using such a strategy one could explore the compensatory capacities of the brain, the neuronal and metabolic reserves of cerebral activity to perform tasks in the face of acute injury or ongoing degeneration.

Psychiatric Disorders

Few cerebral disorders are better suited for study with PET than psychiatric diseases. Despite detailed investigations, no other imaging technique has provided specific insights into the etiology or anatomic locations associated with the many and varied psychiatric syndromes. Many studies have indicated that there are underlying biochemical mechanisms that are affected in these syndromes and result in abnormal states of behavior. The response of patients with these disorders to drug manipulations that correlate with changes in mood support the pervasive biochemical evidence relating psychological and behavioral abnormalities with biochemical mechanisms.

In drug-free patients with bipolar (manic-depressive) mood disorders, measurements of glucose utilization with PET have shown global supratentorial changes in cerebral glucose utilization during different mood states [1]. During the depressive phase of the illness, patients demonstrated reductions in glucose utilization in all supratentorial structures significantly below values found in age- and sex-matched controls. The same patients, when later studied in hypomanic phases of the illness, showed glucose utilization rates that were not different from normals. Although the major changes seen were global, the largest differences occurred in frontal and in the anterior cingulate cortices. Patients with unipolar mood disorders (depression) studied in drug-free states demonstrated global supratentorial glucose metabolic rates that were not different from normal controls. However, these patients did exhibit significantly depressed values of glucose utilization in the striata bilaterally. This reduced striatal metabolism recovered to normal levels in patients who became euthymic spontaneously or by drug therapy.

The results of these studies indicate that PET has the ability to demonstrate functional changes in cerebral biochemistry associated with behavioral disorders. The complex behaviors involved, the difficulties in characterizing those behaviors, and the diagnostic difficulties in obtaining both patient and control groups, make such psychiatric PET studies formidable endeavors. The use of stimulation paradigms (behavioral and pharmacologic) may enhance the specificity and accuracy of such work in the future. This is especially true of pharmacologic challenges in psychiatric populations.

The ability to observe in vivo drug pharmacokinetics can be used to identify the responsiveness of different patient groups to specific pharmacologically active agents. For example, consider a presumed clinically homogeneous population of psychiatric patients in which a specific drug is effective in alleviating symptoms in approximately 15%. Such a therapy would be considered relatively ineffective for the population as a whole, however, for the 15% that responded the therapy was quite effective. Conventional techniques may not be sensitive enough to identify subpopulations with specific pharmacologic sensitivities to different agents. PET studies with either of the two strategies outlined above could provide additional diagnostic information that could potentially distinguish such subgroups and allow for more specific and pathophysiologically appropriate therapies to be selected.

Conclusion and Future Prospects

Technical advances in instrumentation and tracer kinetic methods will progressively increase the number and types of biochemical and physiologic processes that can be determined with PET. Newer instruments will provide not only improved anatomic delineation but increased quantitative accuracy in the analytic measurements that are obtainable in PET studies. Technician operated and PET devoted cyclotron installations are in the process of development. Such installations would reduce the cost of the equipment, both in terms of the initial expenditure and overhead for sophisticated operating staffs. This reduction in cost and complexity can result in a wider distribution of PET installations. At present, emphasis has been placed on the development of ligands and precursors for the study of neurotransmitter systems. The ability to make such measurements should be unique to PET since the requirement for measuring picomolar to nanomolar concentrations would be necessary for such investigations.

As was discussed above, the use of behavioral and pharmacologic stimulation paradigms should increase the specificity and anatomic accuracy of measurements thus far obtained in patient populations with PET. Such studies will expand in the future and provide functional probes in patient populations. Thus, much in the way a cardiologist uses physical exercise to reveal latent abnormalities in coronary perfusion, the neurologist, neurosurgeon, and neuroscientist too can use sensory, motor, cognitive, and pharmacologic tasks to stress regional brain reserve and identify latent abnormalities, the limits of compensatory brain mechanisms, and the means used by the brain to recover or maintain function in the face of injury.

Acknowledgements. My thanks to Jorge Barrio and his chemistry staff for the preparation of FDG in these studies, Norman MacDonald and his staff for cyclotron produced isotopes, Ron Sumida for technical assistance, Lee Griswold for preparing illustrations, and Anita Powers for the preparation of the manuscript. This work was supported in part by DOE contract AM03-76-SF00012, NIH grants R01-6M-248389, P01-NS-15654, M01-RR-00865-11, NIMH grant R01-MH-37916-02, and a grant from the Hereditary Disease Foundation, as well as by NINCDS Teacher Investigator Award 1K07-00588-05-NSPA.

References

1. Baxter LR, Phelps ME, Mazziotta JC, Schwartz JM, Gerner RH, Selin SE, Sumida RM (1985) Cerebral metabolic rate for glucose in mood disorders studied with PET and (F-18)-fluorodeoxy-glucose (FDG). Arch Gen Psychiatry 150:441–447
2. Frost JJ, Wagner HN Jr, Dannals RF, Hayden TR, Links JM, Wilson AA, Burns DH, Wong DF, McPherson RW, Rosenbaum AE, Kuhar MJ, Snyder SH (1985) Imaging opiate receptors in the human brain by positron tomography. J Comput Assist Tomogr 9(2):231–236
3. Kuhl DE, Phelps ME, Markham CH, et al. (1982) Cerebral metabolism and atrophy in Huntington's disease determined by ^{18}FDG and computed tomographic scan. Ann Neurol 12:425–434
4. Kuhl DE, Markham CH, Metter EJ, Riege WH, Phelps ME, Mazziotta JC (1985) Local cerebral glucose utilization in symptomatic and presymptomatic Huntington's disease. In: Sokoloff L (ed) Brain imaging and brain function. Raven, New York, pp 199–209
5. Mazziotta JC, Phelps ME (1984) Positron computed tomography studies of cerebral metabolic responses to complex motor tasks. Neurology [Suppl 1] 34:116
6. Mazziotta JC, Phelps ME, Carson RE, et al. (1982) Tomographic mapping of human cerebral metabolism: Auditory stimulation. Neurology 32:921–937
7. Mazziotta JC, Phelps ME, Carson RE, et al. (1982) Tomographic mapping of human cerebral metabolism: Sensory deprivation. Ann Neurol 12:435–444
8. Mazziotta JC, Phelps ME, Carson RE (1984) Tomographic mapping of human cerebral metabolism: Subcortical responses to auditory and visual stimulation. Neurology 34:825–828
9. Mazziotta JC, Phelps ME, Halgren E (1983) Local cerebral glucose metabolic responses to audio-visual stimulation and deprivation: Studies in human subjects with positron CT. Human Neurobiol 2:11–23
10. Mazziotta JC, Phelps ME, Halgren E, Carson RE, Huang SC, Bayer J (1983) Hemispheric lateralization and local cerebral metabolic blood flow responses to physiologic stimuli. J Cereb Blood Flow Metab [Suppl 1] 3:S246–S247
11. Mazziotta JC, Phelps ME, Miller J, et al. (1981) Tomographic mapping of human cerebral metabolism: Normal unstimulated state. Neurology 31:503–516
12. Mazziotta JC, Phelps ME, Wapenski J (1985) Human cerebral motor system metabolic responses in health and disease. J Cereb Blood Flow Metab [Suppl 1] 5
13. Phelps ME, Huang SC, Hoffman EJ, Selin C, Sokoloff L, Kuhl DE (1979) Tomographic measurement of local cerebral glucose metabolic rate in humans with (F-18)2-fluoro-2-deoxyglucose: Validation of method. Ann Neurol 6:371–388
14. Phelps ME, Kuhl DE, Mazziotta JC (1981) Metabolic mapping of the brain's response to visual stimulation: Studies in man. Science 211:1445–1448
15. Phelps ME, Mazziotta JC (1985) Study of the biochemical basis of human cerebral function with positron computed tomography (PET): Normal and disease states. Science 228:799–809
16. Phelps ME, Mazziotta JC, Huang SC (1982) Study of cerebral function with positron computed tomography. J Cereb Blood Flow Metab 2:113–162
17. Phelps ME, Mazziotta JC, Kuhl DE, et al. (1981) Tomographic mapping of human cerebral metabolism: Visual stimulation and deprivation. Neurology 31:517–529
18. Wagner HN, Burns HD, Dunnals RF, Wong DF, Langstrom B, Dueffler T, Frost JJ, Ravert HT, Links JM, Rosenbloom SB, Lukas SE, Kramer AV, Kuhar MJ (1983) Imaging dopamine receptors in the human brain by positron tomography. Science 22:1264–1266

Functional and Morphological Evaluation of the Cerebral Circulation by Ultrasound

G.-M. von Reutern[1]

Ultrasound was first used in neurology to detect a shift of the intracranial midline. This application is of less importance today because new imaging techniques have become available. Imaging the brain by ultrasound was limited by the acoustic properties of the adult skull [34]. High resolution ultrasound imaging, however, proved to be useful for the examination of newborns and infants using the fontanella as acoustic window [3, 9, 20, 31–33]. In addition, B-mode imaging was successfully applied in neurosurgery during operations [8]. The present paper is confined to the different applications of ultrasound diagnosis in cerebrovascular diseases.

Since Doppler sonography was introduced into medicine the importance of this ultrasound technique has been continuously growing, not only because of its well-known advantages, namely cost effectiveness and harmlessness, but because essential information can be obtained by the method. Ultrasound techniques are the only ones that provide data on both the morphology of vessels and the flow within vessels. This is possible by the combination of the pulse-echo technique (B-mode imaging) with various Doppler techniques. Table 1 shows how each of these two techniques contributes to the evaluation of the cerebral circulation.

Table 1. Contribution of different ultrasound techniques to the evaluation of cerebrovascular circulation

Doppler technique	B-mode imaging
– Localization of stenoses and occlusions	– Course of the vessel
– Local flow disturbances	– Wall motion (lateral, longitudinal)
– Collateral flow	– Local vessel thickness
– Flow volume	– Quality of plaque (homogeneous, inhomogeneous, smooth-irregular surface)
– Vascular resistance and capacitance	

[1] Dept. of Clinical Neurology und Neurophysiology, University of Freiburg, Hansastrasse 9, 7800 Freiburg, Federal Republic of Germany.

Neurology
Ed. by K. Poeck, H. J. Freund, and H. Gänshirt

Basic Technical Principles

Ultrasound sent into the body is reflected at interfaces. The arterial walls are particularly strong reflecting interfaces. The reflections from the blood cells in the vessel are about 40–60 dB weaker than those from the vessel walls. The difference makes it possible to depict the vessel walls as an image. Two basically different methods are available to obtain information from the reflected ultrasound: the pulse-echo method for imaging vessels, and the Doppler method for evaluating the flow.

With the pulse-echo method (Fig. 1), a short train of pulses are sent in rapid sequence, and in the intervals the intensity and transit time of the reflected signals are measured. The return time is a measure of the depth from which the signal is reflected. A-scan refers to the time plotted on the x-axis against intensity on the y-axis. B-scan refers to a two-dimensional image made up of several sound beams. A reflection is shown as a spot with varying brightness according to the intensity of the reflection. Such a sectional image can be achieved by the movement of the transmitter or the parallel use of several transmitters.

With the Doppler method, it is not the transit time of the reflected ultrasound (i.e., the site of a reflector), but the speed of the reflector in relation to the transmitter that is measured by using Doppler effect. If the reflector approaches the transmitter/receiver, then the received frequency is higher than the transmitted frequency. The difference between the two is the Doppler frequency (Doppler shift), which in the insonation of blood vessels is proportional to the velocity of the blood cells and is dependent on the angle of insonation. We distinguish between continuous wave (CW) Doppler and pulsed Doppler. With CW Doppler, the tip of the probe contains separate transmitting and receiving crystals, which continuously transmit and receive. All particles moving within the beam of the ultrasound contribute to the resulting measurement (Fig. 2).

This measurement gives no information as to the depth at which it is made. With pulsed Doppler, a transmitter is used which acts as a receiver in the intervals between the transmitting. The position and size of the sample volume can be selected by means of electronic gating. Only the signal of a particular time interval between

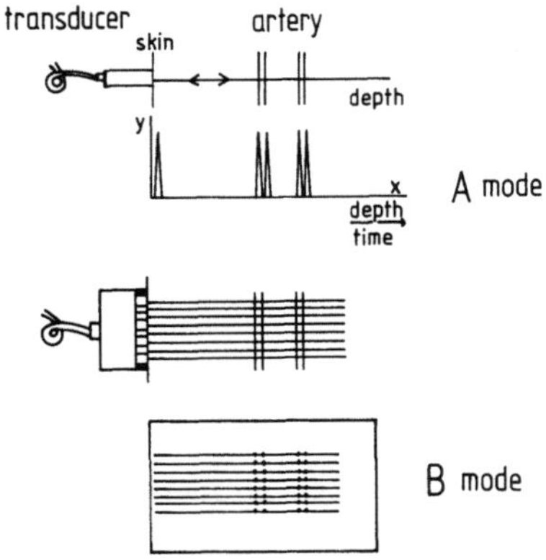

Fig. 1. Echo impulse technique. For explanation see text

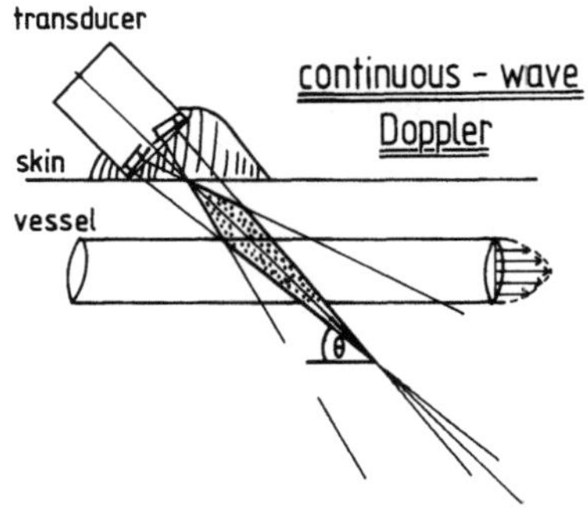

Fig. 2. Schematic representation of CW Doppler sonography. For explanation see text

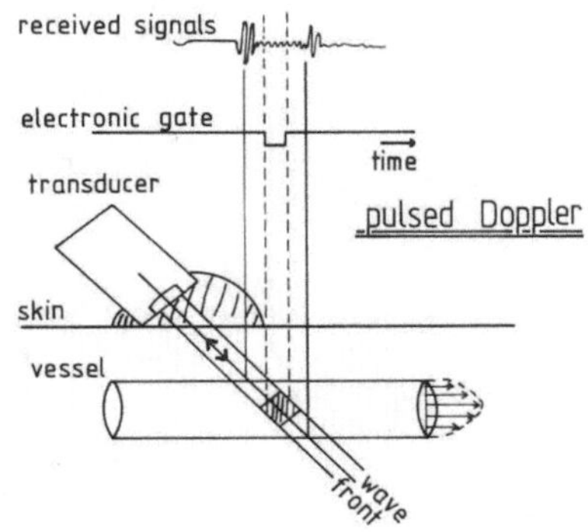

Fig. 3. Schematic representation of pulsed Doppler sonography using electronic gating to define the depth and size of the sample volume

the transmitted pulse is processed. Since the speed of ultrasound in tissue is known, the depth and size of the sample volume can be defined (Fig. 3).

The Doppler signals contain a spectrum of frequencies which correspond to the varied flow velocities of the blood cells. For the cheapest and most common documentation, frequencies are detected by a zero-crossing meter. The continuous registration of an electronically averaged mean value produces the velocity pulse curves (Figs. 5, 7). Independent of this registration, the spectrum is evaluated by the ear of the operator via a loudspeaker. The operator can hear more than the curve can document. In searching for an artery or in following the course of an artery, the operator is guided by the acoustic signal. Less common, because of its expense, is registration of the spectrum in real time. To permit this type of documentation, the frequency is plotted against time. The intensity of a frequency band represents the number of insonated particles flowing at a specific speed. Intensity is reproduced as dot density, gray scale, or color coding (Figs. 6, 8).

Localization of Stenoses and Occlusions

B-mode imaging can localize stenoses of the carotid arteries in the neck. The examination is most useful for the restricted area of the bifurcation, but less reliable for the vertebral arteries, and not practicable for the distal carotid arteries and the intracranial basal arteries. Therefore, the main drawback of B-mode imaging is that this method can be applied only to a short segment of the arteries of interest. On the other hand, with Doppler techniques stenoses and occlusions can be localized from the aortic arch to the intracranial basal arteries.

The examination of the extracranial carotid and vertebral arteries with CW Doppler can still be considered the standard method [6, 23, 30]. The main advantage it offers is the possibility to evaluate the carotid as well as the vertebral artery system [25], which are able to compensate for one another. Because this technique and its criteria are well known, they will not be discussed here. However, with the CW Doppler technique it is not possible to insonate intracranial arteries through the intact bone. This was made possible by Aaslid et al., who introduced the transcranial Doppler method [1].

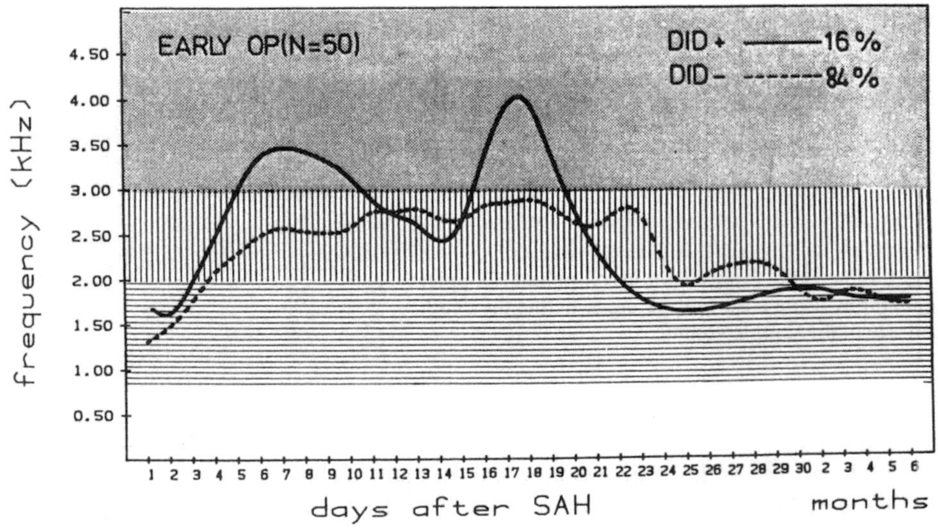

Fig. 4. Follow-up of patients with SAH and early aneurysm operation [14]. Transcranial Doppler sonography of the middle cerebral artery on the operated side. Average of the mean frequency of the envelope curve of the spectrum in 50 patients. Elevated frequencies correspond to vessel narrowing due to spasms. *Full line* represents 8 patients with delayed ischemic deficit (DID), *dotted line* 42 patients without DID. Note the steeper increase of frequencies in the group of symptomatic patients

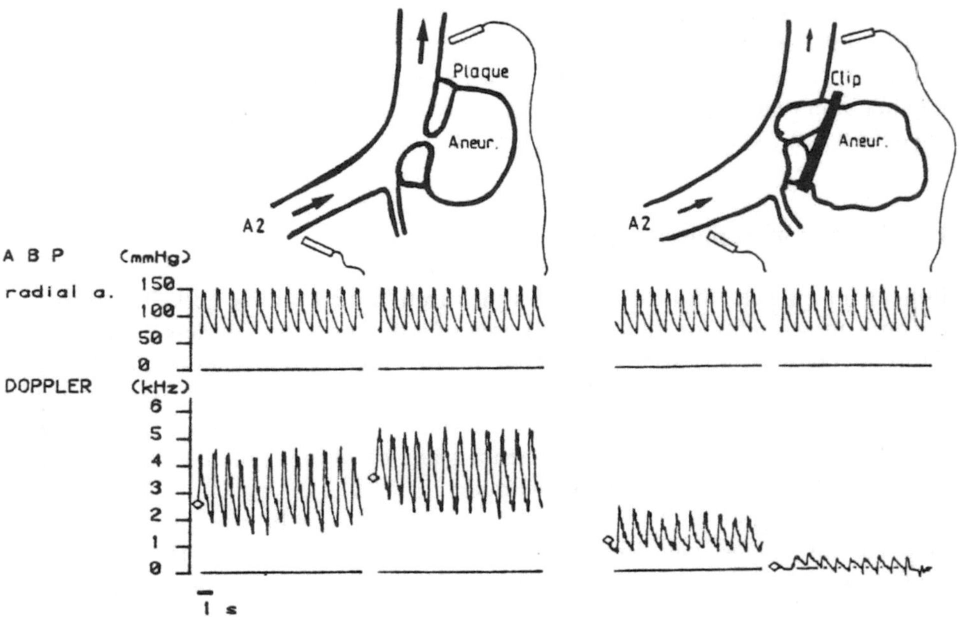

Fig. 5. Intraoperative Doppler sonography with 20 MHz emission frequency [13], recording of the mean frequency (zero-cross meter). Clipping of the aneursym results in a reduction of flow velocity of the parent artery because plaques are pushed in the vessel lumen. ABP, arterial blood pressure

To examine through the temporal bone a pulsed Doppler technique is used with a low emission frequency (2 MHz) combined with a frequency analyzer. Transcranial Doppler should never be applied alone, but only in addition to the complete extracranial evaluation [2]. The following arteries can be reached by the temporal approach: (a) the middle cerebral artery from the origin to the point where it bends toward the sylvian fissure, (b) the horizontal part of the anterior cerebral artery, (c) the pre- and postcommunicating posterior cerebral artery. The intracranial vertebral arteries and the basilar artery are best reached through the occipital foramen. Compression tests (common carotid artery low in the neck) are useful for the differentiation of intracranial arteries, especially those close to the midline [1, 2]. By means of transcranial Doppler it is possible (a) to localize intracranial occlusive disease, (b) to demonstrate the impact of extracranial occlusions on the intracranial flow situation ([2] and Figs. 8, 9), and (c) to follow up spasms after subarachnoid hemorrhage ([14] and Fig. 4).

Small intracranial branches can only be examined during a neurosurgical operation. For this purpose, a pulsed Doppler device with 20 MHz emission frequency and miniaturized probes proved to be suitable because of its high resolution [7, 13]. In extra-intracranial bypass procedures this method facilitates selection of the donor and the recipient arteries, and proof of the patency of the anastomosis and the quality of flow. During aneurysm surgery, clipping of the artery may result in a stenosis. This complication is immediately detected by the direct examination with a microvascular Doppler probe (Fig. 5).

Local Flow Disturbances

Doppler techniques are most suited to describe and to quantify local flow disturbances where a direct insonation is possible (extracranial carotid, vertebral and subclavian arteries, as well as intracranial basal arteries). These disturbances can be caused by (a) physiological diameter variations as in the region of the carotid bifurcation, (b) curvatures, or (c) different degrees of stenoses.

With pulsed Doppler, the flow profile can be examined, which shows the separation of flow lines from the inner wall in curvatures [21] or helical organization of flow in the sinus of the carotid bulb [17, 22, 24]. The nonlaminar flow organization caused by such physiological conditions as a carotid sinus cannot be distinguished from conditions caused by a small plaque or ulceration using Doppler techniques alone. This differentiation is the field of application of the Duplex scan, i.e., combined Doppler sonography and B-mode imaging (Fig. 6).

For clinical purposes, CW Doppler sonography with spectrum analysis is especially valuable because it allows moderate, severe, nearly occluding stenoses, and total occlusions to be differentiated. Direct criteria include: (a) peak frequencies corresponding to the velocity of the central jet stream [29], (b) spectrum broadening corresponding to inhomogenious flow [30], (c) the extension of poststenotic flow disturbances, and (d) the poststenotic flow velocity beyond the area of disturbances. Indirect criteria are the preocclusive reduction of flow velocity and the development of collaterals [18, 28]. Peripheral resistance and blood viscosity are factors influencing these criteria. Nevertheless, Doppler sonography represents the functional de-

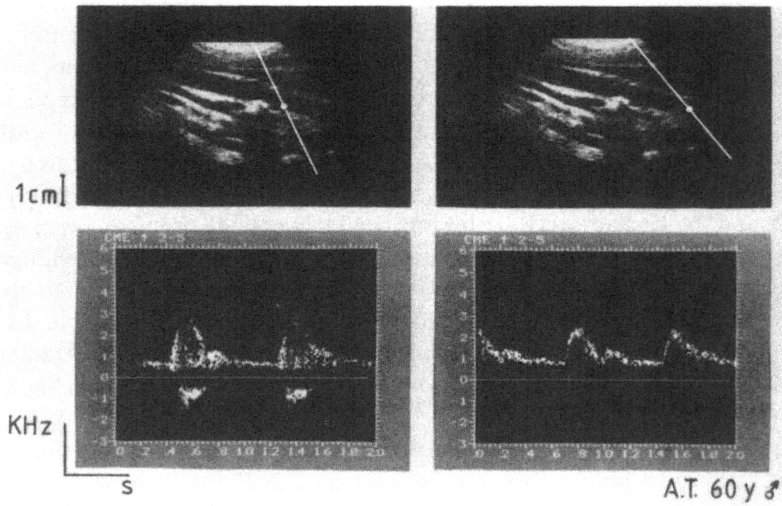

Fig. 6. Duplex scan examination of the carotid bifuraction. This section shows the common and internal carotid artery and a hyperechoic plaque at the origin of the latter. On the *left,* the Doppler sample volume is placed just behind the plaque. The recorded spectrum is broadened with reverse flow components (negative Doppler shift). On the *right,* sample volume 3 cm downstream with normalized spectrum. Similar spectrum changes occur within a large sinus of the internal carotid artery

gree of a stenosis and the impact on flow better than angiography, especially in severe and nearly occluding stenoses, where irregularities often make the measurement of the residual lumen impossible.

Morphology of Vessels

Changes in the mean Doppler shift or flow velocity along the course of an artery reflect changes in the diameter of the vessel. This criterion is useful to detect moderate and severe stenoses, but fails to prove low degrees of the disease (see Chap. on Local flow disturbances, and Fig. 6). The best morphological description of the vessel is achieved by B-mode imaging (Fig. 1) or duplex scanning. Angiography depicts only the inner surface of a perfused vessel, while ultrasound can pick up the thickness of the wall, even if this thickening does not significantly reduce the diameter of the vessel or if the vessel is occluded. Whether ulceration or intraplaque hemorrhage can be detected depends on the resolution of the instrument. If the resolution is very good the overall results of angiography and B-mode imaging seem to be equally reliable when compared with the histopathological findings [15]. In severe stenoses, however, imaging of the intima by ultrasound is often hindered by shadowing behind calcifications. Information about the course of a vessel (abnormal origin and position, coiling and kinking) is of secondary clinical importance, but it helps in interpreting Doppler results, which are dependent on the angle of insonation. Flow disturbances may originate at bending points without significant stenoses. The ob-

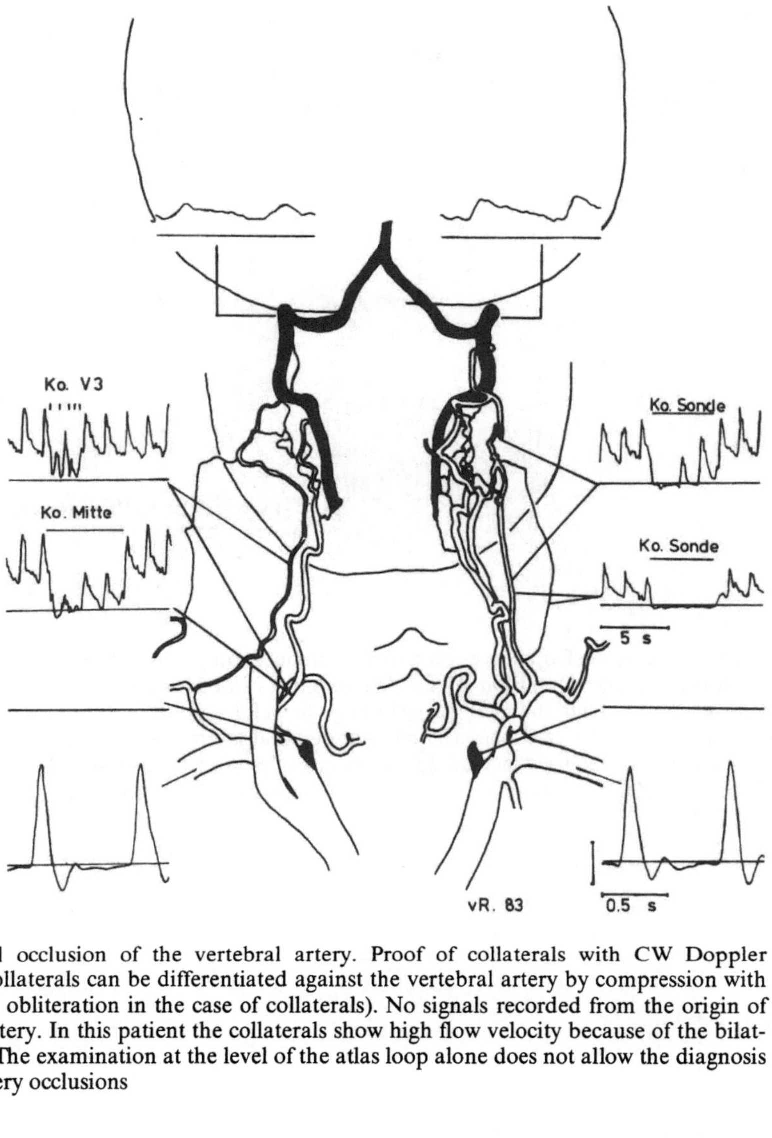

Fig. 7. Bilateral occlusion of the vertebral artery. Proof of collaterals with CW Doppler sonography. Collaterals can be differentiated against the vertebral artery by compression with the probe (—, obliteration in the case of collaterals). No signals recorded from the origin of the vertebral artery. In this patient the collaterals show high flow velocity because of the bilateral occlusion. The examination at the level of the atlas loop alone does not allow the diagnosis of vertebral artery occlusions

servation of the vessel with ultrasound in real time shows diameter and longitudinal pulsations as well as lateral movements with each heart beat or with swallowing. Local stiffness, especially of the bifurcation, enhances longitudinal movements and reduces diameter pulsations.

Collateral Flow

The ophthalmic artery collateral was the first to be examined using Doppler sonography [4, 5, 18]. The objective was to detect stenoses and occlusions of the in-

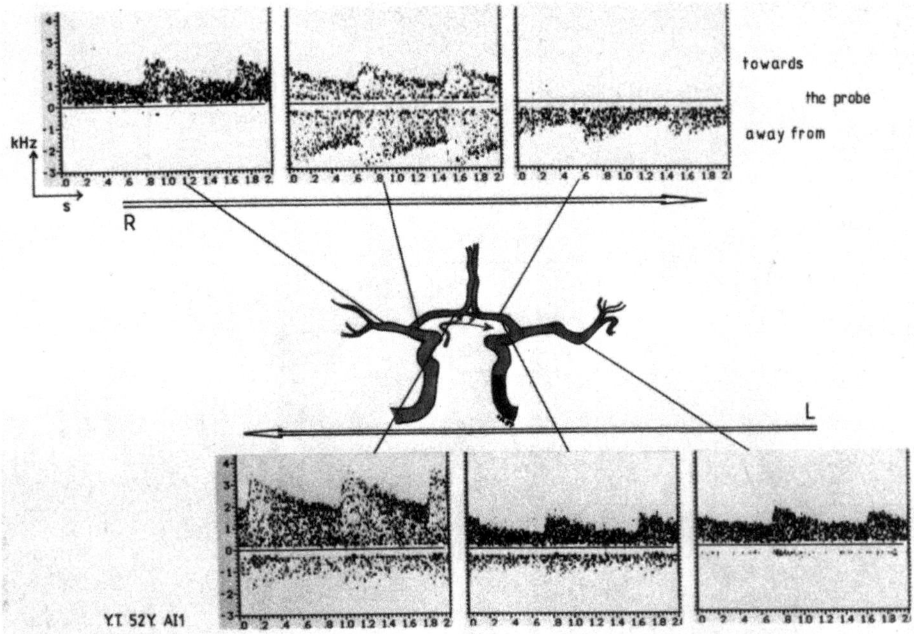

Fig. 8. Intracranial Doppler examination, demonstrating cross-flow via the anterior communicating artery. Occlusion of the left internal carotid artery. Examination at different depths: *above* through the right, *below* through the left temporal bone. Flow towards the probe displayed above the zero line. The anterior cerebral artery shows on the *left* a reverse flow direction and on the *right* increased flow velocity of physiologic direction. Little side difference of the flow velocity of the middle cerebral artery because of collateral compensation

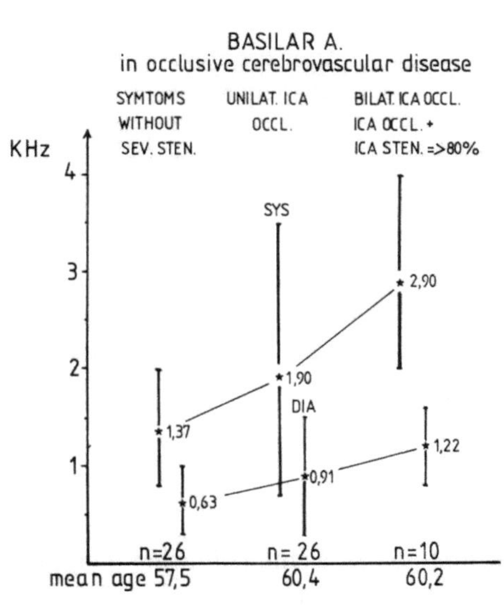

Fig. 9. Flow velocity in the basilar artery with occlusion of the carotid artery. Mean value of maximum peak systolic and late diastolic frequencies, and the range of values. *Left:* patients with cerebrovascular disease, but without occlusion of the carotid artery. *Right:* bilateral occlusions or occlusion with high degree stenosis of the contralateral side. Collateral flow in the basilar artery increases with the severity of carotid obstructions

ternal carotid artery. The Doppler ophthalmic test is no longer needed for that purpose because the direct criteria from the insonation of the neck region provide reliable information on such obstructions [28]. Today, nearly all important collateral pathways can be evaluated by Doppler sonography: the vertebral and occipital artery in subclavian and carotid occlusions [6, 27] and the cervical branches of the thyrocervical and costocervical trunk in occlusions of the vertebral (Fig. 7) and the external carotid artery [25, 26]. Finally, the function of the circle of Willis can be examined using transcranial Doppler sonography, especially the collateral flow through the anterior and posterior communicating artery (Figs. 8 and 9). Only the measurement of peripheral collateral flow through cortical anastomoses between the middle, anterior, and posterior arteries is beyond the capabilities of ultrasound. In general it can be said that Doppler sonography better describes the functional aspects of collateral flow, while angiography with selective catheterization provides more morphological details.

Flow Volume

Flow volume can be calculated from the flow velocity and the diameter of the vessel. Several modes of calculation have been used. The mean flow velocity and the diameter can be calculated from a flow profile using a multigate pulsed Doppler system [10] assuming that the artery is perfectly circular and that the velocity of each sample volume is representative of the velocity of the corresponding half anulus. The mean velocity can also be measured with CW Doppler sonography combined with an A-scan for monitoring the diameter variations by an echo-tracking technique [12, 35] (Fig. 10). Comparative experiments [19] have shown a superiority of the latter method. The clinical value of flow volume measurements is limited, because reliable measurements are restricted to the common carotid artery, which means that today it has not been possible to exactly measure the total cerebral

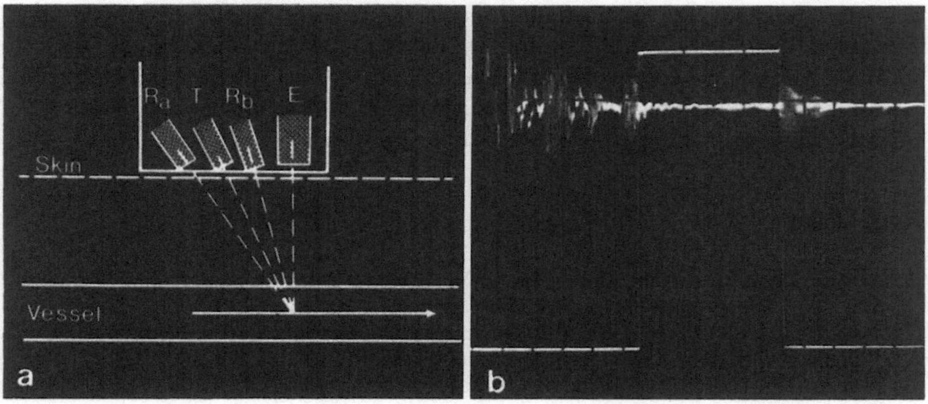

Fig. 10. Measurement of flow volume (QFM). The probe contains one transducer for the diameter measurement with A-mode (display on the right side) and one transmitting as well two receiving crystals with fixed angles in order to calculate the true velocity [19]

blood flow volume. The peripheral resistance of an artery, however, can be estimated from the flow volume and arterial blood pressure [36]. In addition, the capacitance of the intracranial arteries can be calculated by means of a simplified Windkessel model [11]. Peripheral resistance and capacitance correlate with the amount of cerebral artherosclerosis [36]. The possibility of evaluating these general properties of the cerebral arteries in patients has not drawn enough attention among neurologists. These parameters may be of greater importance for the prognosis of a patient than the detection of a localized stenosis.

Discussion

Ultrasound examination techniques can no longer be considered simple screening tests for the detection of carotid artery stenoses. They provide morphologic information on the region from the aortic arch to the intracranial basal arteries as well as functional information about local flow disturbances and collateral flow. Peripheral resistance and capacitance of the arterial bed can also be evaluated. To take advantage of all of these possibilities of the ultrasound method, several specially designed techniques and devices have to be employed. Complete examination is time consuming, but even then the use of ultrasound is more cost effective for the diagnosis of cerebrovascular disease than angiography. Best angiographic results can be obtained if the question to be answered was determined before by ultrasonic diagnosis. Angiography of the intracranial arteries is often indicated for differential diagnostic purposes. Venous digital subtraction angiography does not meet the resolution requirements. Angiography can be performed once or at the most twice on a patient, whereas frequent examinations or even continuous monitoring is possible with ultrasound. This advantage is particularly evident in the case of subarachnoid hemorrhage, where angiography determines the site and the cause of the bleeding and Doppler sonography follows the development of spasms. Although there may be some overlapping indications for ultrasonic and angiographic diagnosis, ultrasonic diagnosis is an essential supplement to CT scan, Xenon rCBF, and PET. As with other methods, the application of ultrasonic methods by inexperienced hands does more harm than good. Unfortunately, this is a common situation, and it is due both to a lack of time for practicing the technique and a lack of willingness to provide sufficient equipment and personnel. From the point of view of the patient, however, such effort and equipment would be a worthwhile investment.

References

1. Aaslid R, Markwalder TM, Nornes H (1982) Noninvasive transcranial Doppler ultrasound recording of flow velocity in basal cerebral arteries. J Neurosurg 57:769–774
2. Arnolds BJ, Reutern von GM (1986) Transcranial Doppler sonography. Examination technique and normal reference values. Ultrasound Med Biol 12:115–123
3. Babcock DS, Han BK (1981) Cranial ultrasonography of infants. Williams and Wilkins, Baltimore
4. Brockenbrough EC (1969) Screening for the prevention of stroke: use of a Doppler flowmeter. Information and Education Resource Support Unit, Washington/Alaska Regional Medical Program

5. Brockenbrough EC (1978) Periorbital Doppler velocity evaluation of carotid obstruction. In: Bernstein EF (ed) Noninvasive diagnostic techniques in vascular disease. Mosby, St. Louis, pp 212–220
6. Büdingen HJ, Reutern von GM, Freund HJ (1982) Doppler-Sonographie der extrakraniellen Hirnarterien. Thieme, Stuttgart
7. Cathignol D, Chapelon JY, Mestas JL (1983) Description et application d'un vélocimètre ultrasonore Doppler pour des petits vaisseaux. Med Biol Eng Comput 21:358–364
8. Chandler WF, Knake JE, McGillicuddy JE, Lillehei KO, Silver TM (1982) Intraoperative use of real-time ultrasonography in neurosurgery. J Neurosurg 57:157–163
9. Dittrich M, Strassburg HM, Dinkel E, Hackelöer BJ (1985) Zerebrale Ultraschalldiagnostik in Pädiatrie und Geburtshilfe. Springer, Berlin Heidelberg New York Tokyo
10. Fish PJ (1981) A method for transcutaneous blood flow measurement – accuracy considerations. In: Kurjak A, Kratochwil A (eds) Recent advances in ultrasound diagnosis. Proceedings 4th European congress on ultrasonics in Med Excerpta Medica. Internat Congr Ser 553. Elsevier North-Holland, Amsterdam, pp 110–115
11. Furuhata H (1982) A non-invasive and quantitative method of measuring the cerebral arteriosclerosis by simulation technique. Jikeikai Med J 29:209–224
12. Furuhata H, Kanno R, Kodairo K, Aoyagi T, Hayashi J, Matsumoto H, Yoshimura S (1978) An ultrasonic blood flow measuring system to detect the absolute volume flow. Jpn J Med Electron Biol Eng [Suppl] 16:334
13. Gilsbach JM (1983) Intraoperative Doppler sonography in neurosurgery. Springer, Wien New York
14. Harders A, Gilsbach JM (1985) Time course of cerebrovascular spasm in early aneurysm operation: transcranial Doppler findings. In: Auer LM (ed) Proceedings of the 2nd International Symposium "Cerebral aneurysm surgery in the acute stage", Graz 1984 (in press)
15. Hennerici M, Reifschneider G, Trockel U, Aulich A (1984) Detection of early aterhosclerotic lesions by duplex scanning of the carotid artery. J Clin Ultrasound 12:455–464
16. Hoeks APG, Ruissen CJ, Hick P, Reneman RS (1985) Transcutaneous detection of relative changes in artery diameter. Ultrasound Med Biol 11:51–59
17. Ku DN, Giddens DP (1983) Pulsatile flow in a model carotid bifurcation. Arteriosclerosis 3:31–39
18. Müller HR (1972) The diagnosis of internal carotid artery occlusion by directional Doppler sonography of the ophthalmic artery. Neurology 22:816–823
19. Müller HR, Radue EW, Saia A, Pallotti C, Buser M (1985) Carotid blood flow measurement by means of ultrasonic techniques: limitations and clinical use. In: Hartmann, Hoyer (eds) Cerebral blood flow and metabolism measurement. Springer, Berlin Heidelberg New York
20. Pape KE, Cusick G, Houang MTW, Blackwell RJ, Sherwood A, Thorburn RJ, Reynolds EOR (1979) Ultrasound detection of brain damage in preterm infants. Lancet 1:1261–1264
21. Peronneau PA, Hinglais JR, Xhaard M, Delouche P, Philippo J (1974) The effects of curvature and stenosis on pulsatile flow in vivo and in vitro. In: Renemann RS (ed) Cardiovascular applications of ultrasound. Proceedings of an international symposium held at Janssen Pharmaceutica, Beerse, Belgium, May 29–30. North-Holland, Amsterdam
22. Phillips DJ, Greene FM Jr, Langlois Y, Roederer GO, Strandness DE Jr (1983) Flow velocity patterns in the carotid bifurcations of young, presumed normal subjects. Ultrasound Med Biol 9:39–49
23. Pourcelot L (1975) Indications de l'ultrasonographie Doppler dans l'étude des vaisseaux périphériques. Année Practicien 25:4671–4680
24. Reneman RS, Merode van T, Hick P, Hoeks APG (1985) Flow velocity patterns in and distensibility of the carotid artery bulb in subjects of various ages. Circulation 71:500–509
25. Reutern von GM (1982) Doppler-Sonographie der hirnversorgenden Arterien mit besonderer Berücksichtigung der direkten Kriterien. In: Kriessmann A, Bollinger A, Keller H (eds) Praxis der Doppler-Sonographie, periphere Arterien und Venen, hirnversorgende Arterien. Thieme, Stuttgart

26. Reutern von GM, Clarenbach P (1980) Value of Doppler examinations of the cervical collateral arteries and the vertebral ostium in the diagnosis of stenoses and occlusions of the vertebral artery. Ultrason 1:153–162
27. Reutern von GM, Pourcelot L (1978) Cardiac cycle dependent alterating flow in vertebral arteries with subclavian artery stenosis. Stroke 9:2229–2236
28. Reutern von GM, Büdingen HJ, Hennerici M, Freund HJ (1976) Diagnose und Differenzierung von Stenosen und Verschlüssen der Arteria carotis mit der Doppler-Sonographie. Arch Psychiatr Nervenkr 222:191–207
29. Spencer MP, Reid JM (1979) Quantitation of carotid stenosis with continuous-wave (C-W) Doppler ultrasound. Stroke 10:326–330
30. Spencer MP, Reid JM (1981) Cerebrovascular evaluation with Doppler ultrasound. Nijhoff, The Hague
31. Strassburg HM, Sauer M (1981) Ultraschalldiagnostik durch die offene Fontanelle des Säuglings. Ultraschall 2:43–49
32. Strassburg HM, Niederhoff H, Sauer M (1982) Die Doppler-sonographische Registrierung der Durchblutung intracranieller Gefäße beim Säugling. Monatsschr Kinderheilkd 130:608–612
33. Volpe JJ (1979) Cerebral blood flow in the newborn infant: relation to hypoxic-ischemic brain injury and periventricular haemorrhage. J Pediatr 94:170–173
34. White DN, Curry GR, Stevenson RJ (1978) The acoustic characteristics of the skull. Ultrasound Med Biol 4:225–252
35. Yoshimura S, Furuhata H, Suzuki N, Kodaira K, Hirota H (1982) A method for the quantitative and noninvasive measurement of blood flow volume in internal and external carotid arteries and vertebral artery. Jikeikai Med J 29:197–208
36. Yoshimura S, Kodaira K, Fujishiro K, Furuhata H (1984) Non-invasive and quantitative measurement of common carotid blood flow volume and estimation of cerebral atherosclerosis using ultrasonic quantitative flow measurement system (QFM). Angéiologie 36:53–66

Application of Digital Subtraction Angiography in Neurological Disorders

M. PEROVITCH[1]

Introduction

The introduction of digital subtraction angiography (DSA) into clinical practice is one of the recent advancements in neuroimaging resulting from the new developments in computer science and applied mathematics. The main impetus for its construction was the need for a less complex and safer modality for the imaging of the vascular system. Although the use of subtraction in cerebral angiography is not a new technique [6, 7], its interface with a digital computer is, however, a novelty of high medical technology. DSA provides dynamic imaging of the brain blood flow through the use of logarithmic enhancement of the iodine signal and digital processing of images. The improved contrast resolution is the major advancement in the digital processing of images, which makes possible the visualization of the brachiocephalic vessels containing a concentration of iodine as low as 2% or even less, contrary to the 40%–60% needed for the standard cerebral angiography [3, 5, 17]. Due to these properties, DSA allows imaging of brain arteries following not only an intraarterial, but also an intravenous injection of contrast media.

The experimental work that led to the introduction of DSA was conducted more or less simultaneously in several laboratories [11, 15, 17]. The transition of DSA from the laboratory to the clinical setting began in 1979 and rapidly gained wide clinical acceptance [3, 5, 14, 23]. In addition to the improved contrast resolution, DSA possessed other attractive qualities. It was less expensive mainly because the cost for the films had been reduced. The decrease of angiographic risks made DSA a more acceptable diagnostic modality. Moreover, DSA significantly reduced the procedure time, as well as the radiation exposure to about 0.1 R compared with 0.2 R minimum with the standard film-screen cerebral angiography [14]. Furthermore, DSA offers a continuous observation on television screens of the flow of the contrast agent through the brain arteries and veins, and the possibility to select the pictures according to their technical and clinical values. It also enables the "playback" of the registered angiograms and their adjustment to the needs of interpretation.

[1] University of Connecticut School of Medicine, Farmington, CT 06032, USA.

Neurology
Ed. by K. Poeck, H. J. Freund, and H. Gänshirt

However, in spite of the appealing qualities of DSA and predictions of some investigators that it could replace other angiographic techniques [14, 15, 23]. its clinical utility has been gradually reduced due to some inherent limitations that have surfaced especially in the past 2 years [21]. Not even the significant upgrading of the equipment for DSA, or the improvements in catheter design, contrast material and automatic injectors, could overcome, so far, these limitations [10, 22].

It is not the purpose of this analysis to deal with detailed physical and technical aspects of DSA, many of which have been already discussed in the literature [18], but rather to give an estimate of the present significance of DSA for the clinical investigation of neurological disorders. In this study, files of 2250 patients (1980–1985) were reviewed in order to establish the diagnostic significance of the digital subtraction angiography. Only the patients who had a complete neurological evaluation were selected. A total of 1200 intravenous and 1050 intraarterial digital subtraction angiographies were evaluated. The research was conducted partially at the Johns Hopkins University and University of Maryland, Baltimore.

Intravenous Digital Subtraction Angiography

Intravenous digital subtraction angiography (IV DSA), introduced first, created considerable enthusiasm, since the arterial imaging could be performed by a simpler venous injection of contrast agents without the need of direct arterial catheterization or puncture. The main advantages of the IV DSA are summarized in Table 1.

Intravenous injection of contrast media for the visualizing of the arterial system has been known and applied for a longer period of time [4, 19]. The recent change in this technique, however, is the introduction of the digital computer in order to enhance the subtracted intravenous arteriography electronically and upgrade arterial images by reducing, at the same time, substantially, the volume and concentration of the used contrast agent [5, 15, 17].

Two contrast injection techniques have been applied for the IV DSA: the peripheral and the central [16]. The second technique, currently used most, consists of catheterization of an antecubital vein using a 5-F curved or straight catheter in the 65 cm and 90 cm lengths with multiple side holes. The catheter is advanced into the superior vena cava close to the right atrium. Following the positioning of the catheter about 30 cc to 40 cc of the 76% or less contrast medium are injected at the rate of 15 cc to 20 cc per second for each run. We tend to inject no more than 150 cc of the contrast medium for a complete examination [17]. The arterial concentration of the contrast agent will be greater following the injection into the superior vena cava

Table 1. Main advantages of the intravenous DSA

1. High contrast resolution
2. Less invasive and safer; lower radiation dose
3. Performed on outpatient basis (in about 90% of cases)
4. Much faster; quick and accurate subtraction and instant replay of images
5. Repeatable at intervals, if necessary
6. Less expensive (about 50% less than the standard cerebral angiography)

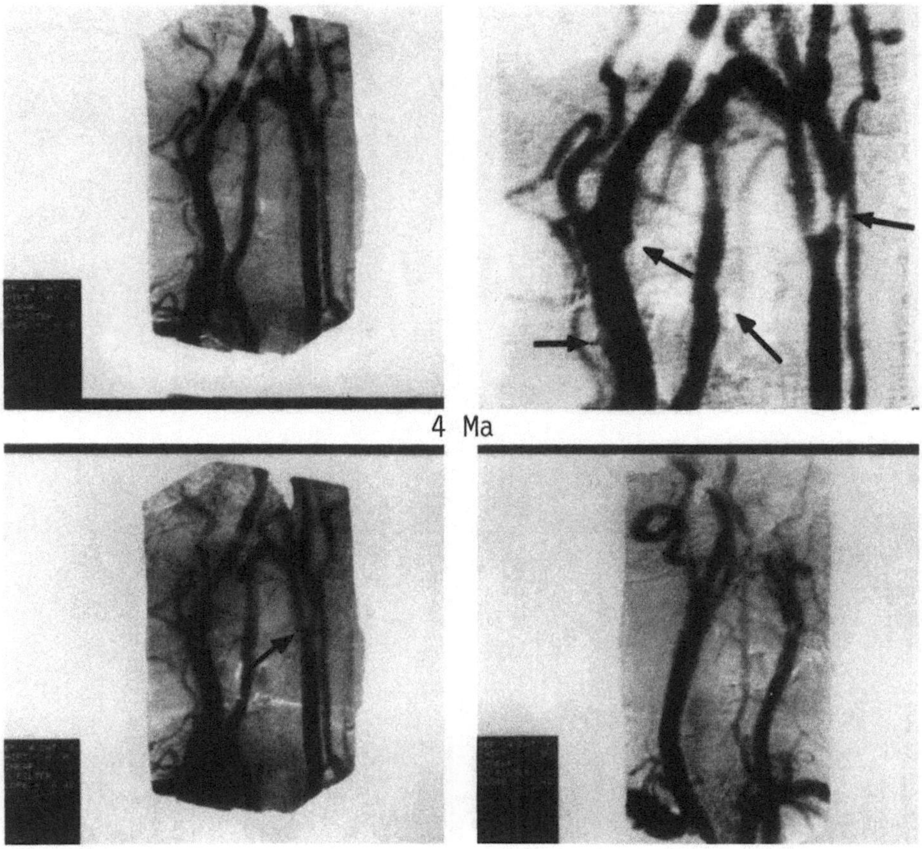

Fig. 1. A IV DSA shows multiple atherosclerotic plaques on the walls of the carotid and vertebral arteries in the neck region, as well as a severe stenosis of the left internal carotid artery. Ulcerative defects, however, cannot be identified

or the atrium itself, and lower if the injection is flushed into the basilic vein. The clear, qualitative superiority of images results from the central injection. Of course, the catheter can be introduced also through the femoral vein and the inferior vena cava to the right atrium. This approach was used exceptionally, in less than 2% of patients in this analysis.

The images of the brachiocephalic arteries were obtained usually at the rate of one frame per second. The rate of exposures, as well as the optimal positioning and the injection of the contrast medium were planned depending upon the specific clinical requirements.

This analysis indicates that the best diagnostic results with IV DSA were obtained in the neck region. If the patient is motionless, which may be difficult in the older and less cooperative, during the contrast medium injection, very good quality angiograms of the carotid and vertebral arteries can be obtained as shown in Fig. 1. Atherosclerotic changes on the walls of these arteries, luminal stenosis, or occlusion

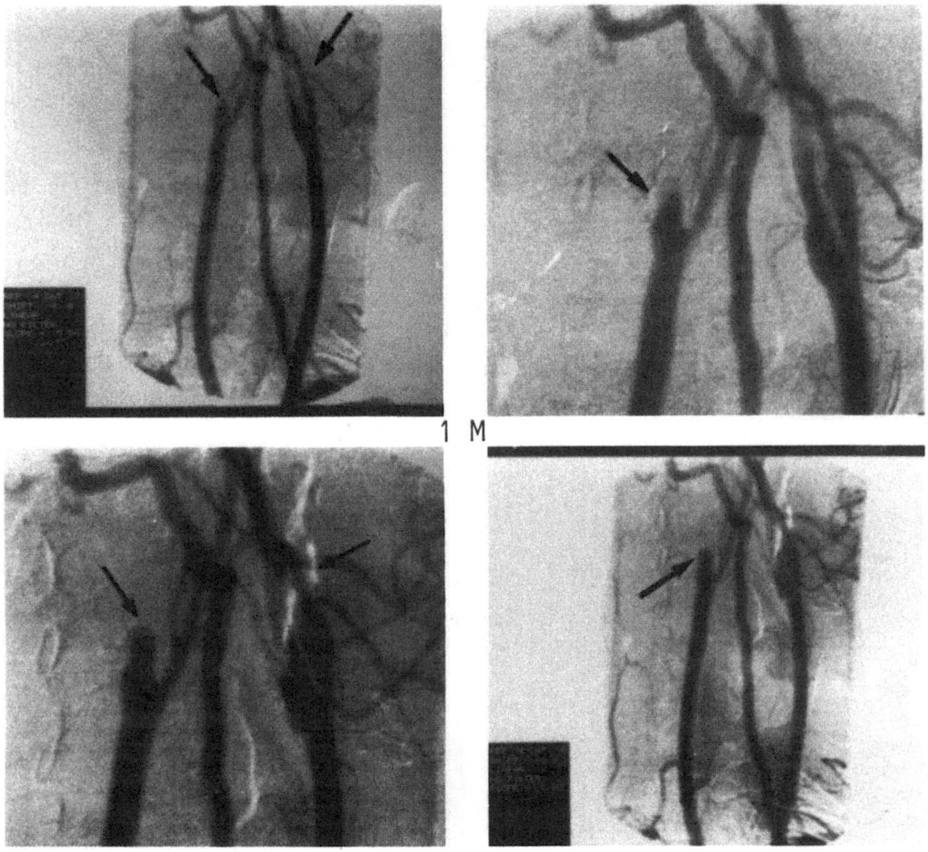

Fig. 2. The occlusion of the right and the stenosis of the left internal carotid arteries are well demonstrated by means of the IV DSA

can be evaluated rather precisely, as seen in Fig. 2, in spite of the small imaging field and small image format for the hard copy. Ulcerative defects, however, may be difficult to discern, if at all.

Moreover, IV DSA proved to be a useful screening procedure, most often performed on an outpatient basis, for the patients with asymptomatic carotid bruits, and for those who are at high risk for developing atherosclerosis associated possibly with transient ischemic episodes. It is also a convenient preoperative examination for cardiac bypass surgery, or a postoperative procedure for evaluation of some carotid endarterectomies. Further on, IV DSA can be of relative diagnostic value in case cerebral angiography with catheterization, or direct puncture, is considered a great risk or cannot be performed.

For visualization of the dural venous sinuses as shown in Fig. 3, as well as of deep brain venous channels as in Fig. 4, IV DSA is the method of choice. It is a simple and fast diagnostic procedure for establishing the presence of the "non-flow" phenomenon in acute brain edema and the state known as "brain death."

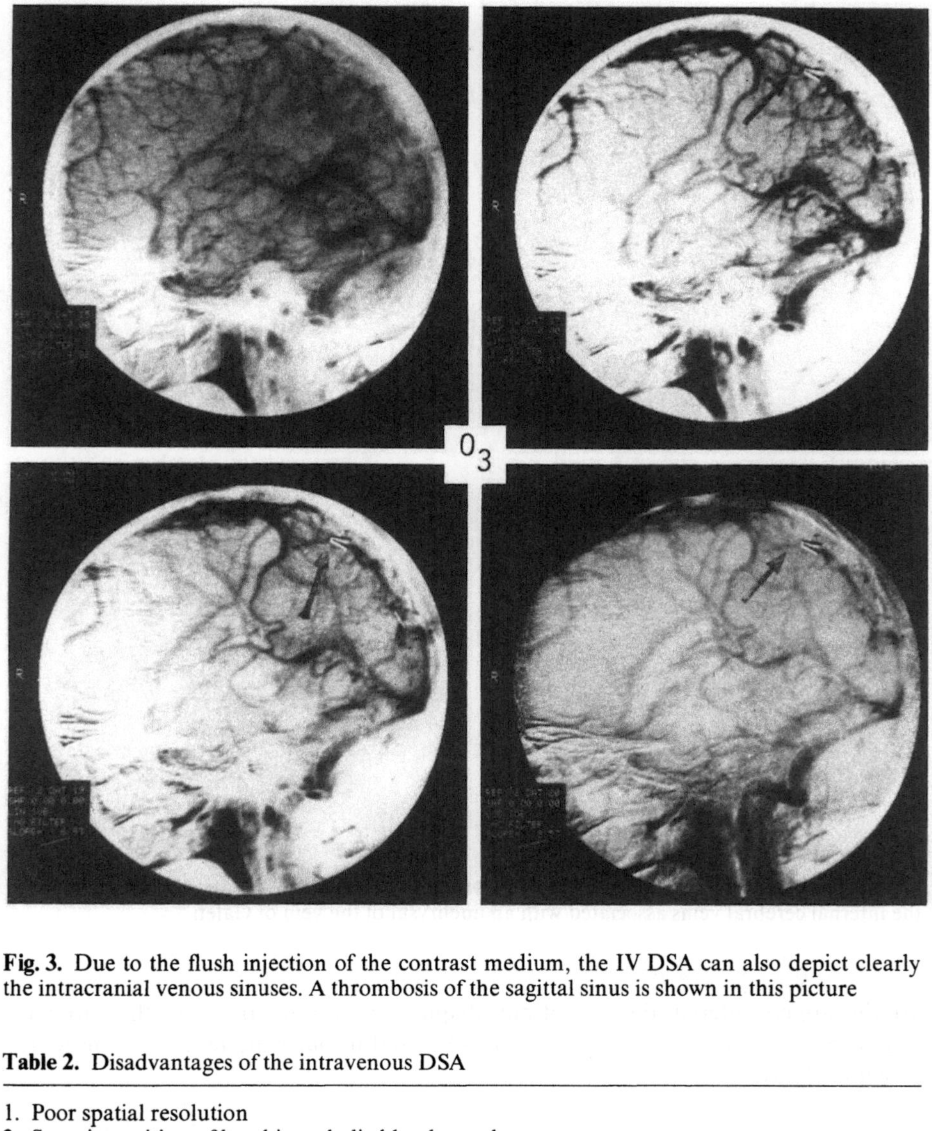

Fig. 3. Due to the flush injection of the contrast medium, the IV DSA can also depict clearly the intracranial venous sinuses. A thrombosis of the sagittal sinus is shown in this picture

Table 2. Disadvantages of the intravenous DSA

1. Poor spatial resolution
2. Superimposition of brachiocephalic blood vessels
3. Patient's motion (swallowing, cough reflex)
4. Poor cardiac output of the patient
5. Arterial intracranial circulation can be examined only superficially
6. Inability to register small vessels (< 1 mm)

It is obvious that IV DSA did not respond to the hope and anticipation that it would replace the more complex intraarterial neurological imaging. This failure was largely due to the limitations presented in Table 2. They have gradually degraded the diagnostic significance of IV DSA to a point that it can be regarded, at present, only as a complementary study. If all examinations of the extra- and intracranial

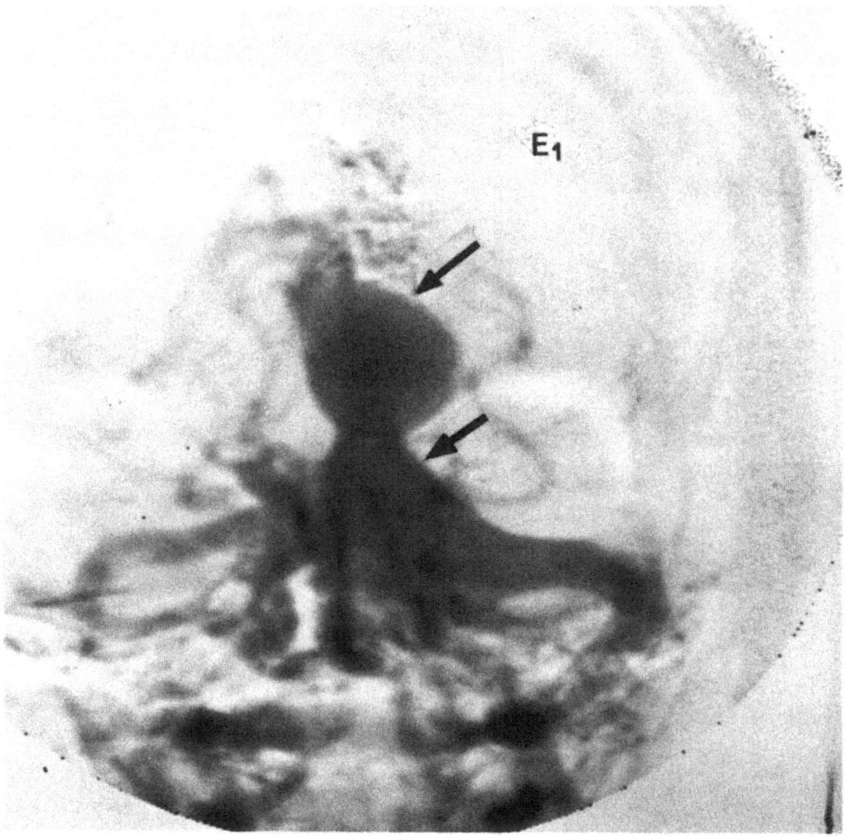

Fig. 4. The magnified frame of this IV DSA provides excellent presentation of an anomaly of the internal cerebral veins associated with an aneurysm of the vein of Galen

arteries are considered, the rate of non-diagnostic examinations with this modality has been reported to be as high as 17%–43%, and in our experience it came to approximately 31% [22].

Intraarterial Digital Subtraction Angiography

It is evident from the foregoing discussion that besides the intravenous DSA there is a second alternative, namely the arterial DSA which has better chances to succeed as a useful neuroimaging technique. It can preserve the advantages of the digital subtraction angiography and, at least partially, avoid the shortcomings of the intravenous DSA. Indeed, in about the past 2 years most of the digital subtraction angiographies analyzed here, have been done through an intraarterial injection of contrast media, whereas the intravenous injection was reserved only for selected patients.

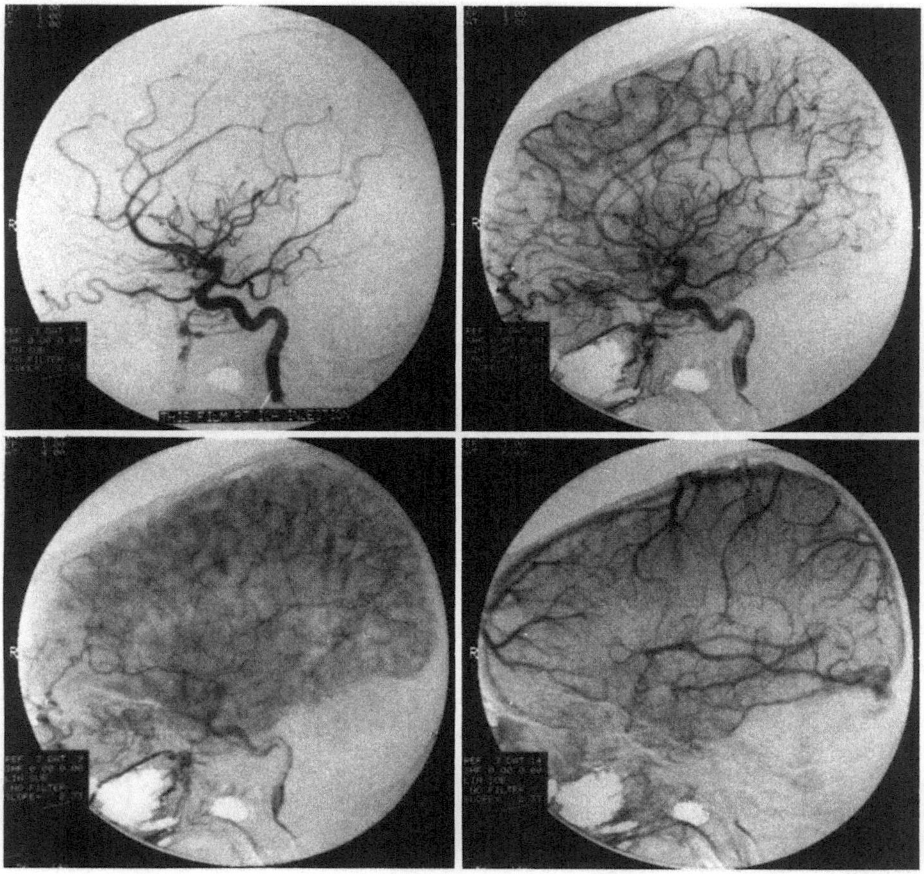

Fig. 5. The superiority of the IA DSA over the IV DSA for the evaluation of the intracranial arterial circulation is emphasized in this illustration

Table 3. Advantages of the intraarterial DSA

1. Faster and less expensive than the standard angiography
2. Safer since less volume of contrast media of lower concentration is injected through smaller catheters
3. Improved spatial resolution in comparison with the intravenous DSA
4. Instant replay of images of very good quality without superimposition of brachiocephalic blood vessels

The main advantages of intraarterial digital subtraction angiography (IA DSA) over intravenous and standard selective angiography are listed in Table 3.

The examination is performed by means of a 5-F, curved or straight, aortic flush catheter with multiple side holes, which is introduced, in our cases, into the aortic arch through the femoral artery. The new 4-F aortic flush catheter may prove to be safer than larger types of catheters, although a lesser amount of the contrast me-

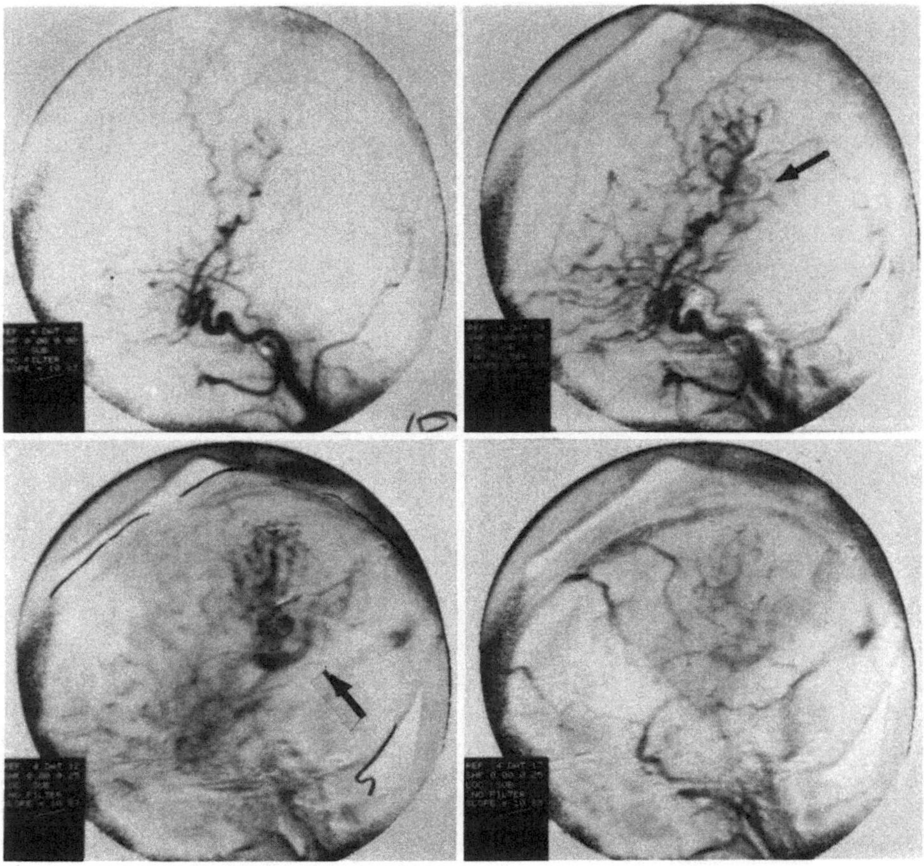

Fig. 6. This case of a subcortical arteriovenous malformation illustrates the diagnostic significance of the IA DSA

dium can be injected in a short period of time. However, the 65 cm long 4-F catheter can provide up to a 38% higher flow rate than the 90 cm one. This is the reason why some investigators advocate the brachial approach for IA DSA [10].

Usually small quantities of a contrast medium, of lower concentration, are injected into the aortic arch in order to visualize first the origin and the neck segments of brachiocephalic arteries. If necessary, selective injections will follow. Obviously, the IA DSA carries some of the well-known risks inherent to the standard selective cerebral angiography [9, 12, 13, 20].

The quality of images of the intracranial circulation that can be obtained by means of the IA DSA is demonstrated in Fig. 5. The vascular network of different intracranial tumors and the arterial aneurysms can be much better assessed using IA DSA than IV DSA. Also the features of arteriovenous malformations, intra- or extracranial, can be evaluated using IA DSA as shown in Fig. 6. It is clear, however, that the exquisite detail obtainable with the standard cerebral film-screen angiography has not been achieved with IA DSA.

Conclusion

In conclusion one can say, on the basis of this analysis, that IV DSA can be used for the evaluation of the bifurcation of the common carotid artery and the intracranial venous circulation. Also, in selected patients, it can be applied as a useful pre- and postoperative screening procedure. Digital imaging has become a complementary technique [1]. It appears that IA DSA could have a more prominent role in future neuroimaging [1, 2, 8]. The possibility of introducing a larger image field, as well as a biplane arrangement will certainly promote a broader application of IA DSA. Furthermore, a 1024 by 1024 matrix could give this method a spatial resolution almost equivalent to that of conventional selective film-screen angiography. Hence, the present qualitative inferiority of digital images can be upgraded.

References

1. Boulos SR, Mehta B, Patel S (1985) Reassessing the role of intravenous DSA. Diagn Imaging 7(5):82–85
2. Brandt-Zawadzki M, Gould R, Norman D, et al. (1982) Digital subtraction cerebral angiography by intra-arterial injection; comparison with conventional angiography. AJNR 3:593–599
3. Carmody RF, Smith JRJ, Seeger JF, et al. (1981) Intravenous cerebral angiography: Early clinical experience. Ariz Med 38:349–350
4. Castellanos A, Pereiras R, Garcia A (1937) La angiocardiografia radio-opaca. Arch Soc Estud Cli (Havana) 31:523
5. Christenson PC, Quitt TW, Sisher HD II, et al. (1980) Intravenous angiography using digital video subtraction intravenous cervicocerebrovascular angiography. AJNR 137:379–386
6. Des Plantes BGZ (1935) Subtraktion: Eine röntgenographische Methode zur separaten Abbildung bestimmter Teile des Objekts. ROEFO 52:69–79
7. Des Plantes BGZ (1961) Subtraktion. Thieme, Stuttgart
8. Foley WD, Milde WM (1985) Hybrid DSA combines time, energy subtraction. Diagn Imaging 7(8):74–76
9. Hessel SJ, Adams DF, Abrams HL (1981) Complications of angiography. Radiology 138:273–281
10. Hicks EM, Becker JG, Holden R (1985) Better catheters, contrast contribute to DSA's growth. Diagn Imaging 7(1):74–80
11. Hillman BJ, Ovitt TW, Nudelman S, et al. (1981) Digital subtraction angiography of renal vascular abnormalities. Radiology 139:277–280
12. Hoogland PH (1983) Arterial digital subtraction angiography (DSA) in neuroradiology: Results and experience. Electromedica 51(3):97–102
13. Kaufman SL, Chang R, Kadir S, et al. (1984) Intra-arterial digital subtraction angiography in diagnostic arteriography. Radiology 151:323–327
14. Karasov GC (1981) Move over for digital radiography. Appl Radiol 10(6):37–42
15. Mistretta CA, Crummy AB, Strother CM (1981) Digital angiography: A perspective. Radiology 139:273–276
16. Modic MT, Weinstein MA, Pavlicek MS, et al. (1983) Intravenous digital subtraction angiography: peripheral versus central injection of contrast material. Radiology 147:711–715
17. Perovitch M (1985) Neuroradiological evaluation of headache. In: Pfaffenrath V, Lundberg P-O, Sjaastad O (eds) Updating in headache. Springer, Berlin Heidelberg New York, pp 76–86
18. Pfeiler M, Marhoff P, Koch R (1985) Effects of X-ray physics and technology in digital radiography. Electromedica 53(2):50–57

19. Robb GP, Steinberg L (1939) Visualization of the chambers of the heart, the pulmonary circulation and great blood vessels in man – a practical method. AJR 41:1–17
20. Sigstedt B, Lunderquist A (1978) Complications of angiographic examination. AJR 130:455–460
21. Turski PA, Zweibel WJ, Strother CM, et al. (1983) Limitations of intravenous digital subtraction angiography. AJNR 3:271–273
22. Vinocur B (1984) Is the party over for intravenous DSA? Diagn Imaging 6(5):76–80
23. Weinstein AM, Modic TM, Buonocore E, Meaney FT (1981) Digital subtraction angiography. Appl Radiol 10(6):53–166

Neuroimaging Using Nuclear Magnetic Resonance and Computerized Tomography in Patients with Multiple Sclerosis, Idiopathic Optic Neuritis, and Systemic Lupus Erythematosus

L. JACOBS, P.R. KINKEL, W.R. KINKEL, F.A. GREEN, and P. COSTELLO[1]

Introduction

There is considerable enthusiasm about the potential of nuclear magnetic resonance (NMR) imaging in the diagnosis and care of patients with diseases of the nervous system. Since its introduction into the clinical environment in the early 1980s, NMR has proven to be equal to or better than CT for imaging a wide variety of central nervous system (CNS) diseases [1]. We compared the NMR and CT findings in three CNS diseases in which computer tomography (CT) has previously proven to be of little or no value, namely, multiple sclerosis, isolated idiopathic optic neuritis, and systemic lupus erythematosis [2–8].

Methods

This report includes data on 173 patients (147 with multiple sclerosis, 15 with isolated idiopathic optic neuritis, and 11 with systemic lupus erythematosus). In all of these patients the diagnoses were definite according to accepted standard clinical and laboratory criteria [9–11].

CT examinations were performed with an EMI 1010 or 1005 scanner (slice thickness 8 mm, matrix 180×180, resolution 1.5 mm). Sections were in the transverse plane oriented 10° (frontal up) from Reid's anatomic baseline. Most patients had both noncontrast and contrast CT examinations. For contrast studies, 30% iothala-

Supported by grants from the Baird, James H. Cummings, Dent, Josephine Goodyear, Margaret L. Wendt, Losasso Family, Samuel and Sarah Slepian Family Foundations, and the Delaware North Companies, all of Buffalo, New York, USA, and the National Institutes of Health (R01NS19649-01)

[1] Dent Neurologic Institute, Millard Fillmore Hospital and State University of New York, School of Medicine at Buffalo, Dept. of Neurology (Drs. Jacobs and Kinkel) and Rheumatology (Drs. Green and Costello), 3 Gates Circle, Buffalo, NY 14209, USA.

Neurology
Ed. by K. Poeck, H. J. Freund, and H. Gänshirt

mate meglumine was administered intravenously at a dosage of 4 ml/kg over 30 min. NMR examinations were performed with a 0.15 Tesla resistive unit (Technicare). The basic principles and techniques of NMR imaging of the head are described elsewhere [12, 13]. The NMR slice thickness was 5–10 mm, intersection interval 0–1 mm, matrix 256×256, and resolution 1.5 mm. Patients were routinely scanned in the horizontal plane and sometimes also in the coronal or sagittal planes. Two pulsing sequences were used: (a) spin-echo (SE) with time to echo (TE) of 30–120 ms and time to repetition (TR) of 500–2120 ms, and (b) inversion recovery (IR) with time to inversion (TI) of 400 ms and TR of 1600 ms.

Results

Multiple Sclerosis (MS)

CT was abnormal in 56 patients (38%); NMR was abnormal in 98 patients (66%). The most common CT abnormality (seen in 42 patients) was one or more areas of decreased densities of white matter. Usually these lesions were bilateral and, located off the ventricular tips or in the centra semiovale above the ventricles (Fig. 1 A). Ten of 117 MS patients who had contrast CT showed one or more enhancing lesions. Hydrocephalus was identified in 20 patients. Posterior fossa lesions were not identified by CT.

NMR identified all of the lesions demonstrated by CT and also revealed one to several additional lesions not seen by CT in patients with abnormal CTs. NMR also revealed one to several lesions in 42 patients whose CTs were completely normal. The NMR abnormalities appeared as areas of low signal intensities on IR and high signal intensities on SE pulsing that were predominantly periventricular in location (Fig. 1 B, C, D). The lesions tended to occur off the ventricular tips; sometimes they completely surrounded the ventricles. Lesions around the temporal horns were often arc-shaped. Often lesions that appeared to be multiple and discrete, separated by normal parenchyma, by IR pulsing appeared larger and confluent by SE pulsing. NMR identified brain-stem lesions in 14 patients: all of these had been missed using CT. SE pulsing almost always identified lesions (supra- and intratentorial) better than IR pulsing. Coronal sections were valuable for assessing the lesions' rostrocaudal extents.

We conducted clinical correlations on 117 NMR lesions in 27 of these patients [6]. Eighty-eight lesions (75%) were clinically silent (bore no relationship to clinical signs). Only six lesions (5%) were definitely related to the clinical signs. All of those lesions were located in the brain stem. Twenty-three lesions (20%) were possibly related to the clinical signs.

Isolated Idiopathic Optic Neuritis (ON)

CT was normal in all 15 of these patients, but NMR was abnormal in eight (53%) [7]. The NMR lesions were best identified on SE images appearing as focal areas of high signal intensities predominantly in the periventricular white matter (Fig. 2). NMR identified 2–7 lesions in six patients; in two patients only one lesion was identified. Lesions of the cerebellum and brain stem were identified in three patients. All of

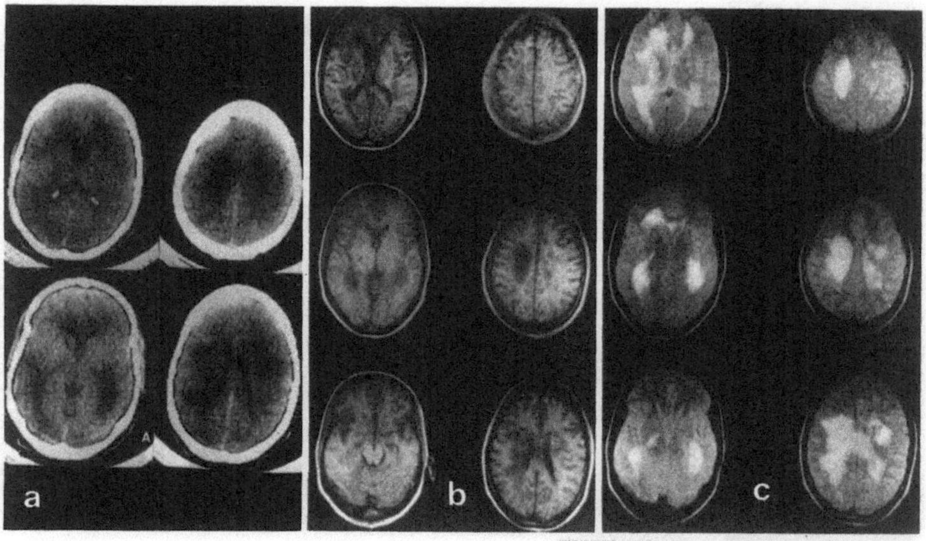

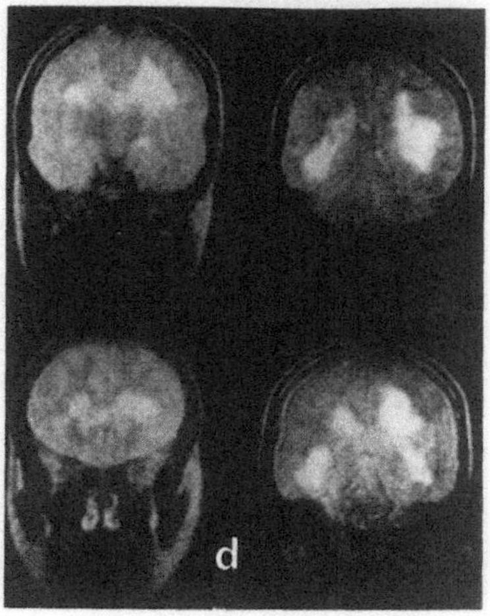

Fig. 1 a–d. CT and NMR examinations of an MS patient. **a** CT (non-contrast) shows areas of decreased densities of cerebral white matter. NMR examinations by IR pulsing (**b**) and SE-120 pulsing in the horizontal (**c**) and coronal (**d**) planes. White matter lesions appear as low signal (*dark*) in **b** and high signal (*bright*) in **c** and **d**. Levels scanned: ventral (*bottom*) to dorsal (*top*) in **a–c**; anterior (*bottom, left*) to posterior (*top, right*) in **d**

these lesions were clinically silent. None of the patients had clinical symptoms or signs suggesting the brain lesions.

Systemic Lupus Erythematosus (SLE)

CT was normal in all 11 of these patients, but NMR was abnormal in four (36%) [8]. The lesions were best visualized on SE images appearing as high signal intensities often located at the corticomedullary junctions appearing linear in horizontal and wedge-shaped in coronal sections (Fig. 3A, B). In three patients at least one of the lesions appeared as a thin band extending perpendicularly from the cortex into the subcortical white matter. The lesions were usually poorly visualized (decreased signal) or missed on IR images. Most of these lesions could be related (at least partially) to previous or current CNS symptoms and signs.

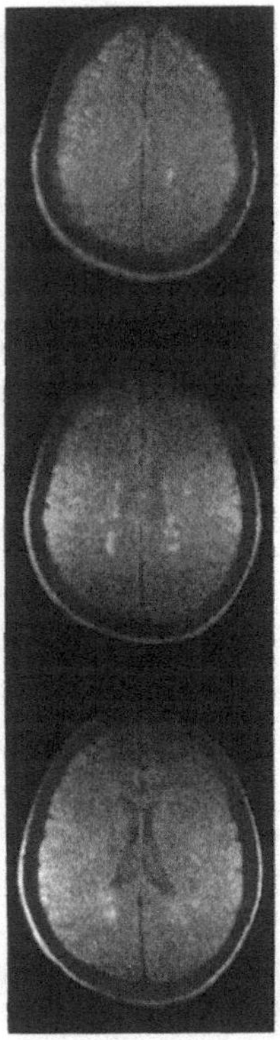

Fig. 2. NMR (SE-90) examination of patient with isolated idiopathic ON. White matter lesions appear bright. Levels: ventral (*bottom*) to dorsal (*top*)

Comment

This study demonstrates an obvious superiority of NMR to CT for imaging the brain in these three diseases [6–8]. Our findings, from the standpoint of imaging, in MS have also been reported by other investigators who studied smaller series of patients [14–17]. In a recent report NMR was found to be more sensitive for making the initial diagnosis of MS not only than CT, but also evoked potentials and cerebrospinal fluid analysis [16]. We feel that NMR may also be more sensitive than the clinical examination in many of these patients as so many of the lesions imaged were clinically silent [6].

The lesions identified in the patients with isolated idiopathic ON had patterns, locations, and extents similar to those seen in MS. It is possible that those lesions are clinically silent MS plaques. Isolated ON may be the first manifestation of MS. However, there is controversy as to the actual percentage of patients who experience isolated ON who will later develop definite MS; the rate of such conversion from ON to MS has ranged from 13%–85% [18]. When, if ever, our ON patients with discernible brain lesions will develop overt MS is purely speculative. An autopsy study has shown that a proportion of patients harbor classic MS brain lesions that remain clinically silent during their entire lives [19]. What can be said is that over half of the

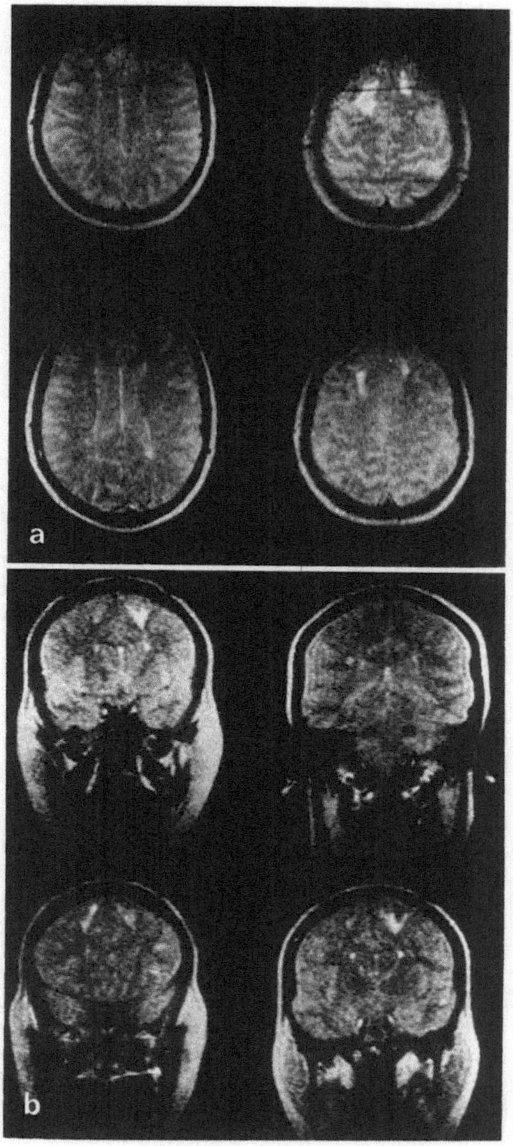

Fig. 3 a, b. NMR (SE-120) of SLE patient. **a** Horizontal, **b** coronal planes. Lesions appear bright. Levels: ventral (*bottom, left*) to dorsal (*top, right*) in **a** and anterior (*bottom, left*) to posterior (*top, right*) in **b**

patients with isolated idiopathic ON harbor one or more clinically silent brain lesion which supports the idea that ON is often one manifestation of a multicentric disease.

There have been two other reports of brain lesions being identified by NMR in patients with SLE [4, 5]. In both, some of the lesions were also seen by CT. All of the lesions identified by NMR in our patients were missed by CT [8]. The lesions disappeared with steroid therapy in one of our patients, as was also observed in another study. It is possible that these lesions represent inflammation in and around the walls of penetrating vessels of the brain which is known to occur in a proportion of SLE patients.

References

1. diMonda R (1985) NMR issues for 1985 and beyond, vol 4. American Hospital Association, Chicago
2. Jacobs L, Kinkel WR (1976) Computerized axial transverse tomography in multiple sclerosis. Neurology 26:390–391
3. Hershey LA, Gado MH, Trotter JL (1979) Computerized tomography in the diagnostic evaluation of multiple sclerosis. Ann Neurol 5:32–39
4. Vermess M, Bernstein RM, Bydder GM, Steiner RE, Young IR, Hughes GRV (1983) Nuclear magnetic resonance (NMR) imaging of the brain in systemic lupus erythematosus. J Comput Assist Tomogr 7:461–467
5. Aisen AM, Gubrielson TO, McCune WJ (1985) MR imaging of systemic lupus erythematosis involving the brain. AJNR 6:197–201
6. Jacobs L, Kinkel WR, Polachini I, Kinkel RP (1985) Correlations of magnetic resonance imaging, computerized tomography and clinical profiles in multiple sclerosis. Neurology
7. Jacobs L, Kinkel PR, Kinkel WR (1985) Silent brain lesions in patients with isolated idiopathic optic neuritis: A clinical and nuclear magnetic imaging study. Science (in press)
8. Kinkel WR, Green FA, Kinkel PR, Jacobs L (1985) Magnetic resonance imaging in patients with systemic lupus erythematosus and signs of central nervous system involvement. Neurology [suppl 1] 35:216
9. Brown JR, et al. (1979) The design of clinical studies to assess therapeutic efficacy in multiple sclerosis. Neurology 29:3–23
10. Perkins GD, Rose FC (1979) Optic neuritis and its differential diagnosis. Oxford University Press, New York, pp 246–248
11. Tan EM, et al. (1982) The 1982 revised criteria for the classification of systemic lupus erythematosus. Arthritis Rheum 25:1217–1277
12. Pykett IL, et al. (1983) Techniques and approaches to proton imaging of the head. Comput Radiol 7:1–17
13. Wehrili FW, McFall JR, Newton T (1983) Parameters determining the appearance of NMR images. In: Newton T, Potts DG (eds) Modern neuroradiology, vol 2. Clinical, New York, pp 81–117
14. Lukes SA, et al. (1983) Nuclear magnetic resonance imaging in multiple sclerosis. Ann Neurol 13:592–601
15. Runge VM, et al. (1984) Magnetic resonance imaging of multiple sclerosis: A study of pulse-technique efficacy. AJNR 5:691–702
16. Gebarski SS, et al. (1985) The initial diagnosis of multiple sclerosis: Clinical impact of magnetic resonance imaging. Ann Neurol 17:469–474
17. Jackson JA, et al. (1985) Magnetic resonance imaging in multiple sclerosis: Results in 32 cases. AJNR 6:171–176
18. Kurtzke JR (1985) Optic neuritis or multiple sclerosis. Arch Neurol 42:704–709
19. Gilbert JJ, Sadler M (1983) Unsuspected multiple sclerosis. Arch Neurol 40:533–536

CT and MRI Diagnoses of Intracranial Tumours Compared with the Results of Stereotactic Biopsy

F. MUNDINGER [1], K. WEIGEL [1], R. FÜRMAIER [2], and B. VOLK [3]

Introduction

Ever since the introduction into medical diagnostics of various image-producing techniques, such as scintiscanning, angiography, computed tomography (CT) or, most recently, nuclear spin tomography, there have been repeated attempts to derive a histological diagnosis of intracranial processes from the shape of presentation, from the pattern of the blood vessels, or from the storage behaviour towards different contrast media. The dangers of false diagnosis involved in such procedures become especially clear when the CT findings are evaluated and compared with the histological results [2, 3, 5, 7, 10, 12].

Not only malignant gliomas but metastases, former haemorrhages, abscesses and even lesions following a disseminating encephalomyelitis were found hidden in the intracerebral processes, all of which appeared as ring structures in the CT scan, and we were only able definitively to prove this histologically through the use of stereotactic biopsy. A reliable morphological diagnosis can therefore not be obtained even with the use of the CT scan [9, 12].

The introduction of nuclear spin tomography renewed the hope that one could formulate a histological diagnosis without biopsy, especially in cases of deeply situated cerebral growths. Here expectations were focused on the different signal behaviour of the single tissue structures, and there were attempts to associate the signal changes with distinct types of tissue. In order to explore how far these procedures are justified and can be used as a basis for suitable therapy, we wish to present a comparative study of CT, magnetic resonance imaging (MRI) and histological findings.

[1] Department of Stereotaxy and Neuronuclear Medicine, Neurosurgical Clinic, Freiburg University.
[2] Gartenstrasse 28, 7800 Freiburg/Breisgau, Federal Republic of Germany.
[3] Department of Neuropathology, Freiburg University.

Neurology
Ed. by K. Poeck, H. J. Freund, and H. Gänshirt

Table 1. Evaluation criteria of MRI

Technical	Proton density Relaxation times (T1, T2) Flow phenomenon
Anatomical	Displacement Ring structure Perifocal reaction Edema Cyst formation

Table 2. Evaluation criteria of CT with enhancement

Imaging	Hypodensity Hyperdensity Isodensity
Anatomical	Calcification Displacement Perifocal edema Cyst formation Ring structure

Cases and Methods

Since 1976 we have evaluated 1320 cases by using CT information about intracerebral lesions as a base for the stereotactic technique. The CT findings are demonstrated in Tables 3–7 as compared to the stereotactically confirmed histology of the lesions. In addition, we examined 109 patients by applying the magnetic resonance (MR) technique between April 1984 and August 1985. However, due to differences in MRI recording techniques and measuring times, and also to incomplete information on measuring techniques, we were only able to evaluate 66 cases comparatively.

In a series of 45 patients we established the optimum MRI recording times and relaxation times (T1 and T2) on the basis of many previous examinations (the system used was the Superconductive Magnet System GYREX 5000, ELSCINT GmbH, Wiesbaden, FRG). In a second series we had to depend on evaluation of pictures recorded by different MRI instruments with different measuring times. Only in 21 cases was the quality sufficiently high for proper evaluation. The evaluation criteria of MR and CT images are listed in Tables 1 and 2.

Results

A comparison of CT findings and stereotactically confirmed histology reveals very clearly the different appearance in the CT scan of tumours of similar dignity and character (Table 3). In the CT scan of 910 cases of glial tumours, 32% appear with a hypodense change and 67% with a hyperdensity. It is very interesting that 73% of

Table 3. Comparison of CT findings and histology determined by stereotactic biopsies

Histology	Cases *n*	Hypodense *n*	Hyperdense *n*	Ring structure *n*
Glial tumours	910	294	614	233
Non-glial tumours	286	48	233	43
Non-tumours	124	51	72	33
Total	1320	393	919	309

Table 4. Breakdown of data given in Table 3, for glial tumours

Histology	Cases	Hypodense		Hyperdense		Ring structure	
	n	*n*	%	*n*	%	*n*	%
Astrocytoma I	170	44	26	124	73	20	12
Astrocytoma II	345	188	54	157	46	37	11
Astrocytoma III	186	28	15	158	85	72	39
Glioblastoma IV	152	11	7	141	93	90	59
Oligodendroglioma	57	23	40	34	60	14	24
Total	910	294		614		233	

Table 5. Breakdown of data given in Table 3, for some non-glial tumours

Histology	Cases	Hypodense		Hyperdense		Ring structure	
	n	*n*	%	*n*	%	*n*	%
Epidermoid	8	6	75	2	25	1	12
Craniopharyngeoma	56	28	50	23	41	1	2
Colloid cyst	10	–		10	100	–	
Metastasis	84	5	6	79	94	32	37
Unclass. tumour	10	1	10	9	90	3	30
Total	168	40		123		38	

Table 6. Breakdown of data given in Table 3, for other non-glial tumours

Histology	Cases	Hypodense		Hyperdense		Ring structure	
	n	*n*	%	*n*	%	*n*	%
Ependymoma	20	2	10	18	90		
Papilloma	9	1	10	8	90	–	
Medulloblastoma	6	–		6	100	–	
PNET	24	–		24	100	2	8
Meningeoma	14	1	7	13	93	1	7
Germinoma	35	1	3	34	97	2	6
Teratoma	10	3	30	7	70	1	10
Total	118	8		110		6	

grade I gliomas appear with hyperdense changes but only 26% with a hypodensity (Table 4; see also Tables 5, 6).

In cases of anaplastic gliomas, 85% showed a hyperdensity and 15% a hypodensity. The group of non-tumorous lesions also had a different appearance in the CT scan (Table 7). The difficulty of CT differentiation between gliomas, metastases, ab-

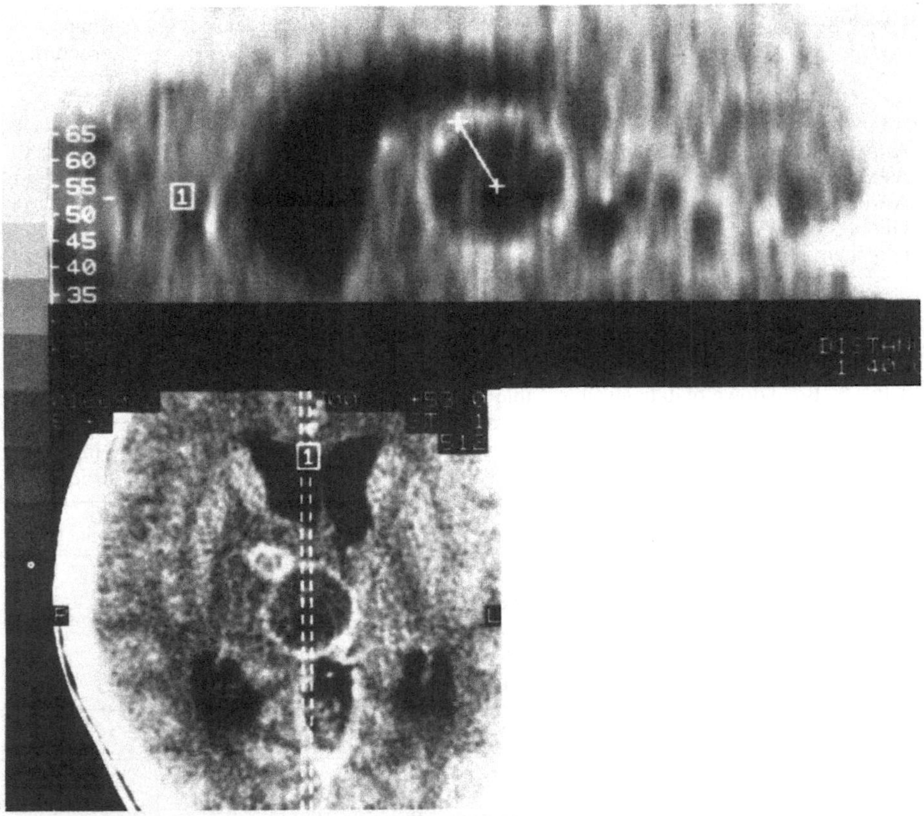

a

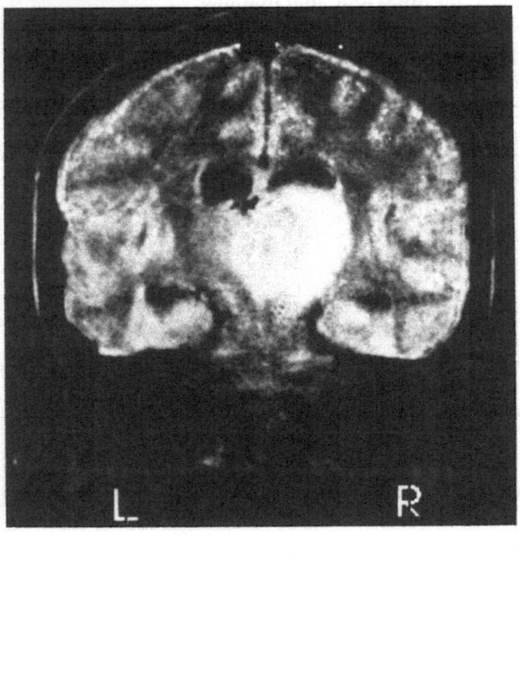

b

Fig. 1 a, b. Subject, 10 years old. **a** CT image showing a ring structure in the rostral parts of the right thalamus with a moderate perifocal oedema, compression of the third ventricle and an occlusive hydrocephalus. An abscess was revealed by the CT stereotactic puncture. +—+ Line of stereotactic probe; [1] front of head. **b** The coronal section in the MRI also shows a ring structure in the right thalamus with a perifocal oedema in the lateral part of the basal ganglia

Table 7. Breakdown of data given in Table 3, for non-tumours

Histology	Cases	Hypodense		Hyperdense		Ring structure	
	n	*n*	%	*n*	%	*n*	%
Haemorrhages	36	5	14	31	86	10	28
Glioses	73	44	60	28	38	10	14
Abscesses	15	2	13	13	87	13	87
Total	124	51		72		33	

Table 8. MRI findings and histology of 66 cases

Histology	Cases *n*	T1 (↑)	T2 (↑↑)	Edema	Cyst
Glioses	8	1	6	4	–
Gliomas I+II	28	15	24	13	2
Gliomas III+IV	13	4	11	8	2
PNET	5	–	5	1	1
Craniopharyng.	3	–	3	–	2
Hypoph. adenoma	1	–	1	1	–
Metastases	2	1	2	1	–
Chondrosarcoma	1	–	–	1	–
Teratomas	2	1	1	1	1
Abscesses	2	–	2	1	–
Normal tissue	1	1	–	–	–
Total	66	23	55	31	8

(↑↑) intensity or prolongation of spin echo

Table 9. CT findings and histology of the same 66 cases as shown in Table 8

Histology	Cases	Hypo-dense	Hyper-dense	Edema	Cyst	Ring structure
	n	*n*	*n*	*n*	*n*	*n*
Glioses	8	4	4	2	–	–
Gliomas I+II	28	19	10	12	2	4
Gliomas III+IV	13	4	10	10	2	4
PNET	5	–	5	2	1	1
Craniopharyng.	3	2	1	–	3	–
Hypoph. adenoma	1	–	1	1	–	–
Metastases	2	–	2	1	–	–
Chondrosarcoma	1	–	1	1	–	1
Teratomas	2	2	–	–	1	1
Abscesses	2	–	2	–	–	1
Normal tissue	1	–	–	–	–	–
Total	66	31	36	29	9	11

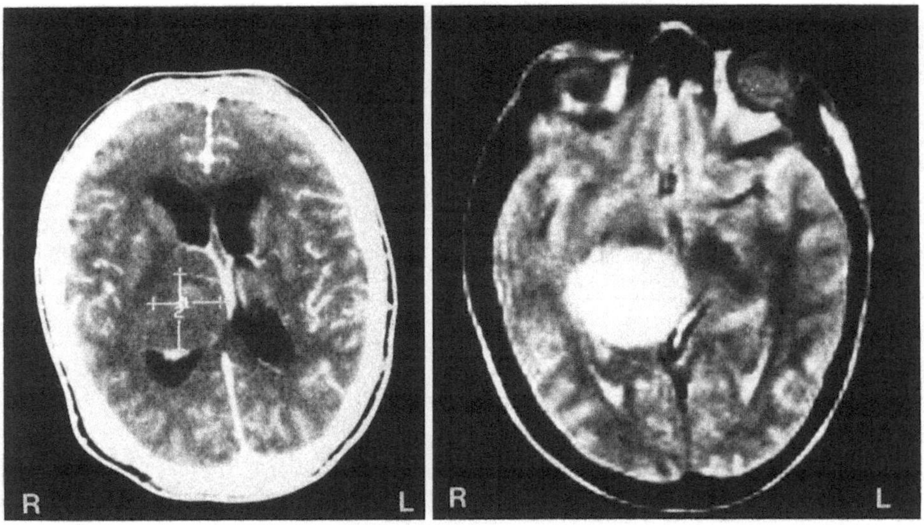

Fig. 2a,b. Subject, 50 years old. **a** CT image showing increased volume of the right pulvinar with a hinted ring structure in the centre, compression of the third ventricle, and a beginning occlusive hydrocephalus. The histology, confirmed by the CT stereotactic technique, was that of a glioblastoma. +—1—+ First diameter, +—2—+ second diameter. **b** The axial section in the MRI shows a sharply delineated area for increased spin echo with a moderate perifocal reaction. A ring structure was not observed

scesses and haemorrhages is especially demonstrated by a comparison of the ring structures in the CT scan and the histology confirmed by the stereotactic technique (Figs. 1a and 2a). Similar differences in the appearance of cerebral lesions can be seen with the MR technique in cases of tumours of comparable dignity and character (Figs. 1b and 2b).

In the MRI, only the T2 signal could be interpreted relatively reliably, especially regarding differences between tumour parts and surrounding reactions. Evaluation of the MRI findings (Table 8) showed an increased T2 intensity in 24 cases among a total of 28 low-grade gliomas; in 13 cases a perifocal edema and in 2 cases a cystic change was revealed. In the CT pictures of the same cases (Table 9), 19 showed a hypodense area and 10 a hyperdensity, with a ring structure in 4 cases.

The histological verification was performed using the stereotactic technique and showed in these 28 cases a fibrillary or pilocytic astrocytoma. Among 13 cases of malignant gliomas we found 4 with hypodense changes and 10 with hyperdensity in the CT pictures. In the MR images, however, an increased T2 intensity was found in 11 cases, and a perifocal edemateous reaction in only 8 out of 12 cases.

Discussion

CT findings in a series of 1309 cases, all of which were histologically confirmed by the CT- or MRI-guided stereotactic technique [1, 5, 6, 11], showed a hyperdensity in cases of tumorous lesions, but also in cases of haemorrhages,glioses and abscesses.

Table 10. Possibility of evaluation by CT scan and MRI in relation to the histological findings

	CT	MRI
Histology of lesions	–	–
Dignity	(+)	(+)
Localisation	+	+
Size, configuration	(+)	(+)
Perifocal oedema	(+)	+
Calcification	+	(+)
Necrosis	(+)	(+)
Cyst formation	(+)	+
Ring structure	+	+
Displacement	+	+

+ possible; (+) reduced possibility; – impossible

Ring structures were above all to be seen in malignant gliomas, metastases and haemorrhages (Tables 3–7).

A comparison of MR and CT images (Tables 8, 9) clearly shows that differing signals in MR can be obtained from histologically similar tissues [2, 4, 10]. Correlation of histology with the CT findings is not possible. In 31 cases we found a hypodense and, in parts, growth-like representation of the changes, and in 11 cases a distinct ring structure which we found in malignant gliomas, metastases, and haemorrhages too. Using the computed tomogram, we were able to prove a perifocal reaction in 29 cases in all, whereas with an MRI evaluation, a clear perifocal edema was revealed in 31 cases.

These difficulties are pointed out in 2 cases with a ring structure revealed by CT and MRI. In the first case an abscess was recognized neither in the CT scan nor in the MRI (Fig. 1). The other case also shows a ring structure in the thalamic region with a perifocal edematous reaction. Using the stereotactic technique, we determined the presence of a malignant glioma grade IV (Fig. 2).

Evaluation of the series of MRI examinations performed under comparable physical conditions showed very clearly that histological evaluation of an intracerebral lesion cannot even today be replaced by a nuclear spin technique. It appears to us very urgent that uniform MRI measuring units be established in order to make possible more accurate comparisons in the future. Particularly in processes of the midline or functionally important areas of the brain, CT- or MRI-guided stereotactic techniques, with their gradual step-by-step sample taking method, provide good, reliable assistance in attempts at correlation, without entailing significant risks to the patient [6, 8].

Our evaluations show that even nuclear spin tomography cannot replace histological diagnosis, and neither can X-ray transmitted computed tomography. Only the location of a lesion and a perifocal reaction can be demonstrated by the CT scan or MRI, thus providing an important prerequisite for a stereotactic probe or resection (Table 10). We therefore strongly advise against performing extensive therapy on the basis of evidence from the image-producing procedures alone, without having previously performed an exact histological confirmation [6, 7, 9, 12].

Conclusion

In spite of the improved quality of modern CT and MRI, and in spite of the improved ability to differentiate changes in intracranial structures, we are convinced that in the classification of the histology and dignity of intracranial lesions, a biopsy is indispensable.

References

1. Birg W, Mundinger F (1973) Computer calculations of target parameters for a stereotactic apparatus. Acta Neurochir (Wien) 29:123–229
2. Birg W, Mundinger F, Mohadjer M, Weigel K, Fürmaier R. X-ray and MR-stereotaxy for functional and nonfunctional neurosurgery. IX Meeting of the World Society Stereotactic and Functional Neurosurgery, Toronto, 4–7 July 1985. Appl Neurophysiol (in press)
3. Bradley WG (1985) Note and impression from meeting: third annual meeting of the society of magnetic resonance in medicine, New York, 13–17 Aug 1984. J Comput Assist Tomogr 9(1):220–224
4. Heafner MD, Schut L, Packer RJ et al (1985) Discrepancy between computed tomography and magnetic resonance imaging in a case of medulloblastoma. Neurosurgery 17:487–489
5. Hueftle MG, Han JS, Kaufman B, Benson JE (1985) MR imaging of brain stem gliomas. J Comput Assist Tomogr 9(2):263–267
6. Kleihues P, Volk B, Anagnostopoulos J, Kiessling M (1984) Morphologic evaluation of stereotactic brain tumor. Acta Neurochir [Suppl 1] (Wien) 33:117–181
7. Mundinger F (1982) CT stereotactic biopsy of brain tumours. In: Voth D, Gutjahr P, Langmaid C (eds) Tumours of the central nervous system in infancy and childhood. Springer, Berlin Heidelberg New York, pp 234–246
8. Mundinger F, Birg W (1982) Stereotactic brain surgery with the aid of computed tomography (CT-stereotaxy). In: Driessen W, Brock M, Klinger M (eds) Computerized tomography, brain metabolism, spinal injuries. Springer, Berlin Heidelberg New York, pp 17–24 (Advances in neurosurgery, vol 10)
9. Mundinger F, Birg W (1984) CT stereotaxy in the clinical routine. Neurosurg Rev 7:219–224
10. Mundinger F, Fürmaier R, Volk B, Weigel K (1985) Der Vergleich von CT- und MRI-Befunden intracranieller Tumoren mit dem stereotaktischen Biopsie-Ergebnis. 36. Jahrestagung der Deutschen Gesellschaft für Neurochirurgie, Berlin, 12–15 May 1985
11. Riechert T, Mundinger F (1956) Beschreibung und Anwendung eines Zielgerätes für stereotaktische Hirnoperationen (2. Modell). Acta Neurochir (Wien) 3:308–337
12. Weigel K, Mohadjer M, Mundinger F (1984) CT-stereotaxy for differential diagnosis and radiotherapy of intracranial metastases. In: Piotrowski W, Brock M, Klinger M (eds) CNS metastases. Neurosurgery in the aged. Springer, Berlin Heidelberg New York Tokyo, pp 87–93 (Advances in neurosurgery, vol 12)

Autoradiographic Distributions of Neurotransmitter Receptors in the Brain of Patients with Parkinson's Disease and MPTP-induced Monkey Parkinsonism

S. Kito, R. Miyoshi, K. Mizuno, K. Nitta, H. Matsubayashi, and Y. Yamamura [1]

Parkinson's disease is a slowly progressive degenerative disorder which is pathologically characterized by neuronal loss of the substantia nigra. Biochemically, deficiency of dopamine in the striatum resulting from degeneration and loss of dopaminergic neurons in the substantia nigra has been confirmed. In addition, from experiments using autopsied human materials [1–6], abnormalities have been reported in the dopaminergic as well as in the following systems: acetylcholine, GABA, serotonin, noradrenaline, and peptide-containing neurons. Recently, it was discovered that 1-methyl-4-phenyl-1,2,3,6-tetrahydropyridine (MPTP), a by-product in the synthesis of MPPP (1-methyl-4-phenyl-4-propionoxy-piperidine), is selectively toxic to the zona compacta of the substantia nigra [7]. In this paper, we report on observed distributions of neurotransmitter receptors in brains of patients with Parkinson's disease and those of primate models with MPTP-induced parkinsonism.

Materials and Methods

Autopsied human brains of two parkinsonian patients and two neurologically intact persons were used in these experiments. Two parkinsonian patients took similar courses of the disease and both of them had been medicated with L-dopa, anticholinergic drugs, and bromocriptine until 2 months before death. As primate models, four male adult Japanese monkeys were used. MPTP was administered intravenously to three monkeys over a period of 5–10 days. One other monkey was used as a control. Seven days after the last injection of MPTP, animals were anesthetized and brains were rapidly removed.

Thus obtained brains were sagittally bisected into hemispheres, and one hemisphere was used for conventional histopathologic observations and the other one for in vitro macroautoradiography of neurotransmitter receptors. The autoradiographic

[1] Third Department of Internal Medicine, Hiroshima University School of Medicine, 1-2-3, Kasumi, Minami-ku, Hiroshima 734, Japan.

Neurology
Ed. by K. Poeck, H. J. Freund, and H. Gänshirt

Table 1. Experimental conditions used in the in vitro labeling of receptors for autoradiographic studies

Receptor	Ligand	Buffer	Ligand concentration/ blank	Incubation (time/ temperature)	Rinses (time/ temperature)
Dopamine	^{3}H-Lisuride	Tris HCl 25 mM pH 7.4[a]	3 nM/10^{-4} M spiperone	60 min/25° C	3 min/25° C
	^{3}H-Spiperone	Tris HCl 0.17 M pH 7.7[b]	0.4 nM/1 μM spiperone	30 min/25° C	5 min × 2/25 °C
mAchR	^{3}H-QNB	phosphate buffer 0.1 M pH 7.4	2 nM/1 μM atropine	60 min/25° C	5 min × 2/4° C
Substance P	^{3}H-Substance P	Tris HCl 50 mM pH 7.4[c]	2 nM/5 μM substance P	30 min/25° C	1 min × 4/4° C

[a] Containing 5 mM Na_2EDTA, 0.02% ascorbic acid, and 10 μM pargyline.
[b] Containing 120 mM NaCl, 5 mM KCl, 2 mM $CaCl_2$, 1 mM $MgCl_2$, and 0.001% ascorbic acid.
[c] Containing 0.2 g/l bovine serum albumin, 40 mg/l bacitracin, 2 mg/l chymostatin, 4 mg/l leupeptin, and 3 mM $MnCl_2$.

technique was the one originally established by Young and Kuhar [8]. The radioactive ligands used were ^{3}H-lisuride and ^{3}H-spiperone (dopamine-receptor ligands), ^{3}H-QNB (a muscarinic acetylcholine receptor antagonist), and ^{3}H-substance P. We performed saturation experiments of these ligands on cryostat sections through the striatum of normal rats and decided optimal experimental conditions for autoradiography (Table 1). As for autoradiography of ^{3}H-spiperone binding sites, 0.3 μM ketanserin, a selective antagonist of 5-HT_2 receptor, was added into the incubation medium in order to observe dopamine-specific binding sites.

Results

Human Brains of Parkinson's Disease

Pathological findings of two patients were consistent with those of Parkinson's disease, i.e., in the substantia nigra, pigmented neurons were markedly decreased and a few remaining neurons were atrophic. There were Lewy bodies in the substantia nigra with mild rarefaction of the granular layer and Torpedoe in the cerebellum of case 2.

Computer-modeled Scatchard plots of saturation experiments of ^{3}H-lisuride binding sites revealed that there were two binding sites, i.e., high and low affinities whose Kd values were 0.62 nM and 54.2 nM, respectively. Lisuride, a dopaminergic ergot alkaloid, has been widely used as a therapeutic drug against Parkinson's disease and hyperprolactinemia. Pharmacologically, lisuride is known to have complicated pharmacokinetics toward monoamine neurons, i.e., it acts not only as a

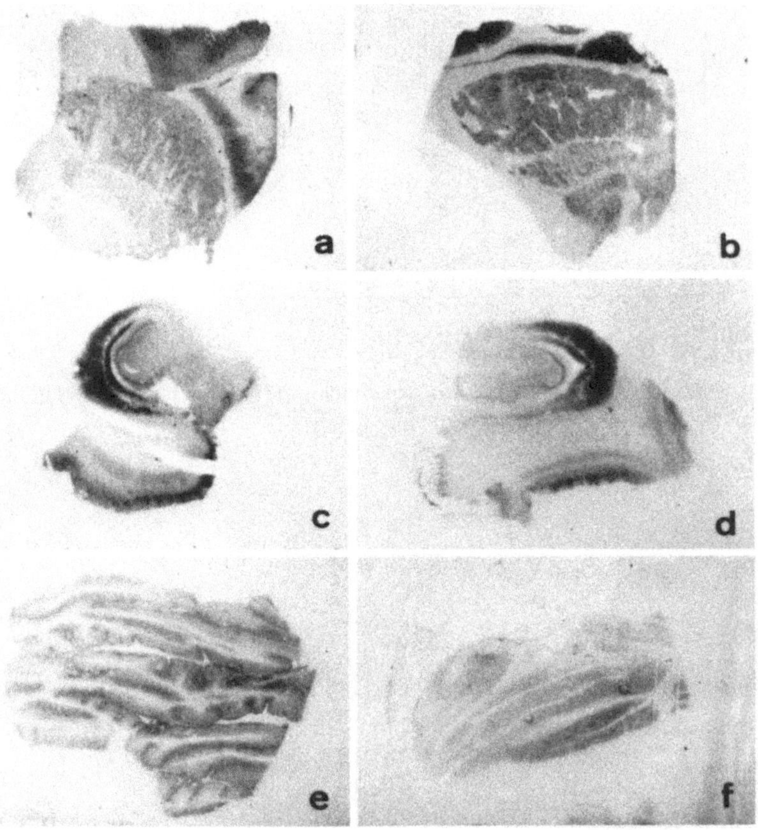

Fig. 1a–f. Autoradiograms of ^{3}H-lisuride high affinity binding sites in human brains. **a, c** and **e** are pictures of nonneurological disorder, and **b, d** and **f** are those of Parkinson's disease. **a** and **b** are autoradiograms of the putamen and globus pallidus; **c** and **d** are the hippocampal formation and **e** and **f** are the cerebellum. In a parkinsonian brain, ^{3}H-lisuride binding sites were increased in the globus pallidus and decreased in the parahippocampal gyrus and cerebellum

dopamine D_2 receptor agonist [9, 10], but also is associated with both serotonergic [11] and adrenergic [12] receptors. The autoradiographic technique was applied to ^{3}H-lisuride high affinity binding sites. Autoradiograms of ^{3}H-lisuride high affinity binding sites of the hemisphere of case 1 are shown in Fig. 1. Figure 1a and 1b shows the putamen and globus pallidus. In a parkinsonian brain (Fig. 1b), the specific ^{3}H-lisuride binding sites were increased in the globus pallidus. Figure 1c and 1d shows the hippocampal formation. The density of ^{3}H-lisuride binding sites was decreased in the parahippocampal gyrus in a brain of Parkinson's disease (Fig. 1d). The cerebellum is shown in Fig. 1e and 1f. In the brain of a neurologically indifferent case (Fig. 1e), ^{3}H-lisuride binding sites were richly observed. However, in a parkinsonian brain (Fig. 1e), they were markedly decreased with loss of structure-dependent distribution of receptors. The presence of primarily β_2 receptors is sug-

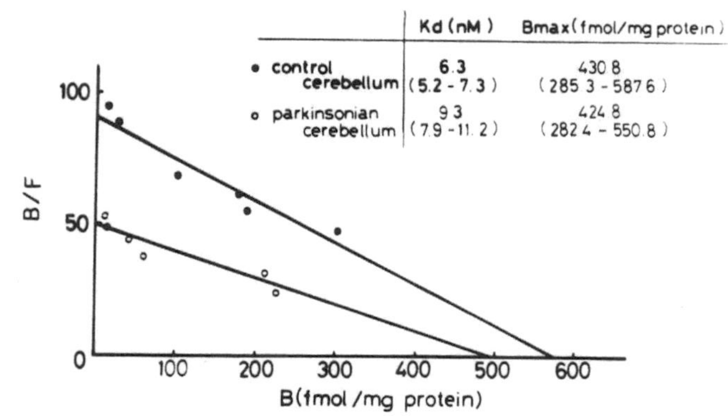

Fig. 2. Scatchard plots of saturation experiments of ^{3}H-DHA binding sites in the cerebellum of a control brain (●) and a parkinsonian brain (○)

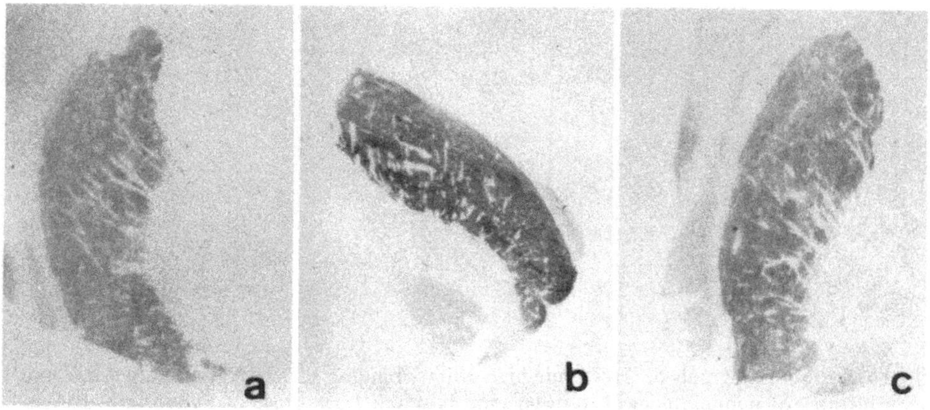

Fig. 3a–c. Autoradiograms of ^{3}H-QNB binding sites in the putamen and globus pallidus of human brains. **a** shows a picture of a control brain, and **b** and **c** show those of parkinsonian brains. In the putamen of parkinsonian brains, ^{3}H-QNB binding sites were increased

gested in the cerebellum. To confirm this alteration through binding experiments more specific to β_2 receptor, we performed saturation experiments using ^{3}H-dihydroalprenolol (^{3}H-DHA) as a radioactive ligand. In the parkinsonian cerebellum, a tendency of the affinity of ^{3}H-DHA binding sites to decrease was observed (Fig. 2). In the cerebral cortex, ^{3}H-lisuride binding sites were decreased in the pre- and postcentral gyri, while increased in the cingulate gyrus (data not shown).

Autoradiograms of ^{3}H-QNB binding sites are shown in Fig. 3. The specific ^{3}H-QNB binding sites existed at a high concentration in the putamen, while they were much less observed in the globus pallidus. In parkinsonian brains of the two cases (Fig. 3b and 3c), ^{3}H-QNB binding sites were increased in the putamen.

In addition, autoradiography of ^{3}H-substance P binding sites was performed. Saturation experiments of ^{3}H-substance P binding sites with use of cryostat sections

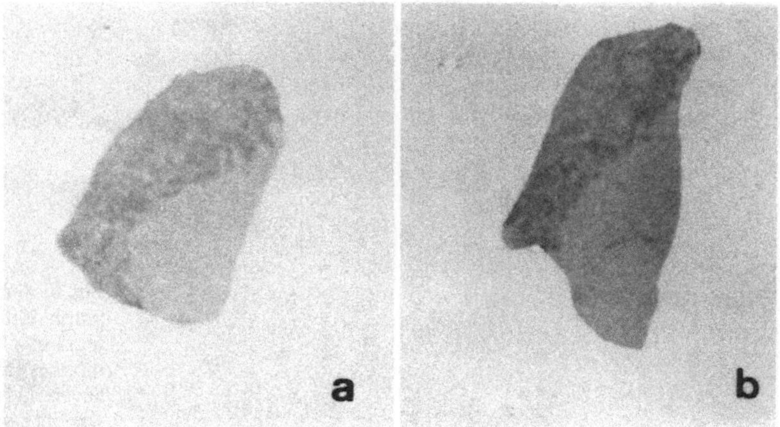

Fig. 4a, b. Autoradiograms of ^{3}H-substance P binding sites in the putamen and globus pallidus of human brains. **a** shows a picture of a control brain, and **b** shows that of a parkinsonian brain. In the globus pallidus of two parkinsonian brains, an increase of ^{3}H-substance P binding sites was observed

through the striatum of normal rats revealed that ^{3}H-substance P binding sites had a single affinity binding site whose Kd value was 0.86 nM. For autoradiography, cryostat sections were incubated with 2 nM ^{3}H-substance P, where the difference between total binding and nonspecific binding was the largest. Autoradiographic pictures of ^{3}H-substance P binding sites are shown in Fig. 4. In the globus pallidus of a parkinsonian brain (Fig. 4b), ^{3}H-substance P binding sites were increased.

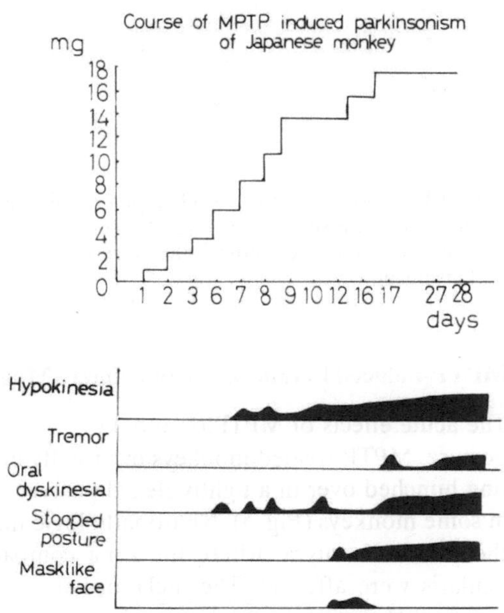

Fig. 5. Clinical course of MPTP-induced parkinsonism of a Japanese monkey

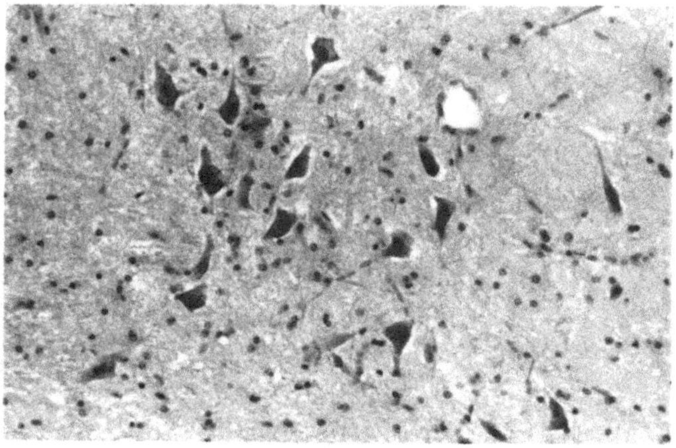

Fig. 6. A microphotograph of the substantia nigra of a MPTP-treated monkey (H.E. stain). Severe nerve cell loss was observed

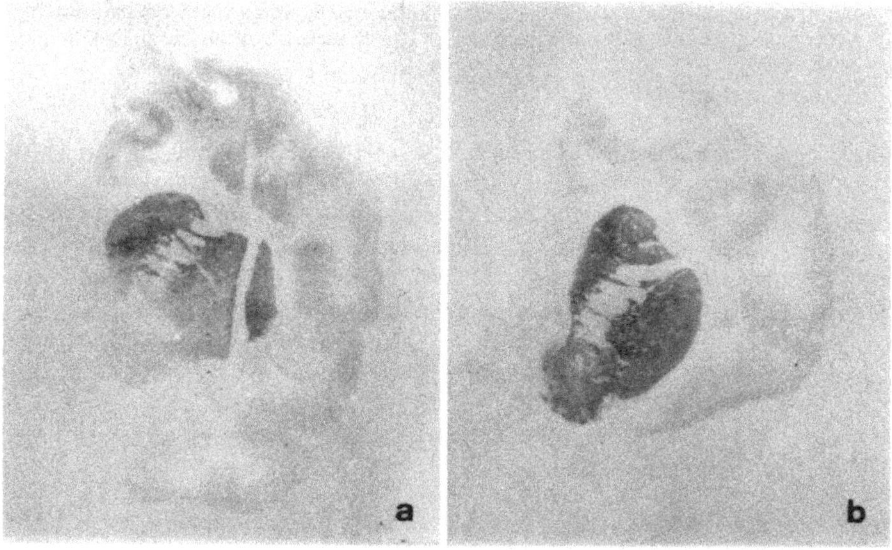

Fig. 7 a, b. Autoradiograms of ^{3}H-spiperone binding sites on sections through the striatum of monkey brains. **a** shows a picture of a control monkey and **b** shows that of an MPTP-treated monkey. ^{3}H-spiperone binding sites were increased in the striatum in brains of MPTP-treated parkinsonism

MPTP-Induced Parkinsonism of Primate Models

The acute effects of MPTP on monkeys included alterations of motor behavior and posture. MPTP-treated monkeys eventually became profoundly akinetic, usually sitting hunched over in a tightly flexed posture. Tremor and oral dyskinesia were seen in some monkeys (Fig. 5). Neuropathologic findings of these monkeys were found in the substantia nigra, where the zona compacta and, to a lesser degree, zona reticularis were affected. The melanin-laden neurons were reduced in number and

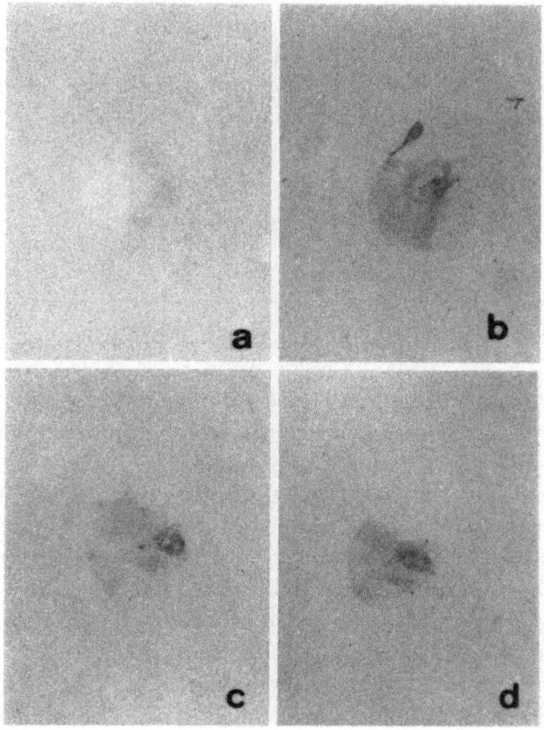

Fig. 8 a–d. Autoradiograms of ^{3}H-QNB binding sites in the medulla oblongata of monkeys. **a** shows a picture of a control brain and **b, c** and **d** show those of parkinsonian brains. A hot spot of ^{3}H-QNB binding sites was observed in all the experimental parkinsonian brains

those surviving also showed atrophy of variable degrees. There was slight to moderate gliosis in these regions (Fig. 6).

Autoradiograms of ^{3}H-spiperone binding sites on sections through the striatum of monkey brains are shown in Fig. 7. There were far fewer binding sites in the cerebral cortex after addition of katanserin. In parkinsonian brains, ^{3}H-spiperone binding sites were increased in the striatum.

As for muscarinic acetylcholine receptors, there were no differences between control brains and parkinsonian brains in the basal ganglia. However, a marked increase of ^{3}H-QNB binding sites was observed in the medulla oblongata, probably in the spinal tractus nucleus of the trigeminal nerve (Fig. 8 b). Since we performed in vitro macroautoradiography using unfixed tissues, we could not identify the individual nucleus precisely. Such a ^{3}H-QNB binding hot spot was observed in all the three diseased monkeys, while ^{3}H-QNB binding sites were weakly observed in a control brain (Fig. 8 a). Significance of these findings was left for further studies.

^{3}H-Substance P binding sites in monkey brains were richly observed in the striatum, globus pallidus, and granular layer of the hippocampus. However, the densities of these areas showed no changes and no abnormal distributions were observed.

Discussion

In the parkinsonian brain, abnormalities of various neurotransmitter systems have been reported [1–6]. We performed in vitro autoradiography of dopamine, muscarinic acetylcholine, and substance P receptors, and studied alterations of these binding sites.

Brains of Patients with Parkinson's Disease

In a parkinsonian human brain, the density of ^{3}H-lisuride high affinity binding sites was not changed in the putamen, while it was increased in the globus pallidus, although both the putamen and globus pallidus are receiving dopaminergic neurons from the substantia nigra. An increase of ^{3}H-lisuride binding sites in the globus pallidus may be due to denervation supersensitivity of receptors resulting from a decreased dopamine concentration. In addition, abnormal distributions of ^{3}H-lisuride binding sites were extended not only to the basal ganglia, but also to the cerebral cortex and cerebellum. It is known that ^{3}H-lisuride binds both adrenergic [12] and serotonergic [11] receptors, as well as dopaminergic receptors. Since the cerebral cortex and cerebellum are little innervated by dopamine neurons, it is considered that abnormal distributions in the cerebral cortex and cerebellum are due to alterations of either adrenergic or serotonergic receptors. Therefore, it is concluded that in patients with Parkinson's disease, abnormalities of adrenergic and serotonergic receptor systems also reach wide areas of the brain. ^{3}H-Lisuride binding sites were markedly decreased in the cerebellum. It is suggested that catecholamine receptors in the cerebellum are primarily β_2 receptors. So, we performed saturation experiments of ^{3}H-DHA using the cerebellar homogenate of the same case. In the parkinsonian cerebellum, a tendency of the affinity of ^{3}H-DHA binding sites to decrease was observed, though statistically not significant. Nevertheless, this finding partly supports the above-mentioned autoradiographic decrease of ^{3}H-lisuride binding sites in the parkinsonian cerebellum. The fact that ^{3}H-lisuride binds not only β_2 adrenergic receptors, but also other catecholamine receptors may explain some discrepancy between these findings.

It was reported by Reisine et al. [5] that the specific binding sites of ^{3}H-QNB were increased in the putamen. According to the authors, the enhanced ^{3}H-QNB binding observed in the putamen coupled with the decrease in choline acetyltransferase activity implies a possible denervation supersensitivity for acetylcholine in this brain area. In our autoradiographic study, it was confirmed that ^{3}H-QNB binding sites were increased in the putamen in parkinsonian brains.

Substance P has been found from striatopallidal and striatonigral neuronal pathways [13–15], where it may act as a neurotransmitter. In 1984, Tenovuo et al. suggested that substance P might play a role in pathophysiology of Parkinson's disease [6]. They measured the amount of substance P immunoreactivity in the postmortem parkinsonian brain by radioimmunoassay and obtained the result that the amount of substance P immunoreactivity was significantly decreased in the substantia nigra and putamen. Taking their result into consideration, a receptor supersensitivity resulting from decrease of substance P in the putamen may cause increase of ^{3}H-substance P binding sites in the globus pallidus.

MPTP-Induced Parkinsonism of Primate Models

As for the change of dopamine receptors in MPTP-induced parkinsonism of primate models, an increase of ^{3}H-spiperone binding sites in the striatum was observed as having been confirmed autoradiographically by us in human brains of parkinsonian patients.

Alterations of ^{3}H-QNB and ^{3}H-substance P binding sites in the basal ganglia which were observed in human parkinsonian brains were not shown in MPTP-induced parkinsonism of primate models. In our experiments, animals were killed 7 days after the last administration of MPTP. This survival period may be too short to compare with human cases, where duration of the illness was longer than 5 years. However, it is assumed that at an early stage of Parkinson's disease, the dopaminergic system may be exclusively affected and other neurotransmitter systems are relatively preserved. Changes of various neurotransmitter systems with the passage of time after MPTP administration will be the next target of our investigations.

References

1. Bokobza B, Ruberg M, Scatton B, Javoy-Agid F, Agid Y (1984) [^{3}H]spiperone binding, dopamine and HVA concentrations in Parkinson's disease and supranuclear palsy. Eur J Pharmacol 99:167–175
2. Llorens-Cortes C, Javoy-Agid F, Agid Y, Taquet H, Schwartz JC (1984) Enkephalinergic markers in substantia nigra and caudate nucleus from parkinsonian subjects. J Neurochem 43:874–877
3. Lloyd KD, Shemen L, Hornykiewicz O (1977) Distribution of high affinity sodium-independent [^{3}H]gamma-aminobutyric acid ([^{3}H]GABA) binding in the human brain: alterations in Parkinson's disease. Brain Res 127:269–278
4. Mayeux R, Stern Y, Cote L, Williams JBW (1984) Altered serotonin metabolism in depressed patients with Parkinson's disease. Neurology 34:642–646
5. Reisine TD, Fields JZ, Yamamura HI, Bird ED, Spokes E, Schreiner PS, Enna SJ (1977) Neurotransmitter receptor alterations in Parkinson's disease. Life Sci 21:335–344
6. Tenovuo O, Rinne UK, Viljanen MK (1984) Substance P immunoreactivity in the postmortem parkinsonian brain. Brain Res 303:113–116
7. Burns RS, Chiueh CC, Markey SP, Ebert MH, Jacobowitz DM, Kopin IJ (1983) A primate model of parkinsonism: selective destruction of dopaminergic neurons in the pars compacta of the substantia nigra by N-methyl-4-phenyl-1,2,3,6-tetrahydropyridine. Proc Natl Acad Sci USA 80:4546–4550
8. Youg III W, Kuhar MJ (1979) A new method for receptor autoradiography: [^{3}H] opioid receptors in rat brain. Brain Res 179:255–279
9. Fuxe K, Agnati LF, Kohler C, Andersson K, Eneroth P, Calza L, Ogren SO (1983) Heterogeneity of brain dopamine systems: possible discrimination of different types of dopamine systems and receptors by ergot drugs. In: Calne DB (ed) Lisuride and other dopamine agonists. Raven, New York, pp 11–31
10. Spano PF, Govoni S, Uzumaki H, Bosio A, Memo M, Lucchi L, Carruba M, Trabucchi M (1983) Stimulation of D_2 dopamine receptors by dopaminergic ergot alkaloids: studies on the mechanism of action. In: Agonoli A (ed) Aging brain and ergot alkaloids. Raven, New York, pp 165–177
11. Rosenfeld MR, Makman MH (1981) The interaction of lisuride, an ergot derivative, with serotonergic and dopaminergic receptors in rabbit brain. J Pharmacol and Exp Ther 216:526–531
12. Cote TE, Eskay RL, Frey EA, Crewe CW, Munemura M, Tsuruta K, Brouwn EM, Kebabian JW (1983) Actions of lisuride on adrenoceptors and dopamine receptors. In: Calne DB (ed) Lisuride and other dopamine agonists. Raven, New York, pp 45–53

13. Hong JS, Yang HYT, Racagni G, Costa E (1977) Projections of substance P containing neurons from neostriatum to substantia nigra. Brain Res 122:541–544
14. Kanazawa I, Emson PC, Cuello AC (1977) Evidence for the existence of substance P containing fibers in striato-nigral and pallido-nigral pathways in rat brain. Brain Res 119:447–453
15. Morz EA, Brownstein MJ, Leeman SE (1977) Evidence for substance P in the striato-nigral tract. Brain Res 125:305–311

Economics of Modern Brain Imaging Techniques

F. AICHNER [1]

Introduction

In many member countries of the World Health Organization (WHO) about 12%–15% of the national expenditure is directed toward health care. Controlling the costs of medical techniques has become synonymous with controlling a handful of large expensive and potentially dramatic aids to diagnosis and treatment such as CT, MRI, and PET scanners, but the introduction of new medical technology is only one of the factors increasing the costs of medical care. Others, of more importance, include access to care, inflation, the increased proportion of aging population, and medical payment policies.

Indeed, there has been an explosion of new techniques like computed tomography (CT), magnetic resonance imaging (MRI), positron emission tomography (PET), digital subtraction angiography (DSA), ultrasound imaging, computerized electroencephalography (EEG), and single photon emission tomography (SPECT). The development of these new techniques has increased worldwide need for imaging methods tremendously. Between 1978 and 1983 the financial expenses for imaging systems in the whole world are supposed to double from 6 billion German marks (DM) to 11 billion DM (1983). The introduction of MRI has further increased these expenses. The decrease of conventional radiology and the growth of the new techniques such as ultrasound, CT, and MRI became apparent [2].

As medical enthusiasm mounted, however, public resistance to these expensive new technologies became evident, particularly among those responsible for funding health care. There is a growing conviction that medical technologies are major contributors to escalating costs. But, it become known, that the high technologies actually account for far less of the annual growth in medical expenditures than do the collective expenses of thousands of small tests and procedures that are more frequently used by physicians and that individually cost little.

For 1978, the Bureau of Radiologic Health (USA) estimated that approximately 186000000 diagnostic radiology examinations and 800000 nuclear medicine examinations were performed. If these examinations had an average cost of $ 45 (US), the total national cost of these imaging procedures was approximately $ 8.4 billion. To-

[1] Department of Neurology, University Hospital, Medical School, Innsbruck, Austria.

Neurology
Ed. by K. Poeck, H. J. Freund, and H. Gänshirt

tal health care costs in the USA for 1978 have been estimated at $ 180 billion. Thus the costs or charges for CT comprise only 5%–8% of diagnostic imaging costs and 0.2%–0.3% of US health care costs. If the annual operating costs of CT, coronary bypass surgery, renal dialysis, etc. were reduced by half, the net savings would equal less than 1% of a year's bill for health care [4].

In the Federal Republic of Germany the health costs for 1976 have been estimated at $ 48 billion, the costs for medical technologies come to 0.8%, while the total health costs for 1981 mounted to $ 70 billion. However, the portion for medical technology in 1981 is only 0.6% [8].

The health value of a new diagnostic technology is determined by its effect on the diagnostic process, the therapy, the course of the disease, and the outcome. At least three important questions must be asked about each potential application of new technologies. First is it an accurate diagnostic method. Second, can it truly yield additional important information. Third, will it supplant existing noninvasive and invasive diagnostic methods? The implications of costs, diffusion, and planning can only be understood through continuing analysis of the impact of the new technologies on medical diagnosis and treatment.

With these reflections in mind, several modern neuroimaging technologies are discussed in the material that follows.

Computed Tomography

In 1983, 6900 CT scanners were counted in the USA, Europe, and Japan (which had the highest CT density of these three regions [8]). CT equipment acquaintance costs are $ 800000, maintenance costs come to $ 300000 per year, while examination costs vary between $ 150 and $ 350 depending on procedures per day, working days per year, and whether the patients are private or publicly insured.

Economic analysis reveals that CT leads to marked reduction of health expenses, since patient admission time is shortened. The morbidity and mortality of the diagnostic evaluation of neurologic patients has decreased significantly. There is ample documentation of the reduced use of nuclear medicine scans, plain radiographs, air studies, and angiograms in medical centers where CT is available. If CT had not been available, the cost of alternate imaging procedures for evaluation of the central nervous system would have been more than $ 1130 million. It is estimated that in 1978 CT reduced this cost by $ 459 million [4]. CT has resulted in dramatic changes in therapy [1]. Fineberg et al. [7] reported that CT led to a change in therapy in 20% of cases. Ambrose and co-workers [3] found a 94% reduction in craniotomies in patients having CT after acute head trauma. CT also influenced the choice of therapy in patients with stroke and intracranial bleeding.

Without marked changes in therapeutic efficacy of brain tumors, it is unlikely that CT will statistically improve survival of patients with brain neoplasma in the next years.

Magnetic Resonance Imaging

MRI is certainly one of the highest-priced technologies that we have ever seen because of the equipment costs, construction problems, and the inability to charge at this time.

The total cost of equipment required for MR-proton imaging is $ 1 700 000–$ 2 350 000. This includes transportation, installation, and room shielding. The cost of construction is $ 750 000. The personnel required for clinical operation are two physicians, one technologist, one receptionist, and one nurse; their annual salaries run to $ 240 000. The estimated annual MRI operating costs and total annual costs are $ 884 000 for resistive magnet and $ 1 264 000 for superconducting magnet [11] (Table 1). Evens, in making a break-even point analysis for CT and NMR in 1983 [5], assumed 3000 patients per year for CT and 1500 patients per year for MRI. The break-even point analysis revealed for MRI examination a cost of $ 775 [6].

In the NMR guideline report of 1983 [11] the charge calculated to economically "break even" with MRI is $ 442 using a resistive magnet and $ 632 using a superconducting magnet (Table 2). Increasing patient throughpout is very important and will reduce the break even point per patient. The MRI market in October 1984 is shown in Table 3, the estimated MRI world market is demonstrated on Table 4.

The main positive effects of MR on health expenses consist in the replacement of other diagnostic procedures, shortening of hospital stay, and shifting from inpatient care to outpatient care. MR cost may not compare unfavorably with those of CT, and increased cost may still be justified if more information can be obtained or if the need for other tests or length of hospitalization could be reduced. At the present, the consensus seems to be that MRI and its cousin CT work complementarily in this and other imaging applications. In reviewing the evaluation of abnormalities related to brain stem, temporal lobe, and spinal cord it is said MRI is far more sensitive and accurate than CT, cisternography, pneumoencephalography, or myelography. The scientific investigation of MRI in regard to its influences on therapeutic plans should be actively supported.

Positron Emission Tomography

PET is likely to remain primarily a research tool because of the high costs of the method currently $ 4 000 000 for equipment and $ 300 000 per annum for staff and maintenance. At present PET scan of CBF and metabolism is used primarily for research purposes; its cost effectiveness as compared to that of the practical clinical applications of two other methods (^{133}Xe and SPECT) for measuring CBF is still unknown. The cost at present is about $ 1000 for each measurement using PET, versus $ 75 per each measurement with ^{133}Xe and stable Xenon CT and $ 300 using SPECT.

However, PET scanning is the only method currently available that provides quantitative regional information for brain metabolism and receptor binding [9].

Table 1. Estimated annual MRI operating costs and total annual costs (US dollars) [11]

	Resistive	Superconducting
Annual operating costs	312000	478200
Annualized equipment costs	572000	786000
Total annual costs	884000	1264000

Table 2. MRI cost per procedure for break-even operation (in US dollars) [11]

Cost per scan	Resistive	Superconducting
2000 Scans annually	442	632
3000 Scans annually	305	431

Table 3. The MRI market: clinical installations, October 1984 (Source: *Diagnostic Imaging*)

Company	World	USA	Europe	Others	Planned	World market share (%)
Technicare	58	49	7	2 (J)	–	36
Picker	28	11	12	5 [a]	6	18
Diasonics	22	18	4	0	–	14
Siemens	15	7	7	1 (J)	19	9
Fonar	8	5	1	2 [b]	7	5
Philips	8	4	4	0	9	5
Bruker	4	2	1	1 (J)	–	3
Elscint	4	2	1	1 (IL)	–	3
General Electric	4	3	1	0	9	3
M & D technology	3	0	3	0	–	2
Toshiba	5	0	0	5 (J)	–	3
Total	159	101	41	17	50	100

[a] Two in Japan, one in Canada, Saudi Arabia, and Singapore
[b] One in Mexico, one in Japan

Table 4. Estimated MRI market of the world (source: Office of Technology Assessment, Washington, D.C.)

Year	Deliveries per year	Cumulative deliveries	Average sales price (millions of US dollars)	Sales/year (millions of US dollars)
1982	15	15	1.3	20
1983	75	90	1.3	100
1984	200	290	1.5	300
1985	400	690	1.6	650
1986	650	1340	1.7	1150
1987	950	2290	1.85	1750
1988	1250	3540	2.0	2500

Digital Subtraction Angiography (DSA)

A digital angiography diagnostic facility has relatively high expenses, totalling between $ 750000 and $ 1000000. Such expenses are not unique to diagnostic radiology but relate to current costs of professional staff, space, equipment, and overhead. Totally new equipment costs more than digital equipment added to currently available equipment. An add-on approach can reduce total costs by $ 130000 per year and reduce the technical component of the break-even charge by $ 60–$ 80 per procedure depending upon volume [5]. The procedure volume is important in establishing a total break-even charge, which will vary between $ 968 and 419 per patient procedures if 4–12 examinations are performed in a standard working day. The total cost of each procedure is about one quarter that of conventional angiography. DSA is emerging as an alternative to conventional arteriography in neurology. Major advantages include its greater safety and lower cost. The main shortcomings of DSA are its sensitivity to patient motion and its decreased spatial resolution. The potential value of DSA as a clinical research tool is significant. DSA is safer than conventional angiography, it is technically easier, demands less staff, and procedures can be carried out on an outpatient basis.

Doppler and Duplex Sonography

Ultrasound is a cheap, cost-effective, and noninvasive method for detecting and screening of carotid and vertebral occlusive disease in the neck and cerebral basal zone identifying patients at high risk from stroke. The cost of continuous wave (CW) Doppler sonography devices are $ 3000–$ 7000; the cost of Duplex sonography is $100000–$ 125000.

Approaches to Controlling the Costs of Modern Brain Imaging Techniques

Disquit over rising costs has come to dominate discussions of the health care system. One of the major causes of the cost spiral in the view of many policy makers is the excessive and inefficient use of innovations such as CT and MR.

Regulating the escalating costs is generally viewed as the least contentious way to control expenses in the 1980s and 1990s. In the following some forms of technology control are discussed with the aim to reduce costs by controlling big, expensive technologies [10, 12].

We must find a way to pay for medical care that is neutral with regard to the use of technology. Present reimbursement systems steer physicians away from a low technology-intensive choice of practice, for the following reasons. First, using technologies results in far more income than using one's head or hands for the same time spent; second, technology reimbursement seems to increase more rapidly than increases in payments for physician–patient interaction, and third, physicians may be able to triple their income by applying a higher technology style to the same practice by adding a number of procedures and tests to standard work-ups.

Medical education on the value of the discerning use of medical technologies is necessary. The teaching of a discerning, less costly use of medical technologies is still missing. Training in technologic restraint is important for both the generalist and the specialist. Medical schools have to deliver educational programs for reducing over-utilization of diagnostic tests. Medical educators must instill in medical students the importance of a restrained use of technologies in patient care. As patients become better informed, less responsible physicians will have greater difficulties in carrying out inappropriate procedures.

Methods must be developed for sharing technology-related savings between insurers, hospitals, and physicians. The voluntary efforts of hospitals to reduce rates of increase in expenditures have produced savings through administrative decisions, rather than clinical decisions. Insurers could foster such efforts by permitting hospitals and physician groups to use some technology-related savings for other important medical programs. Insurers should design reimbursement plans to encourage hospital staff and private physicians to reduce the collective costs of their standard use of technology.

Precisely because these three approaches are interactive, rising costs will best be controlled if all are tackled simultaneously and each pulls its respective way. This is a large and undramatic agenda that will require time to effect. One of the further approaches to controlling the costs of medical technology is related to population and epidemiologic characteristics. Eliminating truly needless procedures would be a clear-cut way to save money without relinquishing potential medical benefits, but if the overwhelming portion of medical procedures have some medical benefit, then eliminating only those of no value will save little.

The economic concern and controversy associated with the rise of new imaging technologies have been blown out of proportion. While these methods are regarded by many people as expensive procedures, in reality any increase in cost as the result of installation and continued use of neuroimaging procedures is more than compensated for by the savings by the concomitant reduction in other procedures, including angiography and exploratory surgery. A better understanding of the effects of different rationing techniques on patient and physician behavior, and the quality of care, as well as the cost, is required.

References

1. Abrams HL, McNeil BJ (1978) Medical implications of computed tomography. CAT Scanning 298:255–261
2. Aichner F, Gerstenbrand F (1986) The impact of the new technologies in the neurological sciences. In: Battistin L, Gerstenbrand F (eds) PET and NMR: new perspectives in neuroimaging and in clinical neurochemistry. Liss, New York
3. Ambrose J, Gooding MR, Uttley D (1976) EMI scan in the management of head injuries. Lancet 1:847–848
4. Evens RG (1980) The economics of computed tomography: comparison with other health care costs. Radiology 136:509–510
5. Evens RG (1983) Cost of digital angiography in 1983. Impaçt on planning and charges. In: Felix R, et al. (eds) Contrast media in digital radiography. Excerpta Medica, Amsterdam, pp 396–402
6. Evens RG (1984) Economic cost of nuclear magnetic resonance imaging. J Comput Assist Tomogr 8:200–203

7. Fineberg HV, Baumann R, Sosman M (1977) Computerized cranial tomography: some effects on diagnostic and therapeutic plans. JAMA 238:224–227
8. Graßmann P (1984) Finanzielle und wirtschaftliche Aspekte medizinischer Großgeräte. Vortrag im Klinikum Großhadern
9. Greitz T, Ingvar DH, Widén L (1985) The metabolism of the human brain studied with positron emission tomography. Raven, New York
10. Moloney TW, Rogers E (1979) Medical technology – a different view of the contentious debate over costs. N Engl J Med 301:1413–1419
11. NMR – Nuclear magnetic resonance guideline report (1983) American Hospital Association Technology Series vol. 2, No 8
12. Schwartz WB, Joskow PL (1978) Medical efficacy vs economic efficacy: a conflict in values. N Engl J Med 299:1462–1464

Subject Index

MIX
Papier aus verantwortungsvollen Quellen
Paper from responsible sources
FSC® C105338

If you have any concerns about our products,
you can contact us on
ProductSafety@springernature.com

In case Publisher is established outside the EU,
the EU authorized representative is:
Springer Nature Customer Service Center GmbH
Europaplatz 3, 69115 Heidelberg, Germany

Printed by Libri Plureos GmbH
in Hamburg, Germany